Cognitive Neuroscience: Behavioral and Psychological Perspectives

Cognitive Neuroscience: Behavioral and Psychological Perspectives

Edited by Nell Croft

hayle
medical

New York

Hayle Medical,
750 Third Avenue, 9th Floor,
New York, NY 10017, USA

Visit us on the World Wide Web at:
www.haylemedical.com

ISBN: 978-1-63241-666-7

Cataloging-in-Publication Data

Cognitive neuroscience : behavioral and psychological perspectives / edited by Nell Croft.
   p. cm.
Includes bibliographical references and index.
ISBN 978-1-63241-666-7
1. Cognitive neuroscience. 2. Neuropsychology. 3. Neurosciences. I. Croft, Nell.
RC341 .C66 2019
612.8--dc23

Table of Contents

Permissions

List of Contributors

Index

Preface

Cognitive neuroscience is the scientific field concerned with the study of the biological basis of cognition. Its focus lies in the neural connections underlying all mental processes. Some of the methods used in cognitive neuroscience involve a number of experimental procedures from cognitive psychology, electrophysiology, behavioral and cognitive genomics, etc. Cognitive psychology and computational neuroscience are two theoretical approaches. Modern neuroscience explores the interactions between the different areas of the brain by applying diverse approaches and technologies for understanding brain functions. Advances in data analysis methods and non-invasive functional neuroimaging have extended the frontiers of cognitive neuroscience. Brain mapping technologies such as PET and fMRI allow the observation of brain function. This book covers in detail some existing theories and innovative concepts revolving around cognitive neuroscience. Some of the diverse topics covered in this book address the behavioral and psychological perspectives of cognitive neuroscience and the recent advances in this field. It includes contributions of experts and scientists, which will provide innovative insights into this field.

This book unites the global concepts and researches in an organized manner for a comprehensive understanding of the subject. It is a ripe text for all researchers, students, scientists or anyone else who is interested in acquiring a better knowledge of this dynamic field.

I extend my sincere thanks to the contributors for such eloquent research chapters. Finally, I thank my family for being a source of support and help.

Editor

A non-targeted metabolite profiling pilot study suggests that tryptophan and lipid metabolisms are linked with ADHD-like behaviours in dogs

Jenni Puurunen[1,2], Sini Sulkama[1,2], Katriina Tiira[1,2], Cesar Araujo[1,2], Marko Lehtonen[3], Kati Hanhineva[4,5] and Hannes Lohi[1,2]*

Abstract

Background: Attention deficit hyperactivity disorder (ADHD) is a prevalent and multifactorial neuropsychiatric disorder in the human population worldwide. Complex etiology and clinical heterogeneity have challenged the research, diagnostics and treatment of the disease. Hyperactive and impulsive behaviour has also been observed in dogs, and they could offer a physiologically relevant model for human ADHD. As a part of our ongoing study to understand the molecular etiology of canine anxiety traits, this study was aimed to pilot an approach to identify metabolic biomarkers in canine ADHD-like behaviours for research, diagnostics and treatment purposes.

Methods: We collected fresh plasma samples from 22 German Shepherds with varying ADHD-like behaviours. All dogs were on the same controlled diet for 2 weeks prior to sampling. A liquid chromatography combined with mass spectrometry (LC–MS)-based non-targeted metabolite profiling was performed to identify plasma metabolites correlating with the ADHD-like behaviour of the dogs.

Results: 649 molecular features correlated with ADHD-like behavioural scores ($p_{raw} < 0.05$), and three of them [sn-1 LysoPC(18:3), PC(18:3/18:2) and sn-1 LysoPE(18:2)] had significant correlations also after FDR correction (pFDR < 0.05). Phospholipids were found to negatively correlate with ADHD-like behavioural scores, whereas tryptophan metabolites 3-indolepropionic acid (IPA) and kynurenic acid (KYNA) had negative and positive correlations with ADHD-like behavioural scores, respectively.

Conclusions: Our study identified associations between canine ADHD-like behaviours and metabolites that are involved in lipid and tryptophan metabolisms. The identified metabolites share similarity with earlier findings in human and rodent ADHD models. However, a larger replication study is warranted to validate the discoveries prior to further studies to understand the biological role of the identified metabolites in canine ADHD-like behaviours.

Keywords: Dog, ADHD, Non-targeted metabolite profiling, Metabolomics

Background

Attention deficit hyperactivity disorder (ADHD) is a multifactorial neuropsychiatric disorder with a high prevalence (5–10 %) among children worldwide. It is also

increasingly reported in adults [1–3]. In general, ADHD is defined by age-inappropriate levels of inattention, impulsivity and hyperactivity [4]. The symptoms can be disabling, interfering with normal everyday life [5]. Moreover, ADHD tends to comorbid with other neuropsychiatric disorders such as anxiety disorders [4]. Although we know that ADHD is highly heritable with mean heritability estimates of 0.7, the exact molecular mechanisms underlying ADHD pathology are still not properly understood due to

*Correspondence: hannes.lohi@helsinki.fi
[1] Department of Veterinary Biosciences and Research Programs Unit, Molecular Neurology, University of Helsinki and Folkhälsan Research Center, Biomedicum Helsinki, P.O.Box 63, 00014 Helsinki, Finland
Full list of author information is available at the end of the article

the genetic complexity and interactions between genetic and environmental factors [3, 4, 6]. However, studies suggest that disruptions in normal functions of dopaminergic, serotonergic and noradrenergic systems may play a key role in ADHD pathogenesis [1, 3, 4].

One potential approach to unravel the biological pathways of ADHD is to utilise animal models, like dogs, which spontaneously show ADHD-like behaviours, such as hyperactivity, impulsivity and inattention. Many young dogs often show hyperactive and impulsive behaviour, but some hunting and working breeds, like the German Shepherd and the Belgian Shepherd, may continue to show these behavioural extremes later in life as well [7]. Due to the physiological similarities, dogs may serve as excellent natural large animal models of human ADHD. Moreover, genetic and pharmacological studies have already suggested that the underlying molecular mechanisms of ADHD behaviours may be shared in dogs and humans [8]. Dogs with high impulsivity scores have been observed to have reduced tolerance for a delay in reward and also lower levels of urinary serotonin and serotonin/dopamine ratio levels, thus, demonstrating convergent validity for canine model of impulsivity [9]. A dopamine transporter polymorphism was also found to associate with high activity levels in Belgian Malinois [10].

One of the challenges in ADHD research lies in the genetic complexity of the disorder. It is expected that multiple small effect genes contribute to ADHD susceptibility [3, 4]. There is a need either for large study cohorts or new natural models with a simpler genetic architecture such as dogs combined with complementary omics approaches. High-throughput technologies, such as metabolomics, may have the potential to facilitate ADHD research. Non-targeted metabolite profiling offers a hypothesis-free approach to detect altered metabolites and pathways in neuropsychiatric disorders. Few successful examples exist and suggest genetic and environmental contributions to diseases [11–13].

In this study, we investigated the association between plasma metabolites and ADHD-like behavioural scores in diet-controlled dogs with varying ADHD-like behaviours in order to identify ADHD-related pathways and biomarker candidates using a LC-qTOF-MS –based approach. Our results reveal associations between ADHD-like behaviours and plasma phospholipids and tryptophan metabolites in dogs.

Methods

Animals and study design
Data on dog ADHD-like behaviour was collected using our validated owner-completed behavioural survey [14]. The questionnaire was advertised to Finnish dog owners and breed clubs of all breeds via Facebook. Both dogs

with hyperactive, impulsive and inattentive behaviours, as well as dogs with no sign of hyperactivity, impulsivity or inattention, were invited to participate in the survey.

The owner-completed behavioural survey included both general questions concerning the details of their dogs' background, daily routines, and everyday behaviour and 13 more specific questions concerning the activity, impulsivity and inattention behaviour of the dog (Additional file 1: Table S1). In the questionnaire, we utilised the previously validated questions on impulsivity and activity levels in dogs [15, 16]. During data collection, the questionnaire was modified three times, resulting in four slightly different versions of the questionnaire (the first survey was a paper version, whereas the three others were online questionnaires). The main questions regarding our target trait, ADHD-like behaviours, were not changed between the versions. The main difference came from adding further background questions to versions three and four (maternal care, place of birth, type of food, extra nutrients, time spent alone/day, daily exercise) to better document the early life experiences and conditions of the dogs. To sort out the dogs with extreme ADHD-like behaviours, factor analysis was used to explore the factorial structure of the questionnaire, and to reveal possible interconnection between the questions concerning activity, impulsivity and inattention. The factor analysis (PROC FACTOR) was performed with SAS (version 9.3) and was conducted using the principal factor method with VARIMAX rotation. Based on the criterion of eigenvalues >1, all 13 questions were grouped into two factors, identified as 'inattention' and 'impulsivity-activity' ('impulsivity-activity' referred to as 'impulsivity' from now on). These two factors were very similar to factors found in the earlier studies [15, 16]. The 'inattention'—factor consisted of questions #1,2,3,4,7,10 and 12, and the 'impulsivity'—factor of questions #5,6,8,9 and 13. Question #11 did not load with either factor and was excluded. Average scores for both inattention and impulsivity factors were calculated for each dog by summing up the points in each individual question and dividing the result by the number of questions in the factor (7 for 'inattention' and 5 for 'impulsivity'). The total ADHD score consisting of the mean of the answers to all the 13 questions concerning the hyperactive, impulsive and inattentive behaviour of the dog was defined for each dog to reflect the total ADHD-like status. All questions had four choices of increasing frequency (never = 1, sometimes = 2, often = 3, very often = 4). Higher scores represented higher ADHD-like behaviours.

Based on the ADHD-like behavioural scores, 22 privately-owned German Shepherds with scores varying from high to low, reflecting the ADHD-like behaviour of the dog, were recruited for the metabolomics study

(Additional file 2: Table S2). Furthermore, the behaviour of the selected dogs was confirmed by owner interviews. The age of the dogs varied from 16 to 91 months, where the mean age was 62 months (median 64.6 months). The data consisted of six males (mean age 58.3 months, ranging from 16 to 86 months) and sixteen females (mean age 63.4 months, ranging from 21 to 91 months). To control the possible effects of diet on the metabolite profiles, all recruited dogs were fed with the same commercial dry food (Royal Canin Maxi Sensible) for 2 weeks prior to sampling with 1 week as a run-in period, during which, the dogs adapted to the diet change. The owners were instructed not to use any other foods or dietary supplements during the two-week period and were asked to report any changes. To investigate the metabolite profiles of the dogs, blood samples were collected from each dog by the same trained person followed by immediate isolation of plasma by a portable centrifuge. Plasma samples were kept on ice during shipping and stored in −20 degrees (max 2 months) prior to metabolomics analysis. Most of the samples were taken at the dog's home and two samples were taken in our laboratory. Samples were collected during the day and in the evening. Most of the dogs (19 out of 22) fasted 12 h before sampling. Samples were collected with the owners' consent under valid ethical licenses (ESAVI/6054/04.10.03/2012 and Royal Canine ethical board 30052016).

Non-targeted LC–MS metabolite profiling analysis

The sample preparation, instrument parameters and pre-processing of raw data were performed in the LC–MS Metabolomics Center at Biocenter Kuopio (University of Eastern Finland), and they are previously presented in detail [17]. Briefly, methanol (300 µl) was used to precipitate the proteins and extract the metabolites from plasma (100 µl). The non-targeted metabolite profiling was carried out using the UHPLC-qTOF-MS system (Agilent Technologies, Waldbronn, Karlsruhe, Germany), which consisted of a 1290 LC system, a Jetstream electrospray ionization (ESI) source and a 6540 UHD accurate-mass quadrupole-time-of-flight (qTOF) mass spectrometry. All samples were analysed using two different chromatographic techniques; i.e., reversed phase (RP) and hydrophilic interaction chromatography (HILIC). In addition, data were acquired in both ionization polarities; i.e., ESI positive (ESI+) and ESI negative (ESI−).

Non-targeted metabolomics data analysis
Data collection and statistical analysis

The LC–MS data was collected using the vendor's software MassHunter Qualitative Analysis B.05.00 (Agilent Technologies), where the ions were extracted to compounds utilising the "Find by molecular feature" algorithm. The data were output as compound exchange format (.cef) files into the Mass Profiler Professional software (MPP 2.2, Agilent Technologies) for compound alignment and data pre-processing. In order to reduce noise and remove insignificant metabolite features, only the features found in at least 50 % of the samples were included in the analysis. This resulted in a dataset comprising 7058 features in four separate analytical runs [1462 in HILIC ESI(+), 1483 in HILIC ESI(−), 2624 in RP ESI(+), and 1489 in RP ESI(−)].

The four datasets were exported into Microsoft Excel (2013), and filtered according to peak area >20,000 to exclude small and insignificant features from further analysis. To investigate the associations between the peak areas of the metabolites and each of the ADHD-like behavioural scores (total, inattention and impulsivity scores), the Spearman correlation analysis was used. The results were adjusted for multiple comparisons by the Benjamini-Hochberg false discovery rate (FDR) correction [18] used in each of the four analytical approaches. Only metabolites with p_{raw} <0.05 were included in the identification analysis, and metabolites with pFDR <0.05 were considered statistically significant. Finally, the remaining features in the lists were inspected in the LC–MS chromatograms and spectra using the MassHunter software to locate chromatographic peaks with poor retention time accuracy and peak symmetry, which were removed from downstream analysis. Peak lists were also investigated to ensure that the molecular ion of a compound was included into automatic MS/MS fragmentation, and if not, targeted MS/MS analysis was performed.

To investigate whether sex, age or fasting status had any effects on the associations between the metabolites and ADHD-like behavioural scores, a partial correlation analysis including sex, age and fasting status as covariates was performed. All the statistical analyses were performed using the R project for Statistical Computing version 3.0.1.

Identification of the molecular features in the LC–MS data

The identification of metabolites was based on the accurate mass and isotope information; i.e., ratios, abundances and spacing, as well as product ion spectra (MS/MS) acquired either in the automatic MS/MS analysis, during the initial data acquisition, or via re-injection of the samples in targeted MS/MS mode. The spectra were compared with the METLIN Metabolite Database [19], the Human Metabolome Database (HMDB) [20], and LipidMaps [21] or fragmentation patterns reported in earlier publications. The identification of lipids was based on their characteristic fragmentation patterns reported in earlier publications [22–25]. Briefly, the key elements for identification were the protonated head group (*m/z*

184.07 for PCs and LysoPCs and m/z 196.03 for LysoPEs), as well as the deprotonated fatty acid fragments visible in the negative ionization mode. For LysoPCs, the product ion at m/z 104 was used to distinguish sn-1 and sn-2 isomers. The MS/MS fragmentation data for all of the identified metabolites is presented in Table 1.

Results

In this study, we used non-targeted LC–MS-based metabolite profiling to create the plasma metabolite profiles of 22 German Shepherds with varying ADHD-like behavioural scores describing the hyperactive, impulsive and inattentive behaviour of the dog. The variation in the dietary profiles was controlled by feeding the same food to all dogs for a 2-week period prior to sampling.

From the LC–MS measurements, we were able to extract 7058 molecular features to downstream statistical analysis. Of these, 649 features correlated with ADHD-like behavioural scores (p_{raw} <0.05). These molecular features were subjected to manual inspection to identify metabolites, resulting in a set of 22 identified and five unidentified metabolites (Table 1).

Tryptophan metabolites are associated with ADHD-like behaviour

Three molecules related to tryptophan metabolism correlated with the ADHD-like behavioural scores (Table 2; Fig. 1). Compounds with m/z 190.086 and retention time (rt) 5.77 min and m/z 190.050 and rt 3.23 min in RP ESI(+) analysis showed identical fragmentation with 3-indolepropionic acid (IPA) (CAS No. 830-96-6) and kynurenic acid (KYNA) (CAS No. 492-27-3), respectively, according to the METLIN database (Table 1). Compound with m/z 176.071 and rt 5.01 in RP ESI(+) analysis was identified as indoleacetic acid (IAA) (CAS No. 87-51-4), based on its MS/MS fragmentation pattern. Higher ADHD-like behavioural scores were associated with lower plasma levels of IPA (total: $r_s = -0.565$, $p_{raw} = 0.006$, pFDR $= 0.381$; inattention: $r_s = -0.618$, $p_{raw} = 0.002$, pFDR $= 0.241$; impulsivity: $r_s = -0.452$, $p_{raw} = 0.035$, pFDR $= 0.560$) and IAA (inattention: $r_s = -0.474$, $p_{raw} = 0.030$, pFDR $= 0.433$) (Table 2; Fig. 1). In contrast, high ADHD-like behavioural scores associated with high plasma levels of KYNA (total: $r_s = 0.511$, $p_{raw} = 0.015$, pFDR $= 0.426$; inattention: $r_s = 0.505$, $p_{raw} = 0.017$, pFDR $= 0.392$; impulsivity: $r_s = 0.498$, $p_{raw} = 0.018$, pFDR $= 0.447$).

More intense ADHD-like behaviour is associated with decreased plasma phospholipids, but increased fatty acids

The majority of the identified metabolites in the plasma of dogs with ADHD-like behaviours were phospholipids, including five phosphatidylcholines (PC) (PC(18:3/18:2), PC(20:5/18:3), PC(20:4/14:0), PC(18:2/16:1) and PC(15:0/18:2)), five lysophosphatidylcholines (LysoPC) (sn-1 LysoPC(18:3), sn-1 LysoPC(14:0), sn-1 LysoPC(15:0), sn-1 LysoPC(17:0) and sn-1 LysoPC(20:3)) and four lysophosphatidylethanolamines (LysoPE) (sn-1 LysoPE(18:2), sn-1 LysoPE(20:5), sn-1 LysoPE(18:1) and sn-1 LysoPE(18:0)) (Table 1). All of these detected phospholipids negatively correlated with the ADHD-like behavioural scores, of which sn-1 LysoPC(18:3), sn-1 LysoPE(18:2) and PC(18:3/18:2) had the strongest associations (Table 2; Fig. 1). The relationships between sn-1 LysoPC(18:3) and all three ADHD-like behavioural scores (total: $r_s = -0.769$, $p_{raw} = 2.93E - 05$, pFDR $= 0.016$; inattention: $r_s = -0.740$, $p_{raw} = 8.26E-05$, pFDR $= 0.030$; impulsivity: $r_s = -0.765$, $p_{raw} = 3.32E-05$, pFDR $= 0.036$), sn-1 LysoPE(18:2) and inattention score ($r_s = -0.697$, $p_{raw} = 3.1E-04$, pFDR $= 0.044$), and PC(18:3/18:2) and total and inattention scores (total: $r_s = -0.804$, $p_{raw} = 1.91E-05$, pFDR $= 0.016$; inattention: $r_s = -0.798$, $p_{raw} = 2.53E-05$, pFDR $= 0.019$) also remained significant after FDR correction. Significant correlations were not due to outliers (Additional file 3: Figure S1).

In addition, two fatty acids were identified as arachidonic acid (C20:4; m/z 303.235) and C18:1 (m/z 283.26428) (Table 1). In contrast to phospholipids, higher ADHD-like behavioural scores were associated with higher plasma levels of C20:4 (total: $r_s = 0.508$, $p_{raw} = 0.016$, pFDR $= 0.163$; inattention: $r_s = 0.579$, $p_{raw} = 0.005$, pFDR $= 0.102$) and C18:1 (total: $r_s = 0.509$, $p_{raw} = 0.016$, pFDR $= 0.426$; inattention: $r_s = 0.532$, $p_{raw} = 0.011$, pFDR $= 0.342$; impulsivity: $r_s = 0.447$, $p_{raw} = 0.025$, pFDR $= 0.492$) (Table 2; Fig. 1).

ADHD-like behavioural scores also correlate with other plasma metabolites

The metabolite with m/z 585.270 and rt 11.35 in the RP ESI(+) analysis correlated positively with all three ADHD-like behavioural scores (total: $r_s = 0.513$, $p_{raw} = 0.015$, pFDR $= 0.426$; inattention: $r_s = 0.580$, $p_{raw} = 0.005$, pFDR $= 0.271$; impulsivity: $r_s = 0.452$, $p_{raw} = 0.035$, pFDR $= 0.560$) and was identified as bilirubin (CAS No. 635-65-4) (Tables 1, 2; Fig. 1). The metabolite with m/z 137.071 and rt 2.22 in the HILIC(+) analysis was identified as 1-methylnicotinamide (CAS No. 3106-60-3). It had a positive association with all three ADHD-like behavioural scores (total: $r_s = 0.647$, $p_{raw} = 0.001$, pFDR $= 0.618$; inattention: $r_s = 0.668$, $p_{raw} = 6.86E-04$, pFDR $= 0.455$; impulsivity: $r_s = 0.571$, $p_{raw} = 0.005$, pFDR $= 0.461$).

The majority of the identified plasma metabolites correlate with all three ADHD-like behavioural scores

Twenty out of the 27 reported metabolites correlated with all three ADHD-like behavioural scores (total,

Table 1 Characteristics of the putatively identified marker metabolites in liquid chromatography-mass spectrometry analysis

Column	Ionization mode	MW	*m/z*	RT (min)	Putative annotation	CID (eV)	MS/MS fragmentation	Identification reference[a]
HILIC	ESI+	231.148	232.155	1.59	Unknown metabolite, putative carnitine	10	232.1531, 85.0290, 173.0782, 95.0856, 60.0803	MS/MS
HILIC	ESI+	136.064	137.071	2.22	1-methylnicotinamide	20	94.0654, 137.0688, 65.0379, 77.0375	MID274
RP	ESI+	189.043	190.050	3.23	Kynurenic acid (KYNA)	10	190.0496, 144.0443, 172.0426	MID5683
HILIC	ESI−	165.079	164.071	3.91	Phenylalanine	10	164.0713, 103.0565, 147.0448, 90.0116, 72.0086	MID28
RP	ESI+	175.064	176.071	5.01	Indoleacetic acid	10	130.0656, 176.0780, 51.0227, 158.0587	HMDB 00197
RP	ESI+	189.079	190.086	5.77	3-Indolepropionic acid (IPA)	10	130.0655, 55.0184, 172.0754, 190.0862	MID6602
HILIC	ESI+	220.143	221.150	7.30	Unknown metabolite	10	221.1465, 84.0806, 87.0429, 90.9738, 203.1374	MS/MS
RP	ESI+	467.303	468.310	9.76	sn-1 LysoPC(14:0)	40	184.0741, 86.0970, 125.0017, 60.0814, 104.1076; ESI(−) 10 eV: 227.1995, 452.2768, 512.3016	MS/MS
RP	ESI−	563.323	562.316	9.85	sn-1 LysoPC(18:3)	10	502.2892, 277.2167, 562.3029; ESI(+) 20 eV: 184.0740, 104.1083	MS/MS
RP	ESI+	499.271	500.278	9.87	sn-1 LysoPE(20:5)	10	500.2786, 359.2548; ESI(−) 20 eV: 498.2860, 169.1368, 301.2172	MS/MS
RP	ESI+	481.319	482.326	10.03	sn-1 LysoPC(15:0)	20	184.0751, 104.1059, 482.3264; ESI(−) 10 eV: 241.2097, 466.2915	MS/MS
RP	ESI−	477.287	476.280	10.12	sn-1 LysoPE(18:2)	20	279.2321, 196.0390, 140.0058, 78.9594, 476.2834; ESI(+) 10 eV: 478.2932, 337.2703	MS/MS
RP	ESI−	479.302	478.295	10.29	sn-1 LysoPE(18:1)	10	281.2477, 478.2945, 196.0306; ESI(+) 10 eV: 480.3077, 44.0505, 62.0614, 339.2930, 462.3008	MS/MS
RP	ESI+	545.350	546.357	10.29	sn-1 LysoPC(20:3)	10	546.3626, 104.1084, 184.0740; ESI(−) 10 eV: 530.3529, 305.2466, 590.3485	MS/MS
RP	ESI+	509.350	510.357	10.42	sn-1 LysoPC(17:0)	20	184.0740, 104.1066, 510.3602; ESI(−) 10 eV: 494.3250, 269.2425, 554.3709	MS/MS
RP	ESI−	481.319	480.313	10.65	sn-1 LysoPE(18:0)	10	283.2631, 480.3112, 196.0353; ESI(+) 10 eV: 341.3049, 482.3239, 44.0494, 464.3121	MS/MS
RP	ESI−	304.241	303.235	10.70	Arachidonic acid (C20:4)	10	303.2354, 59.0219, 259.2326	LipidMaps
RP	ESI−	643.406	642.398	10.72	Unknown metabolite, putative GlcCer(d18:1/12:0) or GlcCer(d14:1/16:0)	20	642.3955, 362.1501, 363.1579, 99.9224	Hsu and Turk [25]

Table 1 continued

Column	Ionization mode	MW	m/z	RT (min)	Putative annotation	CID (eV)	MS/MS fragmentation	Identification reference[a]
RP	ESI+	282.257	283.264	10.94	C18:1	10	283.2847, 43.0540, 71.0867, 149.1310, 57.0704, 101.0773	LipidMaps
RP	ESI−	647.438	646.431	10.94	Unknown metabolite, putative Cer(d18:1/24:1)	40	99.9224, 364.1699, 281.2448, 365.1777, 83.9307, 320.1746, 646.4291	Hsu and Turk [25]
RP	ESI+	584.263	585.270	11.35	Bilirubin	10	299.1388, 585.2677	MID81
RP	ESI−	847.538	846.532	11.56	PC(20:5/18:3)	40	303.2314, 102.9687, 301.2127; ESI(+) 20 eV: 184.0735, 802.5399	MS/MS
RP	ESI−	797.523	796.516	11.59	Unknown PC	10	736.4868, 796.5069; ESI(+) 20 eV: 184.0733, 752.5218	MS/MS
RP	ESI−	799.538	798.531	11.81	PC(20:4/14:0)	20	738.5067, 303.2318, 227.1970, 798.5315; ESI(+) 10 eV: 754.5405, 184.0726	MS/MS
RP	ESI−	825.555	824.547	11.83	PC(18:3/18:2)	20	764.5239, 824.5378, 277.2097, 279.2388, 45.0065; ESI(+) 20 eV: 184.0740, 780.5574, 86.0961	MS/MS
RP	ESI−	801.553	800.547	12.04	PC(18:2/16:1)	20	740.5268, 279.2323, 253.2152, 800.5403; ESI(+) 10 eV: 756.5574, 184.0733	MS/MS
RP	ESI+	743.549	744.556	12.08	PC(15:0/18:2)	10	744.5577, 184.0743; ESI(−) 20 eV: 728.5133, 788.5291, 241.2161, 279.2331	MS/MS

Metabolites with uncertain identity are also included. The characteristics include the identification references together with parameters for the LC–MS analysis, including the chromatography (column), ionization mode in the mass spectrometry (Ionization mode), *MW* molecular weight, identified ion (*m/z*), *RT* retention time, *CID* collision-induced dissociation energy, *MS/MS fragments* fragment ions in the tandem mass spectrometry

LysoPC lysophosphatidylcholine, *LysoPE* lysophosphatidylethanolamine, *PC* phosphatidylcholine

[a] Identification of metabolites is based on manual MS/MS spectral interpretation, METLIN ID when MS/MS spectrum available, commercial standard compound or some fragmentation patterns published earlier [25]

inattention and impulsivity) (Table 2; Fig. 1). Twenty-two metabolites correlated with the total ADHD score and 26 with the inattention score. The metabolites sn-1 LysoPC(14:0), sn-1 LysoPC(18:1) and unknown PC with *m/z* 796.516 correlated only with the inattention score. The impulsivity score correlated with 21 metabolites, and phenylalanine was found to specifically correlate only with the impulsivity score.

Age, sex and fasting have minor effects on the association between metabolites and ADHD-like behavioural scores

Since there were differences in the fasting status of the dogs (Additional file 2: Table S2), we wanted to determine whether this had any effects on the observed correlations between the plasma metabolites and ADHD-like behavioural scores. Also, the possible effects of age and sex were analysed. Correlation coefficients and p-values adjusted for age, sex and fasting are represented in Table 3 together with the original p-values. Most of the associations between the metabolites and ADHD-like behavioural scores remained after controlling for age, sex and fasting status (age, sex and fasting adjusted *p* value < 0.05). However, age, sex and fasting had significant effects on associations between IPA and the impulsivity score (original p = 0.035, adjusted p = 0.058), sn-1 LysoPC(14:0) and the inattention score (original p = 0.049, adjusted p = 0.102), sn-1 LysoPC(17:0) and the inattention score (original p = 0.041, adjusted p = 0.055), unknown PC with *m/z* 796.516 and the inattention score (original p = 0.029, adjusted p = 0.087), IAA and the inattention score (original p = 0.03, adjusted p = 0.062), phenylalanine and the impulsivity score (original p = 0.049, adjusted p = 0.063), and unknown metabolite with *m/z* 221.150

Table 2 Associations between the plasma metabolites and ADHD-like behavioural scores (total ADHD, inattention, impulsivity)

Putative annotation	Total ADHD			Inattention			Impulsivity		
	r_s	p_{raw}	pFDR	r_s	p_{raw}	pFDR	r_s	p_{raw}	pFDR
Putative carnitine	0.505	0.017	0.990	0.450	0.036	0.990	0.509	0.016	0.797
1-methylnicotinamide	0.647	0.001	0.618	0.668	6.86E-04	0.455	0.571	0.005	0.461
Kynurenic acid (KYNA)	0.511	0.015	0.426	0.505	0.017	0.392	0.498	0.018	0.447
Phelynalanine	0.403	ns	ns	0.337	ns	ns	0.425	0.049	0.989
Indoleacetic acid	−0.404	ns	ns	−0.474	0.030	0.433	−0.349	ns	ns
3-Indolepropionic acid (IPA)	−0.565	0.006	0.381	−0.618	0.002	0.241	−0.452	0.035	0.560
Unknown metabolite *m/z* 221.150	0.443	0.039	0.990	0.520	0.013	0.873	0.287	ns	ns
sn-1 LysoPC(14:0)	−0.390	ns	ns	−0.424	0.049	0.510	−0.360	ns	ns
sn-1 LysoPC(18:3)	−0.769	2.93E-05	0.016	−0.740	8.26E-05	0.030	−0.765	3.32E-05	0.036
sn-1 LysoPE(20:5)	−0.544	0.009	0.409	−0.615	0.002	0.241	−0.447	0.037	0.560
sn-1 LysoPC(15:0)	−0.623	0.002	0.330	−0.602	0.003	0.241	−0.659	8.46E-04	0.320
sn-1 LysoPE(18:2)	−0.630	0.002	0.093	−0.697	3.1E-04	0.044	−0.549	0.008	0.230
sn-1 LysoPE(18:1)	−0.382	ns	ns	−0.530	0.011	0.117	−0.218	ns	ns
sn-1 LysoPC(20:3)	−0.508	0.016	0.426	−0.489	0.021	0.409	−0.516	0.014	0.437
sn-1 LysoPC(17:0)	−0.451	0.035	0.491	−0.438	0.041	0.473	−0.441	0.038	0.566
sn-1 LysoPE(18:0)	−0.562	0.006	0.146	−0.574	0.005	0.102	−0.539	0.01	0.232
Arachidonic acid (C20:4)	0.508	0.016	0.163	0.579	0.005	0.102	0.355	ns	ns
Unknown metabolite, putative GlcCer(d18:1/12:0) or GlcCer(d14:1/16:0)	0.504	0.017	0.163	0.524	0.012	0.117	0.447	0.037	0.302
C18:1	0.509	0.016	0.426	0.532	0.011	0.342	0.477	0.025	0.492
Unknown metabolite, putative Cer(d18:1/24:1)	0.509	0.016	0.163	0.536	0.010	0.117	0.461	0.031	0.283
Bilirubin	0.513	0.015	0.426	0.580	0.005	0.271	0.452	0.035	0.560
PC(20:5/18:3)	−0.555	0.009	0.150	−0.621	0.003	0.087	−0.415	ns	ns
Unknown PC *m/z* 796.516	−0.413	ns	ns	−0.465	0.029	0.173	−0.299	ns	ns
PC(20:4/14:0)	−0.558	0.007	0.148	−0.557	0.007	0.110	−0.485	0.022	0.281
PC(18:3/18:2)	−0.804	1.91E-05	0.016	−0.798	2.53E-05	0.019	−0.731	2.52E-04	0.137
PC(18:2/16:1)	−0.518	0.013	0.163	−0.500	0.018	0.137	−0.486	0.022	0.281
PC(15:0/18:2)	−0.578	0.005	0.381	−0.568	0.006	0.305	−0.525	0.012	0.416

Spearman correlation coefficients (r_s) with statistical significance (p_{raw} and pFDR)

and the total ADHD score (original p = 0.039, adjusted p = 0.069).

Discussion

ADHD is a prevalent and severe neuropsychiatric disorder, but yet poorly characterised for underlying genes and molecular networks. Genetic complexity and clinical heterogeneity have challenged the research, warranting new approaches to identify novel biomarkers and pathways. An alternative approach would be a study of a physiologically relevant large animal model with natural ADHD-like behaviours such as the dog [15]. Here, we applied a methodologically well-controlled pilot non-targeted metabolite profiling of canine ADHD-like behaviours in order to investigate the correlation between the plasma metabolite profiles and ADHD-like behavioural scores of German Shepherds with varying ADHD-like behaviours.

We report 27 metabolites that correlated with at least one of the three ADHD-like behavioural scores (total, inattention, impulsivity). The identified ADHD-like behaviour-related candidate metabolites indicate alterations in tryptophan and phospholipids metabolisms. The same pathways have been suggested in human ADHD [26–30], and the possible important overlap in the human and canine pathways warrants a larger replication study in dogs prior to further conclusions of the metabolic similarity of the ADHD models.

We found three interesting metabolites in the tryptophan pathway, IPA, IAA and KYNA. Lower plasma IPA and IAA levels were associated with higher ADHD-like behavioural scores. IPA is a microbial deamination product of dietary tryptophan with antioxidant capacity [31, 32], produced solely by enteric bacteria (including *Clostridium sporogenes*) in the intestines [33–35] (Fig. 2).

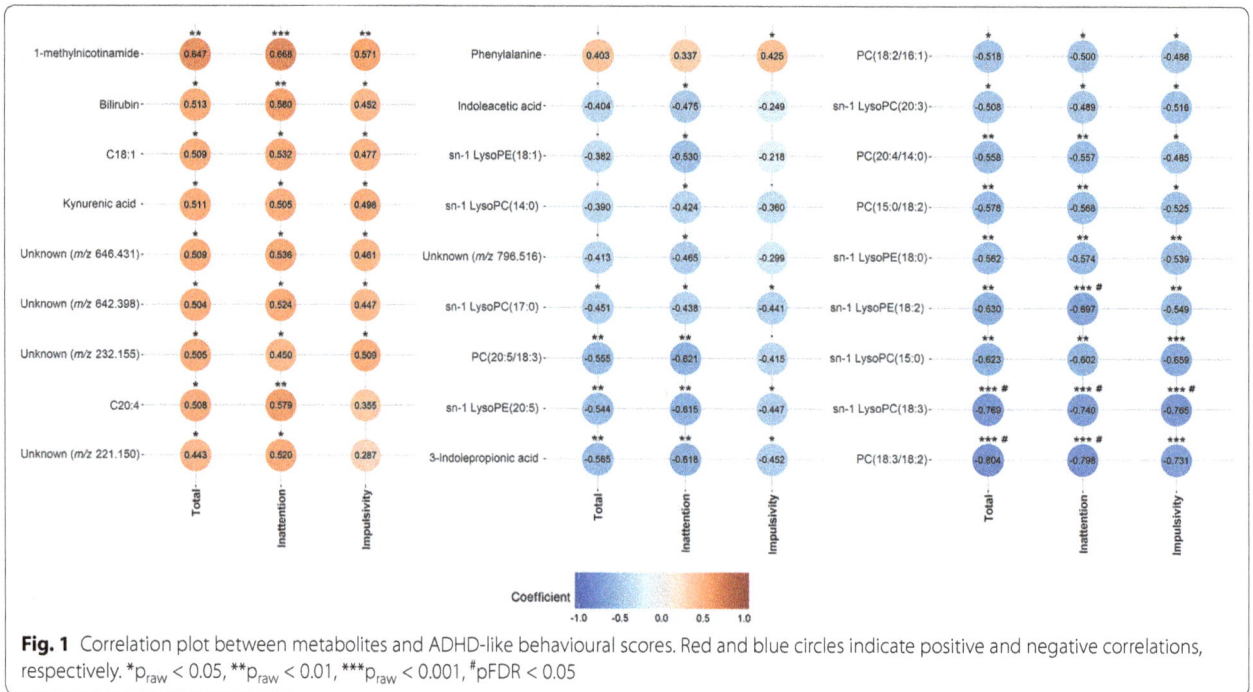

Fig. 1 Correlation plot between metabolites and ADHD-like behavioural scores. Red and blue circles indicate positive and negative correlations, respectively. $*p_{raw} < 0.05$, $**p_{raw} < 0.01$, $***p_{raw} < 0.001$, $\#pFDR < 0.05$

IAA is a plant hormone of the auxin class synthesised via multiple pathways in the plants [36], but it can also be produced in mammals from tryptophan in tissues, and in the intestines by enteric bacteria (including *Clostridium bartlettii*) [37, 38]. Due to the intestinal bacterial production of both IPA and IAA by bacteria belonging to the same genus (*Clostridium*), negative correlations between the ADHD-like behavioural scores and these metabolites suggest differences in intestinal microbiota of dogs with different ADHD-like behaviours, since there were no differences in the diets (and intake of tryptophan) of the dogs. Gut microbiota may have a bidirectional effect on the nervous and the immune systems [39–41]. Since IPA is capable of crossing the blood–brain barrier (BBB) and is known to have neuroprotective actions in the central nervous system (CNS) [35], decreased IPA may predispose dogs to neurological and behavioural abnormalities due to oxidative stress, for example. Alternatively, stress caused by hyperactive and impulsive behaviour may lead to altered gut microbiota and result in changed plasma IPA. Changes in the gut microbiota have been suggested in neuro behavioural disorders such as mood disorders and autism [40].

The third metabolite in the tryptophan pathway, KYNA, was positively correlated with the ADHD-like behavioural scores. KYNA is a neuroactive metabolite produced in the kynurenine pathway of tryptophan metabolism [42, 43]. It acts as an endogenous antagonist of the cholinergic nicotinic α7-receptor (α7nAChR) and the glutamatergic *N*-methyl-D-aspartate receptor (NMDAR) in the CNS and as an agonist of a particular G-protein coupled receptor, GPR35, in immune cells and in the gastrointestinal (GI) tract [44]. Interestingly, altered levels of KYNA have been proposed in schizophrenia [45, 46], depression [47] and bipolar disorder [48]. A recent study demonstrated a reduction in serum KYNA levels in adult ADHD patients, when compared with controls [26]. Interestingly, our data showed a positive relationship between the plasma KYNA levels and ADHD-like behavioural scores in adult dogs, indicating that dogs with more intense ADHD-like behaviour had higher KYNA levels. KYNA is mainly produced via tryptophan catabolism in various tissues, but enteric bacteria in the intestines are also capable of converting dietary tryptophan into KYNA [49, 50] (Fig. 2). Higher plasma KYNA levels may be due to increased bacterial production of KYNA in the intestines or increased catabolism of tryptophan via the kynurenine pathway in the tissues resulting, for example, from inflammation or oxidative stress [51]. Thus, there may be less tryptophan available for transport into the brain for serotonin synthesis. Serotonin, in turn, is an important neurotransmitter, regulating impulsivity and social behaviour [52]. Decreased serotonin levels have been reported in ADHD patients [52]. Thus, the positive correlation between the plasma KYNA levels and ADHD-like behavioural scores may indirectly reflect decreased serotonin levels with

Table 3 Age, sex and fasting-adjusted associations between the plasma metabolites and ADHD-like behavioural scores

Putative annotation	Total ADHD			Inattention			Impulsivity		
	Original	Adjusted		Original	Adjusted		Original	Adjusted	
	p	r_s	p	p	r_s	p	p	r_s	p
Putative carnitine	0.017	0.560	0.013	0.036	0.527	0.02	0.016	0.526	0.021
1-methylnicotinamide	0.001	0.642	0.003	6.86E-04	0.671	0.002	0.005	0.576	0.010
Kynurenic acid (KYNA)	0.015	0.519	0.023	0.017	0.486	0.035	0.018	0.543	0.016
Phelynalanine	ns	ns	ns	ns	ns	ns	0.049	0.435	0.063
Indoleacetic acid	ns	ns	ns	0.030	−0.448	0.062	ns	ns	ns
3-Indolepropionic acid (IPA)	0.006	−0.578	0.010	0.002	−0.655	0.002	0.035	−0.442	0.058
Unknown metabolite m/z 221.150	0.039	0.426	0.069	0.013	0.475	0.040	ns	ns	ns
sn-1 LysoPC(14:0)	ns	ns	ns	0.049	−0.387	0.102	ns	ns	ns
sn-1 LysoPC(18:3)	2.93E-05	−0.782	7.54E-05	8.26E-05	−0.765	1.34E-04	3.32E-05	−0.785	6.86E-05
sn-1 LysoPE(20:5)	0.009	−0.569	0.011	0.002	−0.615	0.005	0.037	−0.499	0.030
sn-1 LysoPC(15:0)	0.002	−0.640	0.003	0.003	−0.598	0.007	8.46E-04	−0.701	8.0E-04
sn-1 LysoPE(18:2)	0.002	−0.670	0.002	0.003	−0.703	8.0E-04	0.008	−0.645	0.003
sn-1 LysoPE(18:1)	ns	ns	ns	0.011	−0.493	0.032	ns	ns	ns
sn-1 LysoPC(20:3)	0.016	−0.550	0.015	0.021	−0.555	0.014	0.014	−0.561	0.013
sn-1 LysoPC(17:0)	0.035	−0.463	0.046	0.041	−0.447	0.055	0.038	−0.499	0.030
sn-1 LysoPE(18:0)	0.006	−0.610	0.006	0.005	−0.622	0.004	0.01	−0.600	0.007
Arachidonic acid (C20:4)	0.016	0.502	0.029	0.005	0.555	0.014	ns	ns	ns
Unknown metabolite, putative GlcCer(d18:1/12:0) or GlcCer(d14:1/16:0)	0.017	0.514	0.024	0.012	0.547	0.015	0.037	0.473	0.041
C18:1	0.016	0.508	0.026	0.011	0.524	0.021	0.025	0.505	0.028
Unknown metabolite, putative Cer(d18:1/24:1)	0.016	0.506	0.027	0.010	0.529	0.020	0.031	0.488	0.034
Bilirubin	0.015	0.511	0.025	0.005	0.544	0.016	0.035	0.515	0.024
PC(20:5/18:3)	0.009	−0.601	0.008	0.003	−0.615	0.007	ns	ns	ns
Unknown PC m/z 796.516	ns	ns	ns	0.029	−0.404	0.087	ns	ns	ns
PC(20:4/14:0)	0.007	−0.559	0.013	0.007	−0.538	0.017	0.022	−0.531	0.019
PC(18:3/18:2)	1.19E-05	−0.804	9.91E-05	2.53E-05	−0.785	1.89E-04	2.52E-04	−0.767	3.24E-04
PC(18:2/16:1)	0.013	−0.529	0.020	0.018	−0.537	0.018	0.022	−0.476	0.039
PC(15:0/18:2)	0.005	−0.604	0.006	0.006	−0.578	0.010	0.012	−0.590	0.008

Spearman correlation coefficients (corrected r_s) from partial correlation analysis including age, sex and fasting status as covariates together with statistical significance (adjusted p). Original p values are also shown (original p)

characteristic behavioural symptoms in dogs with higher ADHD-like behavioural scores.

We observed strong and negative correlations between ADHD-like behavioural scores and fifteen phospholipids, including five PCs, five LysoPCs, four LysoPEs and one unknown PC. The blood lipid composition is affected by nutrition and fasting [53], and we, therefore, changed the diet of all study dogs and controlled fasting in the statistical analysis. Thus, the observed difference suggests alterations in the endogenous phospholipid metabolism or in the absorption of dietary lipids between the study groups. Phospholipids are important signalling molecules and major components of cell membranes regulating membrane fluidity, charge and receptor function [54, 55]. The adequate amount of brain phospholipids and their right fatty acid composition is especially important to ensure optimal membrane functionality in the brain [55]. Regarding this, the lower plasma phospholipids may have negative effects on the physiology and behaviour of dogs with more intense ADHD-like behaviour.

Phospholipids are composed of hydrophobic and hydrophilic parts, which are joined together by glycerol [56]. The hydrophilic part consists of a phosphate group combined with a characteristic head group (choline in PCs and ethanolamine in PEs), whereas the hydrophobic part consists of different kinds of combinations of fatty acids, PCs containing two fatty acids, whereas LysoPCs and LysoPEs contain only one fatty acid [56]. Thus, the composition of phospholipids depends on the availability of free fatty acids, which are incorporated into phospholipids. Interestingly, both human [27, 28, 30, 57] and rodent [58–61] studies have suggested that the omega-3

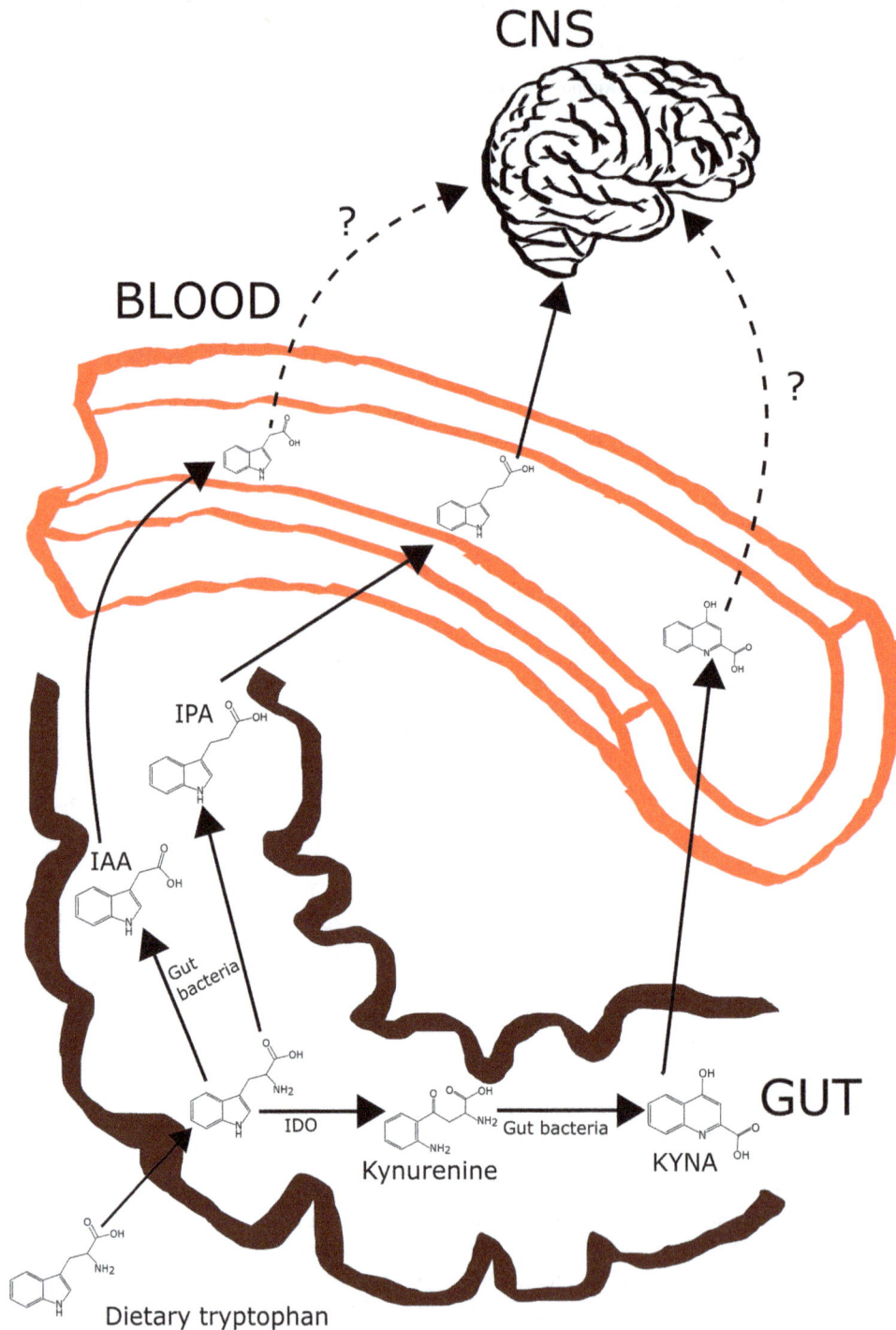

Fig. 2 Simplified illustration of the possible metabolic pathways of dietary tryptophan in the intestines. Dietary tryptophan can be degraded in the intestines by enteric bacteria to produce IAA and IPA or KYNA via kynurenine. From the intestines, IPA, IAA and KYNA are transferred to circulation. IPA is known to cross BBB, and thus, can migrate to CNS and act there, but the ability of IAA and KYNA to cross BBB is uncertain. In addition to the degradation of dietary tryptophan in the intestines, KYNA and IAA can also be synthetised from tryptophan in various other tissues in the body, but IPA is solely produced in the intestines by enteric bacteria. *BBB* blood–brain barrier, *CNS* central nervous system, *IAA* indoleacetic acid, *IDO* indoleamine 2,3-dioxygenase, *IPA* 3-indolepropionic acid, *KYNA* kynurenic acid

polyunsaturated fatty acid (PUFA) status may contribute to the etiology of ADHD. Both children and adult ADHD patients have been demonstrated to have decreased proportions of long chain PUFAs (LC-PUFAs) and especially omega-3 PUFAs, like eicosapentaenoic acid (EPA; 20:5 n-3) and docosahexaenoic acid (DHA; 22:6 n-3), in plasma lipids when compared with control subjects [28, 29, 62–65].

It has been suggested that the relationship between decreased omega-3 PUFAs and ADHD would lie in dopamine neurotransmission, as rodent studies have proposed that chronic omega-3 PUFA deficiency is associated with significantly decreased concentrations of endogenous dopamine and reduced dopamine-2 (D_2) receptor binding in the frontal cortex [59, 61], accompanied by attentional and behavioural problems when compared to rodents fed with diet containing adequate levels of PUFAs [66]. In this study, ADHD-like behavioural scores negatively correlated with plasma phospholipids containing combinations of omega-3 (18:3 n-3 (ALA), 20:5 n-3 (EPA)) and omega-6 (18:2 n-6 (LA)) fatty acids. Our results are not directly comparable to those findings made in ADHD patients, but indicate that phospholipid abnormalities could contribute to canine ADHD-like behaviours too. In contrast to phospholipids, ADHD-behavioural scores were positively associated with plasma levels of free fatty acids C20:4 and C18:1. This may refer to an increased breakdown of phospholipids or problems in the phospholipid synthesis, rather than problems in the intestinal absorption of dietary fatty acids.

Our study also suggests the involvement of oxidative stress in canine ADHD-like behaviours. The ADHD-like behavioural scores showed a positive relationship with fatty acid C20:4, an oxidative stress marker, but a negative relationship with the antioxidant IPA. Impaired balance between the oxidant and antioxidant systems and increased levels of oxidative stress have already been demonstrated in ADHD, although precise mechanisms remain to be characterised [67–70].

We have previously demonstrated the promise of the metabolomics approach in canine fear research [17], and now, we have applied this approach to study canine ADHD-like behaviours with better optimised methodology and preparation of the study cohort. Instead of whole blood, we used fresh plasma samples from dogs that had undergone a controlled diet change before the sampling. However, we have several limitations in our study. First, our sample size is small for conclusive results. Second, we must acknowledge that the behavioural survey is based on the owner reports of the behaviours and activity levels of the dogs, and no behavioural

testing was performed to verify the owner reports. Thirdly, fasting control was incomplete, as some dogs failed it. Finally, the time of sampling varied from daytime to evening and should be less variable in the future to better control possible variations due to the circadian rhythm.

Conclusions

Our metabolomics study suggests associations between canine ADHD-like behaviours and tryptophan and phospholipid metabolisms. A replication study with a larger sample size is needed to validate our findings and to confirm the overlap in the affected pathways between human ADHD and canine ADHD-like behaviours.

Abbreviations
ADHD: attention deficit hyperactivity disorder; BBB: blood-brain barrier; CNS: central nervous system; ESI: electrospray ionization; HILIC: hydrophilic interaction; IAA: indoleacetic acid; IPA: 3-indolepropionic acid; KYNA: kynurenic acid; LC: liquid chromatography; LysoPC: lysophosphatidylcholine; LysoPE: lysophosphatidylethanolamine; MS: mass spectrometry; PC: phosphatidylcholine; RP: reversed phase.

Authors' contributions
HL, SS and KT designed the experiment, JP, ML and KH performed the experiment, JP analysed the data. HL, ML, CA and KH contributed to reagents/materials/analysis tools. JP and HL wrote the manuscript with others' contributions. All authors read and approved the final manuscript.

Author details
[1] Department of Veterinary Biosciences and Research Programs Unit, Molecular Neurology, University of Helsinki and Folkhälsan Research Center, Biomedicum Helsinki, P.O.Box 63, 00014 Helsinki, Finland. [2] The Folkhälsan Research Center, Helsinki, Finland. [3] School of Pharmacy, University of Eastern Finland, Kuopio, Finland. [4] Institute of Public Health and Clinical Nutrition, University of Eastern Finland, Kuopio, Finland. [5] LC–MS Metabolomics Center, Biocenter Kuopio, Kuopio, Finland.

Acknowledgements
We would like to thank Petra Jaakonsaari for technical assistance in sample collection and Miia Reponen for maintaining the LC–MS-qTOF instrument. Royal Canin is thanked for donating food for the participating dogs and The German Shepherd breed club and owners are thanked for participation.

Competing interests
The authors declare that they have no competing interests.

Funding
This study was funded partly by the ERCStG, ERANET-NEURON Mental Disorders, the Finnish Kennel Club, the Academy of Finland, the Orion-Farmos Research Foundation, the Sigrid Juselius Foundation, the Jane and Aatos Erkko Foundation, Biocenter Finland and the Dog Health Research Fund, University of Helsinki.

References

1. Biederman J. Attention-deficit/hyperactivity disorder: a selective overview. Biol Psychiatr. 2005;57(11):1215–20.
2. Polanczyk G, de Lima MS, Horta BL, Biederman J, Rohde LA. The worldwide prevalence of ADHD: a systematic review and metaregression analysis. Am J Psychiatr. 2007;164(6):942–8.
3. Faraone SV, Mick E. Molecular genetics of attention deficit hyperactivity disorder. Psychiatr Clin North Am. 2010;33(1):159–80.
4. Tarver J, Daley D, Sayal K. Attention-deficit hyperactivity disorder (ADHD): an updated review of the essential facts. Child Care Health Dev. 2014;40(6):762–74.
5. Hoegl T, Heinrich H, Barth W, Losel F, Moll GH, Kratz O. Time course analysis of motor excitability in a response inhibition task according to the level of hyperactivity and impulsivity in children with ADHD. PLoS ONE. 2012;7(9):e46066.
6. Li Z, Chang SH, Zhang LY, Gao L, Wang J. Molecular genetic studies of ADHD and its candidate genes: a review. Psychiatr Res. 2014;219(1):10–24.
7. Lindsay S. Handbook of applied dog behavior and training. Iowa: Iowa State University Press; 2001.
8. Hejjas K, Vas J, Topal J, Szantai E, Ronai Z, Szekely A, et al. Association of polymorphisms in the dopamine D4 receptor gene and the activity-impulsivity endophenotype in dogs. Anim Genet. 2007;38(6):629–33.
9. Wright HF, Mills DS, Pollux PM. Behavioural and physiological correlates of impulsivity in the domestic dog (Canis familiaris). Physiol Behav. 2012;105(3):676–82.
10. Lit L, Belanger JM, Boehm D, Lybarger N, Oberbauer AM. Differences in behavior and activity associated with a poly(a) expansion in the dopamine transporter in Belgian Malinois. PLoS ONE. 2013;8(12):e82948.
11. Theodoridis GA, Gika HG, Want EJ, Wilson ID. Liquid chromatography-mass spectrometry based global metabolite profiling: a review. Anal Chim Acta. 2012;711:7–16.
12. Zhou B, Xiao JF, Tuli L, Ressom HW. LC-MS-based metabolomics. Mol BioSyst. 2012;8(2):470–81.
13. Kaddurah-Daouk R, Krishnan KR. Metabolomics: a global biochemical approach to the study of central nervous system diseases. Neuropsychopharmacology. 2009;34(1):173–86.
14. Tiira K, Lohi H. Reliability and validity of a questionnaire survey in canine anxiety research. Appl Anim Behav Sci. 2014;155:82–92.
15. Vas J, Topál J, Péch É, Miklósi Á. Measuring attention deficit and activity in dogs: a new application and validation of a human ADHD questionnaire. Appl Anim Behav Sci. 2007;103:105–17.
16. Lit L, Schweitzer JB, Iosif AM, Oberbauer AM. Owner reports of attention, activity, and impulsivity in dogs: a replication study. Behav Brain Funct. 2010;6(1):1.
17. Puurunen J, Tiira K, Lehtonen M, Hanhineva K, Lohi H. Non-targeted metabolite profiling reveals changes in oxidative stress, tryptophan and lipid metabolisms in fearful dogs. Behav Brain Funct. 2016;12(1):1.
18. Benjamini Y, Hochberg Y. Controlling the false discovery rate: a practical and powerful approach to multiple testing. J R Stat Soc. 1995;57(1):289–300.
19. The METLIN metabolite database. https://metlin.scripps.edu/index.php. Accessed 8 Aug 2015.
20. The Human Metabolome Database. http://www.hmdb.ca/. Accessed 8 Aug 2015.
21. LIPID Metabolites And Pathways Strategy (LIPID MAPS). http://www.lipidmaps.org/. Accessed 8 Aug 2015.
22. Murphy RC, Axelsen PH. Mass spectrometric analysis of long-chain lipids. Mass Spectrom Rev. 2011;30(4):579–99.
23. Xu F, Zou L, Lin Q, Ong CN. Use of liquid chromatography/tandem mass spectrometry and online databases for identification of phosphocholines and lysophosphatidylcholines in human red blood cells. Rapid Commun Mass Spectrom. 2009;23(19):3243–54.
24. Xia YQ, Jemal M. Phospholipids in liquid chromatography/mass spectrometry bioanalysis: comparison of three tandem mass spectrometric techniques for monitoring plasma phospholipids, the effect of mobile phase composition on phospholipids elution and the association of phospholipids with matrix effects. Rapid Commun Mass Spectrom. 2009;23(14):2125–38.
25. Hsu FF, Turk J. Characterization of ceramides by low energy collisional-activated dissociation tandem mass spectrometry with negative-ion electrospray ionization. J Am Soc Mass Spectrom. 2002;13(5):558–70.
26. Aarsland TI, Landaas ET, Hegvik TA, Ulvik A, Halmoy A, Ueland PM, et al. Serum concentrations of kynurenines in adult patients with attention-deficit hyperactivity disorder (ADHD): a case-control study. Behav Brain Funct. 2015;11(1):1.
27. Antalis CJ, Stevens LJ, Campbell M, Pazdro R, Ericson K, Burgess JR. Omega-3 fatty acid status in attention-deficit/hyperactivity disorder. Prostaglandins Leukot Essent Fatty Acids. 2006;75(4–5):299–308.
28. Stevens LJ, Zentall SS, Deck JL, Abate ML, Watkins BA, Lipp SR, et al. Essential fatty acid metabolism in boys with attention-deficit hyperactivity disorder. Am J Clin Nutr. 1995;62(4):761–8.
29. Widenhorn-Muller K, Schwanda S, Scholz E, Spitzer M, Bode H. Effect of supplementation with long-chain omega-3 polyunsaturated fatty acids on behavior and cognition in children with attention deficit/hyperactivity disorder (ADHD): a randomized placebo-controlled intervention trial. Prostaglandins Leukot Essent Fatty Acids. 2014;91(1–2):49–60.
30. Spahis S, Vanasse M, Belanger SA, Ghadirian P, Grenier E, Levy E. Lipid profile, fatty acid composition and pro- and anti-oxidant status in pediatric patients with attention-deficit/hyperactivity disorder. Prostaglandins Leukot Essent Fatty Acids. 2008;79(1–2):47–53.
31. Karbownik M, Reiter RJ, Garcia JJ, Cabrera J, Burkhardt S, Osuna C, et al. Indole-3-propionic acid, a melatonin-related molecule, protects hepatic microsomal membranes from iron-induced oxidative damage: relevance to cancer reduction. J Cell Biochem. 2001;81(3):507–13.
32. Hwang IK, Yoo KY, Li H, Park OK, Lee CH, Choi JH, et al. Indole-3-propionic acid attenuates neuronal damage and oxidative stress in the ischemic hippocampus. J Neurosci Res. 2009;87(9):2126–37.
33. Attwood G, Li D, Pacheco D, Tavendale M. Production of indolic compounds by rumen bacteria isolated from grazing ruminants. J Appl Microbiol. 2006;100(6):1261–71.
34. Wikoff WR, Anfora AT, Liu J, Schultz PG, Lesley SA, Peters EC, et al. Metabolomics analysis reveals large effects of gut microflora on mammalian blood metabolites. Proc Natl Acad Sci USA. 2009;106(10):3698–703.
35. Zhang LS, Davies SS. Microbial metabolism of dietary components to bioactive metabolites: opportunities for new therapeutic interventions. Genome Med. 2016;8(1):1.
36. Zhao Y. Auxin biosynthesis and its role in plant development. Annu Rev Plant Biol. 2010;61:49–64.
37. Weissbach H, King W, Sjoerdsma A, Udenfriend S. Formation of indole-3-acetic acid and tryptamine in animals: a method for estimation of indole-3-acetic acid in tissues. J Biol Chem. 1959;234(1):81–6.
38. Russell WR, Duncan SH, Scobbie L, Duncan G, Cantlay L, Calder AG, et al. Major phenylpropanoid-derived metabolites in the human gut can arise from microbial fermentation of protein. Mol Nutr Food Res. 2013;57(3):523–35.
39. de Theije CG, Bavelaar BM, Lopes da Silva S, Korte SM, Olivier B, Garssen J, et al. Food allergy and food-based therapies in neurodevelopmental disorders. Pediatr Allergy Immunol. 2014;25(3):218–26.
40. Petra AI, Panagiotidou S, Hatziagelaki E, Stewart JM, Conti P, Theoharides TC. Gut-microbiota-brain axis and its effect on neuropsychiatric disorders with suspected immune dysregulation. Clin Ther. 2015;37(5):984–95.
41. Collins SM, Surette M, Bercik P. The interplay between the intestinal microbiota and the brain. Nat Rev Microbiol. 2012;10(11):735–42.
42. Myint AM, Kim YK. Network beyond IDO in psychiatric disorders: revisiting neurodegeneration hypothesis. Prog Neuropsychopharmacol Biol Psychiatr. 2014;48:304–13.
43. Zunszain PA, Anacker C, Cattaneo A, Choudhury S, Musaelyan K, Myint AM, et al. Interleukin-1beta: a new regulator of the kynurenine pathway affecting human hippocampal neurogenesis. Neuropsychopharmacology. 2012;37(4):939–49.
44. Moroni F, Cozzi A, Sili M, Mannaioni G. Kynurenic acid: a metabolite with multiple actions and multiple targets in brain and periphery. J Neural Transm. 2012;119(2):133–9.
45. Wonodi I, Schwarcz R. Cortical kynurenine pathway metabolism: a novel target for cognitive enhancement in Schizophrenia. Schizophr Bull. 2010;36(2):211–8.
46. Sathyasaikumar KV, Stachowski EK, Wonodi I, Roberts RC, Rassoulpour A, McMahon RP, et al. Impaired kynurenine pathway metabolism in the prefrontal cortex of individuals with schizophrenia. Schizophr Bull. 2011;37(6):1147–56.

47. Myint AM, Kim YK, Verkerk R, Scharpe S, Steinbusch H, Leonard B. Kynurenine pathway in major depression: evidence of impaired neuroprotection. J Affect Disord. 2007;98(1–2):143–51.

48. Savitz J, Dantzer R, Wurfel BE, Victor TA, Ford BN, Bodurka J, et al. Neuroprotective kynurenine metabolite indices are abnormally reduced and positively associated with hippocampal and amygdalar volume in bipolar disorder. Psychoneuroendocrinology. 2015;52:200–11.

49. Kuc D, Zgrajka W, Parada-Turska J, Urbanik-Sypniewska T, Turski WA. Micromolar concentration of kynurenic acid in rat small intestine. Amino Acids. 2008;35(2):503–5.

50. Wu W, Nicolazzo JA, Wen L, Chung R, Stankovic R, Bao SS, et al. Expression of tryptophan 2,3-dioxygenase and production of kynurenine pathway metabolites in triple transgenic mice and human Alzheimer's disease brain. PLoS ONE. 2013;8(4):e59749.

51. Patrick RP, Ames BN. Vitamin D and the omega-3 fatty acids control serotonin synthesis and action, part 2: relevance for ADHD, bipolar disorder, schizophrenia, and impulsive behavior. FASEB J. 2015;29(6):2207–22.

52. Banerjee E, Nandagopal K. Does serotonin deficit mediate susceptibility to ADHD? Neurochem Int. 2015;82:52–68.

53. Dougherty RM, Galli C, Ferro-Luzzi A, Iacono JM. Lipid and phospholipid fatty acid composition of plasma, red blood cells, and platelets and how they are affected by dietary lipids: a study of normal subjects from Italy, Finland, and the USA. Am J Clin Nutr. 1987;45(2):443–55.

54. Muller CP, Reichel M, Muhle C, Rhein C, Gulbins E, Kornhuber J. Brain membrane lipids in major depression and anxiety disorders. Biochim Biophys Acta. 2015;1851(8):1052–65.

55. Conquer JA, Tierney MC, Zecevic J, Bettger WJ, Fisher RH. Fatty acid analysis of blood plasma of patients with Alzheimer's disease, other types of dementia, and cognitive impairment. Lipids. 2000;35(12):1305–12.

56. Alberts B, Johnson A, Lewis J, et al. Molecular Biology of the Cell. 4th ed. London: Garland Science; 2002.

57. Richardson AJ, Puri BK. The potential role of fatty acids in attention-deficit/hyperactivity disorder. Prostaglandins Leukot Essent Fatty Acids. 2000;63(1–2):79–87.

58. Chalon S. Omega-3 fatty acids and monoamine neurotransmission. Prostaglandins Leukot Essent Fatty Acids. 2006;75(4–5):259–69.

59. Delion S, Chalon S, Herault J, Guilloteau D, Besnard JC, Durand G. Chronic dietary alpha-linolenic acid deficiency alters dopaminergic and serotoninergic neurotransmission in rats. J Nutr. 1994;124(12):2466–76.

60. Zimmer L, Delpal S, Guilloteau D, Aioun J, Durand G, Chalon S. Chronic n-3 polyunsaturated fatty acid deficiency alters dopamine vesicle density in the rat frontal cortex. Neurosci Lett. 2000;284(1–2):25–8.

61. Zimmer L, Hembert S, Durand G, Breton P, Guilloteau D, Besnard JC, et al. Chronic n-3 polyunsaturated fatty acid diet-deficiency acts on dopamine metabolism in the rat frontal cortex: a microdialysis study. Neurosci Lett. 1998;240(3):177–81.

62. Chen JR, Hsu SF, Hsu CD, Hwang LH, Yang SC. Dietary patterns and blood fatty acid composition in children with attention-deficit hyperactivity disorder in Taiwan. J Nutr Biochem. 2004;15(8):467–72.

63. Bekaroglu M, Aslan Y, Gedik Y, Deger O, Mocan H, Erduran E, et al. Relationships between serum free fatty acids and zinc, and attention deficit hyperactivity disorder: a research note. J Child Psychol Psychiatr. 1996;37(2):225–7.

64. Young GS, Maharaj NJ, Conquer JA. Blood phospholipid fatty acid analysis of adults with and without attention deficit/hyperactivity disorder. Lipids. 2004;39(2):117–23.

65. Hawkey E, Nigg JT. Omega-3 fatty acid and ADHD: blood level analysis and meta-analytic extension of supplementation trials. Clin Psychol Rev. 2014;34(6):496–505.

66. Frances H, Monier C, Bourre JM. Effects of dietary alpha-linolenic acid deficiency on neuromuscular and cognitive functions in mice. Life Sci. 1995;57(21):1935–47.

67. Ceylan MF, Sener S, Bayraktar AC, Kavutcu M. Changes in oxidative stress and cellular immunity serum markers in attention-deficit/hyperactivity disorder. Psychiatr Clin Neurosci. 2012;66(3):220–6.

68. Ceylan M, Sener S, Bayraktar AC, Kavutcu M. Oxidative imbalance in child and adolescent patients with attention-deficit/hyperactivity disorder. Prog Neuropsychopharmacol Biol Psychiatr. 2010;34(8):1491–4.

69. Selek S, Bulut M, Ocak AR, Kalenderoglu A, Savas HA. Evaluation of total oxidative status in adult attention deficit hyperactivity disorder and its diagnostic implications. J Psychiatr Res. 2012;46(4):451–5.

70. Kul M, Unal F, Kandemir H, Sarkarati B, Kilinc K, Kandemir SB. Evaluation of Oxidative Metabolism in Child and Adolescent Patients with Attention Deficit Hyperactivity Disorder. Psychiatr Investig. 2015;12(3):361–6.

2

Logical fallacies in animal model research

Espen A. Sjoberg*

Abstract

Background: Animal models of human behavioural deficits involve conducting experiments on animals with the hope of gaining new knowledge that can be applied to humans. This paper aims to address risks, biases, and fallacies associated with drawing conclusions when conducting experiments on animals, with focus on animal models of mental illness.

Conclusions: Researchers using animal models are susceptible to a fallacy known as false analogy, where inferences based on assumptions of similarities between animals and humans can potentially lead to an incorrect conclusion. There is also a risk of false positive results when evaluating the validity of a putative animal model, particularly if the experiment is not conducted double-blind. It is further argued that animal model experiments are reconstructions of human experiments, and not replications per se, because the animals cannot follow instructions. This leads to an experimental setup that is altered to accommodate the animals, and typically involves a smaller sample size than a human experiment. Researchers on animal models of human behaviour should increase focus on mechanistic validity in order to ensure that the underlying causal mechanisms driving the behaviour are the same, as relying on face validity makes the model susceptible to logical fallacies and a higher risk of Type 1 errors. We discuss measures to reduce bias and risk of making logical fallacies in animal research, and provide a guideline that researchers can follow to increase the rigour of their experiments.

Keywords: Argument from analogy, Confirmation bias, Type 1 error, Animal models, Double-down effect, Validity

---

Logical fallacy

A logical fallacy is a judgment or argument based on poor logical thinking. It is an error in reasoning, which usually means that either the line of reasoning is flawed, or the objects in the premise of the argument are dissimilar to the objects in the conclusion [1]. Scientists are not immune to logical fallacies and are susceptible to making arguments based on unsound reasoning. For instance, a common fallacy is *affirming the consequent*. This involves the following line of reasoning: *if A is true, then X is observed. We observe X, therefore A must be true.* This argument is fallacious because observing X only tells us that there is a possibility that A is true: the rule does not specify that A follows X, even if X always follow A.[1] Studies that have explicitly investigated this in a scientist sample found that 25–33% of scientists make the fallacy of affirming the consequent and conclude that $X \rightarrow A$ is a valid argument [2, 3].

Making logical fallacies is a human condition, and there is a large range of fallacies commonly committed [1, 4, 5]. In the present paper, we will focus on a select few that are of particular relevance to animal model research, especially in the context of validity and reliability of conclusions drawn from an experiment.

---

*Correspondence: espen.sjoberg@hioa.no
Department of Behavioral Sciences, Oslo and Akershus University College of Applied Sciences, St. Olavs Plass, P.O. Box 4, 0130 Oslo, Norway

[1] If you struggle to follow this line of reasoning, a concrete example makes it easier: *If it is wine, then the drink has water in it. Water is in the drink. Therefore, it must be wine.* Nowhere does the rule specify that only wine contains water as an ingredient, so simply making this observation does not allow us to conclude that it is wine.

Confirmation and falsification

The fallacy of affirming the consequent is connected with a tendency to seek evidence that confirms a hypothesis. Many scientists conduct their experiments under the assumption that their experimental paradigm is a legitimate extension of their hypothesis, and thus their results are used to confirm their beliefs. As an example, imagine a hypothesis that states that patients with bipolar disorder have reduced cognitive processing speed, and we do a reaction time test to measure this. Thus, a fallacious line of reasoning would be: *if bipolar patients have reduced cognitive processing speed, then we will observe slower reaction time on a test. We observe a slower reaction time, and therefore bipolar patients have reduced cognitive processing speed.* This would be affirming the consequent, because the observed outcome is assumed to be the result of the mechanism outlined in the hypothesis, but we cannot with certainty say that this is true. The results certainly suggests this possibility, and it may in fact be true, but the patients may have exhibited slower reaction times for a variety of reasons. If a significant statistical difference between bipolar patients and controls is found, it may be common to conclude that the results support the cognitive processing speed hypothesis, but in reality this analysis only reveals that the null hypothesis can be rejected, not necessarily why it can be rejected [6, 7]. The manipulation of the independent variable gives us a clue as to the cause of the rejection of the null hypothesis, but this does not mean that the alternative hypothesis is confirmed beyond doubt.

Popper [8] claimed that hypotheses could never be confirmed; only falsified. He claimed that we could not conclude with absolute certainty that a statement is true, but it is possible to conclude that it is *not true*. The classic example is the white swan hypothesis: even if we have only observed white swans, we cannot confirm with certainty the statement "all swans are white", but if we observe a single black swan then we can reject the statement. Looking for confirmation (searching for white swans) includes the risk of drawing the wrong conclusion, which in this case is reached through induction. However, if we seek evidence that could falsify a hypothesis (searching for black swans), then our observations have the potential to reject our hypothesis. Note that rejecting the null hypothesis in statistical analyses is not necessarily synonymous with falsifying an experimental hypothesis. Null-hypothesis testing is a tool, and when we use statistical analyses we are usually analysing a numerical analogy of our experimental hypothesis.

When a hypothesis withstands multiple tests of falsification, Popper called it *corroborated* [9]. We could argue that if a hypothesis is corroborated, then its likelihood of being true increases, because it has survived a gauntlet of criticism by science [10]. However, it is important to note that Popper never made any such suggestion, as this would be inductive reasoning: exactly the problem he was trying to avoid! Even if a hypothesis has supporting evidence and has withstood multiple rounds of falsification, Popper meant that it is not more likely to be true than an alternative hypothesis, and cannot be confirmed with certainty [11]. Instead, he felt that a corroborated theory could not be rejected without good reason, such as a stronger alternative theory [12]. Popper may be correct that we cannot confirm a hypothesis with absolute certainty, but in practice it is acceptable to assume that a hypothesis is likely true if it has withstood multiple rounds of falsification, through multiple independent studies using different manipulations (see "Animal model experiments are reconstructions" section). However, in the quest for truth we must always be aware of the possibility, however slight, that the hypothesis is wrong, even if the current evidence makes this seem unlikely.

Confirmation bias

Confirmation bias is the tendency to seek information that confirms your hypothesis, rather than seeking information that could falsify it [13]. This can influence the results when the experimenter is informed of the hypothesis being tested, and is particularly problematic if the experiment relies on human observations that has room for error. The experimenters impact on the study is often implicit, and may involve subtly influencing participants or undermining methodological flaws, something also known as *experimenter bias* [14].

The tendency to express confirmation bias in science appears to be moderated by what field of study we belong to. Physicists, biologists, psychologists, and mathematicians appear to be somewhat better at avoiding confirmation bias than historians, sociologists, or engineers, although performance varies greatly from study to study [3, 15–18]. In some cases, the tendency to seek confirming evidence can be a result of the philosophy of science behind a discipline. For instance, Sidman's [19] book *Tactics of Scientific Research*, considered a landmark textbook on research methods in behavior analysis [20–22], actively encourages researchers to look for similarities between their research and others, which is likely to increase confirmation bias.

Confirmation bias has been shown in animal research as well, but this fallacy is reduced when an experiment is conducted double-blind [23]. Van Wilgenburg and Elgar found that 73% of non-blind studies would report a significant result supporting their hypothesis, while this was only the case in 21% of double-blind studies. An interesting new approach to reduce confirmation bias in animal research is to fully automatize the experiment [24, 25]. This involves setting up the equipment and protocols

Cognitive Neuroscience: Behavioral and Psychological Perspectives

in advance, so that large portions of an experiment can be run automatically, with minimal interference by the experimenter. Along with double-blinded studies, this is a promising way to reduce confirmation bias in animal experiments.

It is important to note that the confirmation bias phenomenon occurs as an automatic, unintentional process, and is not necessarily a result of deceptive strategies [26]. As humans, we add labels to phenomena and establish certain beliefs about the world, and confirmation bias is a way to cement these beliefs and reinforce our sense of identity.[2] Scientists may therefore be prone to confirmation bias due to a lack of education on the topic, and not necessarily because they are actively seeking to find corroborating evidence.

Argument from analogy and animal model research

The issues reported in this paper apply to all of science, and we discuss principles and phenomena that any scientist would hopefully find useful. However, the issues will primarily be discussed in the context of research on animal models, as some of the principles have special applications in this field. In this section, we outline how an animal model is defined, and problems associated with arguing from analogy in animal research.

Defining an animal model

The term "animal model" is not universally defined in the literature. Here, we define an animal model as *an animal sufficiently similar to a human target group in its physiology or behaviour, based on a natural, bred, or experimentally induced characteristic in the animal, and which purpose is to generate knowledge that may be extrapolated to the human target group.* In this article, we focus on translational animal models in the context of behavioural testing, which usually involve a specific species or strain, or an animal that have undergone a manipulation prior to testing.

An animal model can of course model another non-human animal, but for the most part the aim of it is to study human conditions indirectly through animal research. That research is conducted on animals does not necessarily mean that the animal acts as a model for humans. It is only considered an animal model when its function is to represent a target group or condition in humans, e.g. people with depression, autism, or brain injury. The current paper focuses on animal models of mental illness, but animal models as a whole represent a large variety of conditions, and are particularly common

to use in drug trials. See Table 1 for an overview of common animal models of mental illnesses.

It should also be noted that the term "animal model" refers to an animal model that has at least been validated to some extent, while a model not yet validated is referred to as a "putative animal model". That a model is "validated" does not mean that the strength of this validation cannot be questioned; it merely means that previous research has given the model credibility in one way or another.

Arguing from analogy

In research on animal models, scientists sometimes use an approach called the *argument from analogy*. This involves making inferences about a property of one group, based on observations from a second group, because both groups have some other property in common [1]. Analogies can be very useful in our daily lives as well as in science: a mathematical measurement, such as "one meter", is essentially an analogy where numbers and quantities act as representations of properties in nature. When applying for a job, a person might argue that she would be a good supervisor because she was also a good basketball coach, as the jobs have the property of leadership in common. Concerning animal models, arguing from analogy usually involves making inferences about humans, based on an earlier observation where it was found that the animals and humans have some property in common. Arguing from analogy is essentially a potentially erroneous judgment based on similarities between entities. However, this does not make the argument invalid by default, because the strength of the argument relies on: (1) how relevant the property we infer is to the property that forms the basis of the analogy; (2) to what degree the two groups are similar; (3) and if there is any variety in the observations that form the basis of the argument [1].

Animal models themselves are analogies, as their existence is based on the assumption that they are similar to a target group in some respect. If the two things we are drawing analogies on are similar enough so that we will reasonably expect them to correlate, an argument from analogy can be strong! However, when we draw the conclusion that two things share a characteristic, because we have established that they already share another, different characteristic, then we are at risk of making the *fallacy of false analogy* [27].

The false analogy

A false analogy is essentially an instance when an argument based on an analogy is incorrect. This can occur when the basis of similarity between objects do not justify the conclusion that the objects are similar in some

---

[2] Thanks to Rachael Wilner for pointing out this argument.

Table 1 A summary of some available animal models of mental illnesses, where the animals themselves act as the model for the target group

Mental illness	Model	References
Anxiety	Serotonin receptor 1A knockout mice	[114]
	Corticosterone treated mice	[115]
Attention-Deficit/Hyperactivity Disorder	Spontaneously Hypertensive rat	[35]
	Thyroid receptor β1 transgenic mice	[116]
Autism	Valproic Acid rat	[81]
Depression	Corticosterone treated rats and mice	[117]
	Chronic Mild Stress rats and mice	[118]
Obsessive Compulsive Disorder	Quinpirole treated rats	[119]
Post-Traumatic Stress Syndrome	Congenital learned helpless rat	[120]
Schizophrenia	Ventral hippocampus lesioned rats	[121]
	Methylazoxymethanol acetate treated rats	[122]
	Developmental vitamin D deficient rats	[123]

The animals are genetically modified, bred for a specific trait, or manipulated in some physiological fashion (e.g. a lesion or drug injection)

other respect. For instance, if Jack and Jill are siblings, and Jack has the property of being clumsy, we might infer that Jill is also clumsy. However, we have no information to assert that Jill is clumsy, and the premise for our argument is based solely on the observation that Jack and Jill have genetic properties in common. We are assuming that clumsiness is hereditary, and therefore this is probably a false analogy. Note that knowledge gained later may indicate that—in fact—clumsiness is hereditary, but until we have obtained that knowledge we are operating under assumptions that can lead to false analogies. Even if clumsiness was hereditary, we could still not say with absolute certainty that Jill is clumsy (unless genetics accounted for 100% of the variance). This new knowledge would mean that our analogy is no longer false, as Jill's clumsiness can probably at least in part be explained by genetics, but we are still arguing from analogy: we cannot know for certain if Jill is clumsy, based solely on observations with Jack.

The false analogy in animal models

With animal models, the false analogy can occur when one group (e.g. an animal) share some characteristics with another group (e.g. humans), and we assume that the two groups also share other characteristics. For instance, because chimpanzees can follow the gaze of a human, it could be assumed that the non-human primates understand what others perceive, essentially displaying theory of mind [28–30]. However, Povinelli et al. [31] argue that this is a false analogy, because we are drawing conclusions about the inner psychological state of the animal, based on behavioural observations. It may appear that the animal is performing a behaviour that requires complex thinking, while in reality it only reminds us of complex thinking [32], most likely because

we are anthropomorphizing the animal's behaviour [33]—particularly the assumption that the mind of an ape is similar to the mind of a human [30]. A different example would be birds that are able to mimic human speech: the birds are simply repeating sounds, and we are anthropomorphising if we believe the birds actually grasp our concept of language.

Robbins [34] pointed out that homology is not guaranteed between humans and primates, even if both the behavioural paradigm and the experimental result are identical for both species: different processes may have been used by the two species to achieve the same outcome. Since an animal model is based on common properties between the animal and humans, we may assume that new knowledge gained from the animal model is also applicable to humans. In reality, the results are only indicative of evidence in humans.

Arguing from analogy, therefore, involves the risk of applying knowledge gained from the animal over to humans, without knowing with certainty if this application is true. Imagine the following line of reasoning: we find result A in a human experiment, and in an animal model we also find result A, establishing face validity for the animal model. Consequently, we then conduct a different experiment on the animal model, finding result B. If we assume that B also exist in humans, without trying to recreate these results in human experiments, then we are arguing from analogy, potentially drawing a false analogy.

Illustration: argument from analogy in the SHR model of ADHD

An illustration of argument from analogy comes from the SHR (spontaneously hypertensive rat) model of ADHD (Attention-Deficit/Hyperactivity Disorder) [35,

36]. Compared to controls, usually the Wistar Kyoto rat (WKY), the SHRs exhibit many of the same behavioural deficits observed in ADHD patients, such as impulsive behaviour [37–42], inattention [35, 37], hyperactivity [37, 43], and increased behavioural variability [44–47].

One measure of impulsive behaviour is a test involving delay discounting. In this paradigm, participants are faced with the choice of either a small, immediate reinforcer or a larger, delayed reinforcer. Both ADHD patients [48] and SHRs [41] tend to show a preference for the smaller reinforcer as the delay between response and reinforcer increases for the large reinforcer. Research on delay discounting with ADHD patients suggests that they are *delay averse*, meaning that impulsivity is defined as making choices that actively seek to reduce trial length (or overall delay) rather than immediacy [48–56], but this is usually achieved by choosing a reinforcer with a short delay.

There is no direct evidence to suggest that SHRs operate by the same underlying principles as ADHD patients. Studies on delay discounting using SHRs tend to manipulate the delay period between response and reinforcer delivery, but do not compare the results with alternative explanations. This is because the rats cannot be told the details of the procedure (e.g. if the experiment ends after a specific time or a specific number of responses). Therefore, most authors who have investigated delay discounting usually avoid the term delay aversion [57]. However, some authors make the argument from analogy where they assume that the rats show a similar effect to ADHD children: Bizot et al. [58] concluded that *"...SHR are less prone to wait for a reward than the other two strains, i.e. exhibit a higher impulsivity level...* (p. 220)", and Pardey, Homewood, Taylor and Cornish [59] concluded that *"... SHRs are more impulsive than the WKY as they are less willing to wait for an expected reinforcer* (p. 170)." Even though the evidence shows that SHRs preference for the large reinforcer drops with increased delay, we cannot conclude with certainty that this occurs because the SHRs do not want to wait. The experimental setup does not tell us anything conclusive about the animal's motivation, nor its understanding of the environmental conditions. Hayden [60] has argued that the delay discounting task is problematic in measuring impulsivity in animals because it is unlikely that the animals understand the concept of the inter-trial interval. Furthermore, if the SHRs were less willing to wait for a reinforcer, then we may argue that this shows immediacy, and not necessarily delay aversion. In this case, it may instead support the dual pathway model of ADHD, which takes into account both delay aversion and an impulsive drive for immediate reward [56, 61, 62].

Assuming that the rats are delay averse or impulsive is arguing from analogy. The evidence may only suggests that the rats are impulsive, not necessarily why they are impulsive. The results may also not speak to whether the reason for this behaviour is the same in ADHD and SHRs (mechanistic validity—see "Mechanistic validity" section). If we were to manipulate the magnitude of the large reinforcer then we will also find a change in performance [57, 63]. How do we know that the SHRs are sensitive to temporal delays, and not to other changes in the experimental setup, such as the inter-trial interval [60], reinforcer magnitude [63], or the relative long-term value of the reward [64]?

The validity criteria of animal models

Before any further discussion on logical fallacies in animal models, the validity criteria of these models must be addressed. We must also point out that there are two approaches to animal model research: (1) validating a putative animal model, and (2) conducting research on an already validated model.

When asserting the criteria for validating an putative animal model, the paper by Willner [65] is often cited, claiming that the criteria for a valid animal model rests on its face, construct, and predictive validity. This means that the model must appear to show the same symptoms as the human target group (face validity), that the experiment measures what it claims to measure and can be unambiguously interpreted (construct validity), and that it can make predictions about the human population (predictive validity). However, there is no universally accepted standard for which criteria must be met in order for an animal model to be considered valid, and the criteria employed may vary from study to study [66–70]. Based on this, Belzung and Lemoine [71] attempted to broaden Willner's criteria into a larger framework, proposing nine validity criteria that assess the validity of animal models for psychiatric disorders. Tricklebank and Garner [72] have argued that, in addition to the three criteria by Willner [65], a good animal model must also be evaluated based on how it controls for third variable influences (internal validity), to what degree results can be generalized (external validity), whether measures expected to relate actually do relate (convergent validity), and whether measures expected to not relate actually do not relate (discriminant validity). These authors argue that no known animal model currently fulfils all of these criteria, but we might not expect them to; what is of utmost importance is that we recognize the limitation of an animal model, including its application. Indeed, it could be argued that a reliable animal model may not need to tick all the validity boxes as long it has predictive validity, because in the end its foremost purpose is to make empirical predictions about its human target group. However, be aware that arguing from analogy reduces the model's predictive validity, because its predictive capabilities may be limited to the animal studied.

Mechanistic validity

Behavioural similarities between a putative model and its human target group is not sufficient grounds to validate a model. In other words, face validity is not enough: arguably, *mechanistic validity* is more important. This is a term that normally refers to the underlying cognitive and biological mechanisms of the behavioural deficits being identical in both animals and humans [71], though we can extend the definition to include external variables affecting the behaviour, rather than attributing causality to only internal, cognitive events. Whether the observed behaviour is explained in terms of neurological interactions, cognitive processes, or environmental reinforcement depends on the case in question, but the core of matter is that mechanistic validity refers to the *cause of the observed behavioural deficit or symptom*. If we can identify the cause of the observed behaviour in an animal model, and in addition establish that this is also the cause of the same behaviour in humans, then we have established mechanistic validity. This validity criterion does not speak to what has triggered the onset of a condition (trigger validity), or what made the organism vulnerable to the condition in the first place (ontopathogenic validity), but rather what factors are producing the specific symptoms or behaviour [71]. For instance, falling down the stairs might have caused brain injury (trigger validity), and this injury in turn reduced dopamine transmission in the brain, which lead to impulsive behaviour. When an animal model is also impulsive due to reduced dopamine transmissions, we have established mechanistic validity (even if the trigger was different).

The validity of models of conditions with limited etiology

Face validity has been argued to be of relatively low importance in an animal model, because it does not speak about why the behaviour occurs [33, 69], i.e. the evidence is only superficial. However, it could be argued that face validity is of higher importance in animal models of ADHD, because the complete etiology underlying the condition is not yet fully known, and therefore an ADHD diagnosis is based entirely on behavioural symptoms [73].

There is limited knowledge of the pathophysiology on many of the mental illnesses in the *Diagnostic and Statistical Manual of Mental Disorders* [74]; depression and bipolar disorder are examples of heterogeneous conditions where animal models have been difficult to establish [75, 76]. When dealing with a heterogeneous mental disorder, it is inherently harder for animal models to mimic the behavioural deficits, particularly a range of different deficits [75, 77–80]. We could argue, therefore, that mechanistic validity in animal models is difficult, if not impossible, to establish from the outset when our knowledge of causality in humans might be limited.

Models can be holistic or reductionist

Animal models can be approached with different applications in mind: it can aim to act *holistic* or *reductionist*. A holistic approach assumes that the model is a good representation of the target group as a whole, including all or most symptoms and behavioural or neurological characteristics. Alternatively, a reductionist approach uses an animal model to mimic specific aspects of a target group, such as only one symptom. This separation may not be apparent, because animal models are usually addressed as if they are holistic; for instance, the valproic acid (VPA) rat model of autism is typically just labelled as an "animal model of autism" in the title or text [81], but experiments typically investigate specific aspects of autism [82–84]. This does not mean that the model is not holistic, but rather that its predictive validity is limited to the aspects of autism investigated so far. Similarly, the SHR is typically labelled as an "animal model of ADHD" [35], but it has been suggested that the model is best suited for the combined subtype of ADHD [36, 73], while Wistar Kyoto rats from Charles River Laboratories are more suited for the inattentive subtype [85]. The point of this distinction between holistic and reductionist approaches is to underline that animal models have many uses, and falsifying a model in the context of one symptom does not mean the model has become redundant. As long as the model has predictive validity in one area or another, then it can still generate hypotheses and expand our understanding of the target group, even if the model is not a good representation of the target group as a whole. Indeed, an animal model may actually be treated as holistic until it can be empirically suggested that it should in fact be reductionist. However, researchers should take care not to assume that a model is holistic based on just a few observations: this would be arguing from analogy and bears the risk of making applications about humans that are currently not established empirically. The exact applications and limitations of an animal model should always be clearly defined [33, 86].

Animal model experiments are reconstructions

The terms "replicate" and "reproduce" are often used interchangeably in the literature [87], but with regards to animal models their distinction is particularly important. *Replication* involves repeating an experiment using the same methods as the original experiment, while a *reproduction* involves investigating the same phenomenon using different methods [88]. Replications assure that the effects are stable, but a reproduction is needed to ensure that the effect was not due to methodological issues.

We suggest a third term, *reconstruction*, which has special applications in animal models. A reconstruction involves redesigning an experiment, while maintaining the original hypothesis, in order to accommodate different species. When an animal experiment aims to investigate a phenomenon previously observed on humans, we have to make certain changes for several reasons. First, the animals are a different species than humans, and have a different physiology and life experience. Second, the animals do not follow verbal instructions and must often (but not always) be trained to respond. Third, the experimental setup must often be amended so that a behaviour equivalent to a human behaviour is measured. A fourth observation is that animal studies tend to use smaller sample sizes than human experiments, which makes them more likely to produce large effect sizes when a significant result is found [89].

An animal model experiment actively attempts to reconstruct the conditions of which we observed an effect with humans, but makes alterations so that we can be relatively certain that an equivalent effect is observed in the animals (or vice versa, where a human experiment measures an equivalent effect to what was observed in an animal study). This questions the construct validity of the study: how certain are we that the task accurately reflects the human behaviour we are investigating?

Another problem concerned with reconstruction is the standardization fallacy [90]. This refers to the fact that animal experiments are best replicated if every aspect of the experiment is standardized. However, by increasing experimental control we lose external validity, meaning that the results are less likely to apply to other situations [91]. The difficulty is therefore to find a balance between the two, and finding this balance may depend on the research question we seek to answer [33, 92]. One approach is to initially begin with replications, and if these are successful move on to perform reproductions, and eventually reconstructions. This is essentially what van der Staay, Arndt and Nordquist [92] have previously suggested: successful direct replication is followed by extended replication where modifications are made within the procedure, the animal's environment (e.g. housing or rearing), or their gender. Should the effect persevere, then we have systematically established a higher degree of generalization without losing internal validity. At the final stage, quasi-replications are conducted using different species, which is similar to our concept of reconstructions, and it is at this stage that the translational value of the findings are evaluated.

The double-down effect

When we run animal model experiments, we have to use a control group for comparison. When we are evaluating a putative model, we are therefore indirectly evaluating both animal groups for their appropriateness as an animal model for the phenomenon in question, even if we hypothesized beforehand that just one group would be suitable, and this is the *double-down effect*. If we were to discover that the control group, rather than the experiment group, shows the predicted characteristic, then it may be tempting to use hindsight bias to rationalize that the result was predicted beforehand, something that should always be avoided! In actuality, this is an occasion that can be used to map the observable characteristics of the animals, which is called *phenotyping*. This may show that the control group has a property that makes them a suitable candidate as a new putative model. Follow-up studies can then formally evaluate whether this putative animal model has validity. This approach is perfectly acceptable, provided that the initial discovery of the control group's suitability is seen as suggestive and not conclusive, until further study provide more evidence.

When an animal model has already been validated, the double-down effect still applies: we are still indirectly evaluating two animal groups at once, but it is less likely that that the control group will display the animal's characteristic due to previous validation. Failure to replicate previous findings can be interpreted in many ways; it could be an error in measurement, differences in experimental manipulations, or that the animal model is simply not suitable as a model in this specific paradigm (but still viable in others). Should we observe that controls express a phenomenon that was expected of the experimental group, then we should replicate the study to rule out that the finding occurred by chance or through some methodological error. This may lead us to suggest the control group as a putative model, pending further validation.

The double-down effect and the file drawer problem

Since the purpose of animal models is to conduct research on non-human animals, with the aim to advance knowledge about humans, then inevitably the animal model and the human condition it mimics must be similar in some respect. If they were not, then the pursuit of the model would be redundant. Therefore, from the outset, there is likely to be publication bias in favour of data that shows support for a putative animal model, because otherwise it has no applications.

The double-down effect of evaluating two animal groups at once makes animal models particularly susceptible to the *file drawer problem*. This is a problem where the literature primarily reflects publications that found significant results, while null results are published less frequently [93, 94]. This aversion to the null creates what Ferguson and Heene called "undead theories", which are theories that survive rejection indefinitely, because null results that refute them are not published [95]. The origin of this trend is not entirely clear, but it probably came into existence by treating the presence of a phenomenon as more interesting than its absence. Once an effect has been documented, replications may now be published that support the underlying hypothesis.

The file drawer effect is probably related to the *sunk-cost effect*: this is a tendency to continue on a project due to prior investment, rather than switching to a more viable alternative [96]. Thus, if we publish null results, it may seem that previous publications with significant findings were wasteful, and we may feel that we are contributing towards dissent rather than towards finding solutions. It may be in the researcher's interest to find evidence supporting the theory in order to justify their invested time, thus becoming victim of confirmation bias.

Furthermore, if null results are found, they might be treated with more skepticism than a significant result. This is, of course, a fallacy in itself as both results should be treated the same: why would a null result be subjected to more scrutiny than a significant result? When the CERN facility recorded particles travelling faster than the speed of light, the observation appeared to falsify the theory of relativity [97]. This result was met with skepticism [98], and it was assumed that it was due to a measurement error (which in the end it turned out to be). Nevertheless, if the result had supported relativity, would the degree of skepticism have been the same?

In the context of animal studies, the double-down effect makes it more likely that a significant result is found when comparing two animal groups. Either group may be a suitable candidate for a putative animal model, even if only one group was predicted to be suitable beforehand. If any result other than a null result will show support for an animal model (or a putative model), then multiple viable models will be present in the literature, all of which will be hard to falsify (as falsifying one model may support another). Indeed, this is currently the case for animal models, where there are multiple available models for the same human conditions [80, 99–103]. The file drawer problem is a serious issue in science [104], and the trend may often be invisible to the naked eye, but methods such as meta-analyses have multiple tools to help detect publication bias in the literature [105].

Measures to improve animal model research

The main purpose of this paper was to address several risks and fallacies that may occur in animal model research, in order to encourage a rigorous scientific pursuit in this field. We do not intend to discourage researchers from using animal models, but rather hope to increase awareness of potential risks and fallacies involved. In order to make the issues addressed in the paper more overviewable, we have created a list for researchers to confer when designing animal experiment and interpreting their data.

1. *Be aware of your own limitations.* Some of the fallacies and risks addressed in this paper may be unavoidable for a variety of reasons. Nevertheless, the first step towards improving one's research is to be aware of the existence of these risks. When writing the discussion section of a report, it may be necessary to point out possible limitations. Even if they are not explicitly stated, it is still healthy for any scientist to be aware of them.[3]

2. *Establish predictive and mechanistic validity.* If you are attempting to validate a putative animal model, ensure that the experiment is as similar as possible to experiments done on humans. If this is not possible, explain why in the write-up. If the experiment is novel, and the animal model is already validated through previous research, then this principle does not necessarily apply, because the purpose is to uncover new knowledge that may be translated to humans. In such instances, a new hypothesis gains validity in a follow-up experiment on humans.
Remember that there are several criteria available for validating an animal model, but there is no universal agreement on which set of criteria should be followed. However, the two most important criteria are arguably predictive validity and mechanistic validity, because face validity is prone to logical fallacies. Establishing mechanistic validity ensures that the mechanisms causing the observed behaviour are the same in the model and humans, while establishing predictive validity means that knowledge gained from the model is more likely to apply to humans.

3. *Define an a priori hypothesis and plan the statistical analysis beforehand.* It is crucial to have an a priori hypothesis prior to conducting the experiment, otherwise one might be accused of data dredging and reasoning after-the-fact that the results were expected [107, 108]. When validating a putative animal model, this drastically reduces the double-down effect. If the data do not show the predicted pattern then it is perfectly acceptable to suggest a new

---

[3] The author of this manuscript once held a conference talk where he suggested the possibility that one of his own research results may have been influenced by confirmation bias [106]. Never assume that only others are prone to bias—even authors of logical fallacy papers may commit fallacies!.

hypothesis and/or a putative animal model for further research.

When designing the experiment, keep in mind which statistical analysis would be appropriate for analysing the data. If the statistical method is chosen post hoc, then it may not correspond to the chosen design, and one might be accused of data dredging, which involves choosing a statistical procedure that is more likely to produce significant results [107]. Also, keep in mind which post hoc tests are planned, and that the correct one is chosen to reduce familywise error when there are multiple comparisons to be made. It is highly recommended that effect sizes are reported for every statistical test: this will give insight into the strength of the observed phenomenon, and also allow a more detailed comparison between studies [109].

4. *Do a power analysis.* For logistical, practical, or economic reasons, animal model research may be forced to use sample sizes smaller than what is ideal. Nevertheless, one should conduct a power analysis to ascertain how many animals should be tested before the experiment starts. When doing multiple comparisons, it may be difficult to establish the sample size because the power analysis may only grant the sample size of an omnibus analysis (the analysis of the whole, not its individual parts), and not what is required to reach significance with post hoc tests [110]. If all the post hoc analyses are of equal interest, choose the sample size required to achieve power of 0.8 in all comparisons. Alternatively, use a comparison-of-most-interest approach where the sample size is determined by the power analysis of the post hoc comparison that is of highest interest [110]. If a power analysis is not conducted, or not adhered to, it may be prudent to use a sample size similar to previously conducted experiments in the literature, and then do a post hoc power analysis to determine the power of your study. Once the experiment is completed and the data analysed, one must never increase the sample size, because this will increase your chances of finding a significant result (confirmation bias) [109, 111, 112].

5. *Double-blind the experiment.* By doing the experiment double-blind, we severely reduce the risk of confirmation bias. This means that the experimenter is blind to the a priori hypothesis of the study, as well as what group each animal belongs to. However, in some cases it may be difficult or impossible to do this. For instance, if the experimental group has a phenotype that distinguishes them from controls (e.g. white vs. brown rats), then it is difficult to blind the experimenter. For logistical and monetary reasons it may also be impractical to have a qualified

experimenter who is blind to the relevant literature of the study. Also, avoid analysing data prior to the experiment's completion, because if the data are not in line with your predictions then one might implicitly influence the experiment to get the data needed (experimenter bias [14]). Be aware that it is nevertheless perfectly acceptable to inspect the data on occasion without statistically analysing it, just to ensure that the equipment is working as it is supposed to (or state in advance at what point it is acceptable to check the data, in case there are circumstances where you may want to terminate the experiment early).

6. *Avoid anthropomorphizing.* While it is inevitable to describe our results in the context of human understanding and language, we must be careful not to attribute the animals with human-like qualities. Avoid making inferences about the animal's thoughts, feelings, inner motivation, or understanding of the situation. We can report what the animals did, and what this means in the context of our hypothesis, but take care not to make assumptions of the inner workings of the animal.

7. *Avoid arguing from analogy.* No matter how validated an animal model is, we cannot be certain that a newly observed effect also applies to humans. If research on an animal model yields new information that could give insight into the human target group, ensure to mention that the data is suggestive, not conclusive, pending further validation. Remember that the strength of an animal model is to generate new knowledge and hypotheses relevant to the target group, including the assessment of potentially useful treatments, but that these new possibilities are only hypothetical once they are discovered.

8. *Attempt to publish, despite a null result.* If you predicted a specific result based on trends in the literature, but failed to find this result, do not be discouraged from publishing the data (especially if you failed to replicate a result in a series of experiments). This is particularly important if the experiment had a low sample size, as null results from such studies are probably the least likely to be published, thus fuelling the file drawer problem. By making the data available via either an article (for instance through *Journal of Articles in Support of the Null Hypothesis*) or a dataset online, then you are actively contributing to reduce the file drawer problem.

9. *Replicate, reproduce, and reconstruct.* Replicating an experiment in order to establish interval validity and reliability of an animal model is essential. When replicating experiments multiple times, we reduce the risk that the original finding was a chance result. If previous replications have succeeded, then attempt

to include a new hypothesis, experimental manipulation, or follow-up experiment during the study to expand our knowledge of the research question. This process establishes both internal and external validity. Finally, reconstruct the experiment on humans, so that the findings may be attributed across species.

A note on neurological similarities

The principles discussed in this paper have been addressed in a behavioural context, but it should be noted that they also apply to neurological evidence for animal models, though increasing the validity in this case can operate somewhat differently.

When we find neurological elements that are the same in both the animal model and the human target group (that do not exist in controls), we should be careful to draw any conclusions based on this. Just like behavioural evidence, the links are suggestive and not necessarily conclusive. It is risky to assume that the physiological properties shared between humans and animals operate the same way. In drug research, over 90% of drugs that show effectiveness on animal models fail to work on humans, a problem called *attrition* [113]. In the context of animal models of mental illness, Belzung and Lemoine [71] proposed the concept *biomarker validity*, which means that the function of a neurological mechanism is the same in the animal model and humans, even if the biomarker responsible for this function may be different across the species. In other words, the two species may have different biological markers, but as long as they operate the same way, and in turn produce the same symptoms, then this adds validity to the model.

Of course, in reality things are not this simple. Neurological evidence is usually not based on the presence of a single component, but rather multiple elements such as rate of neurotransmitter release, reuptake, polymorphism, neural pathways, drug effectiveness, or a combination of factors. The core message is that we must be aware that finding similar neurological elements in both animals and humans does not mean that they operate the same way. If we make this assumption, we are arguing from analogy.

It should be noted that confirmation bias could also be a problematic issue in neuroscientific research. Garner [113] illustrates this with a car example: if we believe that the gas pedal of a car is the cause of car accidents, then removing the gas pedal from a car will drastically reduce the accident rate of that car, confirming that indeed the gas pedal was the cause of car accidents. In neuroscience, we may knock out a gene or selectively breed strains to add or remove a genetic component. When the hypothesized behaviour is shown (or not shown), we might conclude that we have confirmed our hypothesis. The conclusion could be wrong because it is based on correlation, and thus future replications of this result is likely to make the same logical error [113].

Closing remarks

In this paper, it has been discussed how animal models can be susceptible to logical fallacies, bias, and a risk of getting results that could give a false sense of support for a putative animal model. Researchers should remember that behavioural results found in an animal model of a human condition does not guarantee that this knowledge is applicable to humans. Replicating, reproducing and reconstructing results over numerous studies will drastically reduce the probability that the results are similar by chance alone, although this does not necessarily shed light on why the behaviour occurs. Researchers should therefore be encouraged to investigate mechanistic validity, meaning what underlying processes are causing the behaviour. By simply looking at face validity, we have an increased risk of making errors through comparisons.

Animal models can be very useful for investigating the mechanisms behind a human condition. This new knowledge can help improve our understanding and treatment of this condition, but the researcher must not assume that the observed animal behaviour also applies to humans. Ultimately, animal models only provide solid evidence for the animal used, and indicative evidence of human behaviour. However, this is also the strength of animal models: indicative evidence may open the door to new ideas about human behaviour that were not previously considered. Through reconstructions, it can be established whether or not the phenomenon exists in humans, and if the model has mechanistic validity and predictive validity then this certainly increases the application of the model, as well as its value for the progress of human health.

Abbreviations

ADHD: Attention-Deficit/Hyperactivity Disorder; CERN: European Organization for Nuclear Research; DSM: Diagnostic and Statistical Manual of Mental Disorders; SHR: spontaneously hypertensive rat; VPA: valproic acid rat; WKY: Wistar Kyoto rat.

Acknowledgements

Rachael Wilner gave valuable insight and feedback throughout multiple versions of the manuscript, especially into improving the language and structure of the paper, as well as clarifying several arguments. A conversation with Øystein Vogt was largely inspirational in terms of writing this article. Magnus H. Blystad gave feedback that substantiated several claims, particularly the neurology section. Espen Borgå Johansen offered critical input on several occasions, which lead to some arguments being empirically strengthened. Carsta Simon's feedback improved some of the definitions employed in the article. Other members of the research group *Experimental Behavior Analysis: Translational and Conceptual Research*, Oslo and Akershus University College, is to be thanked for their contribution and feedback, particularly Per Holth, Rasmi Krippendorf, and Monica Vandbakk.

Competing interests

The author declare that he has no competing interests.

References

1. Salmon M. Introduction to logic and critical thinking. Boston: Wadsworth Cengage Learning; 2013.
2. Barnes B. About science. New York: Basil Blackwell Inc.; 1985.
3. Kern LH, Mirels HL, Hinshaw VG. Scientists' understanding of propositional logic: an experimental investigation. Soc Stud Sci. 1983;13:131–46.
4. Tversky A, Kahneman D. Extensional versus intuitive reasoning: the conjunction fallacy in probability judgment. Psychol Rev. 1983;90:293–315.
5. Kahneman D. Thinking, fast and slow. London: Macmillan; 2011.
6. Haller H, Krauss S. Misinterpretations of significance: a problem students share with their teachers. Methods Psychol Res. 2002;7:1–20.
7. Badenes-Ribera L, Frías-Navarro D, Monterde-i-Bort H, Pascual-Soler M. Interpretation of the P value: a national survey study in academic psychologists from Spain. Psicothema. 2015;27:290–5.
8. Popper KR. The LOGIC OF SCIENTIfiC DISCOVery. London: Hutchinson; 1959.
9. Lewens T. The meaning of science. London: Pelican; 2015.
10. Leahey TH. The mythical revolutions of american psychology. Am Psychol. 1992;47:308–18.
11. Law S. The great philosophers. London: Quercus; 2007.
12. Keuth H. The Philosophy of Karl Popper. Cambridge: Cambridge University Press; 2005.
13. Nickerson RS. Confirmation bias: a ubiquitous phenomenon in many guises. Rev Gen Psychol. 1998;2:175.
14. Rosenthal R, Fode KL. The effect of experimenter bias on the performance of the albino rat. Behav Sci. 1963;8:183–9.
15. Inglis M, Simpson A. Mathematicians and the selection task. In: Proceedings of the 28th international conference on the psychology of mathematics education; 2004. p. 89–96.
16. Jackson SL, Griggs RA. Education and the selection task. Bull Psychon Soc. 1988;26:327–30.
17. Hergovich A, Schott R, Burger C. Biased evaluation of abstracts depending on topic and conclusion: further evidence of a confirmation bias within scientific psychology. Curr Psychol. 2010;29:188–209.
18. Mahoney MJ. Scientist as subject: the psychological imperative. Philadelphia: Ballinger; 1976.
19. Sidman M. Tactics of scientific research. New York: Basic Books; 1960.
20. Moore J. A special section commemorating the 30th anniversary of tactics of scientific research: evaluating experimental data in psychology by Murray Sidman. Behav Anal. 1990;13:159.
21. Holth P. A research pioneer's wisdom: an interview with Dr. Murray Sidman. Eur J Behav Anal. 2010;12:181–98.
22. Michael J. Flight from behavior analysis. Behav Anal. 1980;3:1.
23. van Wilgenburg E, Elgar MA. Confirmation bias in studies of nestmate recognition: a cautionary note for research into the behaviour of animals. PLoS ONE. 2013;8:e53548.
24. Poddar R, Kawai R, Ölveczky BP. A fully automated high-throughput training system for rodents. PLoS ONE. 2013;8:e83171.
25. Jiang H, Hanna E, Gatto CL, Page TL, Bhuva B, Broadie K. A fully automated drosophila olfactory classical conditioning and testing system for behavioral learning and memory assessment. J Neurosci Methods. 2016;261:62–74.
26. Oswald ME, Grosjean S. Confirmation bias. In: Pohl R, editor. Cognitive illusions: a handbook on fallacies and biases in thinking, judgement and memory. Hove: Psychology Press; 2004. p. 79.
27. Mill JS. A system of logic. London: John W. Parker; 1843.
28. Premack D, Woodruff G. Does the chimpanzee have a theory of mind? Behav Brain Sci. 1978;1:515–26.
29. Call J, Tomasello M. Does the chimpanzee have a theory of mind? 30 years later. Trends Cogn Sci. 2008;12:187–92.
30. Gomez J-C. Non-human primate theories of (non-human primate) minds: some issues concerning the origins of mind-reading. In: Car-
ruthers P, Smith PK, editors. Theories of theories of mind. Cambridge: Cambridge University Press; 1996. p. 330.
31. Povinelli DJ, Bering JM, Giambrone S. Toward a science of other minds: escaping the argument by analogy. Cogn Sci. 2000;24:509–41.
32. Dutton D, Williams C. A view from the bridge: subjectivity, embodiment and animal minds. Anthrozoös. 2004;17:210–24.
33. van der Staay FJ, Arndt SS, Nordquist RE. Evaluation of animal models of neurobehavioral disorders. Behav Brain Funct. 2009;5:11.
34. Robbins T. Homology in behavioural pharmacology: an approach to animal models of human cognition. Behav Pharmacol. 1998;9:509–19.
35. Sagvolden T. Behavioral validation of the spontaneously hypertensive rat (Shr) as an animal model of attention-deficit/hyperactivity disorder (Ad/Hd). Neurosci Biobehav Rev. 2000;24:31–9.
36. Sagvolden T, Johansen EB, Wøien G, Walaas SI, Storm-Mathisen J, Bergersen LH, et al. The spontaneously hypertensive rat model of ADHD—the importance of selecting the appropriate reference strain. Neuropharmacology. 2009;57:619–26.
37. Sagvolden T, Aase H, Zeiner P, Berger D. Altered reinforcement mechanisms in attention-deficit/hyperactivity disorder. Behav Brain Res. 1998;94:61–71.
38. Wultz B, Sagvolden T. The hyperactive spontaneously hypertensive rat learns to sit still, but not to stop bursts of responses with short inter-response times. Behav Genet. 1992;22:415–33.
39. Malloy-Diniz L, Fuentes D, Leite WB, Correa H, Bechara A. Impulsive behavior in adults with attention deficit/hyperactivity disorder: characterization of attentional, motor and cognitive impulsiveness. J Int Neuropsychol Soc. 2007;13:693–8.
40. Evenden JL. The pharmacology of impulsive behaviour in rats Iv: the effects of selective serotonergic agents on a paced fixed consecutive number schedule. Psychopharmacology. 1998;140:319–30.
41. Fox AT, Hand DJ, Reilly MP. Impulsive choice in a rodent model of attention-deficit/hyperactivity disorder. Behav Brain Res. 2008;187:146–52.
42. Sonuga-Barke EJ. Psychological heterogeneity in Ad/Hd—a dual pathway model of behaviour and cognition. Behav Brain Res. 2002;130:29–36.
43. Berger DF, Sagvolden T. Sex differences in operant discrimination behaviour in an animal model of attention-deficit hyperactivity disorder. Behav Brain Res. 1998;94:73–82.
44. Uebel H, Albrecht B, Asherson P, Börger NA, Butler L, Chen W, et al. Performance variability, impulsivity errors and the impact of incentives as gender-independent endophenotypes for ADHD. J Child Psychol Psychiatry. 2010;51:210–8.
45. Johansen EB, Killeen PR, Sagvolden T. Behavioral variability, elimination of responses, and delay-of-reinforcement gradients in Shr and Wky rats. Behav Brain Funct. 2007;3:1.
46. Adriani W, Caprioli A, Granstrem O, Carli M, Laviola G. The spontaneously hypertensive-rat as an animal model of ADHD: evidence for impulsive and non-impulsive subpopulations. Neurosci Biobehav Rev. 2003;27:639–51.
47. Scheres A, Oosterlaan J, Sergeant JA. Response execution and inhibition in children with AD/HD and other disruptive disorders: the role of behavioural activation. J Child Psychol Psychiatry. 2001;42:347–57.
48. Sonuga-Barke E, Taylor E, Sembi S, Smith J. Hyperactivity and delay aversion—I. The effect of delay on choice. J Child Psychol Psychiatry. 1992;33:387–98.
49. Sonuga-Barke EJ, Williams E, Hall M, Saxton T. Hyperactivity and delay aversion III: the effect on cognitive style of imposing delay after errors. J Child Psychol Psychiatry. 1996;37:189–94.
50. Kuntsi J, Oosterlaan J, Stevenson J. Psychological mechanisms in hyperactivity: I response inhibition deficit, working memory impairment, delay aversion, or something else? J Child Psychol Psychiatry. 2001;42:199–210.
51. Solanto MV, Abikoff H, Sonuga Barke E, Schachar R, Logan GD, Wigal T, et al. The ecological validity of delay aversion and response inhibition as measures of impulsivity in AD/HD: a supplement to the NIMH multimodal treatment study of AD/HD. J Abnorm Child Psychol. 2001;29:215–28.

52. Dalen L, Sonuga-Barke EJ, Hall M, Remington B. Inhibitory deficits, delay aversion and preschool AD/HD: implications for the dual pathway model. Neural Plast. 2004;11:1–11.

53. Bitsakou P, Psychogiou L, Thompson M, Sonuga-Barke EJ. Delay aversion in attention deficit/hyperactivity disorder: an empirical investigation of the broader phenotype. Neuropsychologia. 2009;47:446–56.

54. Tripp G, Alsop B. Sensitivity to reward delay in children with attention deficit hyperactivity disorder (ADHD). J Child Psychol Psychiatry. 2001;42:691–8.

55. Marx I, Hübner T, Herpertz SC, Berger C, Reuter E, Kircher T, et al. Cross-sectional evaluation of cognitive functioning in children, adolescents and young adults with ADHD. J Neural Transm. 2010;117:403–19.

56. Marco R, Miranda A, Schlotz W, Melia A, Mulligan A, Müller U, et al. Delay and reward choice in ADHD: an experimental test of the role of delay aversion. Neuropsychology. 2009;23:367–80.

57. Garcia A, Kirkpatrick K. Impulsive choice behavior in four strains of rats: evaluation of possible models of attention deficit/hyperactivity disorder. Behav Brain Res. 2013;238:10–22.

58. Bizot J-C, Chenault N, Houzé B, Herpin A, David S, Pothion S, et al. Methylphenidate reduces impulsive behaviour in Juvenile Wistar rats, but not in adult Wistar, Shr and Wky rats. Psychopharmacology. 2007;193:215–23.

59. Pardey MC, Homewood J, Taylor A, Cornish JL. Re-evaluation of an animal model for ADHD using a free-operant choice task. J Neurosci Methods. 2009;176:166–71.

60. Hayden BY. Time discounting and time preference in animals: a critical review. Psychon Bull Rev. 2015;23:1–15.

61. Scheres A, Dijkstra M, Ainslie E, Balkan J, Reynolds B, Sonuga-Barke E, et al. Temporal and probabilistic discounting of rewards in children and adolescents: effects of age and ADHD symptoms. Neuropsychologia. 2006;44:2092–103.

62. Sonuga-Barke EJ, Sergeant JA, Nigg J, Willcutt E. Executive dysfunction and delay aversion in attention deficit hyperactivity disorder: nosologic and diagnostic implications. Child Adolesc Psychiatr Clin N Am. 2008;17:367–84.

63. Botanas CJ, Lee H, de la Peña JB, de la Peña IJ, Woo T, Kim HJ, et al. Rearing in an enriched environment attenuated hyperactivity and inattention in the spontaneously hypertensive rats, an animal model of attention-deficit hyperactivity disorder. Physiol Behav. 2016;155:30–7.

64. Sjoberg EA, Holth P, Johansen EB. the effect of delay, utility, and magnitude on delay discounting in an animal model of attention-deficit/hyperactivity disorder (ADHD): a systematic review. In: Association of behavior analysis international 42nd annual convention. Chicago, IL; 2016.

65. Willner P. Validation criteria for animal models of human mental disorders: learned helplessness as a paradigm case. Prog Neuropsychopharmacol Biol Psychiatry. 1986;10:677–90.

66. Geyer MA, Markou A. Animal models of psychiatric disorders. In: Bloom FE, Kupfer DJ, editors. Psychopharmacology: the fourth generation of progress. New York: Raven Press; 1995. p. 787–98.

67. McKinney W. Animal models of depression: an overview. Psychiatr Dev. 1983;2:77–96.

68. Koob GF, Heinrichs SC, Britton K. Animal models of anxiety disorders. In: Schatzberg AF, Nemeroff CB, editors. The American Psychiatric Press textbook of psychopharmacology. 2nd ed. Washington: American Psychiatric Press; 1998. p. 133–44.

69. Sarter M, Bruno JP. Animal models in biological psychiatry. In: D'Haenen H, den Boer JA, Willner P, editors. Biological psychiatry. Chichester: Wiley; 2002. p. 37–44.

70. Weiss JM, Kilts CD. Animal models of depression and schizophrenia. In: Schatzberg AF, Nemeroff CB, editors. The American Psychiatric Press textbook of psychopharmacology. 2nd ed. Washington: American Psychiatric Press; 1998. p. 89–131.

71. Belzung C, Lemoine M. Criteria of validity for animal models of psychiatric disorders: focus on anxiety disorders and depression. Biol Mood Anxiety Disord. 2011;1(1):9. doi:10.1186/2045-5380-1-9.

72. Tricklebank M, Garner J. The possibilities and limitations of animal models for psychiatric disorders. Cambridge: RSC Drug Discovery Royal Society of Chemistry; 2012. p. 534–57.

73. Sagvolden T, Johansen EB. Rat models of ADHD. In: Stanford C, Tannock R, editors. Behavioral neuroscience of attention-deficit/hyperactivity disorder and its treatments. Berlin: Springer; 2012. p. 301–15.

74. Association AP. Diagnostic and statistical manual of mental disorders (Dsm-5®). Arlington County: American Psychiatric Pub; 2013.

75. Nestler EJ, Hyman SE. Animal models of neuropsychiatric disorders. Nat Neurosci. 2010;13:1161–9.

76. Gould TD, Einat H. Animal models of bipolar disorder and mood stabilizer efficacy: a critical need for improvement. Neurosci Biobehav Rev. 2007;31:825–31.

77. Karatekin C. A comprehensive and developmental theory of ADHD is tantalizing, but premature. Behav Brain Sci. 2005;28:430–1.

78. Willcutt EG, Doyle AE, Nigg JT, Faraone SV, Pennington BF. Validity of the executive function theory of attention-deficit/hyperactivity disorder: a meta-analytic review. Biol Psychiatry. 2005;57:1336–46.

79. Einat H, Manji HK. Cellular plasticity cascades: genes-to-behavior pathways in animal models of bipolar disorder. Biol Psychiatry. 2006;59:1160–71.

80. Sontag TA, Tucha O, Walitza S, Lange KW. Animal models of attention deficit/hyperactivity disorder (ADHD): a critical review. ADHD Atten Deficit Hyperact Disord. 2010;2:1–20.

81. Schneider T, Przewłocki R. Behavioral alterations in rats prenatally exposed to valproic acid: animal model of autism. Neuropsychopharmacology. 2005;30:80–9.

82. Mehta MV, Gandal MJ, Siegel SJ. Mglur5-antagonist mediated reversal of elevated stereotyped, repetitive behaviors in the VPA model of autism. PLoS ONE. 2011;6:e26077.

83. Markram K, Rinaldi T, La Mendola D, Sandi C, Markram H. Abnormal fear conditioning and amygdala processing in an animal model of autism. Neuropsychopharmacology. 2008;33:901–12.

84. Snow WM, Hartle K, Ivanco TL. Altered morphology of motor cortex neurons in the VPA rat model of autism. Dev Psychobiol. 2008;50:633–9.

85. Sagvolden T, Dasbanerjee T, Zhang-James Y, Middleton F, Faraone S. Behavioral and genetic evidence for a novel animal model of attention-deficit/hyperactivity disorder predominantly inattentive subtype. Behav Brain Funct. 2008;4:b54.

86. van der Staay FJ. Animal models of behavioral dysfunctions: basic concepts and classifications, and an evaluation strategy. Brain Res Rev. 2006;52:131–59.

87. Gómez O, Juristo N, Vegas S. Replication, reproduction and re-analysis: three ways for verifying experimental findings. In: Proceedings of the 1st international workshop on replication in empirical software engineering research (RESER 2010). Cape Town, South Africa; 2010.

88. Cartwright N. Replicability, reproducibility, and robustness: comments on Harry Collins. Hist Polit Econ. 1991;23:143–55.

89. Slavin R, Smith D. The relationship between sample sizes and effect sizes in systematic reviews in education. Educ Eval Policy Anal. 2009;31:500–6.

90. Würbel H. Behaviour and the standardization fallacy. Nat Genet. 2000;26:263.

91. Richter SH, Garner JP, Würbel H. Environmental standardization: cure or cause of poor reproducibility in animal experiments? Nat Methods. 2009;6:257–61.

92. Josef van der Staay F, Arndt S, Nordquist R. The standardization-generalization dilemma: a way out. Genes Brain Behav. 2010;9:849–55.

93. Rosenthal R. The file drawer problem and tolerance for null results. Psychol Bull. 1979;86:638.

94. Sterling TD. Publication decisions and their possible effects on inferences drawn from tests of significance—or vice versa. J Am Stat Assoc. 1959;54:30–4.

95. Ferguson CJ, Heene M. A vast graveyard of undead theories publication bias and psychological science's aversion to the null. Perspect Psychol Sci. 2012;7:555–61.

96. Arkes HR, Blumer C. The psychology of sunk cost. Organ Behav Hum Decis Process. 1985;35:124–40.

97. Brumfiel G. Particles break light-speed limit. Nature. 2011. doi:10.1038/news.2011.554.

98. Matson J. Faster-than-light neutrinos? Physics luminaries voice doubts. Sci Am. 2011. https://www.scientificamerican.com/article/ftl-neutrinos/. Accessed 13 Feb 2017.

99. Davids E, Zhang K, Tarazi FI, Baldessarini RJ. Animal models of attention-deficit hyperactivity disorder. Brain Res Rev. 2003;42:1–21.

100. Klauck SM, Poustka A. Animal models of autism. Drug Discov Today Dis Models. 2006;3:313–8.

101. Arguello PA, Gogos JA. Schizophrenia: modeling a complex psychiatric disorder. Drug Discov Today Dis Models. 2006;3:319–25.

102. Schmidt MV, Müller MB. Animal models of anxiety. Drug Discov Today Dis Models. 2006;3:369–74.

103. Deussing JM. Animal models of depression. Drug Discov Today Dis Models. 2006;3:375–83.

104. Pautasso M. Worsening file-drawer problem in the abstracts of natural, medical and social science databases. Scientometrics. 2010;85:193–202.

105. Rothstein HR, Sutton AJ, Borenstein M. Publication bias in meta-analysis: prevention, assessment and adjustments. Chichester: Wiley; 2006.

106. Sjoberg EA, D'Souza A, Cole GG. An evolutionary hypothesis concerning female inhibition abilities: a literature review. In: Norwegian behavior analysis society conference. Storefjell, Norway; 2016.

107. Smith GD, Ebrahim S. Data dredging, bias, or confounding: they can all get you into the BMJ and the friday papers. Br Med J. 2002;325:1437–8.

108. Simmons JP, Nelson LD, Simonsohn U. False-positive psychology undisclosed flexibility in data collection and analysis allows presenting anything as significant. Psychol Sci 2011:0956797611417632.

109. Sullivan GM, Feinn R. Using effect size—or why the P value is not enough. J Grad Med Educ. 2012;4:279–82.

110. Brooks GP, Johanson GA. Sample size considerations for multiple comparison procedures in Anova. J Mod Appl Stat Methods. 2011;10:97–109.

111. Royall RM. The effect of sample size on the meaning of significance tests. Am Stat. 1986;40:313–5.

112. Nakagawa S, Cuthill IC. Effect size, confidence interval and statistical significance: a practical guide for biologists. Biol Rev. 2007;82:591–605.

113. Garner JP. The significance of meaning: why do over 90% of behavioral neuroscience results fail to translate to humans, and what can we do to fix it? ILAR J. 2014;55:438–56.

114. Ramboz S, Oosting R, Amara DA, Kung HF, Blier P, Mendelsohn M, et al. Serotonin receptor 1a knockout: an animal model of anxiety-related disorder. Proc Natl Acad Sci. 1998;95:14476–81.

115. David DJ, Samuels BA, Rainer Q, Wang J-W, Marsteller D, Mendez I, et al. Neurogenesis-dependent and -independent effects of fluoxetine in an animal model of anxiety/depression. Neuron. 2009;62:479–93.

116. Siesser W, Zhao J, Miller L, Cheng SY, McDonald M. Transgenic mice expressing a human mutant **B**1 thyroid receptor are hyperactive, impulsive, and inattentive. Genes Brain Behav. 2006;5:282–97.

117. Gourley SL, Taylor JR. Recapitulation and reversal of a persistent depression-like syndrome in rodents. Curr Protoc Neurosci. 2009;Chapter 9:Unit-9.32. doi:10.1002/0471142301.ns0932s49.

118. Willner P. Chronic mild stress (CMS) revisited: consistency and behavioural-neurobiological concordance in the effects of CMS. Neuropsychobiology. 2005;52:90–110.

119. Szechtman H, Sulis W, Eilam D. Quinpirole induces compulsive checking behavior in rats: a potential animal model of obsessive-compulsive disorder (OCD). Behav Neurosci. 1998;112:1475.

120. King JA, Abend S, Edwards E. Genetic predisposition and the development of posttraumatic stress disorder in an animal model. Biol Psychiatry. 2001;50:231–7.

121. Lipska BK, Jaskiw GE, Weinberger DR. Postpubertal emergence of hyperresponsiveness to stress and to amphetamine after neonatal excitotoxic hippocampal damage: a potential animal model of schizophrenia. Neuropsychopharmacology. 1993;9:67–75.

122. Lodge DJ, Behrens MM, Grace AA. A loss of parvalbumin-containing interneurons is associated with diminished oscillatory activity in an animal model of schizophrenia. J Neurosci. 2009;29:2344–54.

123. Kesby JP, Burne TH, McGrath JJ, Eyles DW. Developmental vitamin D deficiency alters Mk 801-induced hyperlocomotion in the adult rat: an animal model of schizophrenia. Biol Psychiatry. 2006;60:591–6.

3

Safety out of control: dopamine and defence

Kevin Lloyd[*] and Peter Dayan

Abstract

We enjoy a sophisticated understanding of how animals learn to predict appetitive outcomes and direct their behaviour accordingly. This encompasses well-defined learning algorithms and details of how these might be implemented in the brain. Dopamine has played an important part in this unfolding story, appearing to embody a learning signal for predicting rewards and stamping in useful actions, while also being a modulator of behavioural vigour. By contrast, although choosing correct actions and executing them vigorously in the face of adversity is at least as important, our understanding of learning and behaviour in aversive settings is less well developed. We examine aversive processing through the medium of the role of dopamine and targets such as D_2 receptors in the striatum. We consider critical factors such as the degree of control that an animal believes it exerts over key aspects of its environment, the distinction between 'better' and 'good' actual or predicted future states, and the potential requirement for a particular form of opponent to dopamine to ensure proper calibration of state values.

Keywords: Dopamine, Defence, D_2 receptor, Striatum

Background

Our comprehension of appetitive Pavlovian and instrumental conditioning at multiple levels of theory and experiment has progressed dramatically over the last few years. We now enjoy a richly detailed picture, encompassing computational questions about the sorts of prediction and optimization that animals perform, and priors over these; algorithmic issues about the nature of different sorts of learning that get recruited and exploited in various circumstances; and implementational details about the involvement of many structures, including substantial pre-frontal cortical areas, the amygdala, the striatum, and also their respective dopaminergic neuromodulation [1–8]. Along with this evolving understanding of discrete choice, there is evidence that the vigour of engagement in actions is also partly determined through dopaminergic mechanisms associated with the assignment of positive valence, ensuring an alignment of incentive and activity [9–16].

By contrast, the case of aversive Pavlovian and instrumental conditioning is rather less well understood. Perhaps the most venerable puzzle concerns the instrumental case of active avoidance: how could it be that the desired absence of an aversive outcome can influence the choice and motivation of behaviour [17–22]? However, implementational considerations about the architecture of control make for extra problems—if, for instance, vigorous engagement in actions associated with active defence requires recruitment of mechanisms normally thought of as being associated with rewards rather than (potential) punishments [23, 24]. Further, there are alternative passive and active defensive strategies that impose seemingly opposite demands on these systems [25, 26].

In this review, we examine aversion through the medium of dopamine and some of its key targets. Dopamine is by no means the only, or perhaps even the most important, implementational facet of negative valence. For instance, as we will see, complex, species-specific, defensive systems provide an elaborate hard-wired mosaic of responsivity to a panoply of threatening cues [27–29]. Furthermore, cortically-based methods of reasoning that can incorporate and calculate with intricate prior expectations over such things as the degree

*Correspondence: klloyd@gatsby.ucl.ac.uk
Gatsby Computational Neuroscience Unit,
25 Howland Street, London, UK

to which environmental contingencies afford control, play a crucial role in modulating these defences [30–32]. Nevertheless, dopamine is well suited to the purpose of elucidating aversion because of the role it plays in the above enigmas via its influence over learned choice and vigour. Of dopamine's targets, our principal focus here is the striatum, with particular attention to D_2 receptors because of their seemingly special role in passive forms of behavioural inhibition [8, 33].

Almost all the elements of this account have been aired in previous analyses of appetitive and aversive neural reinforcement learning, with the role of dopamine also attracting quite some attention [34–40]. Our main aims are to weave these threads together, using the sophisticated view of appetitive conditioning as a foundation for our treatment of the aversive case, and to highlight issues that remain contentious or understudied. The issue of behavioural control will turn out to be key. We first outline a contemporary view of appetitive conditioning. We then use this to decompose and then recompose the issues concerning innate and learned defence.

Prediction and control of rewards

Reinforcement learning (RL) addresses the following stark problem: learn to choose actions which maximize the sum of a scalar utility or reward signal over the future by interacting with an initially unknown environment. Such environments comprise states or locations, and transitions between these states that may be influenced by actions. What make this problem particularly challenging are both the trial-and-error nature of learning—the effect of actions must be discovered by trying them—and the possibility that actions affect not only immediate but also delayed rewards by changing which states are occupied in the future [41].

Two broad classes of RL algorithms address this computational problem: *model-based* and *model-free* methods [41, 42]. Briefly, model-based methods use experience to construct an internal model of the structure of the environment (i.e. its states and transitions) and the outcomes it affords. Prediction and planning based on the model can then be used to make appropriate choices. Assuming the possibility of constant re-estimation, the flexibility afforded by this class of methods to changes in contingency (i.e. to environmental structure) and motivational state (i.e. to outcome values) has led to the suggestion that it is suitable as a model of goal-directed action [43–46]. Model-based estimates can also encompass comparatively sophisticated 'meta-statistics' of the environment, such as the degree to which rewards and punishments are under the control of the agent [32].

By contrast, model-free methods do not construct an internal model, but rather learn simpler quantities in the

service of the same goal. One such is the mean *value* of a state, which summarizes how good it is as judged by the cumulative rewards that are expected to accrue in the future when the subject starts from that state. This is, of course, the quantity that requires optimization. Crucially, the values of successive states satisfy a particular consistency relationship [47], so that states which tend to lead to states of high value will also tend to have high value, and vice-versa for states which tend to lead to low-value states. A broad class of model-free RL methods, known as *temporal difference* (TD) methods, use inconsistencies in the values of sampled successive states—a TD *prediction error* signal—to improve estimates of state values [48].

For selecting appropriate actions, a prominent model-free method is the *actor-critic* [41, 49]. This involves two linked processes. One is the *critic*, which uses the TD error to learn the model-free value of each state. However, future rewards typically depend on the actions chosen, or the behavioural *policy* followed. A policy is a state-response mapping, and is stored in the other component, the *actor*, which determines the relative probabilities of selecting actions. It turns out that the same TD prediction error that can improve the predictions of the critic may also be employed to improve the choices of the actor. There are also other model-free quantities that can be used for action selection. These include the Q value [50] of a state-action pair, which reports the expected long-run future reward for taking the particular initial action at the state.

Such model-free methods have the virtue of being able to learn to choose good actions without estimating a world model. However, summarizing experience by simple state values also means that these methods are relatively inflexible in the face of changes in environmental contingencies. Consequently, model-free RL methods have been suggested as a possible model of habitual actions [44, 45].

Both model-based and model-free methods must balance exploration and exploitation. The former is necessary to learn the possibilities associated with a novel domain; the latter then garners the rewards (or avoids the punishments) that the environment has been discovered to afford. This balance depends sensitively on many factors, including prior expectations about the opportunities and threats in the environment, how much control can be exerted over them, and how fast they change [51]. It also requires careful modelling of uncertainty—for instance, it is possible to quantify the value of exploration of unknown options as a function of the expected worth of the exploitation that they could potentially allow in the future [52, 53]. The excess of this over the expected value given current information is sometimes known as an *exploration bonus*, quantifying optimism in the face of uncertainty [54, 55].

Calculating such bonuses correctly, balancing exploration and exploitation optimally, and even just finding the optimal trajectory of actions in a rich state space, are radically computational intractable; heuristics therefore abound which are differently attuned to different classes of method [51]. Perhaps the most important heuristic is the existence of hard-wired systems that embody pre-specified policies. As we will detail below, these are of particular value in the face of mortal threat—animals will rarely have the luxury of being able to explore to find the best response. However, they are also useful in appetitive cases, obviating learning for actions that are sufficiently evolutionarily stable, such as in food-handling, mating and parenting.

Such hard-wired behaviours may be elicited in the absence of learning by certain stimuli, which are therefore designated *unconditioned stimuli* (USs). Presentation of a US typically inspires what is known as a *consummatory* response, attuned to the particularities of the US. It is through Pavlovian, or classical, conditioning that such innate responses can be attached not only to USs but also to formerly neutral predictors of such outcomes. These predictors are then called *conditioned stimuli* (CSs) since their significance is 'conditioned' by experience. Along with targeted preparation for particular outcomes, CS-elicited *conditioned responses* (CRs) include generic, so-called *preparatory*, actions: typically approach and engagement for appetitive cues, associated with predictions of rewarding outcomes; and inhibition, disengagement and withdrawal for aversive cues, associated with future threats or punishments. The predictions that underpin preparation can be either model-based or model-free [56]. We should note that the long-standing distinction between preparatory and consummatory behaviours [57–59] is not always clear cut; however, it has been usefully invoked—though not always in exactly the same terms—in various related theories of dopamine function [11, 60–66].

The fuller case of RL, in which actions come to be chosen because of their contingent effects rather than being automatically elicited by predictions, corresponds to instrumental conditioning. At least in experimental circumstances such as negative automaintenance [67], automatic, Pavlovian, responses can be placed in direct competition with instrumental choices. Perhaps surprisingly, Pavlovian responses often win [68, 69], leading to inefficient behaviour. A less malign interaction between Pavlovian and instrumental conditioning is called 'Pavlovian-instrumental transfer' (PIT) [45, 70–73]. In this, the vigour of instrumental responding (typically for rewards) is influenced positively or negatively by the presence of

Pavlovian CSs associated with appetitive or aversive predictions, respectively.

We start by considering the implications of Pavlovian and instrumental paradigms for the neural realization of control. We use a rather elaborated discussion of appetitive conditioning and rewards as a foundation, since this valence has received more attention and so is better understood. As a preview, we will see that dopamine in the ventral striatum has a special involvement in model-free learning (reporting the TD prediction error). However, dopamine likely also plays an important role in the expression and invigoration of both model-based and model-free behaviour.

Predicting reward: Pavlovian conditioning
Model-free RL, with its TD prediction errors, has played a particularly central role in developing theories of how animals learn state values, the latter interpreted as the predictions of long run rewards that underpin Pavlovian responses [74–77]. There is by now substantial evidence that the phasic activity of midbrain dopamine neurons resembles this TD prediction error in the case of reward [40, 78, 79]. Neural systems in receipt of this dopamine signal are then prime candidates to represent state values. One particularly important such target is the cortical projection to the ventral striatum (or nucleus accumbens; NAc) [78, 80], the plasticity of whose synaptic efficacies may be modulated by dopamine [81–85]. Note that, by contrast, dorsomedial and dorsolateral striatum, which are also targeted by dopamine cells—though by cells in the substantia nigra (SNc) rather than in the ventral tegmental area (VTA)—have been associated respectively with model-based and model-free instrumental behaviour (see below).

Along with its involvement in plasticity, dopamine, particularly in the NAc, has long been implicated in the intensity of the expression of innate, motivated behaviours (i.e., just those behaviours elicited by Pavlovian predictions) in response to both unconditioned and conditioned stimuli [66, 86, 87]. This is a form of Pavlovian vigour [63, 64, 88–91]. Relevant CSs have been described as acquiring 'incentive salience' [65, 92] or 'incentive motivation' [93], possibly via the way that their onset leads to TD errors that reflect state predictions [94]. Perhaps also related to Pavlovian vigour is the observation that the influence of CSs on instrumental responding in PIT paradigms is sensitive to dopamine signalling too [95–97]. It has recently been shown that dopaminergic projections to ventral striatum corelease glutamate [98–100], though see [101], which may modulate these effects.

The influence of dopamine neurons over the expression of behaviour might extend to model-based as well as model-free predictions, based on other afferent projections to the dopamine system. Model-based values are thought to be stored in, and calculated by, other areas, such as the basolateral amygdala and orbitofrontal cortex [87, 102–109].

Three further details of the ventral striatum and dopamine release in this structure are important. Firstly, anatomically, the NAc is classically subdivided into 'core' (NAcC) and 'shell' (NAcS) subregions [110]. As well as being histochemically distinct, these regions differ in their patterns of connectivity. For example, while NAcC resembles dorsal striatum in projecting extensively to classic basal ganglia output structures, such as the ventral pallidum, NAcS is notable for its projections to subcortical structures outside the basal ganglia, such as lateral hypothalamus and periaqueductal gray (PAG), which are involved in the expression of unlearned behaviours [110–114].

Two related ideas are abroad about the separate roles of these structures. One is that NAcS and NAcC mediate the motivational impact of USs and CSs, respectively [87]. For instance, the projection of NAcS to the lateral hypothalamus is known to play a role in the expression of feeding behaviour [112], requiring intact dopamine signalling within NAcS [115]. Conversely, conditioned approach is impaired by lesions or dopamine depletion of NAcC, but not by lesions of NAcS [116, 117].

The other idea is that NAcS and NAcC are involved in *outcome-specific* and *general* PIT, respectively [118]. The difference concerns whether the Pavlovian prediction is of the same outcome as for the instrumental act (specific PIT), or instead exerts influence according to its valence (general PIT). It has been reported that lesions of NAcS abolished outcome-specific PIT but spared general PIT, while lesions of NAcC abolished general PIT but spared outcome-specific PIT [118].

These ideas are not quite compatible, since both sorts of PIT involve conditioned stimuli. Perhaps, instead, we should think of the NAcC as being more involved in preparatory behaviours, attuned only to the valence (positive or negative) of a predicted outcome but not its particularities, while the NAcS is more involved in consummatory behaviours, which additionally reflect knowledge of the particular expected outcome(s) [118–123]. This is less incompatible with the first idea than it might seem, since outcome-specific PIT presumably relies on representation of the US, even if the US itself is not physically present [56]. This latter interpretation aligns with the distinction between model-free and model-based RL predictions, which would then be associated with NAcC and NAcS, respectively [56].

The second relevant, if somewhat contentious (see below), feature is that, as appears to be the case in the striatum generally, the majority of the principal projection neurons in NAc—medium spiny neurons (MSNs)—may express either D_1 or D_2 receptors, but not both [124, 125]. Briefly, dopamine receptors are currently thought to come in five subtypes, each classified as belonging to one of two families based on their opposing effects on certain intracellular cascades: D_1-like (D_1 and D_5 receptors), and D_2-like (D_2, D_3, and D_4 receptors). D_1 and D_2 receptors are of prime interest here since they are by far the most abundantly expressed dopamine receptors in the striatum and throughout the rest of the brain [126–128]. In the striatum, the majority of D_1 and D_2 receptors are thought to occupy states in which their affinities for dopamine are low and high respectively [129], with the consequence that these receptors are influenced differently by changes in phasic and tonic dopamine release [130]. Furthermore, D_1 and D_2 receptors appear to mediate opposite effects of dopamine on their targets: activation of D_1 receptors tends to excite, and D_2 to inhibit, neurons; this modulation of excitability can then also have consequences for activity-dependent plasticity [131, 132].

In the dorsal striatum, there is substantial evidence for an anatomical segregation between D_1-expressing 'Go' (direct; striatomesencephalic) and D_2-expressing 'NoGo' (indirect; striatopallidal) pathways [131, 133–136]. The effect of these pathways on occurrent and learned choice is consistent with the observations about the activating effect of dopamine [137], as we discuss in more detail below. Equivalent pathways are typically assumed to exist in NAc [138–140] although the segregation here seems more debatable [111, 141–143]. Indeed, D_1-expressing MSNs within NAcC are reported to also project within the striatopallidal ('indirect') pathway [141, 144]; there is evidence for co-expression of D_1 and D_2 receptors, particularly in NAcS [124, 145, 146]; and there are suggestions that D_1 and D_2 receptors can interact to form heteromeric dopamine receptor complexes within the same cell [147, 148], though this appears to be still a matter of question [149]. In functional terms, though, at least in the case of appetitive conditioning, it seems there may be parallel Go and NoGo routes, given evidence that D_1 receptors may be of particular importance in learning Pavlovian contingencies [150–154], while antagonists of either D_1 or D_2 receptors appear to disrupt the expression of such learning [155–159], including the expression of preparatory Pavlovian responses [34, 153]. Unfortunately, given the possible association of core and shell with model-free and model-based systems above, experimental evidence that clearly disentangles the roles of D_1 and D_2 receptors in these respective areas in appetitive conditioning appears to be lacking.

The third detail, which applies equally to ventral and dorsal striatum, concerns the link between the activity of dopaminergic cells and the release of dopamine into target areas. While there is little doubt that phasic release of striatal dopamine can be driven by activity in midbrain dopaminergic cells (e.g. [160]), a range of mechanisms local to the striatum is known to play a role in regulating dopamine release, including a host of other neurotransmitters such as glutamate, acetylcholine, and GABA (for recent reviews, see [161, 162]). Indeed, recent evidence suggests that striatal dopamine release can be stimulated axo-axonally by the synchronous activity of cholinergic interneurons, separate from changes in the activity of dopaminergic cells [163]. Furthermore, it has long been suggested that there is at least some independence between fast 'phasic' fluctuations in extracellular dopamine within the ventral striatum and a relatively constant 'tonic' dopamine level; the former are proposed to be spatially restricted signals driven by phasic bursting of dopamine cells, while the latter is thought to be comparatively spatially diffuse and controlled rather by the number of dopamine cells firing in a slower, 'tonic' mode of activity [164–166]. Evidence for co-release of other neurotransmitters alongside dopamine, such as glutamate and GABA, adds further complexity [98, 100, 167, 168].

Controlling reward: instrumental conditioning

In the instrumental, model-free, actor-critic method, the critic is the Pavlovian predictor, associated with the ventral striatum. The actor, by contrast, has been tentatively assigned to the dorsal striatum [78, 80, 169] based on its involvement in instrumental learning and control [170, 171]. The dorsal striatum is also a target of dopamine neurons, albeit from the substantia nigra pars compacta (SNc) rather than the ventral tegmental area (VTA). At a slightly finer grain, habitual behaviour has been particularly associated with dorsolateral striatum [172–175], while goal-directed behaviour has been associated with dorsomedial striatum, as well as ventromedial prefrontal and orbitofrontal cortices (for recent reviews, see [176, 177]). Recent evidence implicates lateral prefrontal cortex and frontopolar cortex in the arbitration between these two different forms of behavioural control in humans [178], and pre- and infra-limbic cortex in rats [179].

As noted above, the classical view of dorsal striatum is that the projections of largely separate populations of D_1-expressing (dMSNs) and D_2-expressing (iMSNs) medium spiny neurons are organised respectively into a direct (striatonigral) pathway, which promotes behaviour, and an indirect (striatopallidal) pathway, which suppresses behaviour [133, 134]. This dichotomous expression of D_1 and D_2 receptors would then allow dopamine to modulate the balance between the two pathways by differentially regulating excitability and plasticity [131]. In particular, activation of D_1 receptors in dMSNs increases their excitability and strengthens the direct pathway via long-term potentiation (LTP) of excitatory synapses. By contrast, activation of D_2 receptors in iMSNs decreases their excitability and weakens the indirect pathway by promoting long-term depression (LTD) of excitatory synapses.

This effect is then the basis of an elegant model-free account of instrumental conditioning [137, 180–182]. The active selection or inhibition of an action is mediated by the balance between direct and indirect pathways. Phasic increases and decreases in dopamine concentration report whether an action results in an outcome that is better or worse than expected, either via direct delivery of reward, or a favourable change in state. An increase consequent on the outcome being better than expected strengthens the direct pathway, making it more likely that the action will be repeated in the future. By contrast, a decrease consequent on the action being worse than expected strengthens the indirect pathway, making a repeat less likely. Much evidence, including recent optogenetic results, appears to support this basic mechanism [181, 183], although it is important to note that recent results suggest a slightly more nuanced view of the simple dichotomy between direct and indirect pathways—for instance, they are reported to be coactive during action initiation [184], consistent with the idea that they form a centre-surround organisation for selecting actions [185–187].

While it is natural to associate a dopamine TD prediction error with model-free prediction and control, there are hints that this signal shows a sophistication which potentially reveals more model-based influences [56, 188–191]. One such influence is exploration: observations of phasic activity of dopamine neurons in response to novel input which is not rewarding in any obvious sense (e.g. a novel auditory stimulus [192]) have been considered as an optimism-based exploration bonus [193]. It is not clear whether such activations depend, as they normatively should, on factors such as reward/punishment controllability that are typically the preserve of model-based calculations. Further, there remains to be a clear analysis of the role dopamine plays in the dorsomedial striatum's known influence over model-based RL [194, 195].

Instrumental vigour

Along with Pavlovian vigour is the possibility of choosing the alacrity or force of an action based on the contingent effects of this choice. Dopamine has also been implicated in this [12], potentially associated with model-based as well as model-free actions [196].

One idea is that there is a coupling between instrumental vigour and relatively tonic levels of dopamine, in the case that the latter report the prevailing average reward rate [9, 197]. This quantity acts as an opportunity cost for sloth, allowing a need for speed to be balanced against the (e.g., energetic) costs of acting quickly. Experiments that directly test this idea have duly supported dopaminergic modulation of vigour in reward-based tasks [13, 14, 16]. Formally, the average rate of TD prediction errors is just the same as the average rate of rewards, suggesting that nothing more complicated would be necessary to implement this effect than averaging phasic fluctuations in dopamine, at least in the model-free case. It could then be that because phasic fluctuations reflect Pavlovian as well as instrumental TD prediction errors, vigour would also be influenced by Pavlovian predictions—something that is contrary to the original instrumental expectation [9] but which is apparent in cases such as PIT [95]. Tonic dopamine has, of course, been suggested to be under somewhat separate control from phasic dopamine [164–166].

The putative involvement of dopamine in both vigour and valence leads to the prediction of a particular sort of hard-wired misbehaviour, or Pavlovian-instrumental conflict, namely that it might be hard to learn to withhold actions in the face of stimuli that predict rewards if inhibition is successful. This is indeed true, for both animals [67] and humans [24].

Defence

The main intent of this review is to understand how the elements of adaptive behaviour that we have just described apply in the aversive case. Coarsely, we need to (i) examine the complexities of consummatory versus preparatory, and active versus passive, defensive choices in the face of unconditioned aversive stimuli and their conditioned predictors; (ii) consider how instrumental avoidance actions can be learned to prevent threats from arising in the first place; and (iii) consider how the vigour of defensive actions is set appropriately.

The reason that we structured this review through the medium of dopamine is that it seems that many of the same dopaminergic mechanisms that we have just described for appetitive conditioning also operate in the aversive case, subject to a few added wrinkles. This makes for puzzles, both for aversion (how one could get vigorous defensive actions when only potential punishments are present and the reward rate is therefore at best negative) and for dopamine (why dopamine would apparently be released in just such purely aversive circumstances).

We argue that it is possible to generalize to these cases an expanded notion of *safety* (cf. [64]), which itself underpins the popular, two-factor solution to instrumental

avoidance [17, 19–22, 198–201]. Amongst other things, this implies subtleties in the semantics of dopamine, and a need to pay attention to the distinctions between reinforcement versus reward, and better versus good. To anticipate, we suggest that evidence for positive phasic and tonic dopamine responses to aversive unconditioned and conditioned stimuli may be explained in terms of a prediction of possible future safety. Furthermore, we suggest that these dopamine responses, and the consequent stimulation of striatal D_2 receptors in particular, play an important role in promoting, or at least licensing, active defensive behaviours.

Aversive unconditioned stimuli

There is some complexity in the consummatory response to an appetitive unconditioned stimulus (US) depending on how it needs to be handled. However, the response elicited by an aversive US—notably fleeing, freezing, or fighting—appears to depend in a richer way on the nature of the perceived threat, and indeed the species of the animal threatened [27]. Different emphases on the nature of the threat, or 'stressor', and the defensive response, or 'coping strategy', have led to subtly different, yet complementary, analyses of defensive behaviour and its neural substrates, which include the amygdala, ventral hippocampus, medial prefrontal cortex (mPFC), ventromedial hypothalamus, and periaqueductal gray (PAG) [25, 26, 28, 202–208] (for a recent review, see [29]).

For our purposes, the most important distinction is between *active* defensive responses, such as fight, flight, or freeze, and *passive* ones, such as quiescence, immobility, or decreased responsiveness. These need to be engaged in different circumstances, subject particularly to whether or not the stressor is perceived as being escapable or controllable [25]. Thus, active responses are adaptive if the stressor is perceived as escapable, since these may cause the stressor to be entirely removed. Conversely, passive responses may be more adaptive in the face of inescapable stress, promoting conservation of resources over the longer term and potential recovery once the stressor is removed. In other words, active responses entail *engagement* with the environment, while passive responses entail a degree of *disengagement* from the environment [25]. Even freezing involves 'attentive immobility', which can be interpreted as a state of high 'internal' engagement in threat monitoring.

The potential link to dopamine here is the proposal, particularly advocated by Cabib and Puglisi-Allegra [209–211] and fleshed out below, that an increased tonic level of dopamine in NAc, and especially the resulting stimulation of dopamine D_2 receptors in this area, promotes active defence, whereas a decreased tonic level of dopamine in NAc, and the resulting decrease in D_2

stimulation, promotes passive defence. This suggestion has clear parallels in the appetitive case. As there, in addition to the canonical direct and indirect pathways, typically associated with dorsal striatum and the expression of instrumental behaviours via disinhibition of cortically-specified actions [133, 137, 185, 212], we should expect accumbens-related Pavlovian defence to involve disinhibition and release of innate behavioural systems organised at the subcortical level, such as in the hypothalamus and PAG [112, 204, 213, 214].

For dopamine release, studies using microdialysis to measure extracellular concentrations of dopamine have reported elevated levels in response to an aversive US in NAc [215, 216], as well as in PFC [217] and amygdala [218, 219]. Using the higher temporal resolution technique of fast-scan cyclic voltammetry (FSCV), it has been reported that an aversive tail pinch US immediately triggers elevated dopamine release in the NAcC which is time-locked to the duration of the stimulus, while in the NAcS dopamine release is predominantly inhibited during the stimulus and either recovers or exceeds baseline levels following US offset [220, 221].

The substrate for this release is less clear. As we noted, many dopamine neurons appear to be activated by unexpectedly appetitive events. Although most studies report that dopamine neurons are inhibited by an aversive US (e.g., an electric shock, tail pinch, or airpuff), there are long-standing reports suggesting that a relatively small proportion may instead be activated [40]. The dopaminergic nature of some such responses appears to have been confirmed more recently via optogenetics [222] and juxtacellular labelling [223]. It has also been suggested that a particular group of ventrally-located dopamine cells in the VTA that projects to mPFC [224, 225] is more uniformly excited by aversive USs [223, 226]. In the SNc, it has recently been reported that dopamine cells projecting to the dorsomedial striatum show immediate suppression of activity, followed by sustained elevation of activity, in response to a brief electrical shock. By contrast, dopamine cells projecting to dorsolateral striatum display an immediate increase in activity before promptly returning to baseline [227].

In relation to defensive behaviour, pharmacological interventions and lesion studies have long suggested that dopamine plays a role (reviews include [12, 34]). More recent evidence supporting a particular role for NAc D_2 receptors in defence comes from a series of experiments exploiting the ability of local disruptions to glutamate signalling in NAcS to elicit motivated behaviours [228, 229]. Thus, Richard and Berridge [230] have shown that expression of certain active defensive behaviours in rats (escape attempts, defensive treading/burying), which can be elicited by local AMPA blockade caudally in medial NAcS, not only requires endogenous dopamine activity [115], but also intact signalling of both D_1 and D_2 receptors. By contrast, (appetitive) feeding behaviour, elicited by glutamate disruption more rostrally in the medial NAcS, only requires intact signalling of D_1 receptors [230]. This result supports a role for D_1 receptors in active defence—as well as particular subregions of NAcS (though see [231] for evidence that the behaviours elicited from these regions is sensitive to context)—but it also seems to indicate an asymmetry in the involvement of D_2 receptors in modulating the expression of innate appetitive versus defensive behaviours.

Other studies also suggest a role for D_2 stimulation in active defence, though do not necessarily trace this to NAcS. For example, the expression of certain defensive behaviours in cats (ear retraction, growling, hissing, and paw striking), elicitable by electrical stimulation in ventromedial hypothalamus, can also be respectively instigated or blocked by direct microinjection into that area of a D_2 agonist or antagonist [232, 233]. Indeed, as mentioned previously, anatomical connections between NAcS and hypothalamus are known to play an important role in controlling motivated behaviours, with NAcS cast in the role of 'sentinel' allowing disinhibition of appropriate behavioural centres located in the hypothalamus [112, 214].

Such lines of evidence are consistent with promotion of active Pavlovian defences via enhanced dopamine release and increased NAc D_2 stimulation. Evidence for the other side of the proposal—promotion of passive Pavlovian defences via a drop in dopamine release and reduced NAc D_2 stimulation—is provided by experiments in which animals are exposed to chronic (i.e. inescapable) aversive stimuli, such as in animal models of depression [234]. Briefly, not only do animals in these settings show diminished expression of active defensive behaviours such as escape attempts over time [235–237], but it has also been observed that an initial increase in NAc tonic dopamine on first exposure to the stressor gradually gives way to reduced, below baseline, dopamine levels [238–241]. Since modifications of the animal's behaviour over time in such cases are presumably driven by experience of the (unsuccessful) outcomes of its escape attempts, and so more naturally fit with an instrumental analysis, we postpone fuller discussion of these results until considering the issue of instrumental behaviour and controllability below. However, we note that these changes in patterns of defence and dopamine release over time potentially yield an interesting case of a model-based influence on dopamine and perhaps model-free behaviours.

Pain research provides a complementary view. Bolles and Fanselow [205] pointed out that efficacious (active) defence requires inhibition of pain-related behaviours oriented towards healing injuries. Thus, it was hypothesized that activation of a fear motivation system, which promotes defensive behaviours (i.e. fight, flight, or freeze), inhibits—for example, by release of endogenous analgesics—a pain motivation system, which promotes recuperative behaviours (i.e. resting and body-care responses). Similarly, activation of the pain system was hypothesized to inhibit the fear system since (active) defensive behaviours would interfere with recovery via (passive) recuperative behaviours. In this light, it is interesting to note the well-established link between NAc dopamine, and D_2 stimulation in particular, and analgesia [242, 243]. Conversely, reductions in motivation in mouse models of chronic pain—consistent with energy-preserving, recuperative functions—have recently been shown to depend on adaptation of (D_2-expressing) iMSNs in NAc [244], and that this adaptation includes an increase in excitability of iMSNs in medial NAcS [245]. In turn, these results are consistent with previous observations of reduced effortful behaviour caused by blockade of NAc D_2 receptors [246, 247]. Both observations are consistent with reductions of actions involved in active defence being caused by the relative strengthening of a ventral indirect pathway.

While these various lines of evidence point to involvement of accumbens dopamine, and NAc D_2 signalling in particular, in modulating defence, we note some important caveats. As mentioned earlier, the separation of direct and indirect pathways in the accumbens is subject to continuing debate, with evidence that D_1-expressing MSNs in NAc also project within the canonical indirect pathway [141] and that a substantial proportion of NAc MSNs co-express D_1 and D_2 receptors [124]. Furthermore, while D_2 receptors may be more attuned to changes in tonic dopamine levels by virtue of their higher affinity, such changes presumably affect occupancy at both D_1 and D_2 receptors dependent on their affinities [130]. In short, rather than completely separate D_1 and D_2 systems that can be independently switched on and off, the true situation is likely to be more complex. Furthermore, experiments involving dopamine receptor agonists and antagonists can be difficult to interpret, since they may involve certain side-effects—such as the well known extrapyramidal symptoms associated with D_2 antagonists [248]—and placing the system into states not encountered during normal functioning.

From an RL perspective, the roles of dopamine and D_2 receptors raise two salient issues. The first is how to make sense of the apparent asymmetry in the involvement of D_2 receptors in defensive, as opposed to appetitive, behaviours. One possibility starts from the observation that traditional paradigms assessing the interaction of Pavlovian and instrumental conditioning suggest that the Pavlovian defence system is biased towards behavioural

inhibition in the face of threat [249, 250]. This Pavlovian bias may potentially require relatively greater inhibition of the ventral indirect pathway in order to *disinhibit* active defensive responses when required. Of course, this mechanistic speculation merely poses the further question of why the Pavlovian defence system should be biased towards behavioural inhibition in the first place. One dubitable speculation is that this stems from asymmetries in the statistics of rewards and punishments in the environment [251]. However, more work is necessary on this point.

The second, and more fundamental, issue is how to interpret variation, particularly enhancement, of NAc dopamine release in response to an aversive US in the first place, given the apparent tie between dopamine, appetitive prediction errors, and reward rates. This is the extended version of the puzzle of active avoidance to which we referred at the beginning. To answer this, we first consider certain similarities and differences between the unexpected arrival of an appetitive or aversive US [252]. This requires us to be more (apparently pedantically) precise about the appetitive case than previously. Here, the unpredicted arrival of the appetitive US (e.g. food) represents an unexpected improvement in the animal's situation. This improvement stems from the fact that the US predicts that an outcome of positive value is immediately attainable. Indeed, all USs can be thought of as predictors, where these predictions are not learned but rather hard-wired. Thus, as previously noted, an appetitive US will engage innate behaviours such as salivation and approach. In turn, these unconditioned responses can be interpreted as reflecting at least an implicit expectation that the predicted reward is attainable/controllable, or at least potentially so, subject to further exploration. Thus, salivation in response to the presence of a food US can be interpreted as reflecting a tacit belief that the food will be consumable (and both require and benefit from ingestion). As reviewed above, the phasic responses of dopamine cells in response to the unexpected presentation of an appetitive US, along with other observations, encourage a TD interpretation in terms of a response to an unexpected predictor of future reward.

Consider now the arrival of an unexpected aversive US (e.g. the sight of a predator). What this event signifies seems more complex. On the one hand, this surprising event presumably indicates that the present situation is *worse* than originally expected, since the animal is now in an undesirable state of danger: i.e., (a) the aversive US is an 'unpredicted predictor of possible future punishment'. As such, we should expect a negative prediction error. Indeed, at least the net value of the prediction error had better be negative to avoid misassignment of positive values to dangerous states and the consequent development of masochistic tendencies (i.e., the active seeking out of such dangerous states). On the other hand, relative to this new state of danger, the possible prospect of future safety—a positive outcome—comes into play. That is, at the point that the animal would actually manage to eliminate the threat if it can do so, the change in state from danger to safety would lead to an appetitive prediction error—just as with the change in state associated with the unexpected observation of food. Thus, provided the animal has the expectation that it will ultimately be able to achieve safety, i.e., that the situation is controllable, observation of the aversive stimulus should predict this future appetitive outcome, and so (b) lead to an immediate appetitive prediction error. The challenge therefore seems to be that of reconciling (a) and (b), i.e., the role of the aversive US as unpredicted predictor of both danger and possible future safety. To avoid any confusion, note that we discuss learning processes associated with signalling safety below; here, we consider hard-wired assessments of the absence of danger.

One attractive reconciliation comes from appealing to the concept of *opponency* [59, 253, 254]. Here, an aversive process would ensure that the net TD error caused by the unexpected aversive US is negative and that dangerous states are correctly assigned negative value. At the same time, an appetitive process would motivate behaviour towards the comparatively benign state of safety. Indeed, it has previously been proposed that the net prediction error can be decomposed in exactly this way [255], with the phasic activity of dopamine neurons signalling the appetitive component of this signal, while the aversive component is signalled by other means (e.g. by phasic serotonergic activity [23, 249, 252, 256]), such that the net prediction error would actually be negative [252].

A further consideration is the value of exploration. In appetitive contexts, we noted that exploration can be motivated by bonuses associated with the future value of what might be presently discovered. A potential heuristic realization of this was through the phasic activity of dopamine neurons inspired by novel stimuli [192, 193]. Consider the extension of this logic to the unexpected arrival of an aversive US: the animal may have the pragmatic *a priori* belief that safety is controllable, but the unexpected (and therefore 'novel') arrival of an aversive US may nevertheless be attended by uncertainty about how this new situation should be controlled. The issue of how exploration may then be carried out in a benign manner is of course particularly salient here (for a recent view of the issue of safe exploration from the RL perspective, see, e.g. [257]). The idea that a novel stressor elicits exploration in the 'search for effective active coping' has also been suggested by Cabib and Puglisi-Allegra [211]. In their scheme, a novel stressor leads to release of noradrenaline in PFC

and dopamine in NAc; both of these are hypothesized to contribute to an active coping response by encouraging exploration (noradrenaline in PFC) and active removal of the stressor (stimulation of D_2 receptors in NAc). Of particular note is that insufficient exploration can lead to persistent miscalibration [258]. That is, if the subject fails to explore, for instance because it believes the aversive stimulus to be insufficiently controllable, then it would never discover that it actually might be removed. Such a belief could result from a computational-level calculation about generalization from prior experience (as in learned helplessness; [31, 32]). At a different level of explanation, insufficient stimulation of D_2 receptors, leading to a lack of inhibition of passive defensive mechanisms, could readily have the same consequence.

Relevant to the issue of exploration and dopamine's possible involvement is the topic of anxiety. Fear and anxiety can be differentiated both by the behaviours they characteristically involve and their sensitivity to pharmacological challenge [259, 260]. Experimental assays of anxiety typically involve pitting the motivation to approach/explore novel situations against the motivation to avoid potential hazards [261]. According to one influential theory, it is exactly the function of anxiety in such cases of approach-avoidance conflict to move the animal towards potential danger, the better to assess risk [26, 259]. Not only is this thought to involve suppression of incompatible defensive responses, but also stimulation of approach; the associated 'behavioural approach system' is associated with NAc and its modulation by dopamine [259]. It would be interesting to consider a recent Bayesian decision-theoretic view of anxiety [262] that focuses on the opposite aspect, namely behavioural inhibition when there is no information to be gathered, and consider potential anti-correlations with dopaminergic modulation of the NAc.

In addition to evidence that some dopamine cells show phasic excitation in response to an aversive US, we also noted evidence from microdialysis studies for enhanced dopamine release in response to an aversive US over longer periods of time. What is the aversive parallel of the suggestion in the appetitive case that tonic dopamine levels, particularly in NAc, reflect an average reward rate which realizes the opportunity cost for acting slowly [9]? In aversive situations, the average reward rate is never strictly positive but, at least intuitively, time spent not actively engaged in a course of appropriate defensive action could be very costly indeed. For example, if an animal has just detected the presence of a predator, time spent not engaged in a course of defensive action could cost the potential safety that has thereby been missed.

Such considerations indicate the incompleteness of this previous account of tonic dopamine levels. In particular, dovetailing with our suggestions regarding phasic dopamine above, the suggested mapping of tonic dopamine to the average rate of reward needs to be broadened to include the potentially-achievable rate of safety [252] which, assuming a prior expectation of controllability, will be positive. This provides a possible explanation for why increased tonic dopamine concentrations have been observed in microdialysis studies in response to an aversive US. However, if the aversive US is inescapable or uncontrollable, then the potentially-achievable rate of safety reduces to nothing. Thus, the tonic release of dopamine would also be expected to decrease. This is consistent with evidence already mentioned that the initial increase in tonic NAc dopamine level dissipates over time, giving way to an eventual fall below baseline levels [238–241].

Pavlovian conditioned defence

In relation to conditioning in aversive settings, similar complexities arise due to the fact that learning is likely to result in both aversive (i.e. danger-predicting) and appetitive (i.e. safety-predicting) conditioned stimuli, and may promote passive or active defensive strategies. Again, we use dopamine as a medium through which to view these complexities, with its preferential attachment to single sides of these dichotomies.

Fear conditioning

Conditioning in the aversive case, where animals are exposed to cues predictive of aversive outcomes, is generally known as *fear conditioning* due to the constellation of physiological and behavioural responses that the aversive CS comes to evoke. As in the appetitive case, conditioned and unconditioned responses need not be the same. Take, for instance, the case of conditioning a rat to a footshock US [263]. Here, the predominant response of the rat on exposure to the environment where it has received footshocks in the past, i.e. the CR, is to freeze. By contrast, the immediate response elicited by the shock itself, i.e. the UR, is a vigorous burst of activity. Furthermore, there can be model-based, outcome-specific, predictions allowing tailored responses (e.g., [264]) as well as model-free, outcome-general, predictions leading to generic preparatory responses such as behavioural inhibition.

The intricacies of how CR and UR relate to each other, which are arguably greater in the case of fear conditioning where these may be in conflict, may explain some of the difficulties in explicating dopamine's role in fear conditioning. A role for dopamine in fear conditioning seems to be generally accepted, though there is less consensus on the exact nature of this role (reviews include [265–267]).

Electrophysiological studies report that a substantial fraction (35–65 %) of putative dopamine neurons are activated by an aversive CS which is interleaved with an appetitive CS, a fraction that even exceeds the frequency (<15 %) of activations in response to an aversive US [191]. However, it has been suggested that many, though not all, of these activations may reflect 'false aversive responses', arising principally from generalization from appetitive to aversive CSs of the same sensory modality [191]. Additionally, an aversive CS may allow the animal to reduce the impact of an aversive US or avoid it entirely, and so in effect act as an instrumental 'safety signal', predicting a relatively benign outcome given a suitable defensive strategy. For example, a CS which predicts an aversive airpuff may facilitate a well-timed blink, thereby reducing the airpuff's aversiveness [268]. This fits with the idea, mentioned above, that dopaminergic responses may be instigated by predicted safety, or a relative improvement in expected state of affairs.

Regardless of the interpretation of such activations of dopamine cells by aversive CSs, this activity appears to play a role in fear conditioning. For example, Zweifel et al. [269] have recently shown that disruption of phasic bursting by dopamine neurons via inactivation of their NMDA receptors impairs fear conditioning in mice. These mice apparently develop a 'generalized anxiety-like phenotype', which the authors ascribe to the animals' failure to learn the correct contingencies.

Similar to observations in microdialysis studies of an increase in NAcS dopamine following an aversive US, enhanced NAcS dopamine release is also observed following presentation of an aversive CS [216]. Such enhanced release in NAcS to the onset of an aversive CS is corroborated by a recent FSCV study [270], though the opposite effect—decreased release—was observed in NAcC. Another recent FSCV study suggests that whether an increase or decrease in NAcC dopamine release is observed following an aversive CS depends critically on the animal's ability to avoid the predicted US [271]. Thus, Oleson et al. [271] found that, when trained in a fear conditioning paradigm—where the aversive US (a shock) was necessarily inescapable—presentation of the CS led to a decrease in NAcC dopamine. By contrast, in a conditioned avoidance paradigm—where the animal could potentially avoid the shock—both decreases *and* increases in NAcC dopamine were observed: an *increase* on trials in which animals successfully avoided shock, but a *decrease* on trials in which animals failed to avoid shock.

Dopamine receptor subtypes appear to play distinct roles. There is some consensus that D_1 receptor agonists and antagonists respectively promote or impede learning and expression in fear conditioning paradigms, while the effect of D_2 manipulations is less clear [265, 267]. One study found that fear-potentiated startle could be restored in dopamine-deficient mice by administration of L-Dopa immediately following fear conditioning, but required intact signalling of D_1 receptors but not of D_2 receptors (although other members of the D_2-like family of receptors were reportedly required; [272]). Consistent with this finding, it has been reported recently that striatal-specific D_1 receptor knock-out mice, but not striatal-specific D_2 receptor knock-out mice, exhibit strongly impaired contextual fear conditioning [273]. Combined with evidence from previous fear conditioning studies [267, 274–277], as well as extensive evidence from the conditioned avoidance literature (see below), it appears that D_2 receptor manipulations affect only the *expression* of conditioned fear, rather than the learning of the association between aversive CS and US. This is consistent with experimental results in appetitive Pavlovian conditioning reviewed above, which suggest that D_1 receptors are particularly important in learning the CS-US contingency, while both D_1 and D_2 receptors are involved in modulating expression of this learning. Further, it has been reported recently that disruption of dopamine signalling in NAcC, but not NAcS, attenuated the ability of an aversive CS to block secondary conditioning of an additional CS, suggesting differential involvement of these areas [278].

Safety conditioning

The situation in which a CS predicts the *absence* of a US is usually known as 'conditioned inhibition' [279, 280]. In the particular case where the predicted absence is of an aversive US, the CS is called a *safety signal* [281, 282]. In considering aversive USs, we previously discussed hard-wired signals for safety—i.e., the absence of danger or threat. By contrast, here we consider previously neutral stimuli whose semantic association with safety is learned.

Such safety signals are capable of inhibiting fear and stress responses, and are known to have rewarding properties. For example, safety signals have been shown to act as conditioned reinforcers of instrumental responses [283]. This is consistent with the proposal of Konorski [59] and subsequent authors [199, 284, 285] that aversive and appetitive motivation systems reciprocally inhibit each other. The idea is that inhibition of the aversive system by a safety signal leads to disinhibition of the appetitive system, and so a safety signal is functionally equivalent to a CS that directly excites the appetitive system.

Neuroscientific study of safety signals is, however, at a relatively early stage (for reviews, see [281, 282]). Studies have identified neural correlates of learned safety in the amygdala [286–288] and striatum [286, 289].

Involvement of dopamine within NAcS in mediating the ability of the safety signal to inhibit fear, and consequently its ability to act as a conditioned reinforcer, is suggested by a recent study [290]. In particular, it was found that both infusion of d-amphetamine, an indirect dopamine agonist, and blockade of D_1/D_2 receptors in NAcS—but not in NAcC—disrupted the fear-inhibiting properties of a safety signal. While this finding implicates a role of NAcS in mediating the impact of the safety signal, why these manipulations had similar, as opposed to contrasting, effects is not clear.

Instrumental defence: learning to avoid

The final form of learning we consider in detail is instrumental avoidance. This is a rich paradigm that involves many of the behaviours and learning processes that we have discussed so far: innate defence mechanisms, fear conditioning, safety conditioning, and instrumental learning (cf. [291]). Furthermore, a role of dopamine in active avoidance, and D_2 receptors in particular, has long been suggested by the fact that dopamine antagonists interfere with avoidance learning [34, 292]. Indeed, such interference led to this paradigm being used to screen dopamine antagonists for antipsychotic activity [10, 12, 248]. Finally, the two-factor theory of active avoidance [17, 200, 201] that we discuss below was actually the genesis of the explanation we have been giving for the ready engagement of dopamine in the case of aversion.

The problem of avoidance and two-factor theory

A typical avoidance learning experiment involves placing an animal (e.g., a rat) in an environment in which a warning signal (e.g., a tone) predicts future experience of an aversive US (e.g., a shock) unless the animal performs a timely instrumental avoidance response (e.g., shuttling to a different location, or pressing a lever). That animals successfully learn to avoid under such conditions posed a problem that concerned early learning theorists [18]: how can the nonoccurrence of an aversive event—a ubiquitous condition—act as a behavioural reinforcer?

A solution to this 'problem of avoidance' has long been suggested in the form of a two-factor theory [17, 59, 200, 293–296]. The name 'two-factor' refers to the hypothesis that two behavioural factors or processes—Pavlovian and instrumental—are involved in the acquisition of conditioned avoidance. Firstly, the warning signal comes to elicit a state of fear through its predictive relationship with the aversive US. Thus, the first factor of the theory refers to the Pavlovian process of fear conditioning. This Pavlovian process then allows the second factor to come into play: if the animal now produces an action leading to the cessation of the warning stimulus, the animal enters a state of relief, or reduced fear, capable of reinforcing the avoidance response. Thus, the second factor refers to an instrumental process by which the avoidance response is reinforced through fear reduction or relief. Such an account can also include stimuli dependent on the avoidance response and which are anticorrelated with the aversive US, thereby becoming predictive of safety [201]. As discussed, these safety signals (SS) themselves are thought to be capable of inhibiting conditioned fear [280], thereby both preventing Pavlovian fear responses (e.g., freezing) which may interfere with the instrumental avoidance response and reinforcing safety-seeking behaviours in fearful states or environments [294, 296], consistent with theories of opponent motivational processes [59, 285].

Avoidance, innate defence, and controllability

As mentioned above, the importance of innate defensive behaviours in the avoidance context has long been noted. Bolles [27], highlighting the importance of such 'species-specific defense reactions', argued that if an avoidance behaviour is rapidly acquired, this is because the required avoidance response coincides with the expression of an innate defensive response by the animal, rather than reflecting a learning process; how difficult the animal finds the avoidance task will depend on the extent to which the avoidance response is compatible with its innate defensive repertoire. In turn, which innate behaviour the animal selects will be sensitive to relevant features of the avoidance situation, such as whether there is a visible escape route or not, reminiscent of Tolman's [297] notion of behavioural support stimuli [206, 298].

Just as in the appetitive case, conflict between such Pavlovian behaviours and instrumental contingencies can lead to apparently maladaptive behaviour, albeit in rather unnatural experimental settings. Thus, Seymour et al. [299] highlight experiments in which self-punitive behaviour arises when an animal is (instrumentally) punished for emitting Pavlovian responses in response to that punishment. In one such unfortunate case, squirrel monkeys were apparently unable to decrease the frequency of painful shocks delivered to them by suppressing their shock-induced tendency to pull at a restraining leash attached to their collar; pulling on the restraining leash was exactly the action that hastened arrival of the next shock [300].

Similarly, just as it has been suggested that the animal's appraisal of whether a threat is escapable or not is crucial in determining its defensive strategy in general (e.g., [25]), it was famously shown that the controllability of an aversive US is crucial in determining subsequent avoidance learning performance [301, 302]. In particular, dogs exposed to inescapable shocks in a first environment showed deficits in initiating avoidance or escape responses in a second environment, even though the aversive US was now escapable. This, of course, led to the concept of 'learned helplessness' [237]. Huys and Dayan [32] presented a model-based account of learned helplessness, arguing that the generalization between environments affected the value of exploration, thereby leading to persistent miscalibration.

The issue of model-free versus model-based influences has received rather less attention in aversive than appetitive contexts. However, sensitivity to revaluation of aversive USs in the context of instrumental avoidance has been demonstrated in rats [303, 304] and humans [305, 306], indicating model-based influences under at least some avoidance conditions. Fernando et al. [303] have recently reported that revaluation of a shock US induced by pairing shock with systemic analgesics (morphine or D-amphetamine), leading rats subsequently to decrease their rate of avoidance responding, could also be achieved by pairing the shock with more selective infusions of a mu-opioid agonist into either NAcS or PAG. Involvement of NAcS and related structures in revaluation in this instance is consistent with the idea that the shell is involved in model-based prediction [56].

Dopamine, D_2 receptors, and active avoidance

Two-factor theories of avoidance fit well with the idea that the striatum, in interaction with dopamine, implements an actor-critic algorithm [21, 22, 78, 80, 169, 307]. Thus, an initial period of learning by the critic (in the ventral striatum) of negative state values (i.e., fear conditioning) allows subsequent instrumental training of an avoidance response by the actor (in the dorsal striatum), since actions leading to the unexpected non-delivery of the aversive US are met with a positive prediction error ('better than expected'), as signalled by dopamine neurons in the midbrain.

It was the abilities of certain antipsychotic drugs and neurotoxic lesions to produce active avoidance learning deficits [248, 292] that suggested a critical role for dopamine in the acquisition of conditioned avoidance. Furthermore, localised neurotoxic lesions suggested that dopamine projections to both dorsal and ventral striatum were required for acquisition of active avoidance [308, 309], corroborated by more recent work on selective restoration of dopamine signalling in dopamine-deficient mice [310]. This is consistent with complementary roles of actor (ventral striatum) and critic (dorsal striatum) in adapting behaviour.

Dopamine's action on D_2 receptors appears of particular importance for this. Evidence from active avoidance studies suggests that while blocking D_2 receptors leaves fear conditioning intact, instrumental learning of the avoidance response requires intact D_2 signalling [292, 311, 312]. From the perspective of the actor-critic, one might conclude that blockade of D_2 receptors therefore does not interfere with the learning of negative state values by the critic but does interfere with the learning of the actor [22]. The finding that D_2 receptor blockade leaves conditioning to aversive stimuli intact in the active avoidance setting is consistent with evidence from fear conditioning studies (see above). Furthermore, that D_2 blockade also disrupts instrumental learning is consistent with dopamine's modulation of direct and indirect pathways in the dorsal striatum, as in Frank's [137] model, since this would be expected to lead to a relative strengthening of the indirect, 'NoGo' pathway and impede acquisition of the appropriate 'Go' response (albeit leaving this model without a means of implementing the preserved fear conditioning). However, this would raise the question of why D_2 receptors within dorsal striatum should be implicated more strongly in learning than are those in ventral striatum. A pertinent observation might be a distinction between the longevity of the effects of tying optogenetic stimulation of (D_1-expressing) dMSNs and (D_2-expressing) iMSNs in the dorsomedial striatum [183] of mice. These authors triggered activation of one or other pathway when the mouse made contact with one of two touch sensors. dMSN stimulation increased preference for its associated lever, whereas iMSN stimulation decreased it. However, whereas the positive preference persisted in extinction throughout a test period, the negative preference rapidly disappeared. Furthermore, it was noted that stimulation of iMSNs elicited brief, immediate freezing followed by an 'escape response', though these behavioural changes were not thought sufficient to explain the bias away from the laser-paired trigger.

Nevertheless, while many findings accord well with an actor-critic account of avoidance learning, there are at least two omissions in such accounts that require correction. Firstly, similar to Bolles' complaints about two-factor theory, actor-critic accounts have largely ignored the role for innate (i.e., Pavlovian) defence mechanisms. Secondly, the key factor of controllability has not been fully integrated with actor-critic models.

Indeed, disruption of innate defensive behaviour by D_2 blockade occurs as well as disruption of instrumental learning of the active avoidance response. There are suggestions that suppression of conditioned avoidance may rely more on disruption of D_2 signalling within ventral, rather than dorsal, striatum [248], consistent with interference with Pavlovian ('critic') rather than instrumental ('actor') processes. For example, post-training injection of a D_2 antagonist into NAcS, but not into dorsolateral striatum, leads to a relatively immediate suppression of a conditioned avoidance response [313]. As we saw above, NAcS, under dopaminergic modulation, is implicated in controlling expression of innate defensive behaviours,

and D_2 activation appears to promote active defensive strategies. Similarly, there is evidence that D_2 blockade leads to enhanced freezing responses—arguably, a more passive form of defence—following footshock, interfering with rats' ability to emit avoidance responses [34, 274], though there remains some doubt about whether fear-induced freezing is an important factor in the disruption of conditioned avoidance [248]. In their review of the role of dopamine in avoidance learning, and defence more generally, Blackburn and colleagues [34] suggest that D_2 blockade does not disrupt defensive behaviour globally but rather 'changes the probability that a given class of defensive response will be selected' ([34], p. 267), in particular increasing the probability of freezing.

In relation to controllability, we have already referred to evidence that exposure to chronic, inescapable stress abolishes stress-induced increases in the concentration of accumbens dopamine [238–241]. Such evidence has led Cabib and Puglisi-Allegra [209–211] to suggest that whether an increase or decrease in accumbens dopamine levels is observed in response to stress depends on whether the stressor is appraised as controllable (increase) or not (decrease). This dissipation of the dopamine response does not appear to be explained by dopamine depletion, since subsequent release from the chronic stressor leads to a large, rapid increase in dopamine concentration [239]. Similarly, Cabib and Puglisi-Allegra [209], using a yoked paradigm in which one of a pair of animals (the 'master') has some control over the amount of shock experienced by means of an escape response while the other ('yoked') animal does not, found evidence consistent with elevated and inhibited NAc dopamine in master and yoked animals, respectively, after an hour of shock exposure.

More recently, Tye et al. [314] used optogenetics to assess the effects of exciting or inhibiting identified VTA dopamine cells in certain rodent models of depression involving inescapable stressors (tail suspension, forced swim, and chronic mild stress paradigms). While optogenetic inhibition of these dopamine cells could induce behaviour that has been related to depression, such as reduced escape attempts, optogenetic activation of the same cells was found to rescue depression-like phenotypes (e.g., promoting escape-related behaviours) induced by chronic stress. Furthermore, it was observed that chronic stress led to a reduction in measures of phasic VTA activity. This latter observation contrasts with studies using repeated social defeat stress, where phasic VTA activity has typically been observed to increase in 'susceptible' animals [315–317]. Apparently contradictory findings regarding stress-induced changes in VTA dopamine activity, and indeed the effects of manipulating this via optogenetic stimulation, might stem from the subtleties of the different paradigms used, but may also reflect heterogeneity in the properties of different VTA dopamine cells, such as between those projecting to mPFC versus NAc (for a recent discussion of these issues, see [318]).

While there is evidence from microdialysis studies that support a link between controllability, defensive strategy, and tonic NAc dopamine, it should be noted that not all such evidence points in this direction. For example, Bland et al. [319] measured both dopamine and serotonin release in NAcS of rats in the yoked pairs paradigm referred to previously. While they did report a trend for increased dopamine release relative to no-shock controls, this increase was neither significant nor differed between master and yoked animals. By contrast, serotonin levels were found to be significantly increased in yoked animals during and after stress exposure, relative to master and no-shock control animals [319]. Experiments using the same paradigm but taking measurements from mPFC found elevated levels of both dopamine and serotonin in yoked animals compared to master and no-shock controls [320].

These latter studies and others [321–323] highlight that consideration of other neuromodulators, notably serotonin, is crucial for a fuller understanding of defensive behaviour. A role of serotonin has long been suggested both in the particular case of active avoidance [312, 324] and in defence more generally [249, 250]. As mentioned, one suggestion is that the putative opponency between appetitive and aversive motivation systems [59, 254, 285] is at least partly implemented in opponency between dopamine and serotonin, respectively [23, 249–251, 256]. A specific computational model of this idea was suggested by Daw et al. [255], and Dayan [252] has more recently considered such opponency in the particular case of active avoidance. However, a modulatory role of controllability in the active avoidance setting has not yet been fully integrated into RL models.

Conclusions

Here, we have discussed unconditioned/conditioned, Pavlovian/instrumental, and passive/active issues associated with aversion. We used dopamine, and particularly its projection into the striatum and the D_2 system, as a form of canary, since the way that dopamine underpins model-free learning, and model-free and model-based vigour, turns out to be highly revealing for the organization of aversive processing. Our essential explanatory strategy rested on three concepts: safety, opponency, and controllability.

When under threat, safety is a desirable state. We suggested that the prospect of possible future safety underlies positive dopamine responses—both tonic and phasic—in response to aversive stimuli. Indeed, the interpretation of these responses is very similar to the more obviously appetitive case involving rewards, since safety is an appetitive outcome. Thus, phasic activation of dopamine cells in response to an aversive stimulus can be interpreted in TD terms as an 'unpredicted predictor of future safety'. Similarly, increased levels of tonic dopamine in conditions of stress, particularly in NAc, can be interpreted as signalling a potentially-achievable rate of safety.

Of course, what makes safety a more subtle concept is that it is relative; it is defined in opposition to danger. Dangerous states are not, in general, good states, which is why, in opposition to an appetitive process directed at safety in such states, there should be an aversive system which signals the disutility of occupying dangerous states. Therefore, positive dopamine responses which putatively signal the appetitive component of a TD prediction error in such states can only be part of the story—an *opponent* signal is required, marking the value of the path that will (hopefully) not be taken, and providing a new baseline against which to measure outcomes. This results in a form of counterfactual learning signal, a quantity that has also been investigated in purely appetitive contexts, and may have special relevance to the dorsal, rather than the ventral, striatum [325–328].

Unfortunately, while the notion of opponent appetitive and aversive processes is long-standing [59, 253, 254, 285], we still know relatively little about their neural realization. As mentioned, one idea is that this opponency maps to dopamine (appetitive) and serotonin (aversive) signalling [23, 249–251, 256], and specific computational models of this idea have been advanced [252, 255]. Recent attention to electrophysiological recordings from identified serotonergic cells in conditions of reward and punishment is particularly welcome in this regard, albeit offering no comfort to these theoretical ideas [329], and we look forward to further work which leverages advances in neuroscientific techniques to clarify the neural substrate of opponency.

Whether safety is appraised as achievable or not appears to be crucial, hence our appeal to the concept of controllability. We reviewed evidence that tonic levels of dopamine are modulated downwards over time with chronic exposure to aversive stimuli. Further, we reviewed evidence that dopamine, and NAc D_2-receptor stimulation in particular, modulates active versus passive defensive strategies (or perhaps better, defensive versus recuperative behaviours). Modulation of dopamine in this way raises pressing questions about controllability at both more and less abstract levels. Indeed, even formalizing an adequate concept of behavioural control in the first instance is nontrivial [32].

The concept of controllability brings model-based and model-free considerations back into focus since, at least intuitively, this concept seems to imply explicit knowledge of action-outcome statistics in the current environment. In relation to dopamine, this is consistent with evidence that a model-based system could potentially influence model-free learning and performance via the dopaminergic TD signal. However, implementation of heuristics aimed at optimizing the exploration-exploitation trade-off, such as possibly instantiated in a dopaminergic exploration bonus, may provide a model-free proxy for controllability. Thus, further work is required to disentangle the relative contributions of model-based and model-free systems in modulating dopamine signals which, in turn, modulate defensive strategy.

We have focused on dopamine in the accumbens at the expense of other areas—notably the amygdala and mPFC—which are of clear relevance to the themes discussed. For example, intact dopamine signalling in the amygdala, as well as in the striatum, appears to be necessary for acquisition of active avoidance behaviour [310], with the central nucleus particularly implicated in mediating conditioned freezing responses that may interfere with active responding [330]. Indeed, there is evidence that D_2 receptors are particularly prevalent in the central amygdala [265, 331], and a recent review [332] suggests that a key role of D_2 receptors in the central nucleus is to modulate reflex-like defensive behaviours organised in the brain stem. This clearly relates to the proposed importance of D_2 in modulating Pavlovian defence discussed here. Similarly, it is known that stress-induced increases in accumbens dopamine release is constrained by activation of D_1 receptors in mPFC, with both mPFC dopamine depletion or blockade of D_1 receptors leading to enhanced stress-induced accumbens release of dopamine (see [211], and references therein). Furthermore, mPFC is thought to be a key player in the appraisal of whether a stressor is under the animal's control [323].

Throughout the review, we have highlighted various issues that merit experimental and theoretical investigation. Experimentally, the most pressing issue is perhaps heterogeneity in the dopamine system—arriving at a clearer view of the potentially separate roles and activation of different groups of dopamine neurons, and reconciling activation and release. Technical advances have allowed increasingly sophisticated attacks on this issue, though a consensus regarding the degree of heterogeneity, both in terms of activity [333, 334] and connectivity [227, 335, 336], has yet to emerge. To the extent that dopamine neurons with different affective receptive fields project to different targets, there is no need for a shared semantics for their activation [23]. However, if reward and punishment-activated dopamine neurons are interdigitated in the way suggested by some experiments [333], then there is a need for a functional analysis as to how downstream systems might be able to interpret the apparently confusing patterns of dopamine release. One speculation in the former case, e.g. if dopamine cells in the ventral versus dorsal VTA showing different responses to aversive stimuli [223] also differentially project to more ventral versus dorsal regions of striatum, respectively, is that this reflects competing objectives to (a) shape (instrumental) policy *retrospectively*, by assigning (dis)credit to actions that may have led to aversive outcomes, and (b) to promote suitable (Pavlovian) behaviour *prospectively* in light of possible future safety.

Similarly, it would be important to understand the true degree of separation between putative direct and indirect pathways in the core and shell of the accumbens. Heterogeneity in the serotonin system, and its interactions with dopamine in the case of aversion, would also merit investigation. A recent revealing analysis of active avoidance in the zebrafish, showing the critical involvement of a pathway linking the lateral habenula to the median raphe [324] is of importance, particularly since most of the recent studies of optogenetically tagged or manipulated 5-HT neurons have focused instead on the dorsal raphe [329, 337–339]. Integrating the whole array of data on patience, satiety, motor action, behavioural inhibition and aversion associated with 5-HT is a major task.

From a more behavioural viewpoint, it would be interesting to get a clearer view of the scope of model-based aversive conditioning. For instance, take the experiment showing that D_2 blockade does not arrest learning aversive predictions even though it does avoidance responses [311]: it is not clear why model-based predictions would not be capable of generating appropriate avoidance behaviour as soon as the D_2 antagonist is washed out—rather leaving it to be acquired slowly, as if it was purely model-free.

Another important experimental avenue is to try and integrate the processing of costs (and indeed, for humans, outcomes such as financial losses) with that of actual punishment. Costs, which could be either physical or mental [340–342], also exert a negative force on behaviour, and indeed also have a slightly complicated relation to dopamine activation and release [12, 16, 343, 344].

From a more theoretical viewpoint, perhaps the most urgent question concerns pinning down the different facets of controllability, the way that these determine operations such as exploration, and relative model-based and model-free influences. Entropy and reachability of outcomes were considered by [32], but other definitions are possible. Work on learned helplessness suggests a key role for the mPFC in suppressing otherwise exuberant 5-HT activity in animals who have the benefit of behavioural control—but what exactly mPFC is reporting is unclear.

A further direction is to construct a more comprehensive theory of aversive vigour [252] looked at this in a rather specific set of experimental circumstances. The direct predictions arising even from this have not been thoroughly tested; but a more general theory, also tied to controllability, would be desirable.

Finally, we have noted various structural asymmetries between appetitive and aversive systems, ascribing many of them to asymmetric priors about the structure of rewards and punishments in environments [23]. It would be important to examine these claims in more detail, and indeed look at the effect of changing the statistics of environments to determine the extent of lability.

In conclusion, we have attempted to use our evolving and rich view of the nature and source of learned, appetitive behaviour to examine the case of aversion and defence. Along with substantial commonalities between the two, we have discussed some critical differences—notably in the way that aversive behaviour appears to piggy-back on appetitive processing, leading to various intricate complexities that are incompletely understood. Dopamine plays a number of critical and apparently confounded roles; we therefore used it to lay as bare as possible the extent and limits of our current understanding.

Authors' contributions
The authors (KL and PD) contributed equally to this work's conception and completion. Both authors read and approved the final manuscript.

Acknowledgements
This work was supported by the Gatsby Charitable Foundation (KL and PD) and an unrestricted Grant from Google Inc. (KL). We are very grateful to Dominik Bach, Anushka Fernando, Dean Mobbs, and Peter Shizgal for their comments on previous versions of the manuscript.

Competing interests
The authors declare that they have no competing interests.

References
1. Schultz W. Neuronal reward and decision signals: from theories to data. Physiol Rev. 2015;95(3):853–951.
2. Kim HF, Hikosaka O. Parallel basal ganglia circuits for voluntary and automatic behaviour to reach rewards. Brain. 2015;138(7):1776–800.
3. Chase HW, Kumar P, Eickhoff SB, Dombrovski AY. Reinforcement learning models and their neural correlates: an activation likelihood estimation meta-analysis. Cogn Affect Behav Neurosci. 2015;15(2):435–59.
4. Ikemoto S, Bonci A, Neurocircuitry of drug reward. Neuropharmacology. 2014;76:329–41.
5. Lee D, Seo H, Jung MW. Neural basis of reinforcement learning and decision making. Annu Rev Neurosci. 2012;35:287–308.
6. Daw ND, Dayan P. The algorithmic anatomy of model-based evaluation. Philos Trans R Soc Lond B Biol Sci. 2014;369(1655):20130478.
7. O'Doherty JP. Contributions of the ventromedial prefrontal cortex to goal-directed action selection. Ann N Y Acad Sci. 2011;1239(1):118–29.
8. Frank MJ, Claus ED. Anatomy of a decision: striato-orbitofrontal interactions in reinforcement learning, decision making, and reversal. Psychol Rev. 2006;113(2):300–26.
9. Niv Y, Daw ND, Joel D, Dayan P. Tonic dopamine: opportunity costs and the control of response vigor. Psychopharmacology. 2007;191(3):507–20.
10. Salamone JD. The involvement of nucleus accumbens dopamine in appetitive and aversive motivation. Behav Brain Res. 1994;61(2):117–33.
11. Salamone JD, Correa M. Motivational views of reinforcement: implications for understanding the behavioral functions of nucleus accumbens dopamine. Behav Brain Res. 2002;137(1):3–25.
12. Salamone JD, Correa M. The mysterious motivational functions of mesolimbic dopamine. Neuron. 2012;76:470–85.
13. Guitart-Masip M, Beierholm UR, Dolan R, Duzel E, Dayan P. Vigor in the face of fluctuating rates of reward: an experimental examination. J Cogn Neurosci. 2011;23(12):3933–8.
14. Beierholm U, Guitart-Masip M, Economides M, Chowdhury R, Düzel E, Dolan R, Dayan P. Dopamine modulates reward-related vigor. Neuropsychopharmacology. 2013;38:1495–503.
15. Floresco SB. The nucleus accumbens: an interface between cognition, emotion, and action. Annu Rev Psychol. 2015;66:25–52.
16. Hamid AA, Pettibone JR, Mabrouk OS, Hetrick VL, Schmidt R, Vander Weele CM, Kennedy RT, Aragona BJ, Berke JD. Mesolimbic dopamine signals the value of work. Nat Neurosci. 2016;19(1):117–26.
17. Mowrer OH. A stimulus-response analysis of anxiety and its role as a reinforcing agent. Psychol Rev. 1939;46:553–65.
18. Bolles RC. The avoidance learning problem. Psychol Learn Motiv. 1972;6:97–139.
19. Grossberg S. A neural theory of punishment and avoidance, I: qualitative theory. Math Biosci. 1972;15(1):39–67.
20. Johnson JD, Li W, Li J, Klopf AH. A computational model of learned avoidance behavior in a one-way avoidance experiment. Adapt Behav. 2001;9(2):91–104.
21. Maia TV. Two-factor theory, the actor-critic model, and conditioned avoidance. Learn Behav. 2010;38(1):50–67.
22. Moutoussis M, Bentall RP, Williams J, Dayan P. A temporal difference account of avoidance learning. Network. 2008;19(2):137–60.
23. Boureau YL, Dayan P. Opponency revisited: competition and cooperation between dopamine and serotonin. Neuropsychopharmacology. 2010;36(1):74–97.
24. Guitart-Masip M, Duzel E, Dolan R, Dayan P. Action versus valence in decision making. Trends Cogn Sci. 2014;18(4):194–202.
25. Bandler R, Keay KA, Floyd N, Price J. Central circuits mediating patterned autonomic activity during active vs. passive emotional coping. Brain Res Bull. 2000;53(1):95–104.
26. McNaughton N, Corr PJ. A two-dimensional neuropsychology of defense: fear/anxiety and defensive distance. Neurosci Biobehav Rev. 2004;28:285–305.
27. Bolles RC. Species-specific defense reactions and avoidance learning. Psychol Rev. 1970;77(1):32–48.
28. Blanchard RJ, Flannelly KJ, Blanchard DC. Defensive behaviors of laboratory and wild rattus norvegicus. J Comp Psychol. 1986;100(2):101–7.
29. Mobbs D, Kim JJ. Neuroethological studies of fear, anxiety, and risky decision-making in rodents and humans. Curr Opin Behav Sci. 2015;5:8–15.
30. Maier SF, Amal J, Baratta MV, Paul E, Watkins LR. Behavioral control, the medial prefrontal cortex, and resilience. Dialogues Clin Neurosci. 2006;8(4):397–406.
31. Maier SF, Watkins LR. Stressor controllability and learned helplessness: the roles of the dorsal raphe nucleus, serotonin, and corticotropin-releasing factor. Neurosci Biobehav Rev. 2005;29(4):829–41.
32. Huys QJ, Dayan P. A Bayesian formulation of behavioral control. Cognition. 2009;113(3):314–28.
33. Frank MJ, Fossella JA. Neurogenetics and pharmacology of learning, motivation, and cognition. Neuropsychopharmacology. 2011;36(1):133–52.
34. Blackburn JR, Pfaus JG, Phillips AG. Dopamine functions in appetitive and defensive behaviours. Prog Neurobiol. 1992;39:247–79.

35. Brooks AM, Berns GS. Aversive stimuli and loss in the mesocorticolimbic dopamine system. Trends Cogn Sci. 2013;17(6):281–6.
36. Holly EN, Miczek KA. Ventral tegmental area dopamine revisited: effects of acute and repeated stress. Psychopharmacology. 2016;233(2):163–86.
37. Lammel S, Lim BK, Malenka RC. Reward and aversion in a heterogeneous midbrain dopamine system. Neuropharmacology. 2014;76:351–9.
38. McCutcheon JE, Ebner SR, Loriaux AL, Roitman MF. Encoding of aversion by dopamine and the nucleus accumbens. Front Neurosci. 2012;6:137.
39. Pignatelli M, Bonci A. Role of dopamine neurons in reward and aversion: a synaptic plasticity perspective. Neuron. 2015;86(5):1145–57.
40. Schultz W. Dopamine reward prediction-error signalling: a two-component response. Nat Rev Neurosci. 2016;17:183–95.
41. Sutton RS, Barto AG. Reinforcement learning: an introduction. Cambridge: MIT Press; 1998.
42. Kaelbling LP, Littman ML, Moore AW. Reinforcement learning: a survey. J Artif Intell Res. 1996;4:237.
43. Doya K. What are the computations of the cerebellum, the basal ganglia and the cerebral cortex? Neural Netw. 1999;12(7):961–74.
44. Daw ND, Niv Y, Dayan P. Uncertainty-based competition between prefrontal and dorsolateral striatal systems for behavioral control. Nat Neurosci. 2005;8(12):1704–11.
45. Dickinson A, Balleine BW. The role of learning in motivation. In: Gallistel CR, editor. Steven's handbook of experimental psychology. New York: Wiley; 2002. p. 497–533.
46. Dolan RJ, Dayan P. Goals and habits in the brain. Neuron. 2013;80(2):312–25.
47. Bellman RE. Dynamic programming. Princeton: Princeton University Press; 1957.
48. Sutton RS. Learning to predict by the methods of temporal differences. Mach Learn. 1988;3(1):9–44.
49. Barto AG, Sutton RS, Anderson CW. Neuronlike adaptive elements that can solve difficult learning control problems. IEEE Trans Syst Man Cybern. 1983;13:835–46.
50. Watkins CJCH. Learning from delayed rewards. Ph.D. Thesis, University of Cambridge; 1989.
51. Dayan P. Exploration from generalization mediated by multiple controllers. In: Baldassare G, Mirolli M, editors. Intrinsically motivated learning in natural and artificial systems. Berlin: Springer; 2013. p. 73–91.
52. Howard RA. Information value theory. IEEE Trans Syst Sci Cybern. 1966;2:22–6.
53. Gittins JC. Bandit processes and dynamic allocation indices. J R Stat Soc. 1979;41(2):148–77.
54. Sutton RS. Integrated architecture for learning, planning, and reacting based on approximating dynamic programming. In: Porter BW, Mooney RJ, editors. Proceedings of the seventh international conference on machine learning. Morgan Kaufman Publishers, Inc. 1990. p. 216–24.
55. Dayan P, Sejnowski TJ. Exploration bonuses and dual control. Mach Learn. 1996;25(1):5–22.
56. Dayan P, Berridge KC. Model-based and model-free pavlovian reward learning: revaluation, revision, and revelation. Cogn Affect Behav Neurosci. 2014;14:473–93.
57. Craig W. Appetites and aversions as constituents of instincts. Biol Bull. 1918;34(2):91–107.
58. Sherrington C. The integrative action of the nervous system. New Haven: Yale University Press; 1906.
59. Konorski J. Integrative activity of the brain. Chicago: University of Chicago Press; 1967.
60. Baldo BA, Kelley AE. Discrete neurochemical coding of distinguishable motivational processes: insights from nucleus accumbens control of feeding. Psychopharmacology. 2007;191(3):439–59.
61. Cools R. Role of dopamine in the motivational and cognitive control of behavior. Neuroscientist. 2008;14(4):381–95.
62. Blackburn JR. The role of dopamine in preparatory and consummatory defensive behaviours. Ph.D. Thesis, University of British Columbia; 1989.
63. Nicola SM. The flexible approach hypothesis: unification of effort and cue-responding hypotheses for the role of nucleus accumbens dopamine in the activation of reward-seeking behavior. J Neurosci. 2010;30(49):16585–600.
64. Ikemoto S, Panksepp J. The role of nucleus accumbens dopamine in motivated behavior: a unifying interpretation with special reference to reward-seeking. Brain Res Rev. 1999;31:6–41.
65. Berridge KC, Robinson TE. What is the role of dopamine in reward: hedonic impact, reward learning, or incentive salience? Brain Res Rev. 1998;28(3):309–69.
66. Robbins TW, Everitt BJ. Functions of dopamine in the dorsal and ventral striatum. Semin Neurosci. 1992;4:119–27.
67. Williams DR, Williams H. Auto-maintenance in the pigeon: sustained pecking despite contingent non-reinforcement. J Exp Anal Behav. 1969;12:511–20.
68. Breland K, Breland M. The misbehavior of organisms. Am Psychol. 1961;16:681–4.
69. Dayan P, Niv Y, Seymour B, Daw ND. The misbehavior of value and the discipline of the will. Neural Netw. 2006;19(8):1153–60.
70. Colwill RM, Rescorla RA. Associations between the discriminative stimulus and the reinforcer in instrumental learning. J Exp Psychol Anim Behav Process. 1988;14(2):155–64.
71. Estes WK. Discriminative conditioning. I: a discriminative property of conditioned anticipation. J Exp Psychol. 1943;32:150–5.
72. Holland PC. Relations between pavlovian-instrumental transfer and reinforcer devaluation. J Exp Psychol Anim Behav Process. 2004;30(2):104–17.
73. Lovibond PF. Facilitation of instrumental behavior by a pavlovian appetitive conditioned stimulus. J Exp Psychol Anim Behav Process. 1983;9:225–47.
74. Rescorla RA, Wagner AR. A theory of pavlovian conditioning: variations in the effectiveness of reinforcement and nonreinforcement. In: Black AH, Prokasy WF, editors. Classical conditioning II: current research and theory. New York: Appleton-Century-Crofts Ltd; 1972. p. 64–99.
75. Sutton R, Barto AG. Toward a modern theory of adaptive networks: expectation and prediction. Psychol Rev. 1981;88(2):135–70.
76. Sutton RS, Barto AG. Time-derivative models of pavlovian reinforcement. In: Gabriel M, Moore J, editors. Learning and computational neuroscience: foundations of adaptive networks. Cambridge: MIT Press; 1990. p. 497–537.
77. Dayan P, Kakade S, Montague PR. Learning and selective attention. Nat Neurosci. 2000;3:1218–23.
78. Montague PR, Dayan P, Sejnowski TJ. A framework for mesencephalic dopamine systems based on predictive hebbian learning. J Neurosci. 1996;16(5):1936–47.
79. Schultz W, Dayan P, Montague PR. A neural substrate of prediction and reward. Science. 1997;275:1593–9.
80. O'Doherty J, Dayan P, Schultz J, Deichmann R, Friston K, Dolan RJ. Dissociable roles of ventral and dorsal striatum in instrumental conditioning. Science. 2004;304:452–4.
81. Calabresi P, Picconi B, Tozzi A, Di Filippo M. Dopamine-mediated regulation of corticostriatal synaptic plasticity. Trends Neurosci. 2007;30(5):211–9.
82. Chen BT, Hopf FW, Bonci A. Synaptic plasticity in the mesolimbic system. Ann N Y Acad Sci. 2010;1187(1):129–39.
83. Reynolds JNJ, Hyland BI, Wickens JR. A cellular mechanism of reward-related learning. Nature. 2001;413(6851):67–70.
84. Reynolds JNJ, Wickens JR. Dopamine-dependent plasticity of corticostriatal synapses. Neural Netw. 2002;15:507–21.
85. Shen W, Flajolet M, Greengard P, Surmeier DJ. Dichotomous dopaminergic control of striatal synaptic plasticity. Science. 2008;321:848–51.
86. Mogenson GJ, Jones DL, Yim CY. From motivation to action: functional interface between the limbic system and the motor system. Prog Neurobiol. 1980;14:69–97.
87. Cardinal RN, Parkinson JA, Hall J, Everitt BJ. Emotion and motivation: the role of the amygdala, ventral striatum, and prefrontal cortex. Neurosci Biobehav Rev. 2002;26(3):321–52.
88. Di Ciano P, Cardinal RN, Cowell RA, Little SJ, Everitt BJ. Differential involvement of NMDA, AMPA/kainate, and dopamine receptors in the nucleus accumbens core in the acquisition and performance of pavlovian approach behavior. J Neurosci. 2001;21(23):9471–7.
89. Flagel SB, Clark JJ, Robinson TE, Mayo L, Czuj A, Willuhn I, Akers CA, Clinton SM, Phillips PEM, Akil H. A selective role for dopamine in stimulus-reward learning. Nature. 2011;469(7328):53–7.

90. Parkinson JA, Dalley J, Cardinal R, Bamford A, Fehnert B, Lachenal G, Rudarakanchana N, Halkerston K, Robbins T, Everitt B. Nucleus accumbens dopamine depletion impairs both acquisition and performance of appetitive pavlovian approach behaviour: implications for mesoaccumbens dopamine function. Behav Brain Res. 2002;137(1):149–63.

91. Saunders BT, Robinson TE. The role of dopamine in the accumbens core in the expression of pavlovian-conditioned responses. Eur J Neurosci. 2012;36(4):2521–32.

92. Berridge KC. The debate over dopamine's role in reward: the case for incentive salience. Psychopharmacology. 2007;191:391–431.

93. Wise RA. Dopamine, learning and motivation. Nat Rev Neurosci. 2004;5(6):483–94.

94. McClure SM, Daw ND, Montague PR. A computational substrate for incentive salience. Trends Neurosci. 2003;26(8):423–8.

95. Dickinson A, Smith J, Mirenowicz J. Dissociation of pavlovian and instrumental incentive learning under dopamine antagonists. Behav Neurosci. 2000;114(3):468–83.

96. Hall J, Parkinson JA, Connor TM, Dickinson A, Everitt BJ. Involvement of the central nucleus of the amygdala and nucleus accumbens core in mediating pavlovian influences on instrumental behaviour. Eur J Neurosci. 2001;13(10):1984–92.

97. Lex A, Hauber W. Dopamine D1 and D2 receptors in the nucleus accumbens core and shell mediate Pavlovian-instrumental transfer. Learn Mem. 2008;15:483–91.

98. Stuber GD, Hnasko TS, Britt JP, Edwards RH, Bonci A. Dopaminergic terminals in the nucleus accumbens but not the dorsal striatum corelease glutamate. J Neurosci. 2010;30(24):8229–33.

99. Tecuapetla F, Patel JC, Xenias H, English D, Tadros I, Shah F, Berlin J, Deisseroth K, Rice ME, Tepper JM, et al. Glutamatergic signaling by mesolimbic dopamine neurons in the nucleus accumbens. J Neurosci. 2010;30(20):7105–10.

100. Zhang S, Qi J, Li X, Wang HL, Britt JP, Hoffman AF, Bonci A, Lupica CR, Morales M. Dopaminergic and glutamatergic microdomains in a subset of rodent mesoaccumbens axons. Nat Neurosci. 2015;18(3):386–92.

101. Moss J, Ungless MA, Bolam JP. Dopaminergic axons in different divisions of the adult rat striatal complex do not express vesicular glutamate transporters. Eur J Neurosci. 2011;33(7):1205–11.

102. Gläscher J, Hampton AN, O'Doherty JP. Determining a role for ventromedial prefrontal cortex in encoding action-based value signals during reward-related decision making. Cereb Cortex. 2009;19(2):483–95.

103. Gottfried JA, O'Doherty J, Dolan RJ. Encoding predictive reward value in human amygdala and orbitofrontal cortex. Science. 2003;301(5636):1104–7.

104. Hatfield T, Han JS, Conley M, Gallagher M, Holland PC. Neurotoxic lesions of basolateral, but not central, amygdala interfere with pavlovian second-order conditioning and reinforcer devaluation effects. J Neurosci. 1996;16(16):5256–65.

105. Holland PC, Gallagher M. Amygdala circuitry in attentional and representational processes. Trends Cogn Sci. 1999;3(2):65–73.

106. Schoenbaum G, Chiba AA, Gallagher M. Orbitofrontal cortex and basolateral amygdala encode expected outcomes during learning. Nat Neurosci. 1998;1(2):155–9.

107. Schoenbaum G, Chiba AA, Gallagher M. Neural encoding in orbitofrontal cortex and basolateral amygdala during olfactory discrimination learning. J Neurosci. 1999;19(5):1876–84.

108. Valentin VV, Dickinson A, O'Doherty JP. Determining the neural substrates of goal-directed learning in the human brain. J Neurosci. 2007;27(15):4019–26.

109. Dickinson A, Balleine B. Actions and responses: the dual psychology of behaviour. In: Eilan N, McCarthy RA, Brewer B, editors. Spatial representation: problems in philosophy and psychology. Oxford: Blackwell; 1993. p. 277–93.

110. Zahm DS, Brog JS. On the significance of subterritories in the "accumbens" part of the rat ventral striatum. Neuroscience. 1992;50(4):751–67.

111. Humphries MD, Prescott TJ. The ventral basal ganglia, a selection mechanism at the crossroads of space, strategy, and reward. Prog Neurobiol. 2010;90(4):385–417.

112. Kelley AE. Ventral striatal control of appetitive motivation: role in ingestive behavior and reward-related learning. Neurosci Biobehav Rev. 2004;27:765–76.

113. Voorn P, Vanderschuren LJMJ, Groenewegen HJ, Robbins TW, Pennartz CMA. Putting a spin on the dorsal-ventral divide of the striatum. Trends Neurosci. 2004;27(8):468–74.

114. Mogenson G, Swanson L, Wu M. Neural projections from nucleus accumbens to globus pallidus, substantia innominata, and lateral preoptic-lateral hypothalamic area: an anatomical and electrophysiological investigation in the rat. J Neurosci. 1983;3(1):189–202.

115. Faure A, Reynolds SM, Richard JM, Berridge KC. Mesolimbic dopamine in desire and dread: enabling motivation to be generated by localized glutamate disruptions in nucleus accumbens. J Neurosci. 2008;28(28):7184–92.

116. Parkinson JA, Olmstead MC, Burns LH, Robbins TW, Everitt BJ. Dissociation in effects of lesions of the nucleus accumbens core and shell on appetitive pavlovian approach behavior and the potentiation of conditioned reinforcement and locomotor activity by d-amphetamine. J Neurosci. 1999;19(6):2401–11.

117. Parkinson JA, Willoughby PJ, Robbins TW, Everitt BJ. Disconnection of the anterior cingulate cortex and nucleus accumbens core impairs pavlovian approach behavior: further evidence for limbic cortical-ventral striatopallidal systems. Behav Neurosci. 2000;114(1):42–63.

118. Corbit LH, Balleine BW. The general and outcome-specific forms of pavlovian-instrumental transfer are differentially mediated by the nucleus accumbens core and shell. J Neurosci. 2011;31(33):11786–94.

119. Bassareo V, Di Chiara G. Differential responsiveness of dopamine transmission to food-stimuli in nucleus accumbens shell/core compartments. Neuroscience. 1999;89(3):637–41.

120. Loriaux AL, Roitman JD, Roitman MF. Nucleus accumbens shell, but not core, tracks motivational value of salt. J Neurophysiol. 2011;106(3):1537–44.

121. Shiflett MW, Balleine BW. At the limbic-motor interface: disconnection of basolateral amygdala from nucleus accumbens core and shell reveals dissociable components of incentive motivation. Eur J Neurosci. 2010;32(10):1735–43.

122. Saddoris MP, Cacciapaglia F, Wightman RM, Carelli RM. Differential dopamine release dynamics in the nucleus accumbens core and shell reveal complementary signals for error prediction and incentive motivation. J Neurosci. 2015;35(33):11572–82.

123. West EA, Carelli RM. Nucleus accumbens core and shell differentially encode reward-associated cues after reinforcer devaluation. J Neurosci. 2016;36(4):1128–39.

124. Valjent E, Bertran-Gonzalez J, Hervé D, Fisone G, Girault JA. Looking BAC at striatal signalling: cell-specific analysis in new transgenic mice. Trends Neurosci. 2009;32(10):538–47.

125. Tritsch NX, Sabatini BL. Dopaminergic modulation of synaptic transmission in cortex and striatum. Neuron. 2012;76:33–50.

126. Beaulieu JM, Gainetdinov RR. The physiology, signaling, and pharmacology of dopamine receptors. Pharmacol Rev. 2011;63:182–217.

127. Missale C, Nash SR, Robinson SW, Jaber M, Caron MG. Dopamine receptors: from structure to function. Physiol Rev. 1998;78(1):189–225.

128. Vallone D, Picetti R, Borrelli E. Structure and function of dopamine receptors. Neurosci Biobehav Rev. 2000;24:125–32.

129. Richfield EK, Penney JB, Young AB. Anatomical and affinity state comparisons between dopamine D1 and D2 receptors in the rat central nervous system. Neuroscience. 1989;30(3):767–77.

130. Dreyer JK, Herrik KF, Berg RW, Hounsgaard JD. Influence of phasic and tonic dopamine release on receptor activation. J Neurosci. 2010;30(42):14273–83.

131. Gerfen CR, Surmeier DJ. Modulation of striatal projection systems by dopamine. Annu Rev Neurosci. 2011;34:441–66.

132. Surmeier DJ, Ding J, Day M, Wang Z, Shen W. D1 and D2 dopamine-receptor modulation of striatal glutamatergic signaling in striatal medium spiny neurons. Trends Neurosci. 2007;30(5):228–35.

133. Albin RL, Young AB, Penney JB. The functional anatomy of basal ganglia disorders. Trends Neurosci. 1989;12(10):366–75.

134. DeLong MR. Primate models of movement disorders of basal ganglia origin. Trends Neurosci. 1990;13:281–5.

135. Gerfen CR, Engber TM, Mahan LC, Susel Z, Chase TN, Monsma FJ, Sibley DR. D1 and d2 dopamine receptor-regulated gene expression of striatonigral and striatopallidal neurons. Science. 1990;250:1429–32.

136. Kravitz AV, Freeze BS, Parker PRL, Kay K, Thwin MT, Deisseroth K, Kreitzer AC. Regulation of parkinsonian motor behaviours by optogenetic control of basal ganglia circuitry. Nature. 2010;466:622–6.

137. Frank MJ. Dynamic dopamine modulation in the basal ganglia: a neurocomputational account of cognitive deficits in medicated and nonmedicated parkinsonism. J Cogn Neurosci. 2005;17(1):51–72.

138. Carlezone WA Jr, Thomas MJ. Biological substrates of reward and aversion: a nucleus accumbens activity hypothesis. Neuropharmacology. 2009;56:122–32.

139. Grueter BA, Robison AJ, Neve RL, Nestler EJ, Malenka RC. ΔFosB differentially modulates nucleus accumbens direct and indirect pathway function. Proc Natl Acad Sci USA. 2013;110(5):1923–8.

140. Hikida T, Yawata S, Yamaguchi T, Danjo T, Sasaoka T, Wang Y, Nakanishi S. Pathway-specific modulation of nucleus accumbens in reward and aversive behavior via selective transmitter receptors. Proc Natl Acad Sci USA. 2013;110(1):342–7.

141. Kupchik YM, Brown RM, Heinsbroek JA, Lobo MK, Schwartz DJ, Kalivas PW. Coding the direct/indirect pathways by D1 and D2 receptors is not valid for accumbens projections. Nat Neurosci. 2015;18:1230–2.

142. Smith RJ, Lobo MK, Spencer S, Kalivas PW. Cocaine-induced adaptations in D1 and D2 accumbens projection neurons (a dichotomy not necessarily synonymous with direct and indirect pathways). Curr Opin Neurobiol. 2013;23:546–52.

143. Nicola SM, Surmeier DJ, Malenka RC. Dopaminergic modulation of neuronal excitability in the striatum and nucleus accumbens. Annu Rev Neurosci. 2000;23:185–215.

144. Lu XY, Ghasemzadeh MB, Kalivas P. Expression of D1 receptor, D2 receptor, substance P and enkephalin messenger RNAs in the neurons projecting from the nucleus accumbens. Neuroscience. 1997;82(3):767–80.

145. Aizman O, Brismar H, Uhlén P, Zettergren E, Levey AI, Forssberg H, Greengard P, Aperia A. Anatomical and physiological evidence for D_1 and D_2 dopamine receptor colocalization in neostriatal neurons. Nat Neurosci. 2000;3(3):226–30.

146. Bertran-Gonzalez J, Bosch C, Maroteaux M, Matamales M, Hervé D, Valjent E, Girault JA. Opposing patterns of signaling activation in dopamine D_1 and D_2 receptor-expressing striatal neurons in response to cocaine and haloperidol. J Neurosci. 2008;28(22):5671–85.

147. Hasbi A, Fan T, Alijaniaram M, Nguyen T, Perreault ML, O'Dowd BF, George SR. Calcium signaling cascade links dopamine D1–D2 receptor heteromer to striatal BDNF production and neuronal growth. Proc Natl Acad Sci USA. 2009;106(50):21377–82.

148. Rashid AJ, So CH, Kong MM, Furtak T, El-Ghundi M, Cheng R, O'Dowd BF, George SR. D1–D2 dopamine receptor heterooligomers with unique pharmacology are coupled to rapid activation of Gq/11 in the striatum. Proc Natl Acad Sci USA. 2007;104(2):654–9.

149. Frederick A, Yano H, Trifilieff P, Vishwasrao H, Biezonski D, Mészáros J, Urizar E, Sibley D, Kellendonk C, Sonntag K, et al. Evidence against dopamine D1/D2 receptor heteromers. Mol Psychiatry. 2015;20:1373–85.

150. Dalley JW, Lääne K, Theobald DE, Armstrong HC, Corlett PR, Chudasama Y, Robbins TW. Time-limited modulation of appetitive Pavlovian memory by D1 and NMDA receptors in the nucleus accumbens. Proc Natl Acad Sci USA. 2005;102(17):6189–94.

151. Eyny YS, Horvitz JC. Opposing roles of D_1 and D_2 receptors in appetitive conditioning. J Neurosci. 2003;23(5):1584–7.

152. Beninger RJ, Miller R. Dopamine D1-like receptors and reward-related incentive learning. Neurosci Biobehav Rev. 1998;22(2):335–45.

153. Parker JG, Zweifel LS, Clark JJ, Evans SB, Phillips PE, Palmiter RD. Absence of NMDA receptors in dopamine neurons attenuates dopamine release but not conditioned approach during Pavlovian conditioning. Proc Natl Acad Sci USA. 2010;107(30):13491–6.

154. Smith-Roe SL, Kelley AE. Coincident activation of NMDA and dopamine D_1 receptors within the nucleus accumbens core is required for appetitive instrumental learning. J Neurosci. 2000;20(20):7737–42.

155. Bernal SY, Dostova I, Kest A, Abayev Y, Kandova E, Touzani K, Sclafani A, Bodnar RJ. Role of dopamine D1 and D2 receptors in the nucleus accumbens shell on the acquisition and expression of fructose-conditioned flavor-flavor preferences in rats. Behav Brain Res. 2008;190(1):59–66.

156. Fraser KM, Haight JL, Gardner EL, Flagel SB. Examining the role of dopamine D_2 and D_3 receptors in Pavlovian conditioned approach behaviors. Behav Brain Res. 2016;305:87–99.

157. Lopez JC, Karlsson RM, O'Donnell P. Dopamine D2 modulation of sign and goal tracking in rats. Neuropsychopharmacology. 2015;40:2096–102.

158. Ranaldi R, Beninger RJ. Dopamine D1 and D2 antagonists attenuate amphetamine-produced enhancement of responding for conditioned reward in rats. Psychopharmacology. 1993;113(1):110–8.

159. Wolterink G, Phillips G, Cador M, Donselaar-Wolterink I, Robbins T, Everitt B. Relative roles of ventral striatal D1 and D2 dopamine receptors in responding with conditioned reinforcement. Psychopharmacology. 1993;110(3):355–64.

160. Sombers LA, Beyene M, Carelli RM, Wightman RM. Synaptic overflow of dopamine in the nucleus accumbens arises from neuronal activity in the ventral tegmental area. J Neurosci. 2009;29(6):1735–42.

161. Cachope R, Cheer JF. Local control of striatal dopamine release. Front Behav Neurosci. 2014;8:1–7.

162. Rice ME, Patel JC, Cragg SJ. Dopamine release in the basal ganglia. Neuroscience. 2011;198:112–37.

163. Threlfell S, Lalic T, Platt NJ, Jennings KA, Deisseroth K, Cragg SJ. Striatal dopamine release is triggered by synchronized activity in cholinergic interneurons. Neuron. 2012;75:58–64.

164. Grace AA. Phasic versus tonic dopamine release and the modulation of dopamine system responsivity: a hypothesis for the etiology of schizophrenia. Neuroscience. 1991;41(1):1–24.

165. Floresco SB, West AR, Ash B, Moore H, Grace AA. Afferent modulation of dopamine neuron firing differentially regulates tonic and phasic dopamine transmission. Nat Neurosci. 2003;6(9):968–73.

166. Grace AA, Floresco SB, Goto Y, Lodge DJ. Regulation of firing of dopaminergic neurons and control of goal-directed behaviors. Trends Neurosci. 2007;30(5):220–7.

167. Tritsch NX, Ding JB, Sabatini BL. Dopaminergic neurons inhibit striatal output through non-canonical release of GABA. Nature. 2012;490(7419):262–6.

168. Tritsch NX, Granger AJ, Sabatini BL. Mechanisms and functions of GABA co-release. Nat Rev Neurosci. 2016;17:139–45.

169. Suri RE, Schultz W. A neural network model with dopamine-like reinforcement signal that learns a spatial delayed response task. Neuroscience. 1999;91(3):871–90.

170. Balleine BW, Delgado MR, Hikosaka O. The role of the dorsal striatum in reward and decision-making. J Neurosci. 2007;27(31):8161–5.

171. Packard MG, Knowlton BJ. Learning and memory functions of the basal ganglia. Annu Rev Neurosci. 2002;25(1):563–93.

172. Yin HH, Knowlton BJ, Balleine BW. Lesions of dorsolateral striatum preserve outcome expectancy but disrupt habit formation in instrumental learning. Eur J Neurosci. 2004;19(1):181–9.

173. Yin HH, Knowlton BJ, Balleine BW. Inactivation of dorsolateral striatum enhances sensitivity to changes in the action-outcome contingency in instrumental conditioning. Behav Brain Res. 2006;166(2):189–96.

174. Yin HH, Knowlton BJ. The role of the basal ganglia in habit formation. Nat Rev Neurosci. 2006;7(6):464–76.

175. Tricomi E, Balleine BW, O'Doherty JP. A specific role for posterior dorsolateral striatum in human habit learning. Eur J Neurosci. 2009;29(11):2225–32.

176. Balleine BW, O'Doherty JP. Human and rodent homologies in action control: corticostriatal determinants of goal-directed and habitual action. Neuropsychopharmacology. 2010;35:48–69.

177. Doll BB, Simon DA, Daw ND. The ubiquity of model-based reinforcement learning. Curr Opin Neurobiol. 2012;22(6):1075–81.

178. Lee SW, Shimojo S, O'Doherty JP. Neural computations underlying arbitration between model-based and model-free learning. Neuron. 2014;81(3):687–99.

179. Killcross S, Coutureau E. Coordination of actions and habits in the medial prefrontal cortex of rats. Cereb Cortex. 2003;13(4):400–8.

180. Cohen MX, Frank MJ. Neurocomputational models of basal ganglia function in learning, memory and choice. Behav Brain Res. 2009;199:141–56.

181. Collins AGE, Frank MJ. Opponent actor learning (opal): modeling interactive effects of striatal dopamine on reinforcement learning and choice incentive. Psychol Rev. 2014;121(3):337–66.

182. Frank MJ, Loughry B, O'Reilly RC. Interactions between frontal cortex and basal ganglia in working memory: a computational model. Cogn Affect Behav Neurosci. 2001;1:137–60.

183. Kravitz AV, Tye LD, Kreitzer AC. Distinct roles for direct and indirect pathway striatal neurons in reinforcement. Nat Neurosci. 2012;15(6):816–9.

184. Cui G, Jun SB, Jin X, Pham MD, Vogel SS, Lovinger DM, Costa RM. Concurrent activation of striatal direct and indirect pathways during action initiation. Nature. 2013;494:238–42.

185. Mink JW. The basal ganglia: focused selection and inhibition of competing motor programs. Prog Neurobiol. 1996;50(4):381–425.

186. Nelson AB, Kreitzer AC. Reassessing models of basal ganglia function and dysfunction. Annu Rev Neurosci. 2014;37:117–35.

187. Calabresi P, Picconi B, Tozzi A, Ghiglieri V, Di Filippo M. Direct and indirect pathways of basal ganglia: a critical reappraisal. Nat Neurosci. 2014;17(8):1022–9.

188. Daw ND, Gershman SJ, Seymour B, Dayan P, Dolan RJ. Model-based influences on humans' choices and striatal prediction errors. Neuron. 2011;69:1204–15.

189. Bromberg-Martin ES, Matsumoto M, Hong S, Hikosaka O. A pallidus-habenula-dopamine pathway signals inferred stimulus values. J Neurophysiol. 2010;104:1068–76.

190. Nakahara H, Itoh H, Kawagoe R, Takikawa Y, Hikosaka O. Dopamine neurons can represent context-dependent prediction error. Neuron. 2004;41(2):269–80.

191. Schultz W. Updating dopamine reward signals. Curr Opin Neurobiol. 2013;23:229–38.

192. Horvitz JC. Mesolimbocortical and nigrostriatal dopamine responses to salient non-reward events. Neuroscience. 2000;96:651–6.

193. Kakade S, Dayan P. Dopamine: generalization and bonuses. Neural Netw. 2002;15:549–59.

194. Balleine BW. Neural bases of food-seeking: affect, arousal and reward in corticostriatolimbic circuits. Physiol Behav. 2005;86(5):717–30.

195. Yin HH, Ostlund SB, Knowlton BJ, Balleine BW. The role of the dorsomedial striatum in instrumental conditioning. Eur J Neurosci. 2005;22(2):513–23.

196. Cagniard B, Beeler JA, Britt JP, McGehee DS, Marinelli M, Zhuang X. Dopamine scales performance in the absence of new learning. Neuron. 2006;51(5):541–7.

197. Niv Y, Joel D, Dayan P. A normative perspective on motivation. Trends Cogn Sci. 2006;10(8):375–81.

198. Masterson FA, Crawford M. The defense motivation system: a theory of avoidance behavior. Behav Brain Sci. 1982;5(04):661–75.

199. Gray JA. The psychology of fear and stress. Cambridge: Cambridge University Press; 1987.

200. Mowrer OH. On the dual nature of learning: a reinterpretation of "conditioning" and "problem-solving". Harv Educ Rev. 1947;17:102–50.

201. Mowrer OH. Two-factor learning theory reconsidered, with special reference to secondary reinforcement and the concept of habit. Psychol Rev. 1956;63(2):114–28.

202. Canteras NS, Graeff FG. Executive and modulatory neural circuits of defensive reactions: implications for panic disorder. Neurosci Biobehav Rev. 2014;46:352–64.

203. Gross CT, Canteras NS. The many paths to fear. Nat Rev Neurosci. 2012;13(9):651–8.

204. Bandler R, Shipley MT. Columnar organization in the midbrain periaqueductal gray: modules for emotional expression? Trends Neurosci. 1994;17(9):379–89.

205. Bolles RC, Fanselow MS. A perceptual-defensive-recuperative model of fear and pain. Behav Brain Sci. 1980;3:291–323.

206. Fanselow MS. Neural organization of the defensive behavior system responsible for fear. Psychon Bull Rev. 1994;1(4):429–38.

207. Fanselow MS, Lester LS. A functional behavioristic approach to aversive motivated behavior: Predatory imminence as a determinant of the topography of defensive behavior. In: Bolles RC, Beecher MD, editors. Evolution and learning. Hillsdale: Erlbaum; 1988. p. 185–211.

208. Gray JA. The neuropsychology of anxiety: an enquiry into the functions of the septo-hippocampal system. Oxford: Oxford University Press; 1982.

209. Cabib S, Puglisi-Allegra S. Opposite responses of mesolimbic dopamine system to controllable and uncontrollable aversive experiences. J Neurosci. 1994;14(5):3333–40.

210. Cabib S, Puglisi-Allegra S. Stress, depression and the mesolimbic dopamine system. Psychopharmacology. 1996;128:331–42.

211. Cabib S, Puglisi-Allegra S. The mesoaccumbens dopamine in coping with stress. Neurosci Biobehav Rev. 2012;36(1):79–89.

212. Redgrave P, Prescott TJ, Gurney K. The basal ganglia: a vertebrate solution to the selection problem? Neuroscience. 1999;89(4):1009–23.

213. Blanchard DC, Blanchard RJ. Ethoexperimental approaches to the biology of emotion. Annu Rev Psychol. 1988;39:43–68.

214. Swanson LW. Cerebral hemisphere regulation of motivated behavior. Brain Res. 2000;886(1):113–64.

215. Joseph MH, Datla K, Young AMJ. The interpretation of the measurement of nucleus accumbens dopamine by in vivo analysis: the kick, the craving or the cognition? Neurosci Biobehav Rev. 2003;27:527–41.

216. Young AMJ. Increased extracellular dopamine in nucleus accumbens in response to unconditioned and conditioned aversive stimuli: studies using 1 min microdialysis in rats. J Neurosci Methods. 2004;138(1):57–63.

217. Abercrombie ED, Keefe KA, DiFrischia DS, Zigmond MJ. Differential effect of stress on in vivo dopamine release in striatum, nucleus accumbens, and medial frontal cortex. J Neurochem. 1989;52(5):1655–8.

218. Inglis FM, Moghaddam B. Dopaminergic innervation of the amygdala is highly responsive to stress. J Neurochem. 1999;72(3):1088–94.

219. Young AMJ, Rees KR. Dopamine release in the amygdaloid complex of the rat, studied by brain microdialysis. Neurosci Lett. 1998;249(1):49–52.

220. Budygin EA, Park J, Bass CE, Grinevich VP, Bonin KD, Wightman RM. Aversive stimulus differentially triggers subsecond dopamine release in reward regions. Neuroscience. 2012;201:331–7.

221. Park J, Bucher ES, Budygin EA, Wightman RM. Norepinephrine and dopamine transmission in 2 limbic regions differentially respond to acute noxious stimulation. Pain. 2015;156(2):318–27.

222. Cohen JY, Haesler S, Vong L, Lowell BB, Uchida N. Neuron-type-specific signals for reward and punishment in the ventral tegmental area. Nature. 2012;482:85–90.

223. Brischoux F, Chakraborty S, Brierley DI, Ungless MA. Phasic excitation of dopamine neurons in ventral VTA by noxious stimuli. Proc Natl Acad Sci USA. 2009;106(12):4894–9.

224. Lammel S, Hetzel A, Häckel O, Jones I, Liss B, Roeper J. Unique properties of mesoprefrontal neurons within a dual mesocorticolimbic dopamine system. Neuron. 2008;57:760–73.

225. Lammel S, Ion DI, Roeper J, Malenka RC. Projection-specific modulation of dopamine neuron synapses by aversive and rewarding stimuli. Neuron. 2011;70(5):855–62.

226. Mantz J, Thierry A, Glowinski J. Effect of noxious tail pinch on the discharge rate of mesocortical and mesolimbic dopamine neurons: selective activation of the mesocortical system. Brain Res. 1989;476(2):377–81.

227. Lerner TN, Shilyansky C, Davidson TJ, Evans KE, Beier KT, Zalocusky KA, Crow AK, Malenka RC, Luo L, Tomer R, et al. Intact-brain analyses reveal distinct information carried by SNc dopamine subcircuits. Cell. 2015;162(3):635–47.

228. Maldonado-Irizarry CS, Swanson CJ, Kelley AE. Glutamate receptors in the nucleus accumbens shell control feeding behavior via the lateral hypothalamus. J Neurosci. 1995;15(10):6779–88.

229. Reynolds SM, Berridge KC. Fear and feeding in the nucleus accumbens shell: rostrocaudal segregation of gaba-elicited defensive behavior versus eating behavior. J Neurosci. 2001;21(9):3261–70.

230. Richard JM, Berridge KC. Nucleus accumbens dopamine/glutamate interaction switches modes to generate desire versus dread: D1 alone for appetitive eating but D1 and D2 together for fear. J Neurosci. 2011;31(36):12866–79.

231. Reynolds SM, Berridge KC. Emotional environments retune the valence of appetitive versus fearful functions in nucleus accumbens. Nat Neurosci. 2008;11:423–5.

232. Sweidan S, Edinger H, Siegel A. The role of D1 and D2 receptors in dopamine agonist-induced modulation of affective defense behavior in the cat. Pharmacol Biochem Behav. 1990;36(3):491–9.

233. Sweidan S, Edinger H, Siegel A. D2 dopamine receptor-mediated mechanisms in the medial preoptic-anterior hypothalamus regulate affective defense behavior in the cat. Brain Res. 1991;549(1):127–37.

234. Willner P. Animal models of depression: an overview. Pharmacol Ther. 1990;45(3):425–55.

235. Steru L, Chermat R, Thierry B, Simon P. The tail suspension test: a new method for screening antidepressants in mice. Psychopharmacology. 1985;85(3):367–70.

236. Porsolt RD, Le Pichon M, Jalfre M. Depression: a new animal model sensitive to antidepressant treatments. Nature. 1977;266(5604):730–2.

237. Maier SF, Seligman ME. Learned helplessness: theory and evidence. J Exp Psychol Gen. 1976;105(1):3–46.

238. Puglisi-Allegra S, Imperato A, Angelucci L, Cabib S. Acute stress induces time-dependent responses in dopamine mesolimbic system. Brain Res. 1991;554:217–22.

239. Imperato A, Angelucci L, Casolini P, Zocchi A, Puglisi-Allegra S. Repeated stressful experiences differently affect limbic dopamine release during and following stress. Brain Res. 1992;577:194–9.

240. Imperato A, Cabib S, Puglisi-Allegra S. Repeated stressful experiences differently affect the time-dependent responses of the mesolimbic dopamine system to the stressor. Brain Res. 1993;601:333–6.

241. Pascucci T, Ventura R, Latagliata EC, Cabib S, Puglisi-Allegra S. The medial prefrontal cortex determines the accumbens dopamine response to stress through the opposing influences of norepinephrine and dopamine. Cereb Cortex. 2007;17(12):2796–804.

242. Leknes S, Tracey I. A common neurobiology for pain and pleasure. Nat Rev Neurosci. 2008;9(4):314–20.

243. Wood PB. Role of central dopamine in pain and analgesia. Expert Rev Neurother. 2008;8(5):781–97.

244. Schwartz N, Temkin P, Jurado S, Lim BK, Heifets BD, Polepalli JS, Malenka RC. Decreased motivation during chronic pain requires long-term depression in the nucleus accumbens. Science. 2014;345(6196):535–42.

245. Ren W, Centeno MV, Berger S, Wu Y, Na X, Liu X, Kondapalli J, Apkarian AV, Martina M, Surmeier DJ. The indirect pathway of the nucleus accumbens shell amplifies neuropathic pain. Nature Neurosci. 2016;19:220–2.

246. Farrar AM, Segovia KN, Randall PA, Nunes EJ, Collins LE, Stopper CM, Port RG, Hockemeyer J, Müller CE, Correa M, Salamone JD. Nucleus accumbens and effort-related functions: behavioral and neural markers of the interactions between adenosine A2A and dopamine D2 receptors. Neuroscience. 2010;166(4):1056–67.

247. Santerre JL, Nunes EJ, Kovner R, Leser CE, Randall PA, Collins-Praino LE, Cruz LL, Correa M, Baqi Y, Müller CE, et al. The novel adenosine A2A antagonist prodrug MSX-4 is effective in animal models related to motivational and motor functions. Pharmacol Biochem Behav. 2012;102(4):477–87.

248. Wadenberg MG, Hicks PB. The conditioned avoidance response test re-evaluated: is it a sensitive test for the detection of potentially atypical antipsychotics? Neurosci Biobehav Rev. 1999;23:851–62.

249. Deakin JFW, Graeff FG. 5-HT and mechanisms of defence. J psychopharmacol. 1991;5:305–15.

250. Graeff FG, Guimarães FS, De Andrade TG, Deakin JF. Role of 5-HT in stress, anxiety, and depression. Pharmacol Biochem Behav. 1996;54(1):129–41.

251. Dayan P, Huys QJM. Serotonin in affective control. Annu Rev Neurosci. 2009;32:95–126.

252. Dayan P. Instrumental vigour in punishment and reward. Eur J Neurosci. 2012;35(7):1152–68.

253. Grossberg S. Some normal and abnormal behavioral syndromes due to transmitter gating of opponent systems. Biol Psychiatry. 1984;19:1075–118.

254. Solomon RL, Corbit JD. An opponent-process theory of motivation: I. temporal dynamics of affect. Psychol Rev. 1974;81(2):119–45.

255. Daw ND, Kakade S, Dayan P. Opponent interactions between serotonin and dopamine. Neural Netw. 2002;15:603–16.

256. Deakin JFW. Roles of serotonergic systems in escape, avoidance and other behaviours. In: Cooper SJ, editor. Theory in psychopharmacology. vol. 2. 2nd edn., New York: Academic Press; 1983. pp. 149–193.

257. García J, Fernández F. A comprehensive survey on safe reinforcement learning. J Mach Learn Res. 2015;16:1437–80.

258. Huys QJ, Daw ND, Dayan P. Depression: a decision-theoretic analysis. Annu Rev Neurosci. 2015;38:1–23.

259. Gray JA, McNaughton N. The neuropsychology of anxiety: an enquiry into the function of the septo-hippocampal system, vol. 33. Oxford: Oxford University Press; 2003.

260. Blanchard RJ, Yudko EB, Rodgers RJ, Blanchard DC. Defense system psychopharmacology: an ethological approach to the pharmacology of fear and anxiety. Behav Brain Res. 1993;58(1):155–65.

261. Lister RG. Ethologically-based animal models of anxiety disorders. Pharmacol Ther. 1990;46(3):321–40.

262. Bach DR. Anxiety-like behavioural inhibition is normative under environmental threat-reward correlations. PLoS Comput Biol. 2015;11(12):1004646.

263. Fanselow MS. The postshock activity burst. Anim Learn Behav. 1982;10(4):448–54.

264. Jenkins H, Moore BR. The form of the auto-shaped response with food or water reinforcers. J Exp Anal Behav. 1973;20(1):163–81.

265. Abraham AD, Neve KA, Lattal KM. Dopamine and extinction: a convergence of theory with fear and reward circuitry. Neurobiol Learn Mem. 2014;108:65–77.

266. Levita L, Dalley JW, Robbins TW. Nucleus accumbens dopamine and learned fear revisited: a review and some new findings. Behav Brain Res. 2002;137:115–27.

267. Pezze MA, Feldon J. Mesolimbic dopaminergic pathways in fear conditioning. Prog Neurobiol. 2004;74:301–20.

268. Frank MJ, Surmeier DJ. Do substantia nigra dopaminergic neurons differentiate between reward and punishment? J Mol Cell Biol. 2009;1:15–6.

269. Zweifel LS, Fadok JP, Argilli E, Garelick MG, Jones GL, Dickerson TMK, Allen JM, Mizumori SJY, Bonci A, Palmiter RD. Activation of dopamine neurons is critical for aversive conditioning and prevention of generalized anxiety. Nat Neurosci. 2011;14(5):620–6.

270. Badrinarayan A, Wescott SA, Vander Weele CM, Saunders BT, Couturier BE, Maren S, Aragona BJ. Aversive stimuli differentially modulate real-time dopamine transmission dynamics within the nucleus accumbens core and shell. J Neurosci. 2012;32(45):15779–90.

271. Oleson EB, Gentry RN, Chioma VC, Cheer JF. Subsecond dopamine release in the nucleus accumbens predicts conditioned punishment and its successful avoidance. J Neurosci. 2012;32(42):14804–8.

272. Fadok JP, Dickerson TMK, Palmiter RD. Dopamine is necessary for cue-dependent fear conditioning. J Neurosci. 2009;29(36):11089–97.

273. Ikegami M, Uemura T, Kishioka A, Sakimura K, Mishina M. Striatal dopamine D1 receptor is essential for contextual fear conditioning. Sci Rep. 2014;4:3976.

274. Blackburn JR, Phillips AG. Enhancement of freezing behaviour by metaclopromide: implications for neuroleptic-induced avoidance deficits. Pharmacol Biochem Behav. 1990;35(3):685–91.

275. de Souza Caetano KA, de Oliveira AR, Brandão ML. Dopamine D$_2$ receptors modulate the expression of contextual conditioned fear: role of the ventral tegmental area and the basolateral amygdala. Behav Pharmacol. 2013;24(4):264–74.

276. Davis M, Falls WA, Campeau S, Kim M. Fear-potentiated startle: a neural and pharmacological analysis. Behav Brain Res. 1993;58:175–98.

277. de Oliveira AR, Reimer AE, Brandão ML. Dopamine D2 receptor mechanisms in the expression of conditioned fear. Pharmacol Biochem Behav. 2006;84(1):102–11.

278. Li SSY, McNally GP. A role of nucleus accumbens dopamine receptors in the nucleus accumbens core, but not shell, in fear prediction error. Behav Neurosci. 2015;129(4):450–6.

279. Pavlov IP. Conditioned reflexes. Oxford: Oxford University Press; 1927.

280. Rescorla RA. Pavlovian conditioned inhibition. Psychol Bull. 1969;72(2):77–94.

281. Christianson JP, Fernando ABP, Kazama AM, Jovanovic T, Ostroff LE, Sangha S. Inhibition of fear by learned safety signals: a mini-symposium review. J Neurosci. 2012;32(41):14118–24.

282. Kong E, Monje FJ, Hirsch J, Pollak DD. Learning not to fear: neural correlates of learned safety. Neuropsychopharmacology. 2014;39:515–27.

283. Fernando ABP, Urcelay GP, Mar AC, Dickinson A, Robbins TW. Safety signals as instrumental reinforcers during free-operant avoidance. Learn Mem. 2014;21:488–97.

284. Dickinson A, Pearce J. Inhibitory interactions between appetitive and aversive stimuli. Psychol Bull. 1977;84:690–711.

285. Dickinson A, Dearing MF. Appetitive-aversive interactions and inhibitory processes. In: Dickinson A, Boakes RA, editors. Mechanisms of learning and motivation. Hillsdale: Erlbaum; 1979. p. 203–31.

286. Rogan MT, Leon KS, Perez DL, Kandel ER. Distinct neural signatures for safety and danger in the amygdala and striatum of the mouse. Neuron. 2005;46:309–20.

287. Genud-Gabai R, Klavir O, Paz R. Safety signals in the primate amygdala. J Neurosci. 2013;33(46):17986–94.

288. Sangha S, Chadick JZ, Janak PH. Safety encoding in the basal amygdala. J Neurosci. 2013;33(9):3744–51.

289. Pollak DD, Rogan MT, Egner T, Perez DL, Yanagihara TK, Hirsch J. A translational bridge between mouse and human models of learned safety. Ann Med. 2010;42(2):127–34.

290. Fernando ABP, Urcelay GP, Mar AC, Dickenson TA, Robbins TW. The role of nucleus accumbens shell in the mediation of the reinforcing properties of a safety signal in free-operant avoidance: dopamine-dependent inhibitory effects of d-amphetamine. Neuropsychopharmacology. 2014;39:1420–30.

291. Bouton ME. Learning and behavior: a contemporary synthesis. Sunderland: Sinauer Associates Inc; 2007.

292. Beninger RJ. The role of dopamine in locomotor activity and learning. Brain Res Rev. 1983;6:173–96.

293. Dinsmoor JA. Punishment: I. the avoidance hypothesis. Psychol Rev. 1954;61:34–46.

294. Dinsmoor JA. Stimuli inevitably generated by behavior that avoids electric shock are inherently reinforcing. J Exp Anal Behav. 2001;75:311–33.

295. Konorski J. Conditioned reflexes and neuron organization. Cambridge: Cambridge University Press; 1948.

296. Miller NE. Studies of fear as an acquirable drive: I. fear as motivation and fear-reduction as reinforcement in the learning of new responses. J Exp Psychol. 1948;38:89–101.

297. Tolman EC. Purposive behavior in animals and men. New York: Century; 1932.

298. Blanchard RJ, Fukunaga KK, Blanchard DC. Environmental control of defensive reactions to footshock. Bull Psychon Soc. 1976;8(2):129–30.

299. Seymour B, Singer T, Dolan R. The neurobiology of punishment. Nat Rev Neurosci. 2007;8(4):300–11.

300. Morse WH, Mead RN, Kelleher RT. Modulation of elicited behavior by a fixed-interval schedule of electric shock presentation. Science. 1967;157(3785):215–7.

301. Overmier JB, Seligman ME. Effects of inescapable shock upon subsequent escape and avoidance responding. J Comp Physiol Psychol. 1967;63(1):28–33.

302. Seligman ME, Maier SF. Failure to escape traumatic shock. J Exp Psychol. 1967;74:1–9.

303. Fernando A, Urcelay G, Mar A, Dickinson A, Robbins T. Free-operant avoidance behavior by rats after reinforcer revaluation using opioid agonists and d-amphetamine. J Neurosci. 2014;34(18):6286–93.

304. Hendersen RW, Graham J. Avoidance of heat by rats: effects of thermal context on rapidity of extinction. Learn Motiv. 1979;10(3):351–63.

305. Declercq M, De Houwer J. On the role of us expectancies in avoidance behavior. Psychon Bull Rev. 2008;15(1):99–102.

306. Gillan CM, Morein-Zamir S, Urcelay GP, Sule A, Voon V, Apergis-Schoute AM, Fineberg NA, Sahakian BJ, Robbins TW. Enhanced avoidance habits in obsessive-compulsive disorder. Biol Psychiatry. 2014;75(8):631–8.

307. Maia TV, Frank MJ. From reinforcement learning models to psychiatric and neurological disorders. Nat Neurosci. 2011;14(2):154–62.

308. Fibiger HC, Phillips AG, Zis AP. Deficits in instrumental responding after 6-hydroxydopamine lesions of the nigro-striatal dopaminergic projection. Pharmacol Biochem Behav. 1974;2:87–96.

309. Koob GF, Simon H, Herman JP, Le Moal M. Neuroleptic-like disruption of the conditioned avoidance response requires destruction of both mesolimbic and nigrostriatal dopamine systems. Brain Res. 1984;303:319–24.

310. Darvas M, Fadok JP, Palmiter RD. Requirement of dopamine signaling in the amygdala and striatum for learning and maintenance of a conditioned avoidance response. Learn Mem. 2011;18(3):136–43.

311. Beninger RJ, Mason ST, Phillips AG, Fibiger HC. The use of extinction to investigate the nature of neuroleptic-induced avoidance deficits. Psychopharmacology. 1980;69:11–8.

312. Beninger RJ. The role of serotonin and dopamine in learning to avoid aversive stimuli. In: Archer T, Nilsson LG, editors. Aversion, avoidance and anxiety: perspectives on aversively motivated behavior. Hillsdale: Lawrence Erlbaum Associates; 1989. p. 265–84.

313. Wadenberg MG, Ericson E, Magnusson O, Ahlenius S. Suppression of conditioned avoidance behavior by the local application of (-)sulpiride into the ventral, but not the dorsal, striatum of the rat. Biol Psychiatry. 1990;28:297–307.

314. Tye KM, Mirzabekov JJ, Warden MR, Ferenczi EA, Tsai HC, Finkelstein J, Kim SY, Adhikari A, Thompson KR, Andalman AS, Gunaydin L, Witten I, Deisseroth K. Dopamine neurons modulate neural encoding and expression of depression-related behaviour. Nature. 2013;493:537–41.

315. Anstrom KK, Woodward DJ. Restraint increases dopaminergic burst firing in awake rats. Neuropsychopharmacology. 2005;10(10):1832–40.

316. Chaudhury D, Walsh JJ, Friedman AK, Juarez B, Ku SM, Koo JW, Ferguson D, Tsai HC, Pomeranz L, Christoffel DJ, et al. Rapid regulation of depression-related behaviours by control of midbrain dopamine neurons. Nature. 2013;493:532–6.

317. Friedman AK, Walsh JJ, Juarez B, Ku SM, Chaudhury D, Wang J, Li X, Dietz DM, Pan N, Vialou VF, et al. Enhancing depression mechanisms in midbrain dopamine neurons achieves homeostatic resilience. Science. 2014;344(6181):313–9.

318. Hollon NG, Burgeno LM, Phillips PE. Stress effects on the neural substrates of motivated behavior. Nat Neurosci. 2015;18(10):1405–12.

319. Bland ST, Twining C, Watkins LR, Maier SF. Stressor controllability modulates stress-induced serotonin but not dopamine efflux in the nucleus accumbens shell. Synapse. 2003;49:206–8.

320. Bland ST, Hargrave D, Pepin JL, Amat J, Watkins LR, Maier SF. Stressor controllability modulates stress-induced dopamine and serotonin efflux and morphine-induced serotonin efflux in the medial prefrontal cortex. Neuropsychopharmacology. 2003;28:1589–96.

321. Amat J, Matus-Amat P, Watkins LR, Maier SF. Escapable and inescapable stress differentially alter extracellular levels of 5-HT in the basolateral amygdala of the rat. Brain Res. 1998;812:113–20.

322. Amat J, Matus-Amat P, Watkins LR, Maier SF. Escapable and inescapable stress differentially and selectively alter extracellular levels of 5-HT in the ventral hippocampus and dorsal periaqueductal gray of the rat. Brain Res. 1998;797:12–22.

323. Amat J, Baratta MV, Paul E, Bland ST, Watkins LR, Maier SF. Medial prefrontal cortex determines how stressor controllability affects behavior and dorsal raphe nucleus. Nat Neurosci. 2005;8:365–71.

324. Amo R, Fredes F, Kinoshita M, Aoki R, Aizawa H, Agetsuma M, Aoki T, Shiraki T, Kakinuma H, Matsuda M, et al. The habenulo-raphe serotonergic circuit encodes an aversive expectation value essential for adaptive active avoidance of danger. Neuron. 2014;84(5):1034–48.

325. Li J, Daw ND. Signals in human striatum are appropriate for policy update rather than value prediction. J Neurosci. 2011;31(14):5504–11.

326. Kishida KT, Saez I, Lohrenz T, Witcher MR, Laxton AW, Tatter SB, White JP, Ellis TL, Phillips PE, Montague PR. Subsecond dopamine fluctuations in human striatum encode superposed error signals about actual and counterfactual reward. Proc Natl Acad Sci USA. 2016;113(1):200–5.

327. D'Ardenne K, Lohrenz T, Bartley KA, Montague PR. Computational heterogeneity in the human mesencephalic dopamine system. Cogn Affect Behav Neurosci. 2013;13(4):747–56.

328. Lohrenz T, McCabe K, Camerer CF, Montague PR. Neural signature of fictive learning signals in a sequential investment task. Proc Natl Acad Sci USA. 2007;104(22):9493–8.

329. Cohen JY, Amoroso MW, Uchida N. Serotonergic neurons signal reward and punishment on multiple timescales. ELife. 2015;4:06346.

330. Choi JS, Cain CK, LeDoux JE. The role of amygdala nuclei in the expression of auditory signaled two-way active avoidance in rats. Learn Mem. 2010;17(3):139–47.

331. Weiner DM, Levey AI, Sunahara RK, Niznik HB, O'Dowd BF, Seeman P, Brann MR. D1 and d2 dopamine receptor mrna in rat brain. Proc Natl Acad Sci USA. 1991;88(5):1859–63.

332. de la Mora MP, Gallegos-Cari A, Arizmendi-García Y, Marcellino D, Fuxe K. Role of dopamine receptor mechanisms in the amygdaloid modulation of fear and anxiety: structural and functional analysis. Prog Neurobiol. 2010;90(2):198–216.

333. Matsumoto M, Hikosaka O. Two types of dopamine neuron distinctly convey positive and negative motivational signals. Nature. 2009;459:837–41.

334. Fiorillo CD. Two dimensions of value: dopamine neurons represent reward but not aversiveness. Science. 2013;341(6145):546–9.

335. Beier KT, Steinberg EE, DeLoach KE, Xie S, Miyamichi K, Schwarz L, Gao XJ, Kremer EJ, Malenka RC, Luo L. Circuit architecture of vta dopamine neurons revealed by systematic input-output mapping. Cell. 2015;162(3):622–34.

336. Menegas W, Bergan JF, Ogawa SK, Isogai Y, Venkataraju KU, Osten P, Uchida N, Watabe-Uchida M. Dopamine neurons projecting to the posterior striatum form an anatomically distinct subclass. ELife. 2015;4:10032.

337. Miyazaki KW, Miyazaki K, Tanaka KF, Yamanaka A, Takahashi A, Tabuchi S, Doya K. Optogenetic activation of dorsal raphe serotonin neurons enhances patience for future rewards. Curr Biol. 2014;24(17):2033–40.

338. Fonseca MS, Murakami M, Mainen ZF. Activation of dorsal raphe serotonergic neurons promotes waiting but is not reinforcing. Curr Biol. 2015;25(3):306–15.

339. Liu Z, Zhou J, Li Y, Hu F, Lu Y, Ma M, Feng Q, Zhang JE, Wang D, Zeng J, et al. Dorsal raphe neurons signal reward through 5-HT and glutamate. Neuron. 2014;81(6):1360–74.

340. Kool W, McGuire JT, Wang GJ, Botvinick MM. Neural and behavioral evidence for an intrinsic cost of self-control. PLoS One. 2013;8(8):72626.

341. McGuire JT, Botvinick MM. Prefrontal cortex, cognitive control, and the registration of decision costs. Proc Natl Acad Sci. 2010;107(17):7922–6.

342. Dayan P. How to set the switches on this thing. Curr Opin Neurobiol. 2012;22(6):1068–74.

343. Gan JO, Walton ME, Phillips PE. Dissociable cost and benefit encoding of future rewards by mesolimbic dopamine. Nat Neurosci. 2010;13(1):25–7.

344. Hollon NG, Arnold MM, Gan JO, Walton ME, Phillips PE. Dopamine-associated cached values are not sufficient as the basis for action selection. Proc Natl Acad Sci. 2014;111(51):18357–62.

4

Clinical application of DEX/CRH test and multi-channel NIRS in patients with depression

Shinya Kinoshita[1], Tetsufumi Kanazawa[1*], Hiroki Kikuyama[1,2] and Hiroshi Yoneda[1]

Abstract

Background: To reduce the number of patients with depression, biomarkers for clarifying psychiatric disorders are warranted. Numerous candidates have been proposed; however, near-infrared spectroscopy (NIRS) with multi-channel probes and a dexamethasone/corticotropin-releasing hormone (DEX/CRH) test are still surviving for practical demand. Thirty-one outpatients with depressed moods were analyzed using both biological tests.

Results: The non-suppressors, as indicated by the DEX/CRH test, exhibited a high severity on the Hamilton Depression Scale and severe anxiety on the State Trait Anxiety Scale. In addition, a unique response was identified via NIRS in the same group suggested by the DEX/CRH assessment.

Conclusions: The results obtained from these biological tests did not fit well with the category defined by operative diagnostic criteria, such as the Diagnostic and Statistical *Manual* of Mental Disorders or The International Classification of Diseases. Thus, it is critical that the utility evaluations of candidate biomarkers not be assessed by comparisons with the categorized criteria for a specific psychiatric disorder.

Trial registration UMIN000013214, Registered 21 February 2014

Keywords: DEX/CRH test, NIRS, Depression, Biomarker, HAMD

Background

A depressed mental state is caused by non-specific mental disorders, such as a mood disorder, schizophrenia, substance abuse, a personality disorder, or nearly every psychiatric condition. If it is more prolonged than expected, several types of costs related to individuals with depressed moods will increase. A recent analysis indicated a 21.5 % cost increment, $173.2 billion (2005) to $210.5 billion (2010), within 5 years, and this cost will be further increased [9]. Another analysis with regard to the global DALY (disability-adjusted life year) indicated that the cost associated with depression would represent the primary cost of all disorders, including physical disorders, in 2030, and it ranked 3rd in 2004 (http://www.who.int/healthinfo/global_burden_disease/GBD_report_2004update_part4.pdf). These analyses have provided warnings regarding the importance of depression prevention. In addition, to perform effective treatment, a precise assessment based on scientific data comprises a key factor.

Evidence regarding the relationship between depression severity and blood flow measurements scaled by Near-Infrared Spectroscopy (NIRS) is accumulating [30, 36, 41]. NIRS comprises a non-invasive imaging device that uses multiple channels to visualize brain activity. It has been developed as a result of the demand to consider a differential diagnosis in patients with depressed moods despite the administration of antidepressant agents for an extended period. A reliable biological marker is required to identify a specific psychiatric disorder because diagnosis in psychiatry currently relies on expressed symptoms or spoken words. NIRS comprises a device that applies knowledge of neuroscience through the assessment of blood flow in the brain; however, another

*Correspondence: psy052@osaka-med.ac.jp
[1] Department of Neuropsychiatry, Osaka Medical College, 2-7, Daigaku-Cho, Takatsuk, Osaka 569-8686, Japan
Full list of author information is available at the end of the article

potential candidate for a reliable biomarker depends on an endocrine imbalance. Particularly in the assessment of disturbed regulation of the hypothalamic-pituitary-adrenocortical (HPA) system, dexamethasone/corticotropin-releasing hormone (DEX/CRH) has been extensively investigated with a view towards the differential diagnosis of depression prior to the development of NIRS. Originally, the dexamethasone suppression test (DST) was used to diagnosis Cushing's syndrome [22]; this endocrine reaction has also been implemented for the diagnosis of endogenous depression. The current standard method is a DEX/CRH test in combination with the administration of CRH, which has been reported to increase the sensitivity from 60 to 80 % for the classic type of depression [12, 13]. There is an unavoidable burden regarding the application of this method for practical usage; however, these two biological methods have been considerably implemented in previous decades for investigating the biomarkers of depression.

In the current study, we investigated patients with a depressed mental state. Following a diagnosis according to the DSM-IV or psychological assessments, two tests using both endocrine (DEX/CRH) and neuroimaging (NIRS) assessments were applied. The aim of the current work was to identify the relationship between the psychiatric diagnosis based on the expressed symptoms and the assessment of two biomarkers.

Methods

Subjects

The subjects comprised 31 outpatients (15 men and 16 women; mean age: 44.2 years, SD: 12.2 years) with a depressive state, who were recruited from patients who attended the Neuropsychiatry Department of Osaka Medical College. The demographic details of the psychiatric diagnoses are shown in Table 1. We have adopted structured clinical interview for DSM-IV TR (SCID) for clinical assessment [7].

The severity of the index depressive episode was assessed with the 21-item version of the Hamilton depression rating scale (HAMD) [10, 15], on the admission day (DEX/CRH on the 2nd day and NIRS on the 3rd day). Enrolled patients (n = 31) were not strictly limited along with the HAMD score because all of the participants had the difficulty to live their life. Regarding the self-evaluation tool for anxiety, the STAI, the State-Trait Anxiety Inventory [26, 34], was administered to the participants on admission day. The majority of the patients were medicated with antidepressants; however, we did not control for the class of antidepressant medication. In addition, we assessed the psychiatric disorders of patients along with the SCID method; therefore, psychiatric comorbidities were not controlled.

DEX/CRH test

The DEX/CRH test was conducted according to the method described by Zobel et al. [42]. The subjects were pretreated with an oral dose of 1.5 mg of DEX at 2200 h on the 1st admission day. On the next day, a vein was cannulated at 1400 h to collect blood at 1430, 1500, 1530, 1545, and 1600 h via an intravenous catheter. Human CRH (100 μg) was intravenously administered at 1400 h immediately after the initial blood collection. The plasma concentrations of ACTH and cortisol were measured via radioimmunoassay at SRL Corporation (Tokyo, Japan). The detection limits for ACTH and cortisol were 5.0 pg/ml and 1.0 μg/dl, respectively.

The definition of the subtypes of the cortisol suppression pattern followed previously described criteria [19, 14] and included incomplete-suppressors (DEX/CRH-cortisol ≥5 μg/dl, moderate-suppressors (1 μg/dl ≤ DEX/CRH-cortisol <5 μg/dl), and enhanced-suppressors (DEX/CRH-cortisol <1 μg/dl). We also included a non-suppressor group with cortisol >5 μg/dl at the test onset to reduce the number of incomplete suppressors (onset-cortisol <5 μg/dl).

NIRS measurement

The NIRS measurements were performed using a 22-channel ETG-4000 Optical Topography System (Hitachi Medical Corporation, Tokyo, Japan). This machine used two sets of wavelengths of near-infrared light (695 and 830 nm, respectively) to identify differences in the absorption spectrum, which thus enabled the measurement of oxy-Hb and deoxy-Hb [23]. Seventeen emitter probes and 16 detector probes were plugged into a 3 × 11 array. The distance between the pair of emission and detector probes was 3.0 cm; the measuring area between each pair of detector probes was defined as a "channel." Probes were placed on the frontal region of the participant. The lowest probes were positioned along the Fp1–Fp2 line in accordance with the international 10–20 system used in electroencephalography.

Activation task

Changes in the hemoglobin concentration were measured during the verbal fluency task [37]. The cognitive activation task was structured to include a 30-s pre-task period, a 60-s task period, and a 70-s post-task period. For the pre- and post-task baseline periods, the participants were instructed to consecutively repeat five Japanese vowels (a, i, u, e, o) aloud. During the task periods, they were instructed to generate as many Japanese words as possible that began with a designated syllable. The initial syllables were presented in counterbalanced order among the participants with

Table 1 Psychiatric diagnoses assessed by the DSM-IV TR for study patients (n = 31)

SCID	Major depressive disorder	Somatoform disorder	Panic disorder	Bipolar II disorder	Schizophrenia	Obsessive–compusive disorder	Bipolar I disorder	Dysthymic disorder	Psychotic disorder
DSM code	296.2 and 296.3	300.82	300.21	296.89	295.3	300.3	296.53	300.4	298.9
Number	17	2	2	1	1	1	3	1	3

each syllable changing every 20 s (0–20 s: /to/, /na/, /a/; 20–40 s:/se/, /i/, /ki/; 40–60 s: /o/, /ta/, /ha/) during the 60-s task period.

Measurement environment

Each participant was seated in a comfortable chair and instructed to remain still to prevent movement artifacts; specifically, head movements, strong biting, or unnecessary eyebrow movements were minimized during the NIRS measurements. The data that clearly contained motion artifacts, based on both our observations and NIRS recordings, were excluded from further analyses.

Statistical analysis

All statistical analyses were performed with JMP Pro® software (Ver. 11.0, SAS Institute Japan Ltd., Tokyo, Japan). Intergroup comparisons were conducted for HAMD, STAI scores and the gained scores from NIRS instrument according to the Kruskal–Wallis test. A value of $p < 0.05$ was considered statistically significant.

Results

According to the previously described criteria for the division of the DEX/CRH response, the numbers of participants in the four groups divided by the cortisol reaction are indicated in Table 2.

First, the association between the reaction in the DEX/CRH test and the severity of depression determined by the HAMD assessment was investigated. The HAMD was recorded by another clinician in a blind manner. There was a difference in the mean value of the HAMD score between the non-suppressors and the other two main groups, incomplete suppressors and moderate suppressors (Fig. 1 Kruskal–Wallis analysis Chi square 7.37, $p = 0.06$). Second, the STAI, which is a self-evaluation tool for anxiety, significantly represented the characteristic psychological feature of the non-suppressor group compared with the other three groups (Fig. 2 Kruskal–Wallis analysis Chi square 7.58, $p = 0.06$). Moreover, we compared the results of the NIRS assessment with the reaction of the DEX/CRH test. Similar to the HAMD assessment, the NIRS recording was performed by a lab technician in a blind manner. The results indicated that the values of the center of gravity at the frontal lobe in the non-suppressor group, which comprised the

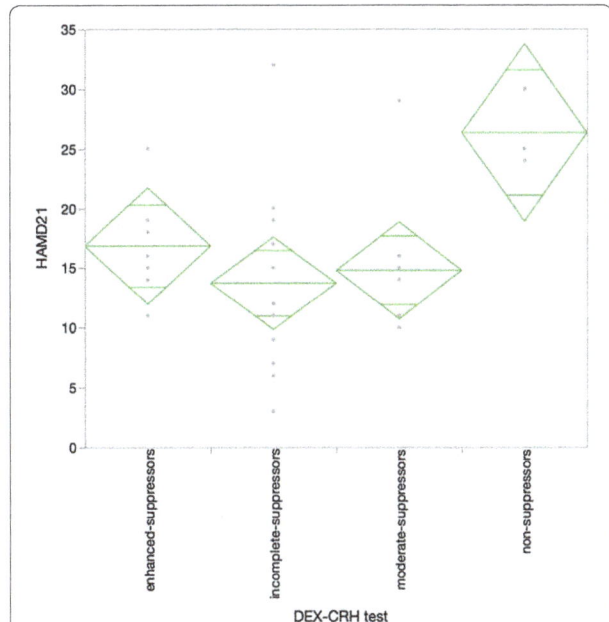

Fig. 1 *Diamond plot* of the HAMD 21 assessment and DEX–CRH test (n = 31). Kruskal–Wallis analysis Chi square 7.37, p = 0.06. Post hoc analysis non-suppressors, 26.3 ± 3.2, vs incomplete suppressors, 13.7 ± 8.2, p = 0.04, vs moderate suppressors, 14.8 ± 5.8, p = 0.03

representative values in NIRS, were significantly different compared with the other three groups by post hoc analysis (Fig. 3 Kruskal–Wallis analysis Chi square 7.02, $p = 0.07$). No significant age difference between the groups that were defined by the two biological methods was found (data not shown).

Discussion

The current sample size is relatively small to provide a definitive conclusion; however, our current work has an advantage in which we employed cases regardless of the diagnosis of psychiatric disorders. Therefore, there is the potential that the novel scientific findings identified from our sample are consistent across diagnoses based on the operative diagnostic criteria, such as the DSM. In addition, this is the first report to assess confirmed cases with depressed mood by two representative assessment methods for depression.

Regarding the DEX/CRH test, it has been reported that 60–80 % of patients with depression exhibited an

Table 2 Number of patients with depression divided by the DEX/CRH test (n = 31)

	DEX/CRH-cortisol	Onset cortisol	Male	Female	Total
Enhanced-suppressors	<1 µg/dl		2	5	7
Moderate-suppressors	1 µg/dl ≤ <5 µg/dl		2	8	10
Incomplete-suppressors	≥5 µg/dl	Onset cortisol <5 µg/dl	8	3	11
Non-suppressors	≥5 µg/dl	Onset cortisol ≥5 µg/dl	3	0	3

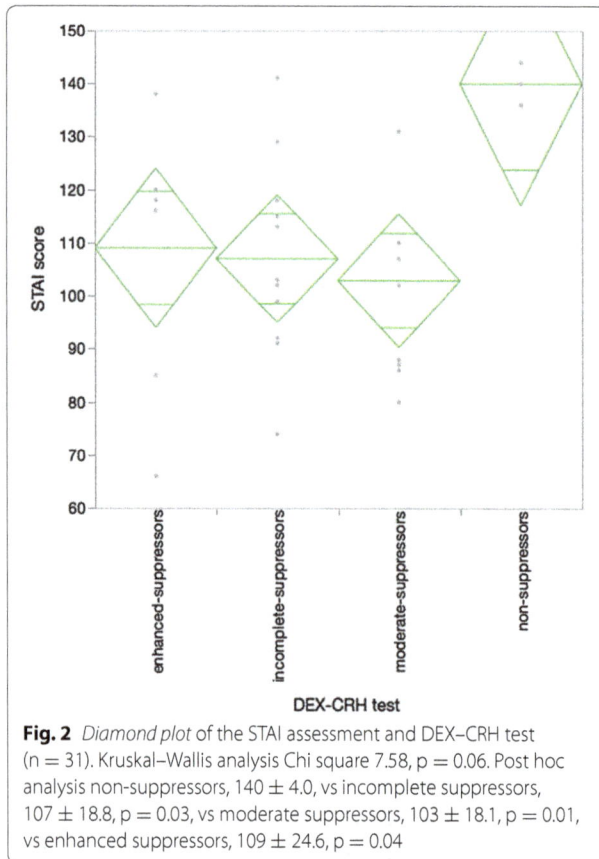

Fig. 2 *Diamond plot* of the STAI assessment and DEX–CRH test (n = 31). Kruskal–Wallis analysis Chi square 7.58, p = 0.06. Post hoc analysis non-suppressors, 140 ± 4.0, vs incomplete suppressors, 107 ± 18.8, p = 0.03, vs moderate suppressors, 103 ± 18.1, p = 0.01, vs enhanced suppressors, 109 ± 24.6, p = 0.04

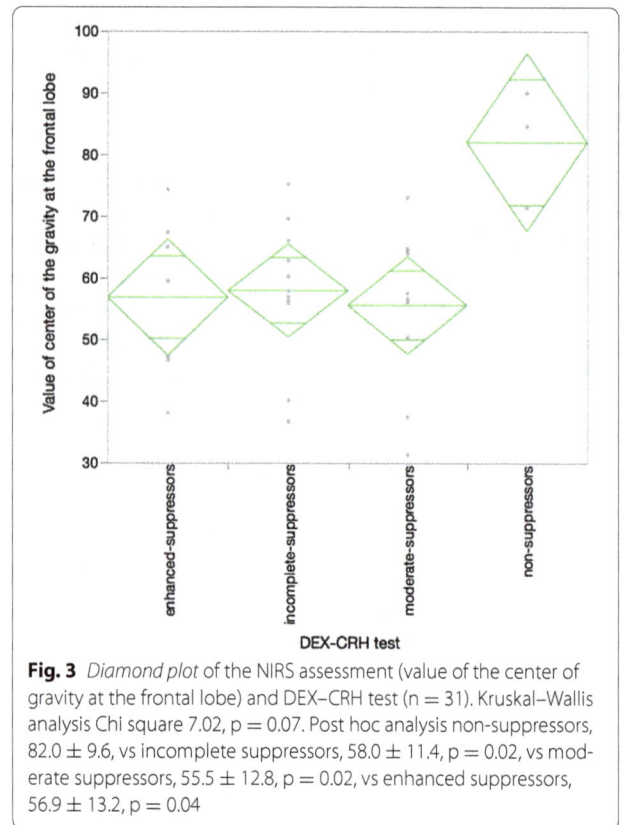

Fig. 3 *Diamond plot* of the NIRS assessment (value of the center of gravity at the frontal lobe) and DEX–CRH test (n = 31). Kruskal–Wallis analysis Chi square 7.02, p = 0.07. Post hoc analysis non-suppressors, 82.0 ± 9.6, vs incomplete suppressors, 58.0 ± 11.4, p = 0.02, vs moderate suppressors, 55.5 ± 12.8, p = 0.02, vs enhanced suppressors, 56.9 ± 13.2, p = 0.04

increased cortisol response prior to the initiation of treatment [18, 42]. It is partly because all participants in this study received medical treatment prior to the assessment, whereas only 11 % (3/31) of the participants in this study exhibited an increase cortisol response (non-suppressors). Moreover, most previous studies utilizing DEX/CRH test have been based on data obtained from inpatients [18, 20], which implies a clinical subgroup with severe symptoms, whereas our current sample consisted of a depression severity at the outpatient level. Moreover, the group that enrolled the largest sample size did not include data for individuals with a HAMD less than 15 [18], whereas the average HAMD score was 15.6 ± 7.5 in our sample. This difference has a significant impact on the interpretation of our data. The percentage of non-suppressors was not high because of the enrolled mild subtype of depression; however, every non-suppressor patient exhibited a high score on the HAMD assessment (average score of HAMD: 27.8) despite inconsistencies in the psychiatric disorders across three patients (two patients: 296.23 major depressive disorder, and one patient: 300.3 obsessive compulsive disorder). Thus, the DEX/CRH approach should again be considered a potentially useful biomarker for dividing the subclasses of depression.

With regard to psychological aspects assessed by STAI, the Kruskal–Wallis analysis indicated there was no significant difference for the divided subgroups regarding the DEX/CRH test; however, a trend was identified particularly for the non-suppressor group (Chi square 7.58, p = 0.06). Anxiety is a non-specific feature of psychiatric disorders. Therefore, the severity of anxiety is not fundamentally considered to be scaled by a biological method. Although the scale is simply based on a self-evaluation scale, our results indicated the potential finding that anxiety across psychiatric disorders, including depression, is represented by a biological scale, such as DEX/CRH. Anxiety-related stimuli cause a systemic response through neural circuits centered on the amygdala, which enhances the increment of cortisol [38]. Therefore, an association between the altered DEX/CRH result and the anxiety scale is reasonable. A previous study demonstrated that individuals with depression and comorbid anxiety (n = 18) related disorders exhibited a significantly lower cortisol level compared with pure depression patients (n = 36) [40]. The non-suppressor group, which showed higher anxiety, more severe depressive symptoms and a distinguished response in the DEX/CRH, should be regarded as one entity in terms of different biological and psychological reactions. Thus, larger sample sizes, especially for the non-suppressor group, are necessary to clarify the association between the STAI scale and DEX/CRH results.

Accumulating evidence supports the relationship between NIRS and the diagnosis of psychiatric disorders [21, 24, 36]. Thus, NIRS is one of the most attractive tools for adopting a biological assessment for clinical practice. One reason is that the device requires only 10–15 min for each individual if VFT is adopted for the assessment. NIRS is sufficiently easy to adopt, even for adolescents, for the evaluation of psychiatric disorders, such as depression, bipolar disorder, and schizophrenia. General interpretation on VFT is a neurocognitive battery for assessing verbal ability or executive control ability. This battery is widely used for assessing these abilities of patients after stroke, patients with Alzheimer's disease or Parkinson's disease [33]. In the current study, we have utilized this battery mainly for recording the measurements of oxy-Hb in the brain, therefore the task performance (the number of words) on each individual were not recorded. The comparison of the performance on VFT between each groups will be of interest. Future work should focus on the task performance across various psychiatric disorders. One of the critical issues regarding the NIRS device is that insufficient data are obtained from the perspective of neuroscience. In an analysis of a larger sample than the current work, our group recently demonstrated that the severity of depression scaled by the HAMD was negatively associated with the integral value of the blood flow at the frontal lobe (n = 43) [16]. This finding was characterized by the point that the assessment was not limited to depressed patients who satisfied the criteria defined by the DSM or ICD. Moreover, several biomarkers, such as DEX/CRH, NIRS and other factors, cannot guarantee the specificity of psychiatric disorders defined by operational diagnostic criteria. The current findings indicated that individuals with a Non-Suppression reaction in the DEX/CRH test exhibited a fairly increased value of the center of gravity at the frontal lobe. A general interpretation regarding the increased value of the center of gravity implies the existence of bipolarity [36]. In specific areas such as the left inferior frontal lobe, [oxy-Hb] was decreased in patients with panic disorders [27, 28]. Although the current work did not focus on a specific channel of NIRS, future research should analyze the data for a specific channel by assessing a larger sample series. Thus, a larger sample size is critical to validate the current work to determine the unknown mechanism of endocrine imbalance and brain response. In addition, the biological data from the mentally healthy controls will serve as a useful reference, although the current design has not been adopted to collect them. Moreover,

the length of the duration of mental illness has a possible effect on the result from the biological assessment. This should be considered in future studies.

Biological assessments embedded in the diagnosis of specific psychiatric disorders are proceeding. Candidate methods have been evaluated using the concordance rate for diagnosis defined by the operative criteria to date; however, a universally accepted biomarker has not been identified. Despite substantial efforts to identify a biological marker, the methodological approach for objective evaluation is incorrect in terms of the fact that the concordance rate between biological assessments and psychiatric diagnoses based on the artificial operative system is not sufficient to satisfy practical demands. For example, a genetic approach has indicated considerable overlap between schizophrenia and bipolar disorder [6, 29]; therefore, the current understanding regarding these disorders has been modified to indicate that the two disorders are related diseases in terms of the genetic aspects [31]. Moreover, recent reports have indicated considerable genetic overlap across several types of psychiatric disorders [4, 8, 11, 25]. According to a recent perspective based on genetic analyses, Craddock and his group have advocated the theory that psychiatric disorders are considered a spectrum [3]. It is true that a decreased frontal lobe is present in the brains of individuals with schizophrenia and bipolar disorder, as well as depression [5, 35]. Regarding therapeutic agents, antidepressants are effective for the improvement of symptoms in schizophrenia and bipolar disorders [32, 39]. Alternatively, antipsychotic agents are used for the treatment of depression [2]. Based on the traditional diagnostic category, it is impossible to explain the differences between psychiatric disorders by genetic or morphological factors or the responsiveness to therapeutic drugs. Our current finding indicates a trend of correlation between the severity of depression and the response to the DEX/CRH test; however, the diagnostic categories did not sufficiently fit the biological assessment. Moreover, our findings also suggest that the current diagnostic criteria are not valid for the assessment of biological markers in psychiatric disorders. Thus, the diagnostic criteria must be updated based on the contributions of biological assessments, such as DEX/CRH or NIRS [1, 17].

Abbreviations
DEX/CRH: dexamethasone/corticotropin-releasing hormone; NIRS: near-infrared spectroscopy; ACTH: adrenocorticotropic hormone; HAMD: Hamilton rating scale for depression; STAI: state-trait anxiety inventory.

Authors' contributions
SK carried out the DEX/CRH test and drafted the manuscript. TK designed the study especially for NIRS and revised the manuscript. HK performed the statistical analysis. YH participated in the design of the study and conducted the study. All authors read and approved the final manuscript.

Author details
[1] Department of Neuropsychiatry, Osaka Medical College, 2-7, Daigaku-Cho, Takatsuk, Osaka 569-8686, Japan. [2] Department of Psychiatry, Shin-Abuyama Hospital, Osaka Institute of Clinical Psychiatry, Osaka, Japan.

Acknowledgements
We are grateful to Drs. Makoto Kawano, Masaki Nishiguchi, Yasuo Kawabata, Shigeru Yamauchi, Hiroyuki Uenishi, Seiya Kawashige, Shinichi Imazu, Katsunori Toyoda, Yoshitaka Nishizawa, Mayuko Takahashi, Tatsushi Okayama, Wakako Odo, Kentaro Ide, Soichiro Maruyama, Seiichiro Tarutani, Emi Minami, Ryosuke Katsura, Yuko Higa, Tomoyoshi Nakano, Yoichiro Kubo, Shota Ouchi, and Tetsuya Togashi for helpful effort to collect the samples. We would like to thank Drs. Nanako Saito, Mai Yoshikawa, and other clinical psychotherapists for collecting the psychological data. We would like to thank Drs. Atsushi Tsutsumi and Jun Koh for the helpful discussion.

Competing interests
The authors declare that they have no competing interests.

Funding
The funding of this research was provided by the department of Neuropsychiatry, Osaka Medical College. No official grant was not used for this work.

References

1. Adam D. Mental health: on the spectrum. Nature. 2013;496:416–8.
2. Berman RM, Fava M, Thase ME, Trivedi MH, Swanink R, Mcquade RD, Carson WH, Adson D, Taylor L, Hazel J, Marcus RN. Aripiprazole augmentation in major depressive disorder: a double-blind, placebo-controlled study in patients with inadequate response to antidepressants. CNS Spectr. 2009;14:197–206.
3. Craddock N, Owen MJ. The Kraepelinian dichotomy—going, going… but still not gone. Br J Psychiatr. 2010;196:92–5.
4. de Rubeis S, He X, Goldberg AP, Poultney CS, Samocha K, Cicek AE, Kou Y, et al. Synaptic, transcriptional and chromatin genes disrupted in autism. Nature. 2014;515:209–15.
5. Drevets WC, Price JL, Simpson JR, Todd RD, Reich T, Vannier M, Raichle ME. Subgenual prefrontal cortex abnormalities in mood disorders. Nature. 1997;386:824–7.
6. Ferreira MA, O'Donovan MC, Meng YA, Jones IR, Ruderfer DM, Jones L, Fan J, et al. Collaborative genome-wide association analysis supports a role for ANK3 and CACNA1C in bipolar disorder. Nat Genet. 2008;40:1056–8.
7. First MB, Spitzer RL, Williams JBW, Gibbon M. Structured clinical interview for DSM-IV-TR (SCID-I)-research version. New York: Biometrics Research, New York State Psychiatric Institute; 2002.
8. Green EK, Grozeva D, Jones I, Jones L, Kirov G, Caesar S, Gordon-smith K, et al. The bipolar disorder risk allele at CACNA1C also confers risk of recurrent major depression and of schizophrenia. Mol Psychiatr. 2010;15:1016–22.
9. Greenberg PE, Fournier AA, Sisitsky T, Pike CT, Kessler RC. The economic burden of adults with major depressive disorder in the United States (2005 and 2010). J Clin Psychiatr. 2015;76(2):155–62.
10. Hamilton M. A rating scale for depression. J Neurol Neurosurg Psychiatr. 1960;23:56.
11. Han K, Holder JLJR, Schaaf CP, Lu H, Chen H, Kang H, Tang J, et al. SHANK3 overexpression causes manic-like behaviour with unique pharmacogenetic properties. Nature. 2013;503:72–7.
12. Heuser I, Yassouridis A, Holsboer F. The combined dexamethasone/CRH test: a refined laboratory test for psychiatric disorders. J Psychiatr Res. 1994;28:341–56.
13. Heuser IJ, Schweiger U, Gotthardt U, Schmider J, Lammers CH, Dettling M, Yassouridis A, Holsboer F. Pituitary-adrenal-system regulation and psychopathology during amitriptyline treatment in elderly depressed patients and normal comparison subjects. Am J Psychiatr. 1996;153:93–9.
14. Hori H, Ozeki Y, Teraishi T, Matsuo J, Kawamoto Y, Kinoshita Y, Suto S, Terada S, Higuchi T, Kunugi H. Relationships between psychological distress, coping styles, and HPA axis reactivity in healthy adults. J Psychiatr Res. 2010;44:865–73.
15. Kalali A, Williams JBW, Kobak KA, Lipschitz J, Engelhardt N, Evans K, Olin J, Rotheman P, Bech P. The new GRID HAM-D: pilot testing and international field trials. Int J Neuropsychopharmacol. 2002;5:S147.
16. Kawano M, Kanazawa T, Kikuyama H, Tsutsumi A, Kinoshita S, Kawabata Y, Yamauchi S, et al. Correlation between frontal lobe oxy-hemoglobin and severity of depression assessed using near-infrared spectroscopy. J Affect Disord. 2016;205:154–8.
17. Koike S, Takizawa R, Nishimura Y, Takano Y, Takayanagi Y, Kinou M, Araki T, Harima H, Fukuda M, Okazaki Y, Kasai K. Different hemodynamic response patterns in the prefrontal cortical sub-regions according to the clinical stages of psychosis. Schizophr Res. 2011;132:54–61.
18. Kunugi H, Ida I, Owashi T, Kimura M, Inoue Y, Nakagawa S, et al. Assessment of the dexamethasone/CRH test as a state-dependent marker for hypothalamic-pituitary-adrenal (HPA) axis abnormalities in major depressive episode: a Multicenter Study. Neuropsychopharmacology. 2006;31:212–20.
19. Kunugi H, Urushibara T, Nanko S. Combined DEX/CRH test among Japanese patients with major depression. J Psychiatr Res. 2004;38:123–8.
20. Kunzel HE, Binder EB, Nickel T, Ising M, Fuchs B, Majer M, Pfennig A, Ernst G, Kern N, Schmid DA, Uhr M, Holsboer F, Modell S. Pharmacological and nonpharmacological factors influencing hypothalamic-pituitary-adrenocortical axis reactivity in acutely depressed psychiatric in-patients, measured by the Dex–CRH test. Neuropsychopharmacology. 2003;28:2169–78.
21. Liu X, Sun G, Zhang X, Xu B, Shen C, Shi L, Ma X, Ren X, Feng K, Liu P. Relationship between the prefrontal function and the severity of the emotional symptoms during a verbal fluency task in patients with major depressive disorder: a multi-channel NIRS study. Prog Neuropsychopharmacol Biol Psychiatr. 2014;54:114–21.
22. Lodish M, Stratakis CA. A genetic and molecular update on adrenocortical causes of Cushing syndrome. Nat Rev Endocrinol. 2016;12:255–62.
23. Maki A, Yamashita Y, Ito Y, Watanabe E, Mayanagi Y, Koizumi H. Spatial and temporal analysis of human motor activity using noninvasive NIR topography. Med Phys. 1995;22:1997–2005.
24. Matsubara T, Matsuo K, Nakashima M, Nakano M, Harada K, Watanuki T, Egashira K, Watanabe Y. Prefrontal activation in response to emotional words in patients with bipolar disorder and major depressive disorder. Neuroimage. 2014;85(Pt 1):489–97.
25. Mccarthy SE, Gillis J, Kramer M, Lihm J, Yoon S, Berstein Y, Mistry M, et al. De novo mutations in schizophrenia implicate chromatin remodeling and support a genetic overlap with autism and intellectual disability. Mol Psychiatr. 2014;19:652–8.
26. Nakazato K, Mizuguchi T. Development and validation of Japanese version of state-trait anxiety inventory. Shinshin-Igaku. 1982;22:107–12.
27. Nishimura Y Tanii H, Hara N, Inoue K, Kaiya H, Nishida A, Okada M, Okazaki Y. Relationship between the prefrontal function during a cognitive task and the severity of the symptoms in patients with panic disorder: a multi-channel NIRS study. Psychiatr Res. 2009;172(2):168–72.
28. Nishimura Y, Tanii H, Fukuda M, Kajiki N, Inoue K, Kaiya H, Nishida A, Okada M, Okazaki Y. Frontal dysfunction during a cognitive task in drug-naive patients with panic disorder as investigated by multi-channel near-infrared spectroscopy imaging. Neurosci Res. 2007;59(1):107–12.
29. O'Donovan MC, Craddock N, Norton N, Williams H, Peirce T, Moskvina V, Nikolov I, et al. Identification of loci associated with schizophrenia by genome-wide association and follow-up. Nat Genet. 2008;40:1053–5.
30. Pu S, Nakagome K, Yamada T, Yokoyama K, Matsumura H, Yamada S, Sugie T, Miura A, Mitani H, Iwata M, Nagata I, Kaneko K. Suicidal ideation is associated with reduced prefrontal activation during a verbal fluency task in patients with major depressive disorder. J Affect Disord. 2015;181:9–17.
31. Purcell SM, Wray NR, Stone JL, Visscher PM, O'Donovan MC, Sullivan PF, Sklar P. Common polygenic variation contributes to risk of schizophrenia and bipolar disorder. Nature. 2009;460:748–52.
32. Saito M, Yasui-furukori N, Nakagami T, Furukori H, Kaneko S. Dose-dependent interaction of paroxetine with risperidone in schizophrenic patients. J Clin Psychopharmacol. 2005;25:527–32.
33. Shao Z, Janse E, Visser K, Meyer AS. What do verbal fluency tasks measure? Predictors of verbal fluency performance in older adults. Front Psychol. 2014;5:772.
34. Spielberger CD. Manual for the state-trait anxiety inventory STAI (form Y) (" self-evaluation questionnaire"); 1983.

35. Stip E, Mancini-marie A, Letourneau G, Fahim C, Mensour B, Crivello F, Dollfus S. Increased grey matter densities in schizophrenia patients with negative symptoms after treatment with quetiapine: a voxel-based morphometry study. Int Clin Psychopharmacol. 2009;24:34–41.
36. Takizawa R, Fukuda M, Kawasaki S, Kasai K, Mimura M, Pu S, Noda T, et al. Neuroimaging-aided differential diagnosis of the depressive state. Neuroimage. 2014;85(Pt 1):498–507.
37. Takizawa R, Kasai K, Kawakubo Y, Marumo K, Kawasaki S, Yamasue H, Fukuda M. Reduced frontopolar activation during verbal fluency task in schizophrenia: a multi-channel near-infrared spectroscopy study. Schizophr Res. 2008;99:250–62.
38. Teicher MH. Biology of anxiety. Med Clin North Am. 1988;72:791–814.
39. Tohen M, Vieta E, Calabrese J, Ketter TA, Sachs G, Bowden C, Mitchell PB, et al. Efficacy of olanzapine and olanzapine-fluoxetine combination in the treatment of bipolar I depression. Arch Gen Psychiatr. 2003;60:1079–88.
40. Veen G, Derijk RH, Giltay EJ, van Vliet IM, Van Pelt J, Zitman FG. The influence of psychiatric comorbidity on the dexamethasone/CRH test in major depression. Eur Neuropsychopharmacol. 2009;19:409–15.
41. Zhang H, Dong W, Dang W, Quan W, Tian J, Chen R, Zhan S, Yu X. Near-infrared spectroscopy for examination of prefrontal activation during cognitive tasks in patients with major depressive disorder: a meta-analysis of observational studies. Psychiatr Clin Neurosci. 2015;69:22–33.
42. Zobel AW, Nickel T, Sonntag A, Uhr M, Holsboer F, Ising M. Cortisol response in the combined dexamethasone/CRH test as predictor of relapse in patients with remitted depression. a prospective study. J Psychiatr Res. 2001;35:83–94.

5

The role of C957T, TaqI and Ser311Cys polymorphisms of the DRD2 gene in schizophrenia

Thelma Beatriz González-Castro[1], Yazmín Hernández-Díaz[1], Isela Esther Juárez-Rojop[2], María Lilia López-Narváez[3], Carlos Alfonso Tovilla-Zárate[4*], Alma Genis-Mendoza[5] and Mariela Alpuin-Reyes[2]

Abstract

Background: The association between the dopamine D2 receptor (*DRD2*) gene and schizophrenia has been studied though no conclusive outcomes have been attained. The aim of this study was to perform a systematic review and meta-analysis to explore the relation between three polymorphisms of the *DRD2* gene (C957T, TaqI and Ser311Cys) and schizophrenia.

Methods: The search was made in PubMed and EBSCO databases (up to February 2016). The systematic review included 34 case–control association studies (34 for C957T, 16 for TaqI and 36 for Ser311Cys). The association analysis comprised the allelic, additive, dominant, and recessive genetic models. The meta-analysis was performed following the preferred reporting items for systematic reviews and meta-analyses (PRISMA) statement.

Results: The meta-analysis showed that TaqI (additive model: OR 0.57, 95% CI 0.30–1.14) and C957T (additive model: OR 0.75, 95% OR 0.58–0.97, recessive model: OR 0.79, 95% CI 0.64–0.98) exert a protective effect against developing schizophrenia. However, the sub-analysis for the C957T variant showed that this polymorphism exhibits a risk factor effect on Chinese individuals (allelic model: OR 1.33, 95% CI 1.04–1.70).

Conclusion: Our meta-analysis suggests an association of the *DRD2* gene and the risk for schizophrenia, given that TaqI and C957T polymorphisms presented a protective effect against schizophrenia, and in the sub-analyses the C957T variant increased the risk for this disorder in the Chinese population.

Keywords: Schizophrenia, *DRD2* gene, Meta-analysis, Systematic review, Polymorphism

Background

Schizophrenia (SZ) is a common and complex multifactorial psychiatric disorder characterized by a variety of symptoms. These symptoms involve multiple psychological domains, including inferential thinking, attention, social interaction, expression of emotions, and volition. Typically, the onset of these symptoms starts manifesting in adolescence or early adulthood [1, 2]. Schizophrenia is a highly heritable and complex multifactorial illness; its heterogeneity is caused by both genetic and environmental factors and their interactions [3, 4]. High genetic risk for schizophrenia has led to considerable research efforts aimed at exploring its association with a number of candidate genes.

Although the biological etiology of schizophrenia is unknown, dopamine system dysfunction has been widely implicated in the pathogenesis of this disorder, and genes involved in dopaminergic pathways are being studied as candidate genes [5, 6]. Particular attention has been focused on the dopamine D2 receptor gene

*Correspondence: alfonso_tovillaz@yahoo.com.mx
[4] División Académica Multidisciplinaria de Comalcalco, Universidad Juárez Autónoma de Tabasco, Ranchería Sur, Cuarta Sección, C.P. 86650 Comalcalco, Tabasco, Mexico
Full list of author information is available at the end of the article

(*DRD2*). This is a transmembrane G protein-linked receptor which activates intracellular signaling by the inhibition of cAMP synthesis [7]. In humans, the *DRD2* gene is localized on chromosome 11 at the q22–q23 locus. This gene presents multiple polymorphisms, about 514 (http://snpper.chip.org/bio/snpper-enter/). From these, we selected three functional variants [8, 9]. The C957T (rs6277) variant constitutes a polymorphism with a synonymous coding C>T transition in exon 7. It has been proposed that this change influences the availability and affinity of the receptors [10–12]. Second, TaqI (rs1800497, C>T) comprises a substitution of an acidic amino acid for a basic one (Glu713Lys), and the two alleles are referred as A2 (cytosine) and A1 (thymine), respectively. The A1 allele is considered the risk allele [13, 14]. Finally, the Ser311Cys (rs1801028, C>G) polymorphism in exon 7 can present two variants, in which the C allele is the normal allele and encodes the amino acid serine (Ser) at codon 311, and the G allele is the risk allele and encodes a cysteine (Cys) [15, 16].

To date, a significant association between SZ and these functional *DRD2* gene polymorphisms (C957T, TaqI and Ser311Cys) has been reported by a number of authors [17–19]. However, several studies have failed to replicate this significant association [14, 20]. At least, two meta-analyses assessing the association between C957T, TaqI and Ser311Cys and schizophrenia have been performed. The first one was carried out by Yao et al. [21] in 2014 and the second by Li et al. [22] in 2015. Given that the dopamine system may contribute to the risk for schizophrenia, we conducted an update meta-analysis of all eligible published case–control studies to evaluate the effect of C957T, TaqI and Ser311Cys polymorphisms of the *DRD2* gene on the overall risk for SZ. The effects of ethnicity were also evaluated in this study.

Methods

The search association between SZ and *DRD2* gene variants was performed according to the following assessments: (1) a meta-analysis of the TaqI polymorphism in subjects with SZ compared to healthy controls, (2) meta-analysis of the C957T polymorphism in subjects with SZ compared to healthy controls, (3) meta-analysis of the Ser311Cys polymorphism in subjects with SZ compared to healthy controls, (4) meta-analysis of the TaqI polymorphism in schizophrenics versus healthy controls in the Caucasian population, (5) meta-analysis of the C957T polymorphism in schizophrenics versus healthy controls in Caucasian and Asian populations, and a further analysis in Chinese and Japanese subjects, (6) meta-analysis of the Ser311Cys polymorphism in schizophrenics versus healthy controls by population. (7) Finally, a

meta-regression method based on age including TaqI, C957T, and Ser311Cys polymorphisms was performed.

The meta-analyses were reported according to the preferred reporting items for systematic reviews and meta-analyses (PRISMA) statement [23, 24]. The PRISMA checklist is included as Additional file 1.

Protocol registration

The protocol of this meta-analysis was registered in PROSPERO (http://www.crd.york.ac.uk/prospero/) with the registration number CRD42015029744.

Publication search

To identify all potentially eligible studies on *DRD2* polymorphisms and schizophrenia risk, we performed a systematic search on PubMed and EBSCO databases that included all papers on the subject published up to February 2016. Relevant studies were identified using the terms: "*DRD2* AND C957T polymorphism AND schizophrenia", "*DRD2* AND rs6277 AND schizophrenia", "*DRD2* AND Ser311Cys polymorphism AND schizophrenia", "*DRD2* AND rs1801028 AND schizophrenia", "*DRD2* AND TaqI polymorphism AND schizophrenia", "*DRD2* AND rs1800497 AND schizophrenia" "DRD AND rs6277", "*DRD2* AND −141CInsDel". References within the retrieved articles and review articles were also screened. Citation lists of retrieved articles were manually examined to ensure search sensitivity.

Inclusion and exclusion criteria

Eligible studies had to meet the following criteria: (1) to be published in peer-reviewed journals, (2) to be designed as case–control studies, (3) to contain independent data, (4) to be association studies in which the frequencies of three genotypes were clearly stated or could be calculated, (5) inclusion of SZ diagnosis in the patient study group, and (6) the articles had to be written in English. Studies were excluded when: (1) they were not case–control studies, (2) they were reviews, comments or editorial articles, (3) they provided insufficient data, and (4) they were repeated studies.

Data extraction

All the available data were extracted from each study by two researchers (Hernández-Díaz and González-Castro) working independently and in accordance with the inclusion criteria listed above. In case of disagreement in the inclusion, a third investigator was involved (Tovilla-Zárate) to resolve the discrepancy and a final decision was reached by the majority of votes. Data such as authors, year of publication, location, ethnic group, number of cases and controls, age, gender, SZ diagnosis of the participants and genotypes were collected.

Publication bias

The possible presence of publication bias was evaluated graphically by drawing funnel plots and statistically by the Egger's standard regression test. In the Egger's test p < 0.10 was considered a statistically significant publication bias. The shape of the funnel plots serve as an indication of any obvious asymmetry for the TaqI, C957T and Ser311Cys variants, which was additionally supported by the Egger's test. Moreover, to strengthen the analysis we evaluated publication bias by using the GRADE approach (Additional file 1). In addition, the 95% confidence interval (95% CI) of the effect size (ES) was also computed; effect size of 0.2 was regarded as small, effect size of 0.5 was considered moderate and ES greater than 0.8 was taken as large.

Quality score assessment

For inclusion in the systematic review, each study was independently assessed by two reviewers (YHD and TBGC) using the Newcastle–Ottawa Assessment Scale (NOS) to estimate the methodological quality [25] (Table 1). The quality score of a given study was based on a score of six as cut-off point to distinguish high from low quality studies.

Statistical analysis

The comprehensive meta-analysis software (CMA, version 2) was used for the statistical analyses. The results are presented as odds ratios (ORs) and were used to assess the strength of the association between TaqI, C957T and Ser311Cys polymorphisms of the *DRD2* gene and SZ risk. Pooled ORs with their corresponding confidence intervals (95% CIs) were calculated for each of the models used: allelic (T vs C), additive (TT vs CC), dominant (TT + CT vs CC), and recessive (TT vs CT + TT). The estimated pooled ORs for each study were calculated using a random-effects model (Dersimonian and Laird method), though the fixed effects model was also considered (Mantel–Haenszel method). Heterogeneity of the studies was assessed with I^2 and Q test statistics to identify significant outcomes. The sources of heterogeneity were also detected by sub-group analyses. Two sub-groups (Caucasian or Asian) according to different descents were analyzed for an ethnic-specific genetic comparison. Sample heterogeneity was analyzed with the Dersimonian and Laird's Q test. Q test results were complemented with graphs to help the visualization of those studies favoring heterogeneity. The reliability of the results was assessed by sensitivity analysis performed for all outcomes to determine whether the results were driven mainly by single studies. In addition, we performed a meta-regression method based on age, to reduce the small sample size problem. We also performed a cumulative meta-analysis to provide a framework for updating the genetic effect of all studies. For the cumulative meta-analysis, studies were sorted chronologically by year of publication. The Hardy–Weinberg equilibrium (HWE) was checked using a Chi square test in each case and control group of the included studies; values of p < 0.05 were considered as showing a significant deviation from HWE. Finally, the strength of agreement between reviewers regarding study selection was evaluated by Kappa statistic.

Results

Characteristics of included studies

On-line literature search supplemented with a manual search resulted in 285 reports comprising 86 case–control studies [1, 10–12, 14–20, 22, 26–69], which were included in this meta-analysis (Table 1); this consisted of 18,692 SZ cases and 22,032 healthy controls. Of the 86 studies, 34 detailed the role of C957T in SZ, 36 examined the association of Ser311Cys with this disorder, and only 16 were available for the meta-analysis approach concerning the TaqI polymorphism and schizophrenia. In the case of TaqI, 12 studies were conducted in Caucasian populations, 2 in Indian, 1 in Iranian and 1 in Turkish populations, with a total of 1969 SZ cases and 1985 healthy controls. With regard to the C957T, 18 studies were conducted in Caucasians, 11 in Asians, 3 studies in Indians, 1 in Brazil and 1 in Turkish populations; in total 8819 SZ cases and 9965 healthy controls were included. Finally, for the Ser311Cys polymorphism, 18 studies were conducted in Asians, 15 in Caucasians and 3 in an Indian population with a total of 7827 SZ cases and 10,014 healthy controls. Characteristics of the 86 studies and the results of the HWE test are shown in Table 1.

TaqI polymorphism and SZ
All populations

Seventeen studies were included to identify the association between TaqI and SZ risk. Following the same pattern of analysis previously established for *DRD2* gene variants, all the genetic models: *allelic* (OR 0.92, 95% CI 0.71–1.19), *additive* (OR 0.59, 95% CI 0.30–1.14), *recessive* (OR 1.34, 95% CI 0.88–2.05) and *dominant* (OR 0.72, 95% CI 0.49–1.06) showed heterogeneity with p < 0.05. Subsequently, when we excluded the studies that favored the presence of the heterogeneity, we then observed the effect of the TaqI polymorphism in all populations using the *additive* genetic model (OR 0.57, 95% CI 0.38–0.86; p value of Q test: 0.32) and found a protective effect in the population as a whole. However, when we analyzed the *recessive model*, a risk effect was encountered (OR 1.50, 95% CI 1.10–2.03; p value of Q test: 0.66); see Table 2). The Egger's test did not yield evidence of publication bias (Fig. 1). To reduce the effect of the small size of the

Table 1 Characteristics of the studies included in this meta-analysis

Author	Location	Nos	Number Cases	Controls	Genotypes Cases A1/A1	A1/A2	A2/A2	Controls A1/A1	A1/A2	A2/A2	p for HWE Cases	Controls
Taq I												
Lafuente [43]	Spain	8	80	188	2	27	51	3	68	117	0.72	0.06
Monakhov [44]	Russia	8	311	364	189	104	18	238	116	10	0.51	0.48
Lafuente [45]	Spain	8	287	243	5	81	157	13	90	184	0.20	0.58
Behravan [17]	Iran	8	38	63	6	21	11	3	39	21	0.01[a]	0.52
Dubertret [46]	France	8	103	83	71	29	3	30	40	13	0.98	0.95
Aslan [14]	Turkey	8	99	109	2	97	0	0	106	3	0.00[a]	0.00[a]
Comings [63]	USA	4	87	69	58	27	2	59	10	0	0.56	0.37
Sanders [65]	USA	4	55	51	38	16	1	36	12	3	0.62	0.20
Campion [79]	France	5	80	80	60	19	1	58	20	2	0.70	0.86
Nöthen [56]	Germany	5	60	60	40	18	2	41	18	1	0.98	0.51
Dollfus [80]	France	6	62	61	41	19	2	11	45	5	0.91	0.00[a]
Jonsson [66]	Sweden	6	104	67	70	30	4	45	18	4	0.74	0.24
Dubertret [52]	France	7	50	50	36	13	1	26	21	3	0.88	0.63
Parsons [81]	Spain	8	119	165	92	24	3	93	68	4	0.39	0.04[a]
Vijayan [1]	India	8	212	194	102	93	17	88	77	29	0.62	0.08
Srivastava [61]	India	8	222	138	123	93	6	21	96	21	0.02[a]	0.00[a]

Author	Location	Nos	Number Cases	Controls	Genotypes Cases CC	CT17	TT	Controls CC	107CT	TT	p for HWE Cases	Controls
C957T												
Jonsson [66]	Sweden	7	173	236	160	12	1	232	4	0	0.23	1.00
Lawford [11]	Australia	6	154	148	48	75	31	27	70	51	0.87	0.73
Hanninen [10]	Finland	7	188	384	59	92	37	104	176	104	0.91	0.102
Kukreti [47]	India	7	101	145	41	38	22	48	64	33	0.03[a]	0.23
Hoenicka [19]	Spain	7	131	364	30	61	40	46	174	144	0.48	0.65
Mo [48]	China	8	174	127	61	96	17	29	69	29	0.02[a]	0.37
Luo [49]	China	6	466	388	409	55	2	351	37	0	0.70	0.98
Monakhov [44]	Russia	8	311	364	99	152	60	78	183	103	0.90	0.91
Gupta [41]	India	8	254	225	104	112	38	76	120	29	0.41	0.09
Betcheva [12]	Bulgaria	8	255	556	58	128	66	192	253	111	0.89	0.09
Dubertret [46]	France	7	144	142	104	37	3	120	21	1	0.92	0.94
Fan [20]	China	8	421	403	366	52	3	368	34	1	0.43	0.55
Tsutsumi [42]	Japan	9	407	384	367	38	1	341	43	2	0.98	0.64
Arinami [27]	Japan	6	260	312	190	66	4	193	102	17	0.79	0.50
Li [82]	England	7	151	145	112	39	0	118	26	1	0.01[a]	0.72
Ohara [32]	Japan	7	170	121	136	34	0	84	36	1	0.37	0.30
Stöber [64]	Germany	7	260	290	207	50	3	236	53	1	0.99	0.21
Breen (1) [83]	England	7	378	292	293	78	7	227	61	4	0.47	0.96
Breen (2)	Scotland	7	151	145	115	33	3	118	26	1	0.71	0.72
Inada [84]	Japan	7	234	94	156	72	6	51	40	3	0.65	0.26
Tallerico [85]	Canada	7	50	51	40	10	0	43	7	1	0.29	0.36
Hori [39]	Japan	7	241	201	162	71	8	142	54	5	0.94	0.96
Himei [40]	Japan	7	190	103	118	69	3	71	27	5	0.06	0.30
Dubertret [52]	France	8	103	83	83	19	1	43	33	7	0.93	0.79
Kapman [86]	Finland	7	93	94	86	7	0	88	6	0	0.60	0.65

Table 1 continued

Author	Location	Nos	Number		Genotypes						p for HWE	
			Cases	Controls	Cases			Controls			Cases	Controls
					CC	CT17	TT	CC	107CT	TT		
Parsons [81]	Spain	8	108	153	88	20	0	135	18	0	0.59	0.28
Lafuente [45]	Spain	8	243	291	208	33	2	235	54	2	0.63	0.75
Luu [67]	China	8	211	201	165	44	2	163	34	4	0.60	0.24
Sanders [57]	Europe	8	1870	2002	1495	354	21	1643	341	18	0.99	0.94
Cordeiro [68]	Brazil	8	229	733	183	38	8	498	206	29	0.00[a]	0.20
Srivastava [61]	India	8	233	224	161	65	7	172	48	4	0.81	0.75
Kurt [87]	Turkey	8	73	60	45	26	2	34	25	1	0.71	0.26
Saiz [88]	Spain	8	272	404	181	76	15	301	98	5	0.08	0.51
Xiao [69]	China	8	120	100	96	22	2	68	28	4	0.62	0.51

[a] Significant p value

Table 2 Analysis of the association studies between the *DRD2* gene TaqI polymorphism and SZ in all populations and in a Caucasian sub-group

Model analysis		Model effects		p value of Q test
		Random OR (95% CI)	Fixed OR (95% CI)	
All populations				
Allelic	With heterogeneity	0.92 (0.71–1.19)	*0.89 (0.80–0.99)*	<0.00
	Without heterogeneity	0.92 (0.79–1.07)	0.92 (0.81–1.05)	0.256
Additive	With heterogeneity	0.59 (0.30–1.14)	*0.51 (0.37–0.71)*	<0.00
	Without heterogeneity	*0.57 (0.38–0.86)*	*0.57 (0.39–0.81)*	0.326
Recessive	With heterogeneity	1.34 (0.88–2.05)	1.17 (0.95–1.44)	<0.00
	Without heterogeneity	*1.50 (1.10–2.03)*	*1.50 (1.10–2.03)*	0.664
Dominant	With heterogeneity	0.72 (0.49–1.06)	*0.72 (0.62–0.84)*	<0.00
	Without heterogeneity	0.85 (0.72–1.01)	0.85 (0.72–1.01)	0.586
Caucasian population				
Allelic	With heterogeneity	0.88 (0.66–1.18)	*0.86 (0.77–0.96)*	<0.00
	Without heterogeneity	0.86 (0.71–1.05)	0.86 (0.71–1.05)	0.551
Additive	With heterogeneity			
	Without heterogeneity	*0.60 (0.36–0.99)*	*0.59 (0.39–0.91)*	0.263
Recessive	With heterogeneity			
	Without heterogeneity	0.90 (0.69–1.18)	0.90 (0.71–1.15)	0.403
Dominant	With heterogeneity	0.76 (0.50–1.14)	*0.77 (0.64–0.93)*	<0.00
	Without heterogeneity	0.89 (0.71–1.11)	0.89 (0.72–1.10)	0.397

Italic values denote significant value, p < 0.05

sample in the analyses, we performed a meta-regression method based on age for the whole population. This analysis revealed a point estimate slope of −0.05365 and p value of 0.01686 (Fig. 2).

Caucasian population
Given that previous studies have reported a positive association between TaqI and SZ risk in Caucasians [46], we

decided to conduct a meta-analysis on the Caucasian population. This sub-group analysis by ethnicity included seven studies which showed no evidence of any association between TaqI and SZ in Caucasian populations. The results for the different genetic models were: *allelic* (OR 0.86, 95% CI 0.71–1.05; p value of Q test: 0.55), *recessive* (OR 0.90, 95% CI 0.69–1.18; p value of Q test: 0.40) and *dominant* (OR 0.89, 95% CI 0.71–1.11; p value of Q test:

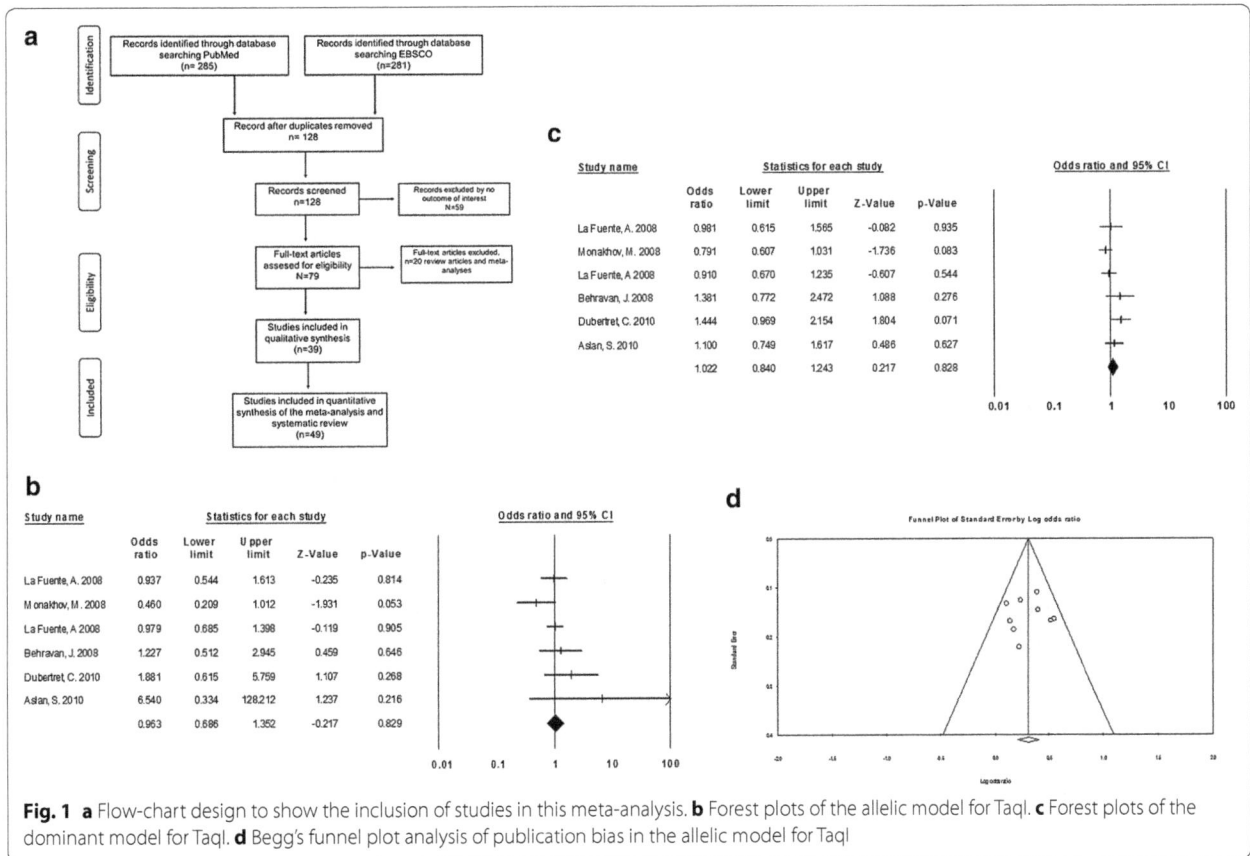

Fig. 1 a Flow-chart design to show the inclusion of studies in this meta-analysis. **b** Forest plots of the allelic model for TaqI. **c** Forest plots of the dominant model for TaqI. **d** Begg's funnel plot analysis of publication bias in the allelic model for TaqI

0.39). However, in the *additive* model we observed a protective effect of TaqI on schizophrenia (OR 0.60, 95% CI 0.36–0.99; p value of Q test: 0.26) (Fig. 3).

C957T polymorphism and schizophrenia
All populations
We performed an analysis in the population as a whole to explore the probable risk role of the C957T polymorphism in schizophrenia. Initially, we conducted a meta-analysis with the four genetic models proposed: *allelic* (OR 0.92, 95% CI 0.81–1.05), *additive* (OR 0.77, 95% CI 0.57–1.05), *recessive* (OR 0.84, 95% CI 0.66–1.06) and *dominant* (OR 0.91, 95% CI 0.78–1.05), in which p of Q test <0.05 indicated heterogeneity. No statistical association was found between the C957T polymorphism and schizophrenia. However, when we discarded the studies favoring heterogeneity, we obtained the following outcomes of statistical association for the models: *additive* (OR 0.75, 95% CI 0.58–0.97; p value of Q test: 0.15) and *recessive* (OR 0.79; 95% CI 0.64–0.98; p value of Q test: 0.21) (Table 3). In addition, the Egger's test revealed no evidence of publication bias (Fig. 4). With regard to the meta-regression based on age, the slope was 0.00849 and the p value 0.38756 (Fig. 2).

Caucasian population
We performed a stratified analysis by ethnicity to measure SZ risk by populations. With regard to Caucasians, the first outcomes with a p of Q test <0.05 showed evidence of heterogeneity in the *allelic* (OR 0.98, 95% CI 0.81–1.18), *additive* (OR 0.85, 95% CI 0.54–1.34), *recessive* (OR 0.89, 95% CI 0.65–1.23) and *dominant* (OR 0.98, 95% CI 0.79–1.21) models. Subsequently, when heterogeneity was discarded, the outcome presented a positive association with schizophrenia in the *allelic* model (OR 0.73, 95% CI 0.60–0.89; p value of Q test: 0.44). However, a slight possibility of an association in the *additive* (OR 0.80, 95% CI 0.66–0.97; p value of Q test <0.00) and *recessive* (OR 0.83, 95% CI 0.71–0.98; p value of Q test <0.00) models could be suggested. But since these findings were in the presence of heterogeneity and using the fixed effects model, we did not consider them for the analysis. For all the analyses in Caucasians, the p value of the Egger's test suggested the non-existence of publication bias (Fig. 5).

Asian population
Finally, for the C957T polymorphism in the Asian population we followed the same pattern of analysis

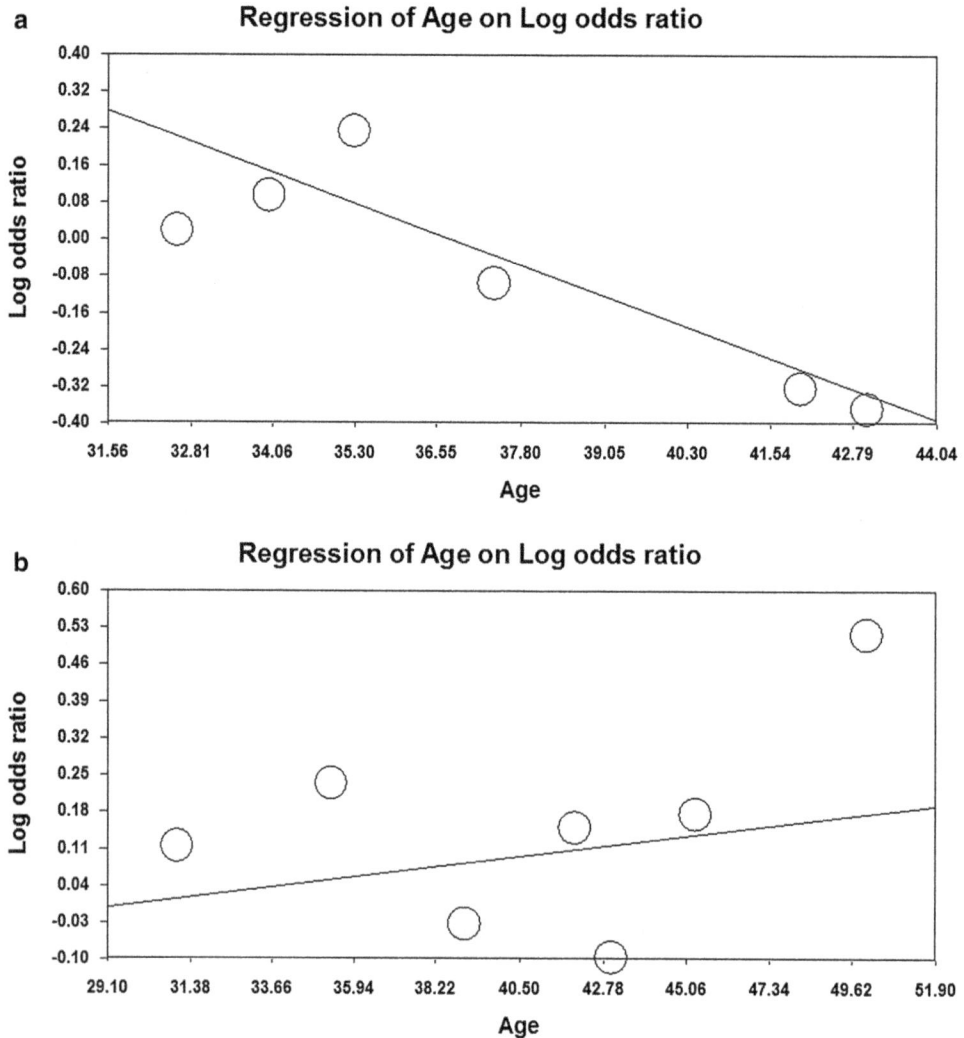

Fig. 2 Meta-regression method based on age in the population as a whole. **a** TaqI polymorphism and **b** C957T polymorphism

as in the previous sub-section. In the initial analysis the outcomes exhibited the presence of heterogeneity (p < 0.05) in the *allelic* (OR 0.84, 95% CI 0.66–1.07) and *dominant* models (OR 0.84, 95% CI 0.64–1.10). After we excluded the studies that favored heterogeneity, the results evidenced an association between the C957T polymorphism and SZ in the four models: *allelic* (OR 0.66, 95% CI 0.52–0.83; p value of Q test: 0.72), *additive* (OR 0.49, 95% CI 0.28–0.86; p value of Q test: 0.20), *recessive* (OR 0.52, 95% CI 0.32–0.83; p value of Q test: 0.33) and *dominant* (OR 0.61, 95% CI 0.50–0.74; p value of Q test: 0.061), using the random effects method. However, we want to emphasize that the outcomes showed the same protective association between C957T and SZ in the all models when we used the fixed effects model.

C957T polymorphism in Chinese and Japanese populations
In order to perform a more comprehensive and comparative meta-analysis we conducted two more sub-analyses, but only for the subjects born in Japan and in China. These sub-analyses helped to compare our findings with previous published met-analyses. Initially, we selected the studies that explored the role of C957T in Japanese schizophrenics and found a relation to SZ in the four models without heterogeneity, viz.: *allelic* (OR 0.69, 95% CI 0.57–0.85; p value of Q test: 0.11), *additive* (OR 0.51, 95% CI 0.27–0.95; p value of Q test: 0.24), *recessive* (OR 0.54, 95% CI 0.29–0.99; p value of Q test: 0.27) and *dominant* (OR 0.58, 95% CI 0.45–0.76; p value of Q test: 0.98), but all the results were for the fixed effects model. Nevertheless, when we used the random effects method we encountered the same pattern only in the *allelic* (OR

a

Study name	Statistics for each study					Odds ratio and 95% CI
	Odds ratio	Lower limit	Upper limit	Z-Value	p-Value	
La Fuente, A 2008	0.981	0.615	1.565	-0.082	0.935	
Monakhov, M 2008	0.791	0.607	1.031	-1.736	0.083	
Lafuente, A 2008	0.910	0.670	1.235	-0.607	0.544	
Dubertret, C. 2010	1.444	0.969	2.154	1.804	0.071	
	0.975	0.761	1.251	-0.196	0.845	

0.01   0.1   1   10   100

b

Funnel Plot of Standard Error by Log odds ratio

c

Study name	Statistics for each study					Odds ratio and 95% CI
	Odds ratio	Lower limit	Upper limit	Z-Value	p-Value	
La Fuente, A 2008	0.937	0.544	1.613	-0.235	0.814	
Monakhov, M 2008	0.460	0.209	1.012	-1.931	0.053	
Lafuente, A 2008	0.979	0.685	1.398	-0.119	0.905	
Dubertret, C. 2010	1.881	0.615	5.759	1.107	0.268	
	0.903	0.617	1.322	-0.523	0.601	

0.01   0.1   1   10   100

d

Funnel Plot of Standard Error by Log odds ratio

Fig. 3 a Forest plots of the allelic model for TaqI in Caucasians. **b** Begg's funnel plot analysis of publication bias of the allelic model for TaqI in Caucasians. **c** Forest plots of the dominant model for TaqI in Caucasians. **d** Begg's funnel plot analysis of publication bias in the dominant model for TaqI in Caucasians

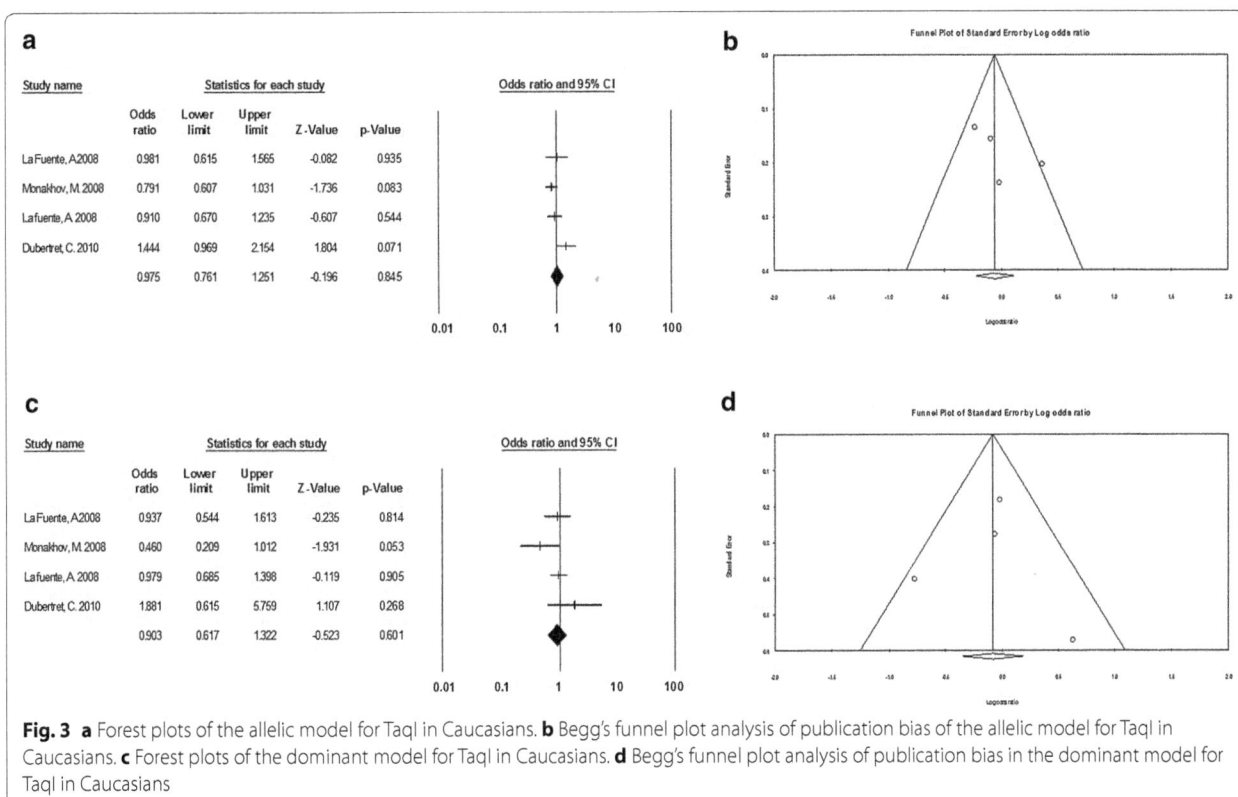

0.71, 95% CI 0.53–0.94) and *dominant* (OR 0.58, 95% CI 0.45–0.76) models. With regard to the Chinese population, we found a similar association to that of the previous sub-analysis. Interestingly, we found a risk effect in the *allelic* (OR 1.33, 95% CI 1.04–1.70; p value of Q test: 0.50) and *dominant* (OR 1.36, 95% CI 1.04–1.77; p value of Q test: 0.69) models, without heterogeneity using the random effects method (Table 4).

Ser311Cys polymorphism and SZ

For this polymorphism the meta-analysis was performed for the overall population. The outcomes in Caucasian and Asian populations were similar to those found for the previous variants. Since the present work showed the same results as in previous studies [21], we will not discuss this polymorphism in the present work. However, we present the details in Additional file 2.

Sensitivity analysis

In addition, a sensitivity analysis was carried out in which one study at a time was excluded to determine whether a specific study was favoring a marked heterogeneity. Nevertheless, the presence of heterogeneity was not explained by just one study. Furthermore, to measure the effects over time on the studies, we performed a

cumulative meta-analysis, in which individual data sets were ordered chronologically (Additional file 3).

Discussion

Schizophrenia is a complex genetic disorder manifesting combined environmental and genetic factors. Several studies have suggested that genetic variants of the *DRD2* gene play a role in SZ etiology [70, 71]. To assess the relationship between the *DRD2* genetic variants and the risk to develop schizophrenia, we conducted a meta-analysis of three *DRD2* polymorphisms: TaqI, C957T and Ser-311Cys. The meta-analysis approach is a powerful tool to summarize contradicting results from different studies and has been used to analyze the role of various genes in schizophrenia [54, 72, 73].

First, we performed the analysis of the TaqI polymorphism to assess the role of this genetic variant in schizophrenia. There was a protective effect in the additive model in the population as a whole and in Caucasians. Also, we found a risk effect when using the recessive model in the combined results of the analysis for all populations. However, various studies have reported that TaqI polymorphism does not play an important role in the psychopathological symptoms of schizophrenia, whereas other researches agree with our results [21, 22, 63, 66]. One of the reasons for this discrepancy could

Table 3 Analysis of association studies between the *DRD2* gene C957T polymorphism and schizophrenia by populations

Model analysis		Random OR (95% CI)	Fixed OR (95% CI)	p value of Q test
All populations				
Allelic	With heterogeneity	0.92 (0.81–1.05)	*0.93 (0.87–0.98)*	<0.00
	Without heterogeneity	1.03 (0.93–1.15)	1.03 (0.93–1.15)	0.595
Additive	With heterogeneity	0.77 (0.57–1.05)	*0.76 (0.65–0.89)*	<0.00
	Without heterogeneity	*0.75 (0.58–0.97)*	*0.74 (0.61–0.91)*	0.151
Recessive	With heterogeneity	0.84 (0.66–1.06)	0.82 (0.72–0.94)	<0.00
	Without heterogeneity	*0.79 (0.64–0.98)*	*0.78 (0.66–0.92)*	0.211
Dominant	With heterogeneity	0.91 (0.78–1.05)	0.94 (0.88–1.01)	<0.00
	Without heterogeneity	0.89 (0.77–1.03)	0.89 (0.78–1.02)	0.308
Caucasian population				
Allelic	With heterogeneity	0.98 (0.81–1.18)	0.98 (0.91–1.05)	<0.00
	Without heterogeneity	1.03 (0.88–1.21)	1.00 (0.87–1.14)	0.252
Additive	With heterogeneity	0.85 (0.54–1.34)	*0.80 (0.66–0.97)*	<0.00
	Without heterogeneity	0.94 (0.63–1.40)	0.90 (0.63–1.27)	0.354
Recessive	With heterogeneity	0.89 (0.65–1.23)	*0.83 (0.71–0.98)*	<0.00
	Without heterogeneity	*0.73 (0.60–0.89)*	*0.73 (0.60–0.89)*	0.440
Dominant	With heterogeneity	0.98 (0.79–1.21)	1.03 (0.93–1.13)	<0.00
	Without heterogeneity	1.04 (0.89–1.21)	1.03 (0.89–1.20)	0.400
Asian population				
Allelic	With heterogeneity	0.84 (0.66–1.07)	*0.82 (0.73–0.93)*	<0.00
	Without heterogeneity	*0.66 (0.52–0.83)*	*0.66 (0.52–0.83)*	0.725
Additive	With heterogeneity			
	Without heterogeneity	*0.49 (0.28–0.86)*	*0.45 (0.29–0.70)*	0.206
Recessive	With heterogeneity			
	Without heterogeneity	*0.52 (0.32–0.83)*	*0.49 (0.32–0.75)*	0.330
Dominant	With heterogeneity	0.84 (0.64–1.10)	*0.85 (0.73–0.99)*	<0.00
	Without heterogeneity	*0.61 (0.50–0.74)*	*0.61 (0.50–0.74)*	0.864

Italic values denote significant value, p < 0.05

be the relative small size of the sample, which limits the statistical power for the detection of a relationship between the TaqI polymorphism and schizophrenia [72]; more studies are needed to further validate these results. Another explanation is the environmental exposure that could trigger the expression of a gene, and this in turn could modify other genes which may then interact with *DRD2* and increase the risk to present the disease. In spite of the contrasting outcomes published, the role of TaqI has been more related to substance abuse, since the less frequent allele (A1 allele) has been associated with some psychiatric disorders such as alcoholism and substance abuse [74, 75]. On the other hand, previous studies have demonstrated that subjects with one or two A1 alleles of the *DRD2* polymorphism at the Taq1 A locus present lower *DRD2* density than those with no A1 allele [76]. Also, other studies have shown that female patients with the A1 allele exhibit greater prolactin response to

nemonapride, a selective antagonist for D2-like dopamine receptors in schizophrenic patients [77]. Due to this association between TaqI and schizophrenia, the A1 allele has been suggested to diminish dopaminergic activity in the central nervous system [78].

For the C957T polymorphism, the comparisons performed in our study showed a significant positive association between this polymorphism and SZ in the overall population and in Caucasian and Asian sub-groups. In this sense, we recognize the existence of two previous meta-analyses [21, 22], in which many differences are observed: first, we identified a protective effect of the T allele of C957T using the additive and recessive models when analyzing the population as a whole, as well as when using the recessive model in Caucasians and the four genetic models in Asians. In contrast, Yao et al. did not observe any association. The differences could be due to the size of the samples. Our

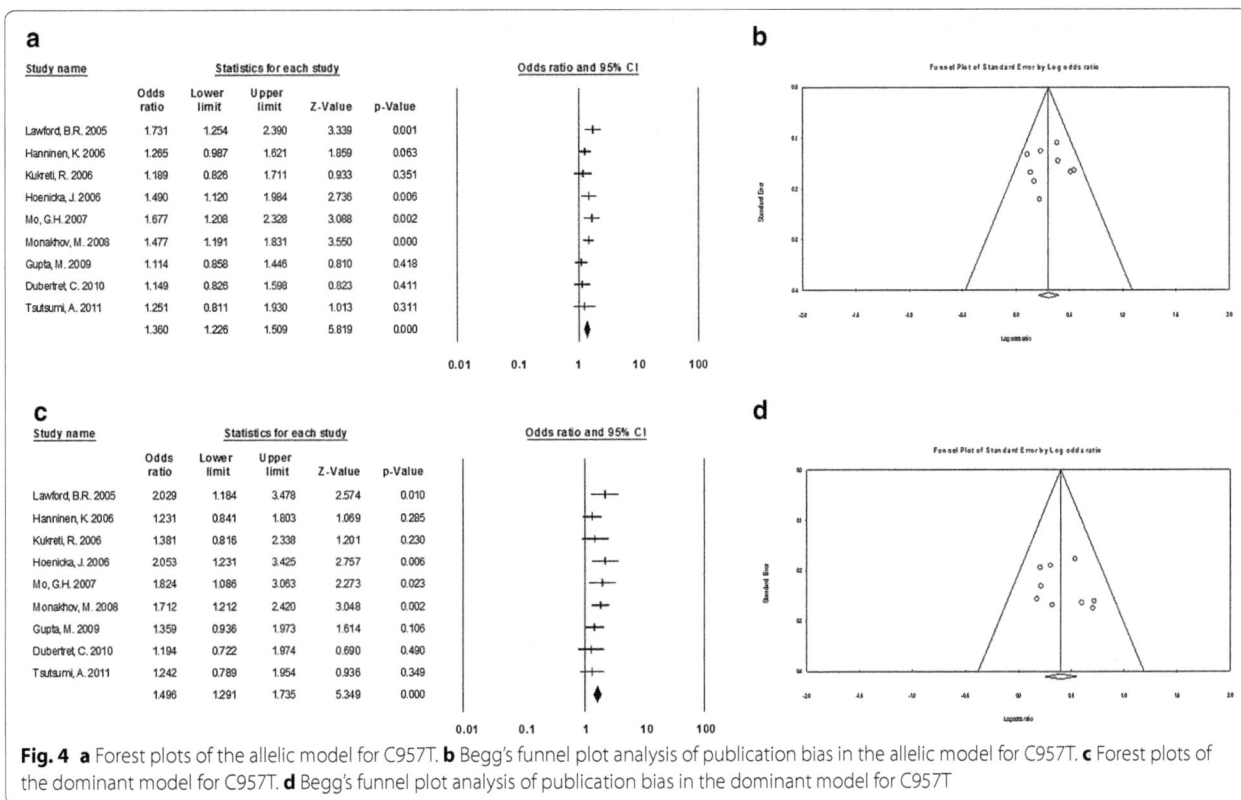

Fig. 4 a Forest plots of the allelic model for C957T. **b** Begg's funnel plot analysis of publication bias in the allelic model for C957T. **c** Forest plots of the dominant model for C957T. **d** Begg's funnel plot analysis of publication bias in the dominant model for C957T

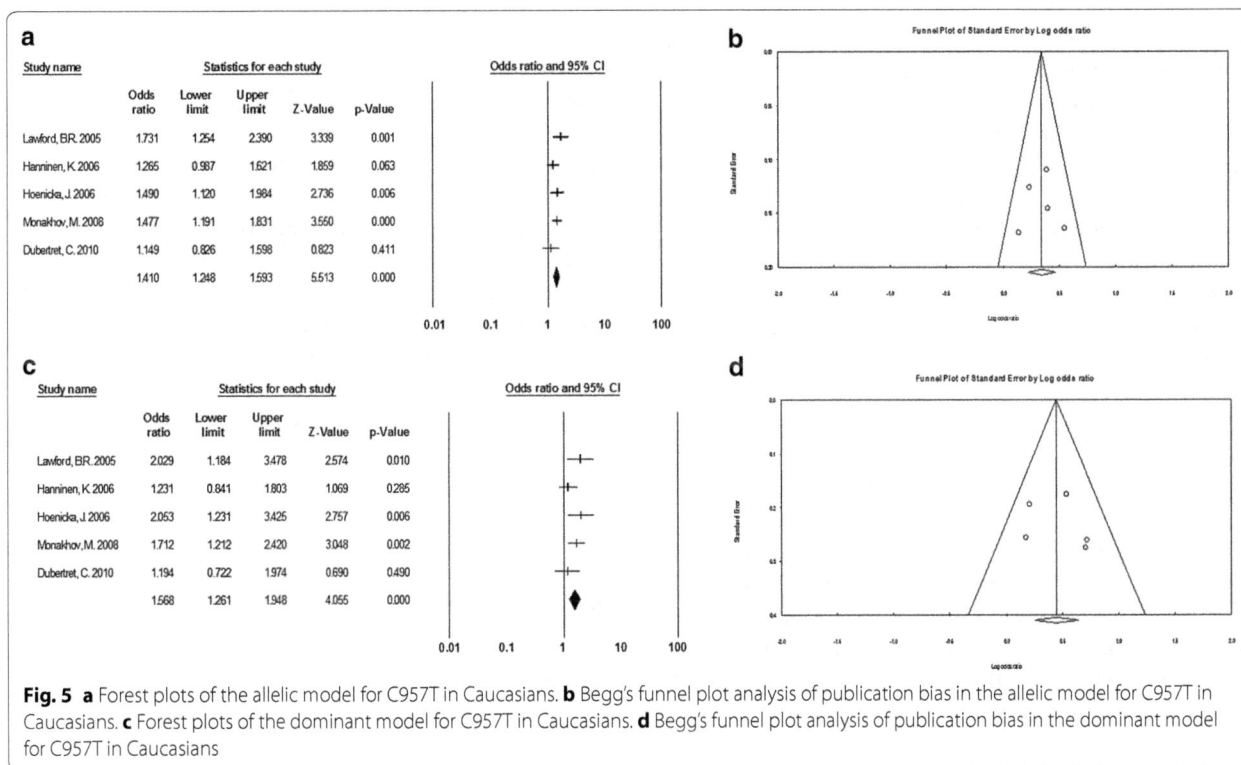

Fig. 5 a Forest plots of the allelic model for C957T in Caucasians. **b** Begg's funnel plot analysis of publication bias in the allelic model for C957T in Caucasians. **c** Forest plots of the dominant model for C957T in Caucasians. **d** Begg's funnel plot analysis of publication bias in the dominant model for C957T in Caucasians

Table 4 Analysis of association studies between the *DRD2* C957T polymorphism and schizophrenia in China and Japan

Model analysis		Model effects		p value of Q test
		Random OR (95% CI)	Fixed OR (95% CI)	
Japan				
Allelic	With heterogeneity	0.79 (0.58–1.07)	*0.78 (0.66–0.93)*	0.017
	Without heterogeneity	*0.71 (0.53–0.94)*	*0.69 (0.57–0.85)*	0.112
Additive	With heterogeneity			
	Without heterogeneity	0.50 (0.24–1.07)	*0.51 (0.27–0.95)*	0.243
Recessive	With heterogeneity			
	Without heterogeneity	0.53 (0.26–1.08)	*0.54 (0.29–0.99)*	0.279
Dominant	With heterogeneity	0.79 (0.55–1.14)	*0.78 (0.64–0.96)*	0.011
	Without heterogeneity	*0.58 (0.45–0.76)*	*0.58 (0.45–0.76)*	0.988
China				
Allelic	With heterogeneity	0.95 (0.62–1.45)	0.92 (0.77–1.11)	<0.00
	Without heterogeneity	*1.33 (1.04–1.70)*	*1.33 (1.04–1.70)*	0.507
Additive	With heterogeneity			
	Without heterogeneity	0.55 (0.21–1.39)	*0.40 (0.22–0.73)*	0.173
Recessive	With heterogeneity			
	Without heterogeneity	0.54 (0.25–1.15)	*0.46 (0.26–0.79)*	0.283
Dominant	With heterogeneity	0.96 (0.62–1.48)	1.02 (0.82–1.28)	<0.00
	Without heterogeneity	*1.36 (1.04–1.77)*	*1.36 (1.04–1.77)*	0.697

Italic values denote significant value, p < 0.05

present study used 8819 SZ patients and 9965 healthy controls compared with 6075 SZ and 6643 controls of the previous meta-analysis by Yao et al. [21]. We included 2792 cases and 3322 controls more. In the Asian population a protective effect was found in all the models we used. As a consequence, we decided to perform an analysis by Asiatic subpopulations. Therefore, we divided the Asian population into Chinese and Japanese samples. In these sub-analyses we encountered unexpected results: the Chinese population showed an increased risk, whereas the Japanese population showed a protective association. This is clear an "allele paradox" between populations that may reflect the difference in the distribution of allele frequencies across the geographical localization. Our results draw attention to the influence of other factors such as the environment, which could be acting with ethnicity in this genetic association.

There are several limitations in this study. First, the sample size for some sub-group analyses was limited; therefore, more studies with larger samples should be included to enhance the reliability and stability of the meta-analysis. Second, a language bias may be present given that only studies published in English were included. Third, due to the limitation of the data, we did

not stratify according to other potential factors which may enhance the risk for the development of SZ, such as gender, age of onset and clinical manifestations.

Conclusions

The meta-analysis indicated that TaqI and C957T polymorphisms show a protective effect against SZ. In the sub-analysis of the C957T polymorphism we observed that this variant may contribute to the occurrence of schizophrenia in Chinese subjects, so the influence of ethnicity could be important in modifying the role of this polymorphism in SZ. Given the limitations of the studies included in the meta-analysis, future studies with larger samples and prospective designs are needed to fully understand the relationship between these polymorphisms and SZ. However, this meta-analysis still provides new insights into the role of the *DRD2* gene in SZ risk.

Abbreviations
DRD2: dopamine D2 receptor; SZ: schizophrenia; NOS: Newcastle–Ottawa Assessment Scale; PRISMA: preferred reporting items for systematic reviews and meta-analyses; HWE: Hardy–Weinberg equilibrium.

Authors' contributions

TBGC, YHD, CATZ conceived the study, participated in its design, and helped to draft the manuscript. IEJR and MLLN helped to perform the statistical analyses and to draft the manuscript. AGM and MAR coordinated and supervised the integration of data. All authors read and approved the final manuscript.

Author details

[1] División Académica Multidisciplinaria de Jalpa de Méndez, Universidad Juárez Autónoma de Tabasco, Jalpa de Méndez, Tabasco, Mexico. [2] División Académica de Ciencias de la Salud, Universidad Juárez Autónoma de Tabasco, Villahermosa, Tabasco, Mexico. [3] Secretaría de Salud, Hospital General de Yajalón, Yajalón, Chiapas, Mexico. [4] División Académica Multidisciplinaria de Comalcalco, Universidad Juárez Autónoma de Tabasco, Ranchería Sur, Cuarta Sección, C.P. 86650 Comalcalco, Tabasco, Mexico. [5] Secretaría de Salud, Instituto Nacional de Medicina Genómica (INMEGEN), Servicios de Atención Psiquiátrica (SAP), Ciudad de México, Mexico.

Acknowledgements

None.

Competing interests

The authors declare that they have no competing interests.

Funding

This research received no grant from any funding agency in the public, commercial or not-for-profit sectors.

References

1. Vijayan NN, Bhaskaran S, Koshy LV, Natarajan C, Srinivas L, Nair CM, Allencherry PM, Banerjee M. Association of dopamine receptor polymorphisms with schizophrenia and antipsychotic response in a South Indian population. Behav Brain Funct. 2007;3:34.
2. Cannon TD. How schizophrenia develops: cognitive and brain mechanisms underlying onset of psychosis. Trends Cogn Sci. 2015;19(15):00233–8.
3. Winchester CL, Pratt JA, Morris BJ. Risk genes for schizophrenia: translational opportunities for drug discovery. Pharmacol Ther. 2014;143(1):34–50.
4. Cannon TD, van Erp TG, Bearden CE, Loewy R, Thompson P, Toga AW, Huttunen MO, Keshavan MS, Seidman LJ, Tsuang MT. Early and late neurodevelopmental influences in the prodrome to schizophrenia: contributions of genes, environment, and their interactions. Schizophr Bull. 2003;29(4):653–69.
5. Moran PM, O'Tuathaigh CM, Papaleo F, Waddington JL. Dopaminergic function in relation to genes associated with risk for schizophrenia: translational mutant mouse models. Prog Brain Res. 2014;211:79–112.
6. Seeman P. Schizophrenia and dopamine receptors. Eur Neuropsychopharmacol. 2013;23(9):999–1009.
7. Sumiyoshi T, Kunugi H, Nakagome K. Serotonin and dopamine receptors in motivational and cognitive disturbances of schizophrenia. Front Neurosci. 2014;8:395.
8. Noble EP. The DRD2 gene in psychiatric and neurological disorders and its phenotypes. Pharmacogenomics. 2000;1(3):309–33.
9. Hoenicka J, Aragues M, Ponce G, Rodriguez-Jimenez R, Jimenez-Arriero MA, Palomo T. From dopaminergic genes to psychiatric disorders. Neurotox Res. 2007;11(1):61–72.
10. Hanninen K, Katila H, Kampman O, Anttila S, Illi A, Rontu R, Mattila KM, Hietala J, Hurme M, Leinonen E, et al. Association between the C957T polymorphism of the dopamine D2 receptor gene and schizophrenia. Neurosci Lett. 2006;407(3):195–8.
11. Lawford BR, Young RM, Swagell CD, Barnes M, Burton SC, Ward WK, Heslop KR, Shadforth S, van Daal A, Morris CP. The C/C genotype of the C957T polymorphism of the dopamine D2 receptor is associated with schizophrenia. Schizophr Res. 2005;73(1):31–7.
12. Betcheva ET, Mushiroda T, Takahashi A, Kubo M, Karachanak SK, Zaharieva IT, Vazharova RV, Dimova II, Milanova VK, Tolev T, et al. Case–control association study of 59 candidate genes reveals the DRD2 SNP rs6277 (C957T) as the only susceptibility factor for schizophrenia in the Bulgarian population. J Hum Genet. 2009;54(2):98–107.
13. Ponce G, Perez-Gonzalez R, Aragues M, Palomo T, Rodriguez-Jimenez R, Jimenez-Arriero MA, Hoenicka J. The ANKK1 kinase gene and psychiatric disorders. Neurotox Res. 2009;16(1):50–9.
14. Aslan S, Karaoguz MY, Eser HY, Karaer DK, Taner E. Comparison of DRD2 rs1800497 (TaqIA) polymorphism between schizophrenic patients and healthy controls: lack of association in a Turkish sample. Int J Psychiatry Clin Pract. 2010;14(4):257–61.
15. Itokawa M, Arinami T, Toru M. Advanced research on dopamine signaling to develop drugs for the treatment of mental disorders: Ser311Cys polymorphisms of the dopamine D2-receptor gene and schizophrenia. J Pharmacol Sci. 2010;114(1):1–5.
16. Kaneshima M, Higa T, Nakamoto H, Nagamine M. An association study between the Cys311 variant of dopamine D2 receptor gene and schizophrenia in the Okinawan population. Psychiatry Clin Neurosci. 1997;51(6):379–81.
17. Behravan J, Hemayatkar M, Toufani H, Abdollahian E. Linkage and association of DRD2 gene TaqI polymorphism with schizophrenia in an Iranian population. Arch Iran Med. 2008;11(3):252–6.
18. Jonsson EG, Sillen A, Vares M, Ekholm B, Terenius L, Sedvall GC. Dopamine D2 receptor gene Ser311Cys variant and schizophrenia: association study and meta-analysis. Am J Med Genet B Neuropsychiatr Genet. 2003;15(1):28–34.
19. Hoenicka J, Aragues M, Rodriguez-Jimenez R, Ponce G, Martinez I, Rubio G, Jimenez-Arriero MA, Palomo T. C957T DRD2 polymorphism is associated with schizophrenia in Spanish patients. Acta Psychiatr Scand. 2006;114(6):435–8.
20. Fan H, Zhang F, Xu Y, Huang X, Sun G, Song Y, Long H, Liu P. An association study of DRD2 gene polymorphisms with schizophrenia in a Chinese Han population. Neurosci Lett. 2010;477(2):53–6.
21. Yao J, Pan YQ, Ding M, Pang H, Wang BJ. Association between DRD2 (rs1799732 and rs1801028) and ANKK1 (rs1800497) polymorphisms and schizophrenia: a meta-analysis. Am J Med Genet Part B Neuropsychiatr Genet. 2015;168(1):1–13.
22. Liu L, Fan D, Ding N, Hu Y, Cai G, Wang L, Xin L, Xia Q, Li X, Xu S, et al. The relationship between DRD2 gene polymorphisms (C957T and C939T) and schizophrenia: a meta-analysis. Neurosci Lett. 2014;583:43–8.
23. Swartz MK. The PRISMA statement: a guideline for systematic reviews and meta-analyses. J Pediatr Health Care. 2011;25(1):1–2. doi:10.1016/j.pedhc.2010.09.006.
24. Moher D, Liberati A, Tetzlaff J, Altman DG. Preferred reporting items for systematic reviews and meta-analyses: the PRISMA statement. Int J Surg. 2010;8(5):336–41.
25. Stang A. Critical evaluation of the Newcastle–Ottawa scale for the assessment of the quality of nonrandomized studies in meta-analyses. Eur J Epidemiol. 2010;25(9):603–5.
26. Itokawa M, Arinami T, Futamura N, Hamaguchi H, Toru M. A structural polymorphism of human dopamine D2 receptor, D2(Ser311→Cys). Biochem Biophys Res Commun. 1993;196(3):1369–75.
27. Arinami T, Itokawa M, Enguchi H, Tagaya H, Yano S, Shimizu H, Hamaguchi H, Toru M. Association of dopamine D2 receptor molecular variant with schizophrenia. Lancet. 1994;343(8899):703–4.
28. Hattori M, Nanko S, Dai XY, Fukuda R, Kazamatsuri H. Mismatch PCR RFLP detection of DRD2 Ser311Cys polymorphism and schizophrenia. Biochem Biophys Res Commun. 1994;202(2):757–63.
29. Nanko S, Hattori M, Dai XY, Fukuda R, Kazamatsuri H. DRD2 Ser311/Cys311 polymorphism in schizophrenia. Lancet. 1994;343(8904):1044.
30. Arinami T, Itokawa M, Aoki J, Shibuya H, Ookubo Y, Iwawaki A, Ota K, Shimizu H, Hamaguchi H, Toru M. Further association study on dopamine D2 receptor variant S311C in schizophrenia and affective disorders. Am J Med Genet. 1996;67(2):133–8.

31. Chen CH, Chien SH, Hwu HG. No association of dopamine D2 receptor molecular variant Cys311 and schizophrenia in Chinese patients. Am J Med Genet. 1996;67(4):418–20.

32. Ohara K, Nakamura Y, Xie DW, Ishigaki T, Deng ZL, Tani K, Zhang HY, Kondo N, Liu JC, Miyasato K, et al. Polymorphisms of dopamine D2-like (D2, D3, and D4) receptors in schizophrenia. Biol Psychiatry. 1996;40(12):1209–17.

33. Fujiwara Y, Yamaguchi K, Tanaka Y, Tomita H, Shiro Y, Kashihara K, Sato K, Kuroda S. Polymorphism of dopamine receptors and transporter genes in neuropsychiatric diseases. Eur Neurol. 1997;1:6–10.

34. Harano M. Ser-311-Cys polymorphism of the dopamine D2 receptor gene and schizophrenia—an analysis of schizophrenic patients in Fukuoka. Kurume Med J. 1997;44(3):201–8.

35. Tanaka T, Igarashi S, Onodera O, Tanaka H, Fukushima N, Takahashi M, Kameda K, Tsuji S, Ihda S. Lack of association between dopamine D2 receptor gene Cys311 variant and schizophrenia. Am J Med Genet. 1996;67(2):208–11.

36. Spurlock G, Williams J, McGuffin P, Aschauer HN, Lenzinger E, Fuchs K, Sieghart WC, Meszaros K, Fathi N, Laurent C, et al. European multicentre association study of schizophrenia: a study of the DRD2 Ser311Cys and DRD3 Ser9Gly polymorphisms. Am J Med Genet. 1998;81(1):24–8.

37. Morimoto K, Miyatake R, Nakamura M, Watanabe T, Hirao T, Suwaki H. Delusional disorder: molecular genetic evidence for dopamine psychosis. Neuropsychopharmacology. 2002;26(6):794–801.

38. Serretti A, Lattuada E, Lorenzi C, Lilli R, Smeraldi E. Dopamine receptor D2 Ser/Cys 311 variant is associated with delusion and disorganization symptomatology in major psychoses. Mol Psychiatry. 2000;5(3):270–4.

39. Hori H, Ohmori O, Shinkai T, Kojima H, Nakamura J. Association analysis between two functional dopamine D2 receptor gene polymorphisms and schizophrenia. Am J Med Genet. 2001;105(2):176–8.

40. Himei A, Koh J, Sakai J, Inada Y, Akabame K, Yoneda H. The influence on the schizophrenic symptoms by the DRD2Ser/Cys311 and −141C Ins/Del polymorphisms. Psychiatry Clin Neurosci. 2002;56(1):97–102.

41. Gupta M, Chauhan C, Bhatnagar P, Gupta S, Grover S, Singh PK, Purushottam M, Mukherjee O, Jain S, Brahmachari SK, et al. Genetic susceptibility to schizophrenia: role of dopaminergic pathway gene polymorphisms. Pharmacogenomics. 2009;10(2):277–91.

42. Tsutsumi A, Glatt SJ, Kanazawa T, Kawashige S, Uenishi H, Hokyo A, Kaneko T, Moritani M, Kikuyama H, Koh J, et al. The genetic validation of heterogeneity in schizophrenia. Behav Brain Funct. 2011;7(43):1744–9081.

43. Lafuente A, Bernardo M, Mas S, Crescenti A, Aparici M, Gasso P, Deulofeu R, Mane A, Catalan R, Carne X. Polymorphism of dopamine D2 receptor (TaqIA, TaqIB, and −141C Ins/Del) and dopamine degradation enzyme (COMT G158A, A-278G) genes and extrapyramidal symptoms in patients with schizophrenia and bipolar disorders. Psychiatry Res. 2008;161(2):131–41.

44. Monakhov M, Golimbet V, Abramova L, Kaleda V, Karpov V. Association study of three polymorphisms in the dopamine D2 receptor gene and schizophrenia in the Russian population. Schizophr Res. 2008;100(1–3):302–7.

45. Lafuente A, Bernardo M, Mas S, Crescenti A, Aparici M, Gasso P, Goti J, Sanchez V, Catalan R, Carne X. −141C Ins/Del polymorphism of the dopamine D2 receptor gene is associated with schizophrenia in a Spanish population. Psychiatr Genet. 2008;18(3):122–7.

46. Dubertret C, Bardel C, Ramoz N, Martin PM, Deybach JC, Ades J, Gorwood P, Gouya L. A genetic schizophrenia-susceptibility region located between the ANKK1 and DRD2 genes. Prog Neuropsychopharmacol Biol Psychiatry. 2010;34(3):492–9.

47. Kukreti R, Tripathi S, Bhatnagar P, Gupta S, Chauhan C, Kubendran S, Janardhan Reddy YC, Jain S, Brahmachari SK. Association of DRD2 gene variant with schizophrenia. Neurosci Lett. 2006;392(1–2):68–71.

48. Mo GH, Lai IC, Wang YC, Chen JY, Lin CY, Chen TT, Chen ML, Liou YJ, Liao DL, Bai YM, et al. Support for an association of the C939T polymorphism in the human DRD2 gene with tardive dyskinesia in schizophrenia. Schizophr Res. 2007;97(1–3):302–4.

49. Luo PF. Association of dopamine D2 receptor polymorphisms with paranoid schizophrenia in the North Chinese population. Beijing: Peking Union Medical College; 2008.

50. Asherson P, Williams N, Roberts E, McGuffin M, Owen M. DRD2 Ser311/Cys311 polymorphism in schizophrenia. Lancet. 1994;343(8904):1045.

51. Crawford F, Hoyne J, Cai X, Osborne A, Poston D, Zaglul J, Dajani N, Walsh S, Bradley R, Solomon R, et al. Dopamine DRD2/Cys311 is not associated with chronic schizophrenia. Am J Med Genet. 1996;67(5):483–4.

52. Dubertret C, Gouya L, Hanoun N, Deybach JC, Ades J, Hamon M, Gorwood P. The 3′ region of the DRD2 gene is involved in genetic susceptibility to schizophrenia. Schizophr Res. 2004;67(1):75–85.

53. Gejman PV, Ram A, Gelernter J, Friedman E, Cao Q, Pickar D, Blum K, Noble EP, Kranzler HR, O'Malley S, et al. No structural mutation in the dopamine D2 receptor gene in alcoholism or schizophrenia. Analysis using denaturing gradient gel electrophoresis. JAMA. 1994;271(3):204–8.

54. Gonzalez-Castro TB, Tovilla-Zarate CA, Hernandez-Diaz Y, Fresan A, Juarez-Rojop IE, Ble-Castillo JL, Lopez-Narvaez L, Genis A, Hernandez-Alvarado MM. No association between ApoE and schizophrenia: evidence of systematic review and updated meta-analysis. Schizophr Res. 2015;169(1–3):355–68.

55. Laurent C, Bodeau-Pean S, Campion D, d'Amato T, Jay M, Dollfus S, Thibault F, Petit M, Samolyk D, Martinez M, et al. No major role for the dopamine D2 receptor Ser→Cys311 mutation in schizophrenia. Psychiatr Genet. 1994;4(4):229–30.

56. Nothen MM, Wildenauer D, Cichon S, Albus M, Maier W, Minges J, Lichtermann D, Bondy B, Rietschel M, Korner J, et al. Dopamine D2 receptor molecular variant and schizophrenia. Lancet. 1994;343(8908):1301–2.

57. Sanders AR, Duan J, Levinson DF, Shi J, He D, Hou C, Burrell GJ, Rice JP, Nertney DA, Olincy A, et al. No significant association of 14 candidate genes with schizophrenia in a large European ancestry sample: implications for psychiatric genetics. Am J Psychiatry. 2008;165(4):497–506.

58. Sasaki T, Macciardi FM, Badri F, Verga M, Meltzer HY, Lieberman J, Howard A, Bean G, Joffe RT, Hudson CJ, et al. No evidence for association of dopamine D2 receptor variant (Ser311/Cys311) with major psychosis. Am J Med Genet. 1996;67(4):415–7.

59. Shaikh S, Collier D, Arranz M, Ball D, Gill M, Kerwin R. DRD2 Ser311/Cys311 polymorphism in schizophrenia. Lancet. 1994;343(8904):1045–6.

60. Sobell J, Sigurdson DC, Heston L, Sommer S. S311C D2DR variant: no association with schizophrenia. Lancet. 1994;344(8922):621–2.

61. Srivastava V, Deshpande SN, Thelma BK. Dopaminergic pathway gene polymorphisms and genetic susceptibility to schizophrenia among north Indians. Neuropsychobiology. 2010;61(2):64–70.

62. Verga M, Macciardi F, Pedrini S, Cohen S, Smeraldi E. No association of the Ser/Cys311 DRD2 molecular variant with schizophrenia using a classical case control study and the haplotype relative risk. Schizophr Res. 1997;25(2):117–21.

63. Comings DE, Comings BG, Muhleman D, Dietz G, Shahbahrami B, Tast D, Knell E, Kocsis P, Baumgarten R, Kovacs BW, et al. The dopamine D2 receptor locus as a modifying gene in neuropsychiatric disorders. JAMA. 1991;266(13):1793–800.

64. Stober G, Jatzke S, Heils A, Jungkunz G, Knapp M, Mossner R, Riederer P, Lesch KP. Insertion/deletion variant (−141C Ins/Del) in the 5′ regulatory region of the dopamine D2 receptor gene: lack of association with schizophrenia and bipolar affective disorder. Short communication. J Neural Transm. 1998;105(1):101–9.

65. Sanders AR, Rincon-Limas DE, Chakraborty R, Grandchamp B, Hamilton JD, Fann WE, Patel PI. Association between genetic variation at the porphobilinogen deaminase gene and schizophrenia. Schizophr Res. 1993;8(3):211–21.

66. Jonsson EG, Nothen MM, Neidt H, Forslund K, Rylander G, Mattila-Evenden M, Asberg M, Propping P, Sedvall GC. Association between a promoter polymorphism in the dopamine D2 receptor gene and schizophrenia. Schizophr Res. 1999;40(1):31–6.

67. Luu SU, Liao HM, Hung TW, Liu BY, Cheng MC, Liao DL, Chen SJ, Chen CH. Mutation analysis of adenosine A2a receptor gene and interaction study with dopamine D2 receptor gene in schizophrenia. Psychiatr Genet. 2008;18(1):43. doi:10.1097/YPG.0b013e3281b1173c.

68. Cordeiro Q, Siqueira-Roberto J, Zung S, Vallada H. Association between the DRD2 −141C insertion/deletion polymorphism and schizophrenia. Arq Neuropsiquiatr. 2009;67(2A):191–4.

69. Xiao L, Shen T, Peng DH, Shu C, Jiang KD, Wang GH. Functional −141C Ins/Del polymorphism in the dopamine D2 receptor gene promoter and schizophrenia in a Chinese Han population. J Int Med Res. 2013;41(4):1171–8.

70. Gejman PV, Sanders AR, Duan J. The role of genetics in the etiology of schizophrenia. Psychiatr Clin N Am. 2010;33(1):35–66.

71. Schwab SG, Wildenauer DB. Genetics of psychiatric disorders in the GWAS era: an update on schizophrenia. Eur Arch Psychiatry Clin Neurosci. 2013;263(2):013–0450.

72. Gonzalez-Castro TB, Tovilla-Zarate CA. Meta-analysis: a tool for clinical and experimental research in psychiatry. Nord J Psychiatry. 2014;68(4):243–50.

73. Li W, Guo X, Xiao S. Evaluating the relationship between reelin gene variants (rs7341475 and rs262355) and schizophrenia: a meta-analysis. Neurosci Lett. 2015;609:42–7.

74. Comings DE, Muhleman D, Ahn C, Gysin R, Flanagan SD. The dopamine D2 receptor gene: a genetic risk factor in substance abuse. Drug Alcohol Depend. 1994;34(3):175–80.

75. Blum K, Braverman ER, Wood RC, Gill J, Li C, Chen TJ, Taub M, Montgomery AR, Sheridan PJ, Cull JG. Increased prevalence of the Taq I A1 allele of the dopamine receptor gene (DRD2) in obesity with comorbid substance use disorder: a preliminary report. Pharmacogenetics. 1996;6(4):297–305.

76. Suzuki A, Mihara K, Kondo T, Tanaka O, Nagashima U, Otani K, Kaneko S. The relationship between dopamine D2 receptor polymorphism at the Taq1 A locus and therapeutic response to nemonapride, a selective dopamine antagonist, in schizophrenic patients. Pharmacogenetics. 2000;10(4):335–41.

77. Mihara K, Suzuki A, Kondo T, Nagashima U, Ono S, Otani K, Kaneko S. No relationship between Taq1 a polymorphism of dopamine D(2) receptor gene and extrapyramidal adverse effects of selective dopamine D(2) antagonists, bromperidol, and nemonapride in schizophrenia: a preliminary study. Am J Med Genet. 2000;96(3):422–4.

78. Noble EP. The D2 dopamine receptor gene: a review of association studies in alcoholism and phenotypes. Alcohol. 1998;16(1):33–45.

79. Campion D, d'Amato T, Bastard C, Laurent C, Guedj F, Jay M, Dollfus S, Thibaut F, Petit M, Gorwood P, et al. Genetic study of dopamine D1, D2, and D4 receptors in schizophrenia. Psychiatry Res. 1994;51(3):215–30.

80. Dollfus S, Campion D, Vasse T, Preterre P, Laurent C, d'Amato T, Thibaut F, Mallet J, Petit M. Association study between dopamine D1, D2, D3, and D4 receptor genes and schizophrenia defined by several diagnostic systems. Biol Psychiatry. 1996;40(5):419–21.

81. Parsons MJ, Mata I, Beperet M, Iribarren-Iriso F, Arroyo B, Sainz R, Arranz MJ, Kerwin R. A dopamine D2 receptor gene-related polymorphism is associated with schizophrenia in a Spanish population isolate. Psychiatr Genet. 2007;17(3):159–63.

82. Li T, Arranz M, Aitchison KJ, Bryant C, Liu X, Kerwin RW, Murray R, Sham P, Collier DA. Case–control, haplotype relative risk and transmission disequilibrium analysis of a dopamine D2 receptor functional promoter polymorphism in schizophrenia. Schizophr Res. 1998;32(2):87–92.

83. Breen G, Brown J, Maude S, Fox H, Collier D, Li T, Arranz M, Shaw D, StClair D. –141 C del/ins polymorphism of the dopamine receptor 2 gene is associated with schizophrenia in a British population. Am J Med Genet. 1999;88(4):407–10.

84. Inada T, Arinami T, Yagi G. Association between a polymorphism in the promoter region of the dopamine D2 receptor gene and schizophrenia in Japanese subjects: replication and evaluation for antipsychotic-related features. Int J Neuropsychopharmacol. 1999;2(3):181–6.

85. Tallerico T, Ulpian C, Liu IS. Dopamine D2 receptor promoter polymorphism: no association with schizophrenia. Psychiatry Res. 1999;85(2):215–9.

86. Kampman O, Anttila S, Illi A, Lehtimaki T, Mattila KM, Roivas M, Leinonen E. Dopamine receptor D2 –141C insertion/deletion polymorphism in a Finnish population with schizophrenia. Psychiatry Res. 2003;121(1):89–92.

87. Kurt H, Dikmen M, Basaran A, Yenilmez C, Ozdemir F, Degirmenci I, Gunes HV, Kucuk MU, Mutlu F. Dopamine D2 receptor gene –141C insertion/deletion polymorphism in Turkish schizophrenic patients. Mol Biol Rep. 2011;38(2):1407–11.

88. Saiz PA, Garcia-Portilla MP, Arango C, Morales B, Arias B, Corcoran P, Fernandez JM, Alvarez V, Coto E, Bascaran MT, et al. Genetic polymorphisms in the dopamine-2 receptor (DRD2), dopamine-3 receptor (DRD3), and dopamine transporter (SLC6A3) genes in schizophrenia: data from an association study. Prog Neuropsychopharmacol Biol Psychiatry. 2010;34(1):26–31.

6

Non-targeted metabolite profiling reveals changes in oxidative stress, tryptophan and lipid metabolisms in fearful dogs

Jenni Puurunen[1], Katriina Tiira[2,3], Marko Lehtonen[4,5], Kati Hanhineva[1,5] and Hannes Lohi[2,3]*

Abstract

Background: Anxieties, such as shyness, noise phobia and separation anxiety, are common but poorly understood behavioural problems in domestic dogs, *Canis familiaris*. Although studies have demonstrated genetic and environmental contributions to anxiety pathogenesis, better understanding of the molecular underpinnings is needed to improve diagnostics, management and treatment plans. As a part of our ongoing canine anxiety genetics efforts, this study aimed to pilot a metabolomics approach in fearful and non-fearful dogs to identify candidate biomarkers for more objective phenotyping purposes and to refer to potential underlying biological problem.

Methods: We collected whole blood samples from 10 fearful and 10 non-fearful Great Danes and performed a liquid chromatography combined with mass spectrometry (LC–MS)-based non-targeted metabolite profiling.

Results: Non-targeted metabolomics analysis detected six 932 metabolite entities in four analytical modes [RP and HILIC; ESI(−) and ESI(+)], of which 239 differed statistically between the test groups. We identified changes in 13 metabolites (fold change ranging from 1.28 to 2.85) between fearful and non-fearful dogs, including hypoxanthine, indoxylsulfate and several phospholipids. These molecules are involved in oxidative stress, tryptophan and lipid metabolisms.

Conclusions: We identified significant alterations in the metabolism of fearful dogs, and some of these changes appear relevant to anxiety also in other species. This pilot study demonstrates the feasibility of the non-targeted metabolomics and warrants a larger replication study to confirm the role of the identified biomarkers and pathways in canine anxiety.

Keywords: Dog, Anxiety, Fear, Non-targeted metabolite profiling, Metabolomics

Background

Anxiety-related disorders, including compulsions, fearfulness, noise phobia, generalized anxiety and separation anxiety, are common but complex and poorly understood behavioural problems in domestic dogs (*Canis familiaris*) [1–3]. Clinical, ethological and pharmacological studies suggest that the underlying biochemical mechanisms are shared in dogs and humans. This is demonstrated, for example, by a successful treatment of the dogs with human anxiolytes [4]. Given the biological similarity of canine and human anxiety, dogs with a particular genomic system could serve as a feasible gene discovery model for human anxiety and improve the molecular understanding of the disease in general. Breed-specificity of many anxieties, such as canine compulsive disorder, suggests genetic susceptibility [4–6]. However, environmental factors, such as negative experiences and poor socialization during puppyhood, affect also behavior [7–9] and complicate gene discoveries, which are still rare [10–14].

One of the challenges in anxiety research concerns objective behavioural measurement to establish valid research cohorts for gene discovery. Current approaches

*Correspondence: hannes.lohi@helsinki.fi
[2] Department of Veterinary Biosciences and Research Programs Unit, Molecular Neurology, University of Helsinki, Biomedicum Helsinki, P.O. Box 63, 00014 Helsinki, Finland
Full list of author information is available at the end of the article

rely on behavioural questionnaires and tests, which appear to correlate well [2] but have intrinsic limitations related to subjectivity and temporality, respectively. There is a need for more objective measures such as physiological biomarkers, which could help not only phenotyping but could also refer to the underlying affected molecular pathways. High-throughput –omics technologies such as metabolomics could facilitate discovery of biomarkers for research, diagnostics and treatment options. Non-targeted metabolite profiling offering a hypothesis-free approach can detect molecular biosignatures and has been successfully applied to identify genetic and environmental contributions to diseases [15–17]. For example, metabolic profiling of schizophrenia has revealed changes in glutamine and arginine metabolism, which may reflect genetic susceptibility to this neuropsychiatric disorder [18].

In this pilot study, we aimed to compare metabolite profiles of fearful and non-fearful dogs to identify fear-related pathways and biomarkers for more objective phenotyping. We have previously developed a validated approach for anxiety phenotyping in dogs [2] to select 10 fearful and 10 non-fearful Great Danes. We analysed whole blood samples using a non-targeted LC-qTOF-MS metabolomics method to compare the metabolic profiles. Our results reveal changes in several anxiety-relevant components in fearful dogs and warrant a larger metabolomics study in canine anxiety to replicate the findings in this pilot study.

Methods

Animals and study design

The dogs were selected from our previously established anxiety research cohort [2], which included a validated owner-filled anxiety questionnaire and a behavioural test for part of the dogs (4 out of 10 controls and 3 out of 10 cases). The questionnaire survey included both general questions concerning dog's behavior in various situations (such as meeting unfamiliar people, dogs, and behavior in new situations, and when exposed to loud sounds) and daily routines, and also several more specific background questions concerning the early experiences of the dog, related to e.g. puppy period and socialization [2]. Based on the data from the questionnaire, several behavioral variables were derived and used to select dogs to the study groups. The variables that we were interested the most were fear towards unfamiliar people (human fear_frequency, human fear_intensity), fearfulness total and noise sensitivity. Human fear_frequency was simply the owner reported frequency of dog showing fearful reaction when meeting a stranger (frequency scoring $0 =$ never; $1 = 0$–40 % of the occasions; $2 = 40$–60 % of the occasions; $3 = 60$–100 % of the occasions: $4 =$ always

when meeting unfamiliar people). Human fear_intensity was calculated as follows: the frequency of showing fearful reaction when meeting unfamiliar people was multiplied with the sum of owner recorded fearful behavioral reactions. Each type of behavior equaled 1, except the avoidance-reaction which was weighted by multiplying it with 5. Fearfulness variable was calculated as a sum of frequencies of showing fearful behavioural reactions towards unfamiliar people (see scoring above 0–4), unfamiliar dogs (0–4) and in new situations (0–4), and thus the score varied between 0 and 12. In addition, we calculated a variable describing the dog's fear of loud noises (noise sensitivity), by calculating a sum of frequencies of showing a fearful reaction towards thunder (see scoring above 0–4), fireworks (0–4) and gunshot (0–4). The behaviour of seven of the dogs was verified by a short 5-min test conducted by same person for all the dogs—not all dogs were tested as some had already died between the blood sampling and behavioral testing, or lived too far. Shortly, test consisted of three parts; meeting an unfamiliar person, exploration in the novel space, and novel object test. More details of the test can be found from Tiira and Lohi, 2014.

We selected 10 fearful and 10 non-fearful Great Danes for the study, and detailed information about all the individual dogs is presented in Table 1. Our criteria for non-fearful dogs was that all the variables (human fear_frequency, human fear_intensity, fearfulness total and noise sensitivity) had to have score 0. In the case group, our main inclusion criterion was that the dog had to show fear towards unfamiliar people at 40–100 % of all situations (human fear_frequency score 2–4). In addition, dog's needed to have fearfulness score >2. Additionally to these criteria, we used matched pairs with approximately same age for blood samples between case and control groups. We aimed, at first, to get only males, however, in order to keep the age of blood sampling approximately same in both control and case groups we also had to include two females for both groups. EDTA-blood samples were collected from each dog and stored in −20 degrees. The blood samples were collected from the privately owned Finnish dogs with owners consent under a valid ethical license (Finnish National Animal Experiment Board, ELLA, license number ESAVI/6054/04.10.03/2012).

Dietary information

The owners were retrospectively asked to report the diet of the dog at the time of blood sampling to help us consider possible nutritional effects on metabolite profiles. Dietary information was collected from 17 out of 20 dogs (two cases and one control missing). Comparison of the diet profiles indicated only minor differences between

Table 1 Demographics of the dogs

	Age (years)	Mean age (SD)	Sex	Fearfulness (total)	Human fear_frequency	Human fear_ intensity	Noise sensitivity	Behavioral test	Diet
1	1.1	3.5 (2.5)	Male	4	3	10	3	No	Not known
2	1.5		Male	10	2	16	2	No	Dry food, raw meat, oils
3	2.4		Male	3	4	21	3	No	Dry food
4	2.8		Male	7	4	28	0	No	Raw food, oils
5	4.2		Male	10	3	30	0	Yes	Not known
6	5.4		Male	6	2	14	5	No	Dry food
7	4.4		Male	8	2	14	4	Yes	Not known
8	9.3		Male	6	3	6	8	No	Dry food
9	1.8		Female	8	4	28	0	No	Dry food, meat, fish
10	1.6		Female	10	4	30	0	Yes	Raw food, oils
11	3.2	3.4 (2.2)	Male	0	0	0	0	No	Raw food, oils
12	4.5		Male	0	0	0	0	No	Dry food
13	3.3		Male	0	0	0	0	Yes	Dry food, oils
14	1.1		Male	0	0	0	0	No	Not known
15	8.5		Male	0	0	0	0	Yes	Dry food
16	4.8		Male	0	0	0	0	Yes	Dry food, meat
17	3.3		Male	0	0	0	0	No	Dry food, oils
18	1.6		Male	0	0	0	0	No	Dry food, oils, vitamin C
19	2		Female	0	0	0	0	Yes	Homemade food, meat, dry food, oils
20	2.1		Female	0	0	0	0	No	Not known

Detailed information, including age, sex, behavioral scores and diet, is provided for each individual dog. Dogs numbered from 1 to 10 are fearful dogs, whereas dogs numbered from 11 to 20 are non-fearful dogs

the test groups. The diets contained equally a mix of raw food, commercial dry foods, homemade food and different dietary supplements in both test groups. However, the dietary profiles varied greatly within the test groups but similar variations were observed in both groups. The basic contents of all commercial dry foods fed to the dogs were rice, chicken meal, pork meal, maize, fish oil, animal fat, vegetable fibre, and beet pulp in addition to minerals, such as calcium (Ca) and phophorus (P), micronutrients, such as iron (Fe), copper (Cu), zinc (Zn) and iodine (I), and vitamins, such as vitamins A, D_3 and E. Interestingly, there were minor differences in the intake of pulses between case and control dogs, since the commercial dry foods eaten by a few control dogs but not cases contained soybean oil, soybean meal and pea bran meal.

Non targeted LC MS metabolite profiling analysis

The non-targeted LC-qTOF-MS-analysis and preprocessing of raw data were performed in the LC–MS Metabolomics Center at Biocenter Kuopio (University of Eastern Finland). For metabolite extraction, 400 µL of acetonitrile was added to 100 µL of whole blood sample,

and mixed in vortex at maximum speed 15 s. The samples were incubated on ice bath for 15 min, and centrifuged at $16000 \times g$ for 10 min in order to collect the supernatant. The supernatants were filtered into HPLC vials using 0.2 µm Acrodisc® Syringe Filters with a PTFE membrane (PALL Corporation, Ann Arbor, MI) prior subjecting to the LC–MS analyses. From every extracted sample, aliquots of 10 µL was taken and combined in one tube, and used as the quality control (QC) sample in the analysis.

The whole blood samples were analysed by the UHPLC-qTOF-MS system (Agilent Technologies, Waldbronn, Karlsruhe, Germany) that consisted of a 1290 LC system, a Jetstream electrospray ionization (ESI) source, and a 6540 UHD accurate-mass qTOF spectrometer. The samples were analyzed using two different chromatographic techniques, i.e. reversed phase (RP) and hydrophilic interaction chromatography (HILIC) to maximize metabolome coverage. The RP chromatography was performed on Zorbax Eclipse XDB-C18 column (100 × 2.1 mm, 1.8 µm, Agilent Technologies, Palo Alto, CA, USA). The temperature of the column was kept on 50 °C, and the flow rates of mobile phases were set as

0.4 mL/min. The mobile phases consisted of water (eluent A) and methanol (eluent B), both containing 0.01 % (v/v) of formic acid. The gradient profile employed was as follows: 2 → 100 % B (0–10 min); 100 % B (10–14.5 min); 100 → 2 % B (14.5–14.51 min); 2 % B (14.51–16.50 min). The injection volume in RP was 2 µl. The HILIC chromatography was performed on Acquity UPLC BEH Amide column (100 × 2.1 mm, 1.7 µm; Waters Corporation, Milford, MA), and the temperature of the column was kept on 45 °C. The flow rate was 0.6 mL/min, and eluents A and B consisted of 50 % v/v and 90 % v/v ACN, respectively, both containing 20 mM ammonium formate. The gradient was as follows: 100 % B (0–2.5 min); 100 → 0 % B (2.5–10 min); 0 → 100 % B (10–10.01 min); 100 % B (10.01–12.5 min). The injection volume in HILIC was 2 µl.

The MS ion source conditions were as follows: ESI source, operated both in positive (+ve) and negative (−ve) ionization mode, drying gas temperature 325 °C with a flow of 10 L/min, sheath gas temperature 350 °C and flow 11 L/min, nebulizer pressure 45 psi, capillary voltage 3500 V, nozzle voltage 1000 V, fragmentor voltage 100 V, and skimmer 45 V. For data acquisition, the mass range was 20–1600 amu with acquisition rate 1.67 spectra/s. In order to get the automatic MS/MS spectrums, four ions with the highest intensities were selected from every precursor scan cycle for fragmentation performed on the QC samples. After two product ion spectra, these ions were excluded, and released again for fragmentation after a 0.25-min hold. The collision energies were 10, 20 and 40 V. If the molecular ion of a compound was not included into automatic MS/MS fragmentation, targeted MS/MS analyses with collision energies 10 and 20 V were conducted. A continuous mass axis calibration was performed by monitoring two reference ions from an infusion solution throughout the runs. In positive mode the reference ions were m/z 121.050873 and m/z 922.009798, and in negative mode m/z 112.985587 and m/z 966.000725. Data acquisition was conducted with MassHunter Acquisition B.04.00 (Agilent Technologies). The QC samples were injected in the beginning and ending of the analysis and also after every 10 samples.

Non-targeted metabolomics data analysis
Data collection and statistical analysis
The LC–MS data was collected using the vendor's software MassHunter Qualitative Analysis B.05.00 (Agilent Technologies), where the ions were extracted to compounds utilizing the "Find by molecular feature" algorithm. The data were output as compound exchange format (.cef-files) into the Mass Profiler Professional software (MPP 2.2, Agilent Technologies) for compound

alignment, data preprocessing, and statistical analysis (Student's t test between the case and control groups). In order to reduce noise and remove insignificant metabolite features, only the features found in at least 60 % of the samples in at least one replicate group (case or control) were included in the analysis. This resulted in a dataset comprising 6 932 features in four separate analytical runs [986 in HILIC ESI(+), 1 071 in HILIC ESI(−), 3 790 in RP ESI(+), and 1 085 in RP ESI(−)].

The pre-processed data from each of the four analytical approaches were subjected to supervised classification algorithm partial least-squares discriminant analysis (PLS-DA; Simca-13, Umetrics, Sweden). The data were log10-transformed, pareto-scaled and the model was validated by the Simca-13 internal cross validation, and the resulting variable importance projection (VIP) values for each metabolite [19, 20], were integrated in the data. The PLS-DA illustrates the differences between case and control groups by investigating those metabolites that are the largest discriminators in the data, and the larger the VIP value is, the more significant contributor the metabolite is in the model.

The data was filtered according to VIP >1 in order to reduce insignificant features from the data, resulting in a dataset comprising 2 114 features in the four analytical runs [308 in HILIC ESI(+), 301 in HILIC ESI(−), 1 162 in RP ESI(+), and 343 in RP ESI(−)]. After adjusting for multiple comparisons by Benjamini-Hochberg false discovery rate (FDR) correction [21] (R project for Statistical Computing version 3.0.1.) within each of the four analytical approaches, the peak lists were filtered according to uncorrected p value <0.05, fold change (FC) ≥±1.2, PLS-DA VIP >1, and feature present in at least seven replicates in either of the groups. This resulted in dataset of 239 entities [45 in HILIC ESI(+), 41 in HILIC ESI(−), 127 in RP ESI(+), and 26 in RP ESI(−)], where the compounds having FDR corrected p value <0.05 were considered as statistically significant differences between control and case groups, whereas those with uncorrected p value <0.05 were regarded nominally significant. In addition, the filtered data were subjected to the K-means cluster algorithm with the Pearson correlation as distance metric followed by the hierarchical cluster analysis and heat-map output for data visualization [22].

Finally, the remaining peaks in the lists were manually inspected in the LC–MS chromatograms and spectra with the MassHunter software to locate peaks with poor retention and peak shape, which were filtered out from further analysis. Peak lists were also looked through to ensure that the molecular ion of a compound was included into data dependent MS/MS analysis, and in case not, targeted MS/MS analysis was performed.

Identification of the differential features in the LC–MS data

The identification of metabolites was based on the accurate mass and MS/MS fragmentation spectra acquired either in the automatic, data dependent MS/MS analysis during the initial data acquisition, or via re-injection of the samples in targeted MS/MS mode. The spectra were compared against The METLIN Metabolite Database (https://metlin.scripps.edu/index.php), Human Metabolome Database (HMDB) (http://www.hmdb.ca/), and LipidMaps (http://www.lipidmaps.org/), or fragmentation patterns reported in earlier publications. The identification of lipids was based on their characteristic fragmentation patterns reported in earlier publications [23–25]. The key elements for identification were the protonated head group (m/z 184.07 for PCs and LysoPCs, and m/z 196.03 for PEs) as well as the deprotonated fatty acid fragments visible in the negative ionization mode (the MS/MS fragmentation data for all of the identified metabolites is presented in Table 1). The identification of plasmalogen was based on the m/z 303 corresponding to arachidonic acid (C20:4), and on the characteristic fragmentation pattern of phosphoethanolamine plasmalogens (PEP) described previously [26].

Results

A non-targeted LC–MS-based metabolomics platform was used to compare the whole blood metabolite profiles of fearful and non-fearful dogs. The two test groups had similar overall dietary profiles with a note that many control dogs were reported to consume more protein-rich food such as soybeans than cases. We detected a total of 6 932 molecular features in the four separate LC–MS runs, of which 239 were differential between the two groups (Student's t-test, p value < 0.05; FC $\geq\pm1.2$; PLS-DA VIP >1). This set of compounds (239) was subjected to manual inspection to identify metabolites and to remove redundant ions as well as poorly retained and integrated peaks. This analysis resulted in a set of 13 known metabolites and 5 unknown features (Table 2).

Several phospholipids were differential between fearful and non-fearful dogs

Majority of the significantly changed metabolites in canine whole blood were identified as phospholipids, including phosphatidylcholines (PC), lysophosphatidylcholines (LysoPC), phosphatidylethanolamine plasmalogen (PEP) and lysophosphatidylethanolamine (LysoPE). Majority of them were decreased in the group of fearful dogs, especially PC(16:0/23:5) (−2.1-fold; Pcorr = 0.0226), PC(18:0/20:4) (−2.0-fold; P = 0.02) and PC(18:0/19:1) (−2.0-fold; P = 0.0376) showed remarkable differences between the two test groups. Additionally, an unknown lipid with m/z 578.312 (−2.8-fold;

P = 0.0103), which exhibited similar fragmentation pattern to LysoPCs, was detected. Furthermore, a metabolite with m/z 748.531 was regarded as a nominally increased in fearful dogs (1.8-fold; P = 0.0447). The fragmentation suggested this compound to be PE(P-18:1/20:4), a phosphatidylethanolamine plasmalogen belonging to subclass of ether-linked lipids that are characterized by an ether linkage at the sn-1 position and an ester-linkage at the sn-2 position on the glycerol backbone of the lipid [26, 27].

Oxidative stress and tryptophan pathways affected in fearful dogs

We found also several metabolites related to oxidative stress and tryptophan pathways that were changed between fearful and non-fearful dogs. Two compounds, m/z values of 137.046 (1.9-fold; P = 0.025) and 212.002 (1.8-fold; P = 0.048), showed identical fragmentations with hypoxanthine (MID 83) and indoxylsulfate (MID 253) in METLIN, respectively. Both of these metabolites are known to promote oxidative stress [28–32], and indoxylsulfate is an indole-derived metabolite of tryptophan [32]. Metabolite with m/z 247.144 (2.2-fold; P = 0.0485) was identified as hypaphorine, a methylated form of tryptophan, based on its similar fragmentation pattern with the previously published spectra [33, 34]. We found also lower levels of tryptophan among fearful dogs (−1.6-fold, Pcorr = 0.0087), although the significance of this finding is questionable since tryptophan was detected in altered levels only in RP analysis and not in HILIC analysis. The latter would be more reliable method to detect amino acids.

Other metabolic changes in fearful dogs

Another particularly clear change in the metabolite profiles of the two test groups was the accumulation of pyrocatechol sulfate, a phenolic metabolite with m/z 188.986 (2.4-fold; P = 0.015). It was identified based on fragmentation match with pyrocatechol standard compound, and additional fragment ion at m/z 79.957 corresponding to sulfate group $[SO_3]^-$ in the molecular structure of the compound. Additionally, a compound with m/z 284.294 and rt 10.59 in the RP ESI(+) analysis was observed to accumulate in case group (1.3-fold; P = 0.0266) and identified as stearamide (MID 34494), a fatty amide found in food packaging materials according to Human Metabolome Database (HMDB).

The most remarkable accumulation in case group was observed for a compound with m/z 312.326 and rt 11.01 in the RP ESI(+) analysis (2.8-fold; P = 0.024). However, this compound remained unidentified due to its unknown fragmentation pattern, although the retention time highly suggests fatty acid structure. The identity of

Table 2 Characteristics for the putatively identified marker metabolites in liquid chromatography-mass spectrometry analysis

	Column	Ionization mode	MW	m/z	RT (min)	Putative annotation	p-value[a]	FDR corrected p-value[b]	Fold change (FC)[c]	CID (eV)	MS/MS fragmentation	Identification reference[d]	VIP
Cluster 1	RP	ESI+	821.577	822.584	10.67	PC(16:0/23:5)	0.0017	0.0226	−2.06	20	822.584, 184.074; ESI(−) 40 eV: 806.556, 343.249, 255.233	MS/MS	2.24
	RP	ESI+	801.587	802.595	11.35	PC(18:0/19:1)	0.0376	0.1316	−1.98	20	184.072, 784.5833, 802.594; ESI(−) 40 eV: 295.229, 283.261, 786.565	MS/MS	1.30
	RP	ESI+	204.09	205.097	2.30	Tryptophan	4.22E−04	0.0087	−1.58	10	188.0698, 146.0599, 144.0806, 130.0613, 132.0788, 159.0881, 205.0947	Standard	0.84
	RP	ESI+	537.295	538.309	10.25	LysoPC(19:0)	0.0488	0.1461	−1.53	20	104.106, 501.236, 560.310 [M + Na]+; ESI(−) 20 eV: 522.323, 297.245	MS/MS	1.68
Cluster 2	RP	ESI−	579.319	578.312	8.79	Unknown LysoPC	0.0103	0.0884	−2.79	20	293.209, 578.310, 518.291; ESI(+) 20 eV: 104.107, 534.319, 184.074	MS/MS	2.08
	HILIC	ESI−	88.016	87.009	1.77	Unknown metabolite	0.0427	0.1108	−2.58	10	44.999, 73.857	MS/MS	1.34
	RP	ESI+	809.592	810.599	12.64	PC(18:0/20:4)	0.0200	0.0965	−2.00	40	184.073, 86.095; ESI(−) 40 eV: 303.234, 283.265, 794.567	MS/MS	1.82
	RP	ESI+	517.316	518.323	8.81	LysoPC(18:3)	0.0472	0.1443	−1.86	40	184.072, 104.104, 86.094, 60.082; ESI(−) 20 eV: 502.2945, 277.2162	MS/MS	1.47
	RP	ESI+	499.270	500.277	9.17	LysoPE(20:5)	0.0416	0.1376	−1.64	10	500.2786, 359.2548; ESI(-) 20 eV: 498.2860, 169.1368, 301.2172	MS/MS	1.28
Cluster 3	RP	ESI+	311.319	312.326	11.01	Unknown metabolite	0.0240	0.1055	2.85	20	312.326, 57.071, 102.095, 100.075, 214.214, 81.068	MS/MS	1.88
	HILIC	ESI−	189.994	188.986	0.69	Pyrocatechol sulfate	0.0150	0.0734	2.36	40	108.024, 79.957, 53.042, 80.965, 109.027	Pyrocatechol standard	1.55

Table 2 continued

Column	Ionization mode	MW	m/z	RT (min)	Putative annotation	p-value[a]	FDR corrected p-value[b]	Fold change (FC)[c]	CID (eV)	MS/MS fragmentation	Identification reference[d]	VIP
	HILIC	ESI+	246.137	247.144	1.42	Hypaphorine	0.0485	0.1719	2.17	10	188.071, 60.081, 146.061, 55.017, 247.206, 144.079, 85.0245, 118.928	Keller et al. [34]	1.29
	RP	ESI−	213.009	212.002	2.43	Indoxylsulfate	0.0480	0.1870	1.78	10	212.007, 80.966, 132.043	MID 253	1.85
	RP	ESI+	370.308	371.315	10.96	Unknown fatty acyl, either di-(2-ethylhexyl) adipate or dioctyl hexanedioate	0.0335	0.1253	1.55	10	129.0557, 111.0459, 147.0635, 101.0612, 57.0694, 241.1772	MS/MS	1.60
	RP	ESI+	315.277	316.285	8.7	Unknown sphingosine, either dehydrophyto-sphingosine, 6-hydroxysphin-gosine, or (4OH,8Z,t18:1) sphingosine	0.0087	0.0619	1.50	40	93.071, 43.055, 57.069, 81.070, 69.069, 67.055, 95.048, 77.040	MID 392	0.68
	RP	ESI+	283.287	284.294	10.59	Stearamide	0.0266	0.1108	1.28	20	284.295, 57.070, 102.091, 88.076, 71.085, 43.054	MID 34494	1.73
Cluster 4	HILIC	ESI+	136.039	137.046	1.43	Hypoxanthine	0.0250	0.1225	1.87	20	137.046, 119.035, 94.040, 110.035, 55.029, 82.038	MID 83	1.60
	RP	ESI−	749.54	748.531	12.51	PE(P-18:1/20:4)	0.0447	0.1866	1.81	20	748.526, 303.234; ESI(+) 20 eV: 361.275, 390.2773, 609.529, 750.551	MS/MS	1.61

Also the most significant non-identified marker metabolites are included. The characteristics include both uncorrected and FDR corrected p values, fold changes, Variable influence on projection (VIP) –values, and identification references together with parameters for the LC-MS analysis, including the chromatography (Column), ionization mode in the mass spectrometry (Ionization mode), molecular weight (MW), identified ion (m/z), retention time (RT), collision induced dissociation energy (CID), and fragment ions in the tandem mass spectrometry (MS/MS fragments). n = 20 dogs (10 fearful and 10 non-fearful dogs). Note that two metabolic features, tryptophan and unknown sphingosine, are included in the table despite their low VIP values, since they otherwise show statistical significance

LysoPC lysophosphatidylcholine, LysoPE lysophosphatidylethanolamine, PC phosphatidylcholine, PE phosphatidylethanolamine

a Student's t-test comparing the fold change against the Control group. P values <0.05 were considered as statistically significant

b Benjamini-Hochberg false discovery rate (FDR) corrected p value

c Average fold change when compared against the Control group, with p values. Fold changes ≥±1.2 were considered as statistically significant. Positive values indicate increased whole blood levels in case dogs vs. control dogs, whereas negative values indicate decreased whole blood levels in case dogs vs. control dogs

d Identification of metabolites is based on manual MS/MS spectral interpretation, METLIN ID when MS/MS spectrum available, commercial standard compound, or some earlier published fragmentation patterns. Keller et al. [34]

three other metabolic markers remain also unclear, since compound with m/z 87.009 (-2.6; P = 0.0427) would match with pyruvate by its mass but its MS/MS fragmentation pattern was not identical with the spectrum in METLIN, whereas the feature with m/z 371.315 (1.6-fold; P = 0.0335) in the RP ESI(+) analysis showed similar fragmentation to two fatty acyls, di-(2-ethylhexyl)adipate and dioctyl hexanedioate, although could not be distinguished from each other. A metabolite with m/z 316.285 and rt 8.7 has MS/MS fragmentation similar to sphingosines, but due to the lack of published spectra, its exact identity remains unclear.

Chemometric analysis of the LC–MS data

The partial least squares discriminant analysis (PLS-DA) analysis yielding variable influence projection (VIP) values for metabolites indicated that the most important discriminator metabolites, i.e. those metabolites with high VIP values, had usually also low p-values and high fold changes, being prominent candidate biomarkers (e.g. PC(16:0/23:5): Pcorr = 0.0226, VIP = 2.24) (Table 2). Moreover, the PLS-DA analysis also clearly visualized the differences between control and case dogs, as exemplified with the data from the RP ESI(+) mode (Fig. 1).

The 239 differential features were also subjected to the K-means cluster algorithm followed by hierarchical cluster analysis giving a heat map as an output (Fig. 2). Four clusters were formed. Cluster 1 contained a set of 70 decreased metabolites among case group, including identified PC(16:0/23:5), PC(18:0/19:1), LysoPC(19:0) and tryptophan. Also cluster 2 included features having lower concentrations in case group but with larger diversity among the samples. The third group clustered 58 compounds increased among fearful dogs, including pyrocatechol sulfate, hypaphorine, indoxylsulfate, stearamide, sphingosine-like molecule, putative fatty acyl, and one unknown feature with sharp and large peak. Cluster 4 indicated hypoxanthine and PE(P-18:1/20:4) together with several unknown metabolites having higher concentrations among fearful dogs. Hierarchical cluster analysis also reveleaD the relatively high degree of heterogeneity between the samples, especially within the control group (Fig. 2).

Discussion

Anxiety-related disorders are common but yet poorly characterized for molecular underpinnings in any species. Research is challenged by clinical and genetic heterogeneity and there is a need for novel biomarkers to pinpoint affected pathways, to improve diagnostics, and to support research. This pilot study with non-targeted metabolomics addressed canine fear to establish methodology and to compare metabolic profiles in fearful and

non-fearful dogs in order to elucidate the molecular phenomena related to anxiety. We identified 13 differential metabolites which indicated decreased phospholipids, elevated levels of the metabolites in oxidative stress pathways, and altered tryptophan metabolism in fearful dogs.

About half of the identified 13 metabolites were phospholipids, including three PCs, two LysoPCs, one LysoPE and one phosphatidylethanolamine plasmalogen. PCs, LysoPCs and LysoPE were all decreased and only plasmalogen elevated in fearful dogs. Phospholipids are major components of cell membranes and important signalling molecules [35]. Together with fatty acids they have been associated with anxiety-related diseases and behavior in humans and mice [17, 35–41]. In schizophrenia patients, for example, lower levels of plasma PEs and PCs have been measured when compared to healthy controls, suggesting an involvement of lipid disorder in schizophrenia [42]. Since the blood lipid composition is strongly affected by nutrition [43], the observed difference in the phospholipid levels could originate from diet. However, our case and control groups had similar diets, and therefore, differences in dietary lipids do not likely explain the differences observed. This suggests endogenous cause, i.e. altered absorption of dietary lipids or disturbed lipid metabolism, for the affected pathways in the fearful dogs.

Plasmalogens are important signalling molecules and free radical scavengers present in the majority of cell membranes [27, 44]. This family of ether-linked phospholipids has been heavily studied due to the potential anti-oxidant properties of plasmalogens [45, 46]. Previous studies of metabolic syndrome [47] and sepsis [48] patients have suggested decreased plasmalogen levels as a marker for oxidative stress. In the present study, fearful dogs had higher levels of PE(P-18:1/20:4) and it could be a secondary response for oxidative stress caused by chronic fear.

Besides plasmalogen, two other oxidative stress-related biomarkers were increased in fearful dogs: hypoxanthine and indoxylsulfate. Hypoxanthine is an oxidative stress stimulator [28, 29] and it effects are mediated by xanthine oxidase (XO), an enzyme which oxidases hypoxanthine to xanthine and further to uric acid. As a by-product of this process a highly deleterious superoxide is generated [30]. Indoxylsulfate promotes also oxidative stress [31, 32]. It is a uremic toxin metabolite of tryptophan that induces endothelial ROS production [32]. Oxidative stress is caused by an accumulation of reactive oxygen species (ROS), when the balance between pro- and anti-oxidant systems of the cell is disturbed [49]. As a result, several cellular components such as DNA, lipids, nucleic acids and proteins are damaged, and the levels of pro-inflammatory cytokines are increased. Oxidative stress has been associated with neuropsychiatric disorders like

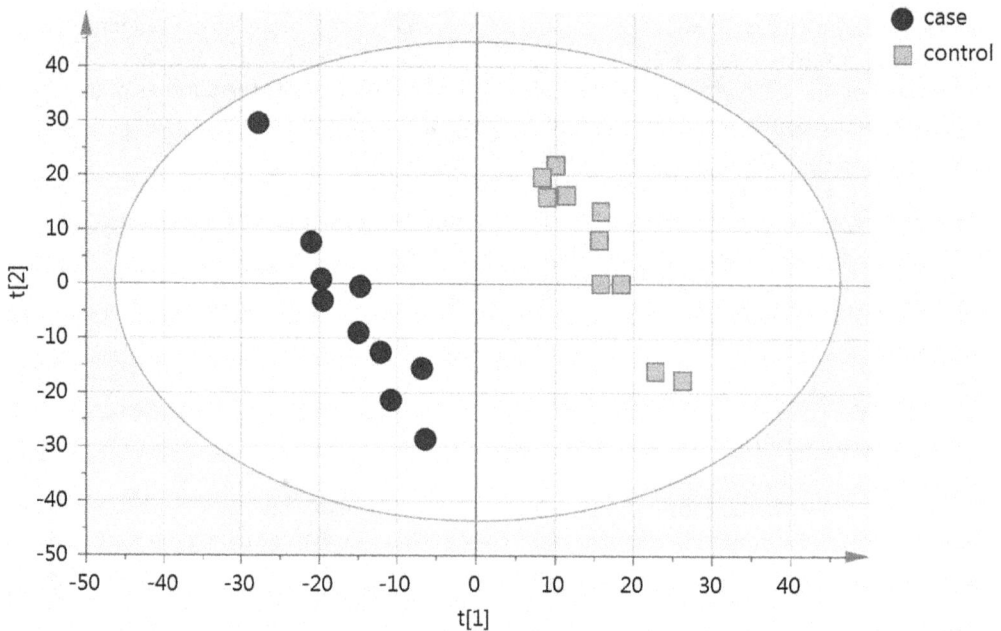

Fig. 1 Partial least squares discriminant analysis (PLS-DA) of the reversed phase positive ESI–MS mode data. The *score plot* shows the individual samples in both case and control groups. Case group (*black circles*); Control group (*grey squares*)

schizophrenia, anxiety, PTSD and social phobia across species [49–55]. There are also evidence that mitochondria-directed antioxidants relieve anxiety in rodents [56]. Further research is required to investigate the cause, whether primary or secondary, and significance of the elevated oxidative stress in the fearful dogs.

The third affected pathway was related to tryptophan metabolism. Fearful dogs had lower levels of tryptophan but increased levels of indoxylsulfate and hypaphorine. The latter two molecules are tryptophan metabolites. Hypaphorine ($C_{14}H_{18}N_2O_2$), an indole alkaloid and a betaine of tryptophan [33, 34] was greatly increased in fearful dogs. Biological functions of this metabolite are not well known and there is no link between hypaphorine and behavior. Since hypaphorine is a biomarker of consumption of pulses like beans and peas, increased hypaphorine could originate from diet. Unexpectedly, we found increase of hypaphorine in fearful dogs although dietary records indicated that control dogs had higher content of pulses in diet. This suggests that it is unlikely that such a significant and systematic difference in cases would result from nutrition solely. Instead, this observed change may refer to endogenic causes related to tryptophan metabolism, since hypaphorine is an N-methylated form of tryptophan. Also the identification of the other tryptophan metabolite indoxylsulfate supports the significance of altered tryptophan metabolism in fearful dogs. However, more research is needed to clarify the

connection between these observed changes in canine anxiety.

This study demonstrates the promise of metabolomics approach in research related to canine anxiety, although we recognize technical and theoretical limitations that could be improved in future studies. First, we used whole blood and not plasma as a starting material. Whole blood challenges experimental conditions, including a sample preparation phase and may result in extra background followed by complications in downstream analyses. The replication study should be performed with fresh plasma samples collected in standardized manner. Second, the extraction conditions in the LC–MS platform were optimized for human samples and more optimal conditions should be investigated for samples of dog origin for higher quality of data. Third, better management of diet profiles of the participating dogs and sampling protocols should be considered in future experiments. The sampling time (morning/evening), the length of the sample storage time in the freezer and dog's physical activity could have had effects on the metabolite profiles and should be controlled in future experiments. Finally, due to our small sample size but high amount of detected metabolic features, most of the observed changes were not significant after correction for multiplicity. Therefore, too far conclusions cannot be drawn from these results, and larger cohorts are needed although require more efforts for preparation given that we research private pets

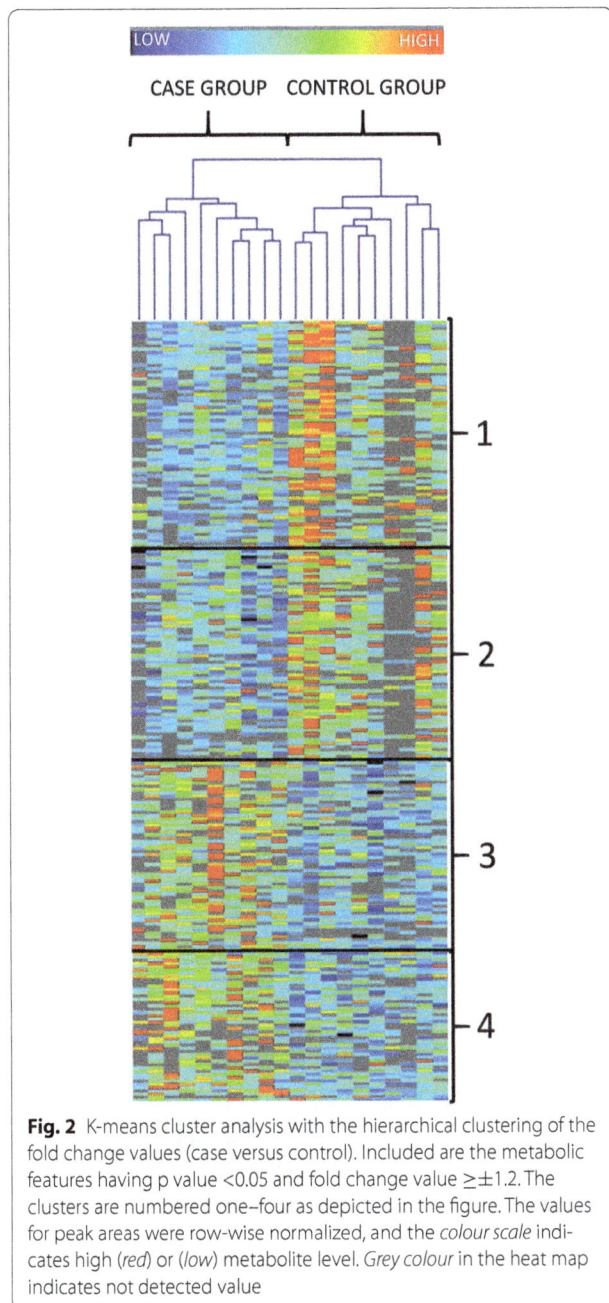

Fig. 2 K-means cluster analysis with the hierarchical clustering of the fold change values (case versus control). Included are the metabolic features having p value <0.05 and fold change value ≥±1.2. The clusters are numbered one–four as depicted in the figure. The values for peak areas were row-wise normalized, and the *colour scale* indicates high (*red*) or (*low*) metabolite level. *Grey colour* in the heat map indicates not detected value

metabolites were differential in the whole blood of fearful dogs, and are involved in oxidative stress, tryptophan and lipid metabolisms. Furthermore, these changes appear relevant to anxiety also in other species. This study demonstrates the power of the non-targeted metabolite profiling approach and encourages for a replication in a larger cohort of dogs with anxiety. Reliable replication of the identified biomarkers and pathways in this study could lead to applications for improved phenotyping and understanding of anxiety across species.

Abbreviations
ESI: electrospray ionization; HILIC: hydrophilic interaction; LC: liquid chromatography; LysoPC: lysophosphatidylcholine; LysoPE: lysophosphatidylethanolamine; MS: mass spectrometry; PC: phosphatidylcholine; PLS-DA: partial least squares discriminant analysis; RP: reversed phase; VIP: variable influence on projection.

Authors' contributions
HL developed the idea, HL and KT designed the experiment, ML and KH performed the experiment, JP analysed the data. HL, ML, KT and KH contributed to reagents/materials/analysis tools. JP and HL wrote the manuscript with KT and KH contributions. All authors read and approved the final manuscript.

Author details
¹ Institute of Public Health and Clinical Nutrition, University of Eastern Finland, Kuopio, Finland. ² Department of Veterinary Biosciences and Research Programs Unit, Molecular Neurology, University of Helsinki, Biomedicum Helsinki, P.O. Box 63, 00014 Helsinki, Finland. ³ The Folkhälsan Research Center, Helsinki, Finland. ⁴ School of Pharmacy, University of Eastern Finland, Kuopio, Finland. ⁵ LC–MS Metabolomics Center, Biocenter Kuopio, Kuopio, Finland.

Acknowledgements
Petra Jaakonsaari, Sini Karjalainen and Ranja Eklund from Lohi laboratory are thanked for technical assistance. Miia Reponen is thanked for maintaining the LC–MS-qTOF instrument, and Maria Lankinen for guidance in statistical analyses. We thank the Great Dane breed club and owners for participation and donating samples for research. This study was funded partly by the ERCStG (260997), the Academy of Finland, the Orion-Farmos Foundation, the Sigrid Juselius Foundation, the Jane and Aatos Erkko Foundation, Biocenter Finland, ERA-Net NEURON II and the Dog Health Research Fund, University of Helsinki. The funding sources had no further role in study design; in the collection, analysis and interpretation of data; in the writing of the report; and in the decision to submit the paper for publication.

Competing interests
The authors declare that they have no competing interests.

not colony dogs. However, despite the heterogeneous background and conditions of this pilot study, we were clearly able to identify several anxiety relevant metabolites in fearful Great Danes and thereafter warrant the future applications of metabolomics investigations.

Conclusions
In summary, the pilot non-targeted metabolite profiling of canine anxieties indicates significant differences between fearful and non-fearful dogs. 13 identified

References
1. Overall KL, Dunham AE, Frank D. Frequency of nonspecific clinical signs in dogs with separation anxiety, thunderstorm phobia, and noise phobia, alone or in combination. J Am Vet Med Assoc. 2001;219(4):467–73.
2. Tiira K, Lohi H. Reliability and validity of a questionnaire survey in canine anxiety research. Appl Anim Behav Sci. 2014;155:82–92.
3. Pineda S, Anzola B, Olivares A, Ibanez M. Fluoxetine combined with clorazepate dipotassium and behaviour modification for treatment of anxiety-related disorders in dogs. Vet J. 2014;199(3):387–91.
4. Overall KL. Natural animal models of human psychiatric conditions: assesment of mechanism and validity. Prog Neuro-Psychopharmacol Biol Psychiat. 2000;24:727–76.

5. Tiira K, Hakosalo O, Kareinen L, Thomas A, Hielm-Bjorkman A, Escriou C, et al. Environmental effects on compulsive tail chasing in dogs. PLoS One. 2012;7(7):e41684. doi:10.1371/journal.pone.0041684(7).

6. Hedhammar Å, Hultin-Jäderlund K. Behaviour and disease in dogs. In: Jensen. P. editors. Behavioral biology of dogs. Oxfordshire: CAB International; 2007. p. 243–262.

7. van der Waaij EH, Wilsson E, Strandberg E. Genetic analysis of results of a Swedish behavior test on German shepherd dogs and Labrador Retrievers. J Anim Sci. 2008;86(11):2853–61.

8. Pierantoni L, Albertini M, Pirrone F. Prevalence of owner-reported behaviours in dogs separated from the litter at two different ages. Vet Rec. 2011;169(18):468.

9. Foyer P, Wilsson E, Wright D, Jensen P. Early experiences modulate stress coping in a population of German shepherd dogs. Appl Anim Behav Sci. 2013;146(1–4):79–87.

10. Wan M, Hejjas K, Ronai Z, Elek Z, Sasvari-Szekely M, Champagne FA, et al. DRD4 and TH gene polymorphisms are associated with activity, impulsivity and inattention in Siberian Husky dogs. Anim Genet. 2013;44(6):717–27.

11. Hejjas K, Kubinyi E, Ronai Z, Szekely A, Vas J, Miklosi A, et al. Molecular and behavioral analysis of the intron 2 repeat polymorphism in the canine dopamine D4 receptor gene. Genes Brain Behav. 2009;8(3):330–6.

12. Millet B, Chabane N, Delorme R, Leboyer M, Leroy S, Poirier MF, et al. Association between the dopamine receptor D4 (DRD4) gene and obsessive-compulsive disorder. Am J Med Genet B Neuropsychiatr Genet. 2003;116B(1):55–9.

13. Kubinyi E, Vas J, Hejjas K, Ronai Z, Bruder I, Turcsan B, et al. Polymorphism in the tyrosine hydroxylase (TH) gene is associated with activity-impulsivity in German shepherd dogs. PLoS One. 2012;7(1):e30271.

14. Hejjas K, Vas J, Topal J, Szantai E, Ronai Z, Szekely A, et al. Association of polymorphisms in the dopamine D4 receptor gene and the activity-impulsivity endophenotype in dogs. Anim Genet. 2007;38(6):629–33.

15. Theodoridis GA, Gika HG, Want EJ, Wilson ID. Liquid chromatography-mass spectrometry based global metabolite profiling: a review. Anal Chim Acta. 2012;711:7–16.

16. Zhou B, Xiao JF, Tuli L, Ressom HW. LC-MS-based metabolomics. Mol BioSyst. 2012;8(2):470–81.

17. Kaddurah-Daouk R, Krishnan KR. Metabolomics: a global biochemical approach to the study of central nervous system diseases. Neuropsychopharmacology. 2009;34(1):173–86.

18. He Y, Yu Z, Giegling I, Xie L, Hartmann AM, Prehn C, et al. Schizophrenia shows a unique metabolomics signature in plasma. Transl Psychiatry. 2012;2:e149.

19. Sugimoto M, Kawakami M, Robert M, Soga T, Tomita M. Bioinformatics tools for mass spectroscopy-based metabolomic data processing and analysis. Curr Bioinform. 2012;7(1):96–108.

20. Brereton RG, Lloyd GR. Partial least squares discriminant analysis: taking the magic away. J Chemometrics. 2014;28(4):213–25.

21. Benjamini Y, Hochberg Y. Controlling the false discovery rate: a practical and powerful approach to multiple testing. J Roy Stat Soc Ser B (Methodol). 1995;57(1):289–300.

22. Saeed AI, Bhagabati NK, Braisted JC, Liang W, Sharov V, Howe EA, et al. TM4 microarray software suite. Methods Enzymol. 2006;411:134–93.

23. Murphy RC, Axelsen PH. Mass spectrometric analysis of long-chain lipids. Mass Spectrom Rev. 2011;30(4):579–99.

24. Xu F, Zou L, Lin Q, Ong CN. Use of liquid chromatography/tandem mass spectrometry and online databases for identification of phosphocholines and lysophosphatidylcholines in human red blood cells. Rapid Commun Mass Spectrom. 2009;23(19):3243–54.

25. Xia YQ, Jemal M. Phospholipids in liquid chromatography/mass spectrometry bioanalysis: comparison of three tandem mass spectrometric techniques for monitoring plasma phospholipids, the effect of mobile phase composition on phospholipids elution and the association of phospholipids with matrix effects. Rapid Commun Mass Spectrom. 2009;23(14):2125–38.

26. Berry KAZ, Murphy RC. Electrospray ionization tandem mass spectrometry of glycerophosphoethanolamine plasmalogen phospholipids. J Am Soc Mass Spectrom. 2004;15(10):1499–508.

27. Wallner S, Schmitz G. Plasmalogens the neglected regulatory and scavenging lipid species. Chem Phys Lipids. 2011;164(6):573–89.

28. Rodrigues AF, Roecker R, Junges GM, de Lima DD, da Cruz JG, Wyse AT, et al. Hypoxanthine induces oxidative stress in kidney of rats: protective effect of vitamins E plus C and allopurinol. Cell Biochem Funct. 2014;32(4):387–94.

29. Mesquita Casagrande AC, Wamser MN, de Lima DD, da Pereira Cruz JG, Wyse AT, Dal Magro DD. In vitro stimulation of oxidative stress by hypoxanthine in blood of rats: prevention by vitamins e plus C and allopurinol. Nucleosides Nucleotides Nucleic Acids. 2013;32(1):42–57.

30. Chen Q, Park HC, Goligorsky MS, Chander P, Fischer SM, Gross SS. Untargeted plasma metabolite profiling reveals the broad systemic consequences of xanthine oxidoreductase inactivation in mice. PLoS One. 2012;7(6):e37149.

31. Muteliefu G, Enomoto A, Jiang P, Takahashi M, Niwa T. Indoxyl sulphate induces oxidative stress and the expression of osteoblast-specific proteins in vascular smooth muscle cells. Nephrol Dial Transplant. 2009;24(7):2051–8.

32. Dou L, Jourde-Chiche N, Faure V, Cerini C, Berland Y, Dignat-George F, et al. The uremic solute indoxyl sulfate induces oxidative stress in endothelial cells. J Thromb Haemost. 2007;5(6):1302–8.

33. Ozawa M, Honda K, Nakai I, Kishida A, Ohsaki A. Hypaphorine, an indole alkaloid from Erythrina velutina, induced sleep on normal mice. Bioorg Med Chem Lett. 2008;18(14):3992–4.

34. Keller BO, Wu BT, Li SS, Monga V, Innis SM. Hypaphorine is present in human milk in association with consumption of legumes. J Agric Food Chem. 2013;61(31):7654–60.

35. Muller CP, Reichel M, Muhle C, Rhein C, Gulbins E, Kornhuber J. Brain membrane lipids in major depression and anxiety disorders. Biochim Biophys Acta. 2015;1851(8):1052–65.

36. Carrie I, Clement M, de Javel D, Frances H, Bourre JM. Phospholipid supplementation reverses behavioral and biochemical alterations induced by n-3 polyunsaturated fatty acid deficiency in mice. J Lipid Res. 2000;41(3):473–80.

37. Bosch G, Beerda B, Hendriks WH, van der Poel AF, Verstegen MW. Impact of nutrition on canine behaviour: current status and possible mechanisms. Nutr Res Rev. 2007;20(2):180–94.

38. DeMar JC Jr, Ma K, Bell JM, Igarashi M, Greenstein D, Rapoport SI. One generation of n-3 polyunsaturated fatty acid deprivation increases depression and aggression test scores in rats. J Lipid Res. 2006;47(1):172–80.

39. Hennebelle M, Champeil-Potokar G, Lavialle M, Vancassel S, Denis I. Omega-3 polyunsaturated fatty acids and chronic stress-induced modulations of glutamatergic neurotransmission in the hippocampus. Nutr Rev. 2014;72(2):99–112.

40. Liu JJ, Galfalvy HC, Cooper TB, Oquendo MA, Grunebaum MF, Mann JJ, et al. Omega-3 polyunsaturated fatty acid (PUFA) status in major depressive disorder with comorbid anxiety disorders. J Clin Psychiatry. 2013;74(7):732–8.

41. Takeuchi T, Iwanaga M, Harada E. Possible regulatory mechanism of DHA-induced anti-stress reaction in rats. Brain Res. 2003;964(1):136–43.

42. Kaddurah-Daouk R, McEvoy J, Baillie RA, Lee D, Yao JK, Doraiswamy PM, et al. Metabolomic mapping of atypical antipsychotic effects in schizophrenia. Mol Psychiatry. 2007;12(10):934–45.

43. Dougherty RM, Galli C, Ferro-Luzzi A, Iacono JM. Lipid and phospholipid fatty acid composition of plasma, red blood cells, and platelets and how they are affected by dietary lipids: a study of normal subjects from Italy, Finland, and the USA. Am J Clin Nutr. 1987;45(2):443–55.

44. Donovan EL, Pettine SM, Hickey MS, Hamilton KL, Miller BF. Lipidomic analysis of human plasma reveals ether-linked lipids that are elevated in morbidly obese humans compared to lean. Diabetol Metab Syndr. 2013;5(1):24.

45. Lessig J, Fuchs B. HOCl-mediated glycerophosphocholine and glycerophosphoethanolamine generation from plasmalogens in phospholipid mixtures. Lipids. 2010;45(1):37–51.

46. Engelmann B, Brautigam C, Thiery J. Plasmalogen phospholipids as potential protectors against lipid peroxidation of low density lipoproteins. Biochem Biophys Res Commun. 1994;204(3):1235–42.

47. Colas R, Sassolas A, Guichardant M, Cugnet-Anceau C, Moret M, Moulin P, et al. LDL from obese patients with the metabolic syndrome show increased lipid peroxidation and activate platelets. Diabetologia. 2011;54(11):2931–40.

48. Brosche T, Bertsch T, Sieber CC, Hoffmann U. Reduced plasmalogen concentration as a surrogate marker of oxidative stress in elderly septic patients. Arch Gerontol Geriatr. 2013;57(1):66–9.

49. Bouayed J, Rammal H, Soulimani R. Oxidative stress and anxiety: relationship and cellular pathways. Oxid Med Cell Longev. 2009;2(2):63–7.

50. Zhang Y, Filiou MD, Reckow S, Gormanns P, Maccarrone G, Kessler, et al. Proteomic and metabolomic profiling of a trait anxiety mouse model implicate affected pathways. Mol Cell Proteomics. 2011;10(12):M111.008110. doi:10.1074/mcp.M111.008110.

51. Filiou MD, Zhang Y, Teplytska L, Reckow S, Gormanns P, Maccarrone G, et al. Proteomics and metabolomics analysis of a trait anxiety mouse model reveals divergent mitochondrial pathways. Biol Psychiatry. 2011;70(11):1074–82.

52. Rammal H, Bouayed J, Younos C, Soulimani R. Evidence that oxidative stress is linked to anxiety-related behaviour in mice. Brain Behav Immun. 2008;22(8):1156–9.

53. Prabakaran S, Swatton JE, Ryan MM, Huffaker SJ, Huang JT, Griffin JL, et al. Mitochondrial dysfunction in schizophrenia: evidence for compromised brain metabolism and oxidative stress. Mol Psychiatry. 2004;9(7):684–97.

54. Filiou MD, Asara JM, Nussbaumer M, Teplytska L, Landgraf R, Turck CW. Behavioral extremes of trait anxiety in mice are characterized by distinct metabolic profiles. J Psychiatr Res. 2014;S0022–3956(14):00216–7. doi:10.1016/j.jpsychires.2014.07.019.

55. Wilson CB, McLaughlin LD, Nair A, Ebenezer PJ, Dange R, Francis J. Inflammation and oxidative stress are elevated in the brain, blood, and adrenal glands during the progression of post-traumatic stress disorder in a predator exposure animal model. PLoS One. 2013;8(10):e76146. doi:10.1371/journal.pone.0076146(10).

56. Stefanova NA, Fursova AZ, Kolosova NG. Behavioral effects induced by mitochondria-targeted antioxidant SkQ1 in Wistar and senescence-accelerated OXYS rats. J Alzheimers Dis. 2010;21(2):479–91.

7

Effects of GABA$_B$ receptors in the insula on recognition memory observed with intellicage

Nan Wu[1,2†], Feng Wang[1,2†], Zhe Jin[3], Zhen Zhang[1,2], Lian-Kun Wang[1,2], Chun Zhang[1,2] and Tao Sun[1,2*]

Abstract

Background: Insular function has gradually become a topic of intense study in cognitive research. Recognition memory is a commonly studied type of memory in memory research. GABA$_B$R has been shown to be closely related to memory formation. In the present study, we used intellicage, which is a new intelligent behavioural test system, and a bilateral drug microinjection technique to inject into the bilateral insula, to examine the relationship between GABA$_B$R and recognition memory.

Methods: Male Sprague–Dawley rats were randomly divided into control, Sham, Nacl, baclofen and CGP35348 groups. Different testing procedures were employed using intellicage to detect changes in rat recognition memory. The expression of GABA$_B$R (GB1, GB2) in the insula of rats was determined by immunofluorescence and western blotting at the protein level. In addition, the expression of GABA$_B$R (GB$_1$, GB$_2$) was detected by RT-PCR at the mRNA level.

Results: The results of the intellicage test showed that recognition memory was impaired in terms of position learning, punitive learning and punitive reversal learning by using baclofen and CGP35348. In position reversal learning, no significant differences were found in terms of cognitive memory ability between the control groups and the CGP and baclofen groups. Immunofluorescence data showed GABA$_B$R (GB1, GB2) expression in the insula, while data from RT-PCR and western blot analysis demonstrated that the relative expression of GB1 and GB2 was significantly increased in the baclofen group compared with the control groups. In the CGP35348 group, the expression of GB1 and GB2 was significantly decreased, but there was no significant difference in GB1 or GB2 expression in the control groups.

Conclusions: GABA$_B$R expression in the insula plays an important role in the formation of recognition memory in rats.

Keywords: GABA$_B$R, Insula, Recognition of memory, Intellicage

Background

The insula in humans is located in the deep side of the lateral fissure, which is also known as the "hidden fifth lobe". The position of the insula is deep, the surrounding structure is complex, and there is contact with the vast majority of brain areas [1]. In recent years, with advances in functional imaging and the development of deep brain electrical technology, the function of the insula has received substantially more attention. Recent studies have suggested that the insular cortex is the key node of the brain salience network (Salience network) [2]. The insula integrates body perception, produces subjective feelings, determines stimulus-driven attentional capture, coordinates neural resources, and causes the body to respond to stimuli. Additionally, studies have found that the insula of rodents plays a central role in the formation of taste and visual recognition memory [3, 4], and the anterior insula is an important area for perception and arousal in humans [5].

*Correspondence: suntao6699@163.com
†Nan Wu and Feng Wang contributed to the work equally and should be regarded as co-first authors
[1] Ningxia Key Laboratory of Cerebrocranial Disease, Incubation Base of National Key Laboratory, Ningxia Medical University, Yinchuan, Ningxia, China
Full list of author information is available at the end of the article

Recognition memory is a subcategory of declarative memory, which is an important index with which to evaluate the level of memory consolidation. Recognition memory includes at least two different memory processes: recollection and familiarity [6]. Recognition memory depends on many memory sub-systems of the brain network, including the visual pathway, temporal lobe medial structure (hippocampus and olfactory cortex) [4], frontal lobe and parietal cortex. Moreover, different brain regions are interrelated, highly integrated, and play different roles in recognition memory [7]. At present, many studies have focused on the role of the medial temporal lobe structure and frontal cortex in recognition memory. Although the structure of the insula has been studied, most studies utilized fMRI (functional magnetic resonance imaging) [5, 8]. The use of stereotactic microinjection technology to study the relationship between the insula and recognition memory is still rare [1].

$GABA_BR$ is a metabotropic receptor of GABA that mediates slow and sustained inhibitory effects. $GABA_BR$ is composed of two subunits, GB1 and GB2. GABA plays a role in relieving stress and calming the excitement of nerves by acting on $GABA_BR$. When GABA binds to $GABA_BR$, the G protein is activated. Then, a reduction in the presynaptic Ca^{2+} influx and inhibition of the release of a neurotransmitter or an increase in postsynaptic membrane K^+ efflux leads to posterior membrane hyperpolarization and has an effect on G protein activation [9]. Post-synaptic, $GABA_BR$ activation can also enhance $GABA_AR$ function that is outside of the synapse to maintain normal network function [10]. Recent studies have shown that $GABA_BR$ participates in many important physiological activities and pathological changes. $GABA_BR$ directly interacts with transcription factors, regulates long-term protein synthesis and metabolic activities, plays a central role in hippocampal neuron hyperactivity [11] and is important for memory consolidation [10, 12]. Moreover, $GABA_BR$ is a key regulator of neurogenesis, synaptic plasticity and the long-term potentiation (LTP), which are important for guiding the regulation of long-term memory [12–14]. The $GABA_BR$ agonist baclofen impairs learning and memory, while the $GABA_BR$ antagonist CGP35348 improves cognitive processing. Baclofen inhibits spatial learning in mice by activating the TREK-$2K^+$ channel through the PKA pathway [15]; it also promotes the disappearance of normal elastic memory traces and disrupts the consolidation of conditioned reward memory [16]. Although the contribution of $GABA_BR$ to memory has been widely recognized, some contradictory conclusions exist due to differences in behavioural tasks, animal strains, gender, drug concentrations, time, and pathways used in experimental animals, so the relationship between the regulation of

learning and memory and $GABA_BR$ expression still warrants further research [14, 17]. Furthermore, the role and mechanism of $GABA_BR$ in the recognition of the insula is not yet clearly understood.

In the present study, we focused on cognitive function in normal rats after treatment with the $GABA_B$ receptor agonist baclofen and the antagonist CGP35348, which were injected into the bilateral insula. Furthermore, by controlling the changes in $GABA_BR$ expression in the insula, we examined the behavioural changes in recognition memory via intellicage.

Methods
Reagents
Primary antibodies against GB_1R and GB_2R were purchased from Abcam (Cambridge, UK). $GABA_B$ receptor agonist Baclofen and antagonist CGP35348 were obtained from Sigma (St. Louis, US). The First Strand cDNA Synthesis Kit was purchased from Thermo Fisher. The PCR primers were designed and synthesized by Sangon Biotech (Shanghai, CN). The BCA Protein Assay Kit and Total Protein Extraction Kit were purchased from Jiangsu KeyGEN BioTECH Corp, Ltd.

Animals
Male Sprague–Dawley rats (6–8 weeks old, 250–300 g) were provided from the Animal Center of Ningxia Medical University. Each rat was singly housed with an alternating 12:12 h light/dark cycle. These rats were randomly divided into a control group (Control), Sham operation group (Sham), saline group (Nacl), Baclofen group (BLF), and CGP 35348 group (CGP), (sham group was similar in operation with saline group, but was injected with drugs and saline), with five animals in each group. All animal use procedures were approved by the Ningxia Medical University Medical Center Animal Care and Use Committee and were conducted in accordance with the National Institutes of Health Guide for the Care and Use of Laboratory Animals. (No. 2016-124).

Model establishment
After an acclimatization period of at least 1 week, the animals received surgical implantation of cannulae aimed at the insular cortex according to a standardized protocol [18].

Surgery
Rats were implanted with bilateral canulas aimed at the granular insular cortex. Before surgery, animals were anesthetized with 10% chloral (4 ml/kg, ip.). The animals were mounted into a stereotaxic frame used to position the 22-gauge stainless steel guide canula in the

granular insulars. Coordinates obtained from the Paxinos and Watson brain atlas (mm from bregma: AP = +1.2; ML = ±5.5; mm from skull surface: DV = −6.5). The guide canula was anchored to the skull using stainless steel screws and acrylic cement [19]. The animals were allowed 14 days for recovery after guide canula surgeries before the behavioural test.

Microinjection procedure

All microinjections were done slowly (1 µl/0.5 min) using a 5 µl Hamilton syringe connected by Pe-20 polyethylene tube. The stainless steel injection needle (50 G) was cut to protrude 0.5 mm beyond the tips of the guide cannulae and left in place for 1 min after injection to allow diffusion of the solution and to prevent back flow. Saline (0.3 nmol/µl), Baclofen (125 ng/µl) [20], and CGP35348 (12.5 µg/µl) [21], were injected bilaterally into the granular insular 30 min before the start of the behavioural test each day.

Implanted signal transponders

After 14 days recovery from guide canula surgeries and 24 h before introduction into intellicage, the rats were anesthetized with 10% chloral (4 ml/kg, ip.) and the transponders were implanted subcutaneously into the scapula of rats using the injector system delivered with the intellicage. The detector was then used to verify their appropriate subdermal location by read-out of the transponder [22].

Intellicage

The intellicage (TSE Systems GmbH,Germany; http://www.newbehavior.com) is an automated group-housing apparatus allowing experimental testing within the home cage. The cage (410 × 190 × 435 cm) is equipped with four operant conditioning chambers located in each corner. Each conditioning chamber contains two water-drinking bottles and is accessible by a small opening containing a transponder reader antenna that registers the microchip of the entering rat. Access to each water bottle is controlled by gated nosepoke holes containing infrared beam-break sensors, which can be programmed to open or remain closed upon visit or nosepoke response. As each rat was implanted with a unique microchip, corner entry and nosepoke data could be integrated with microchip readings collected by each conditioning corner's antenna, allowing data to be separated by each individual rat.

Behavioural test

Two weeks after surgery, rats were transferred to IntelliCages. Learning and memory information were collected from 9:00 a.m. to 12:00 a.m. Drug perfusion was performed half an hour before the experiment. At the end of each trial, rats were removed, fed freely in a single cage and water-cut (7:00 a.m.–9:00 a.m.) (Fig. 1).
Intellicage learning module design:

1. *Free exploration* free exploration to allow rats to become, familiar with the environment for 10 days. All doors can be opened to reach the water bottle. The number of corner visits and nosepokes was monitored to assess rat exploratory power and corner preferences.

2. *Nosepoke learning* for a total of 10 days, all doors were closed and rats must complete the nosepoke to open the door to drink water. The number of corner visits and nosepokes was monitored to assess rat exploratory power and corner preferences. Special attention was directed to determine the least preferred corner of each rat in order to guide the next module design.

3. *Behavioural extinguishment* rats were allowed to explore for 1 day to extinguish the previous learning behaviour, during which time all rats were able to access all corners and vial vents.

4. *Position learning* for a total of 10 days, the rat's least preferred corner of the nosepoke adaptation period was designated as "correct", while the remaining corners were designated as "error". All rats were able to visit all the corners, but only when the corner was "correct", would the door could be opened and drinking allowed. The position learning ability was measured by calculating the number of correct corner visits.

5. *Position reversal learning* for a total of 10 days, the opposite corner of the "correct" corner in the position learning was designated as the new "correct" corner and remaining corners were designated as "error". Rats were able to enter all places freely, The position reversal learning ability was measured by calculating the number of correct corner visits.

6. *Behavioural extinguishment* the same as in step3.

7. *Novelty exploration* for a total of 4 days, the LED lights of one corner were opened randomly. The light shifted in a counter-clockwise direction on each day. All rats were free to enter all corners, the number of corners visited was calculated, and the "novelty object preference" was evaluated.

8. *Behavioural extinguishment* the same as in step3.

9. *Punitive learning* for / days, the leftside of all the corners was assigned as its "correct" (reward) side. Unlike position learning, in this module, rat nosepoke to the "error" side incurred a blow penalty (aversion to irritation).

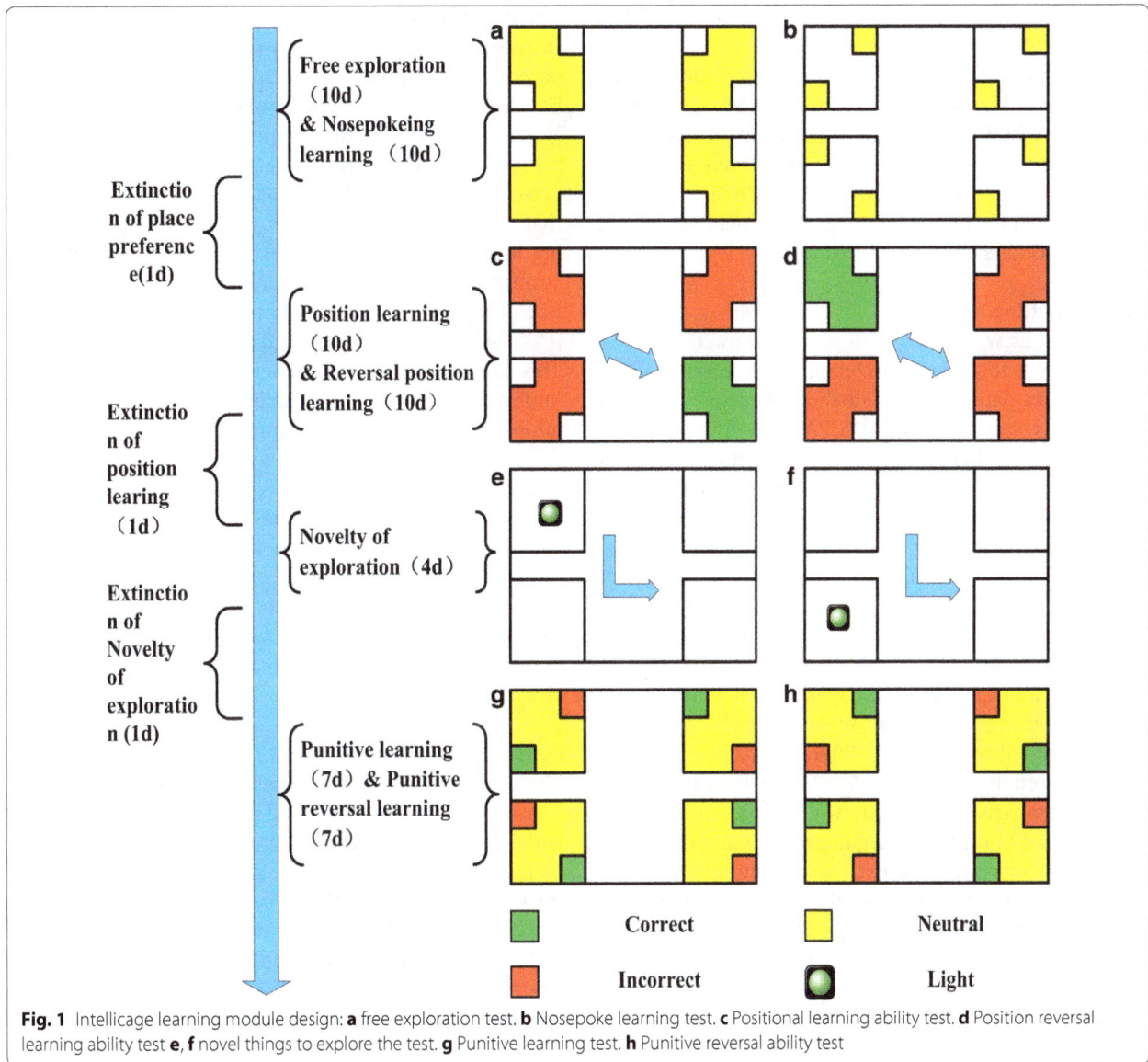

Fig. 1 Intellicage learning module design: **a** free exploration test. **b** Nosepoke learning test. **c** Positional learning ability test. **d** Position reversal learning ability test **e**, **f** novel things to explore the test. **g** Punitive learning test. **h** Punitive reversal ability test

10. Penalty reversal learning: for 7 days, the rightside of all the corners was assigned as the "correct" (reward) side and nosepoke of the "error" side was penalized.

Sample collection

After behavioural tests, the rats were sacrificed following anaesthesia with 10% chloral hydrate and the insular tissues of some rats were collected. The other rats were perfused with 4% Paraformaldehyde solution. The isolated brains were stored in sucrose solution to dehydrate gradiently and embedded in OCT for frozen tissue sections.

Immunofluorescence

The immunofluorescence method of SABC (StreptAvidin Biotin Complex) staining was performed as below.

After antigen retrieval using citric acid buffer, the sections were blocked with serum and incubated with antibodies (GB$_1$, 1:300; GB$_2$, 1:500) at 4 °C overnight. After washing in PBS, donkeyanti-rabbit-FITC (green) fluorescence second antibody drop, room temperature 1 h, PBS wash 10 min × 4 times. The cartridge was dried and directly blocked with anti-quencher. The insular GI areas of immunostained slides were observed and positive cells were quantitatively analyzed using Image J1.48 analysis system. Six fields of view were picked for every slide.

RT-PCR

Total RNA of insular tissues was extracted using TRIzol reagent according to the manufacturer's protocol. First-strand cDNA was generated using M-MLV reverse transcriptase. PCR was performed to detect the mRNA expression of each gene. PCR application conditions were described as followed: denaturation at 94 °C for 3 min, followed by 40 cycles of denaturation at 94 °C for 30 s, annealing at 58 °C for 30 s and extension at 72 °C for 45 s. RT-PCR products were analyzed and visualized on 4% agarose gel containing ethidium bromide (EB). Images were captured by Tanon 3500 digital gel imaging system. The PCR primers used were listed in Table 1.

Western blotting

Insular tissues were lysed with protein extraction kit on ice, and then total protein content was determined by BCA protein determination method. Protein from each sample was separated by SDS/PAGE and transfer on to a PVDF membrane. After blocking with 5% non-fat milk for 1 h, the membranes were immunoblotted with primary antibodies (GB_1, 1:300; GB_2, 1:500) overnight. After incubated with secondary antibody (1:5000), signal detection was performed by Odyssey infrared laser imaging system, followed by gray intensity analysis.

Statistical analysis

All results are expressed as the mean ± SD. Analysis was performed using SPSS 21.0 software. For the behaviour test, the significance of the difference between groups was measured using one-way ANOVA followed by Tukey test for comparison between two groups. For RT-PCR and Western blotting, the significance of the difference between groups was measured using one-way ANOVA followed by Bonferroni's Multiple Comparison test for comparison between two groups. $P < 0.05$ was considered to be statistically significant (*$P < 0.05$, **$P < 0.01$).

Results

Behavioural test

Intellicage

Free exploration: There was no statistically significant difference in terms of the visit [$F_{(4, 245)} = 2.272$, $P > 0.05$] (Fig. 2a) and nosepoke [$F_{(4, 245)} = 0.693$, $P > 0.05$] (Fig. 2b) measures of learning ability between the five groups of rats. The results showed that under normal conditions, the cognitive learning ability of the five groups of rats was basically the same.

Table 1 Specific primers used in real-time PCR analysis

Gene	Primer	Sequence (5′→3′)
GAPDH	FW	GAGTCAACGGATTTGGTCGT
	RV	GACAAGATTCCCGTTCTCAG
GB1	FW	AGATTGTGGACCCCTTGCAC
	RV	AGAAAATGCCAAGCCACGTA
GB2	FW	CACCGAGTGTGACAATGCAAA
	RV	CCAGATTCCAGCCTTGGAGG

Nosepoke learning

In terms of the number of visits and nosepokes, compared with the other three groups, the visit rate of the BLF and CGP groups was decreased [$F_{(4, 245)} = 48.12$, $P < 0.01$]. Furthermore, the number of visits in the BLF group was significantly reduced compared with the CGP group [$q = 5.385$, $P < 0.01$] (Fig. 2c). This finding suggests that baclofen and CGP35348 can inhibit spatial learning in normal rats, but the baclofen inhibitory effect is stronger. Additionally, the number of nosepokes in the BLF group was significantly lower than in the CGP group [$F_{(4, 245)} = 57.15$, $P < 0.01$], [$q = 8.44$, $P < 0.01$] (Fig. 2d). This finding indicates that baclofen and CGP35348 also inhibit the skills of learning ability of normal rats and that inhibition by baclofen was stronger.

Position learning

The correct number of visits of the BLF and CGP groups was significantly lower than those of the other three groups [$F_{(4, 245)} = 56.26$, $P < 0.01$], while there was no significant difference between the BLF group and the CGP group ($q = 3.164$, $P > 0.05$) (Fig. 2e). This indicates that baclofen and CGP35348 can inhibit spatial learning and memory in normal rats.

Position reversal learning

There were no significant differences in the number of correct visits between the BLF and the CGP groups compared with the other three groups, but the number of correct visits for the BLF group was significantly lower than that of the CGP group [$q = 4.45$, $P < 0.05$] (Fig. 2f). This suggests that baclofen and CGP35348 have an effect on learning and memory and that baclofen has a stronger inhibitory effect on the reversal of spatial position learning, which may not affect the spatial learning ability of rats.

Novelty exploration

The learning ability of five groups of rats did not show statistical significance in terms of the number of visits [$F_{(4, 95)} = 1.039$, $P > 0.05$] (Fig. 2g). The results showed that for the five groups of rats the novelty exploration of learning ability was basically the same.

Punitive learning

The number of correct nosepokes in the BLF group and the CGP group was significantly lower than that in the other three groups [$F_{(4, 170)} = 32.20$, $P < 0.01$], and the BLF and CGP groups showed a statistically significant difference in nosepokes [$q = 4.48$, $P < 0.05$] (Fig. 2h). This result indicates that baclofen and CGP35348 could inhibit the spatial and skills learning components of recognition memory in normal rats and that the inhibitory effect of baclofen was stronger.

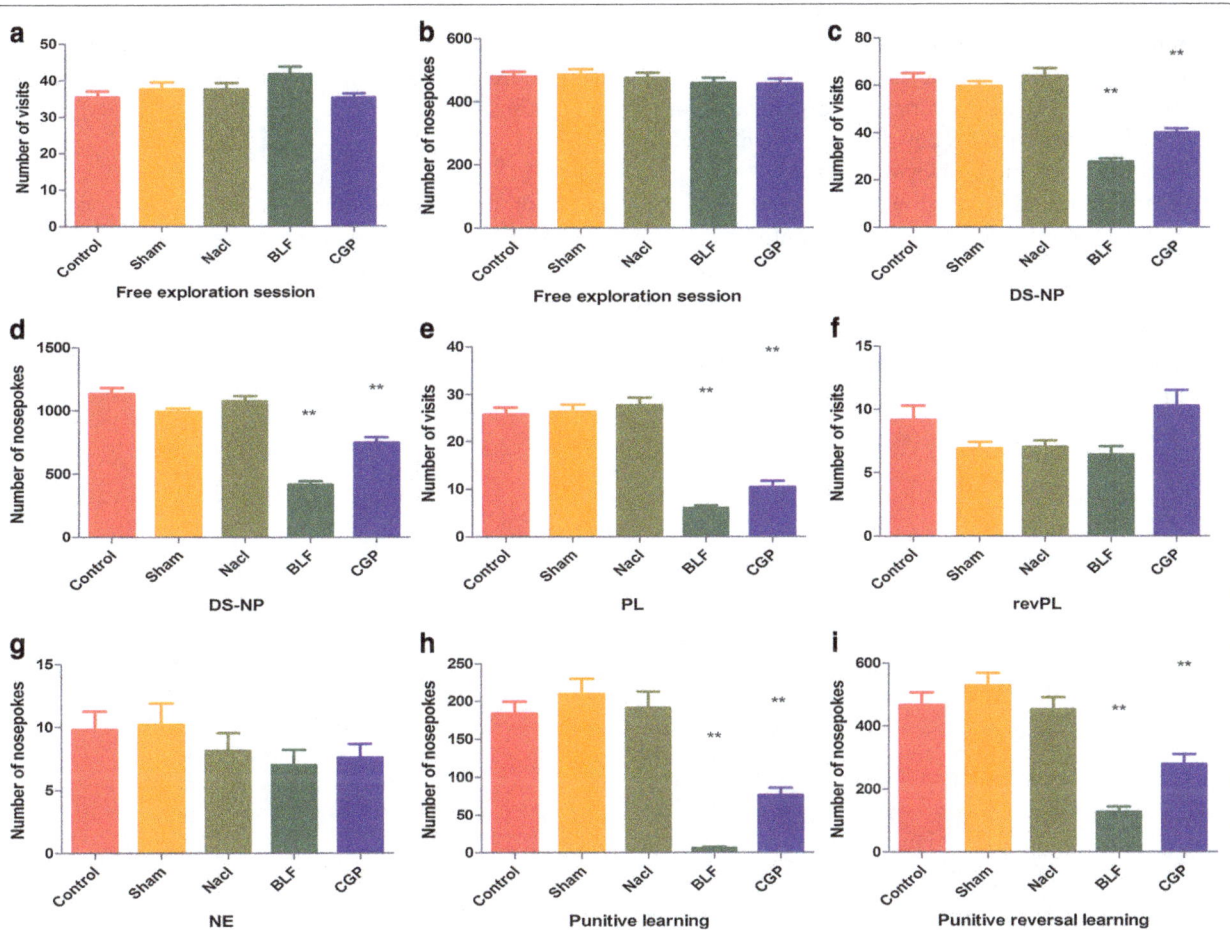

Fig. 2 Behavioural test (**a**). **b** Free exploratory: there was no significant difference in visit and nosepoke between the five groups of rats, indicating that the model preparation had no effect on the basic learning ability of rats. **c** Number of visits in nosepoke learning: In the BLF and CGP groups, the number of visits decreased ($P < 0.01$, compared with the other three groups), and the BLF group decreased significantly ($P < 0.01$, compared with the CGP group). **d** Number of nosepokes in nosepoke learning: The BLF and CGP groups showed decreased numbers of nosepokes ($P < 0.01$, compared with the other three groups). The decreasing trend in the BLF group was more obvious ($P < 0.01$, compared with the CGP group). **e** Number of correct visits in position learning: the number of correct visits decreased in the BLF and CGP groups ($P < 0.01$, compared with the other three groups). **f** Number of correct visits in position reversal learning: There was no statistically significant reduction in the number of correct visits in the BLF and CPG groups compared with the other three groups ($P < 0.01$). **g** Number of visits in novelty exploration: The results showed no significant difference in the visiting times of five groups of rats. **h** Number of correct nosepokes in punitive learning: The BLF and CGP groups exhibited fewer correct nosepokes ($P < 0.05$, compared with the other three control groups), and the number in the BLF group was significantly lower ($P < 0.05$, compared with the CGP group). **i** Number of correct nosepokes in punitive reversal learning: The correct number of nosepokes in the BLF and CGP groups was reduced ($P < 0.01$, compared with the other three groups), and the BLF group had the least number of correct nosepokes ($P < 0.05$, compared with the CGP group)

Punitive reversal learning

The number of correct nosepokes in the BLF and CGP groups was significantly lower than that in the other three groups [$F_{(4, 170)} = 23.01$, $P < 0.01$], while the BLF and CGP groups showed a statistically significant difference in terms of the number of correct nosepokes [$q = 4.46$, $P < 0.05$] (Fig. 2i). This finding indicates that baclofen and CGP35348 had inhibitory effects on spatial and skills learning of recognition memory and that baclofen had a stronger inhibitory effect.

The conversion efficiency of learning and memory:

1. During the first 5 days of position reversal learning, the BLF group showed less frequent visits compared with the other four groups [$F_{(4, 245)} = 5.611$, $P < 0.01$]. In addition, the number of correct visits decreased significantly in the BLF group compared with the CGP group [$q = 4.14$, $P < 0.01$] (Fig. 3a). However, in the second 5 days, the BLF and CGP groups showed the same performance as the control groups in terms of the number of correct visits. The number of correct visits in the BLF group was significantly lower than that in the CGP group [$q = 3.95$,

$P < 0.01$] (Fig. 3b), which indicates that, at the beginning of reversal learning, baclofen inhibits the conversion efficiency of learning more than CGP35348. The response ability of rats to spatial localization transformation is poor, but after a period of learning, Baclofen's inhibition slowly weakens.

2. In the BLF and CGP groups, the number of correct nosepokes decreased significantly from the first 3 days [F $(4, 70) = 25.56$, $P < 0.01$] to the last 3 days of the reversal of learning [F $(4, 70) = 68.17$, $P < 0.01$]. The BLF and CGP groups differed significantly from each other [q $= 5.56$, $P < 0.01$] (Fig. 3c), [q $= 6.76$, $P < 0.01$] (Fig. 3d). This finding indi-

cated that baclofen and CGP35348 could inhibit the learning efficiency of rats. Baclofen produced a more obvious reduction in the reversal of learning efficiency.

Nissl

Nissl staining showed that the target of the insula was in accordance with the experimental requirement (Fig. 4).

Immunofluorescence

Immunofluorescence showed normal expression of GB1 and GB2 in the insula, indicating that the normal rat insula contains GABA$_B$R (Fig. 5).

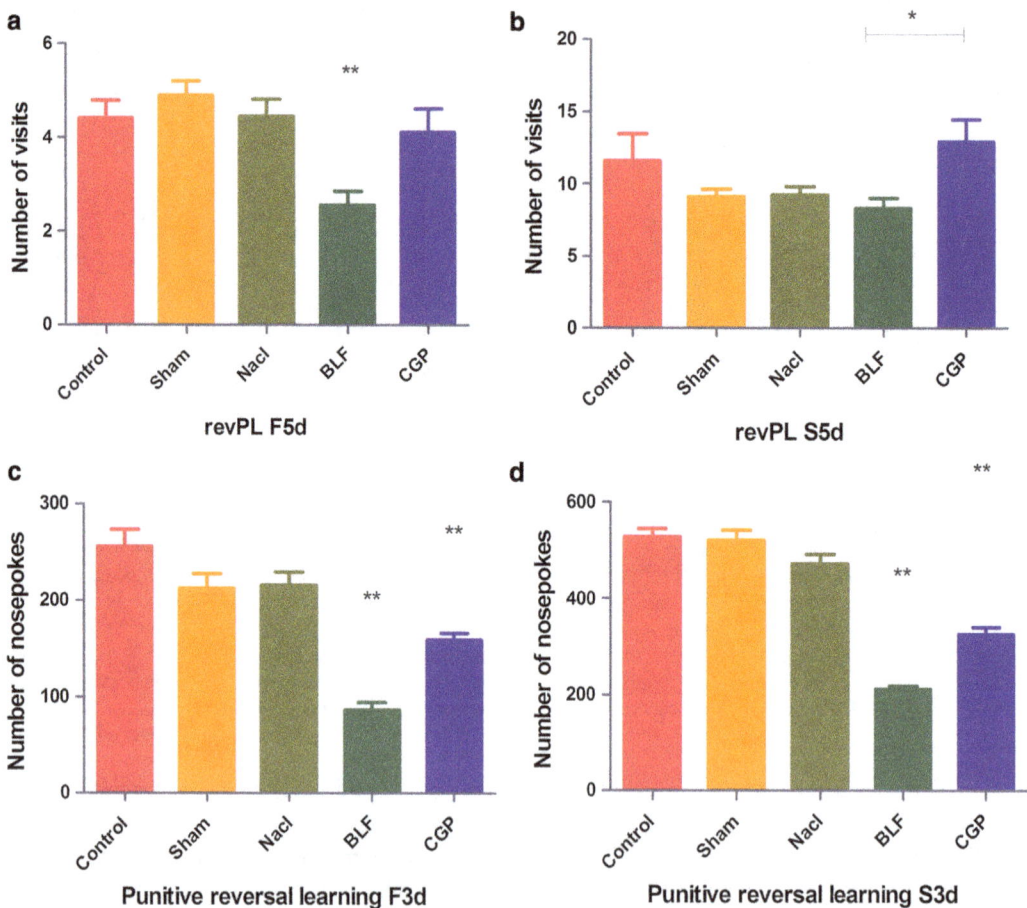

Fig. 3 Reversing learning efficiency change of position reversal learning and penetration reversal learning. **a, b** Position reversal learning: reversing learning efficiency change of position reversal learning: in the BLF group, the learning efficiency was significantly inhibited in the first 5 days ($P < 0.05$, compared with the CGP group). When the CGP group was compared with the other three groups, the difference in learning efficiency was not statistically significant. In the BLF group, learning efficiency was inhibited in the second 5 days ($P < 0.05$), but there was no significant difference in learning efficiency compared with the other three control groups. The results of the CGP group were the same as those of the BLF group. **c, d** Penetration reversal learning: reversing learning efficiency change of penetration reversal learning: Learning efficiency was inhibited in the BLF and CGP groups in the first 3 days, and the difference was statistically significant ($P < 0.01$, compared with the other groups). The learning ability of the animals in the BLF group was worse ($P < 0.01$, compared with the CGP group). The learning efficiency was significantly inhibited in the BLF and CGP groups in the last 3 days, the difference was statistically significant ($P < 0.01$, compared with the other groups), and the learning ability of the BLF group worsened ($P < 0.01$ compared with the CGP group)

RT-PCR

The expression of GB1and GB2 was much higher in the Baclofen group but lower in the CGP group compared to the other groups [GB1F $(4, 20) = 15.51$, $P < 0.01$] [GB2F $(4, 20) = 35.98$, $P < 0.01$] (Fig. 6).

Western blotting

The expression of GB1 and GB2 was much higher in the Baclofen group, but lower in the CGP group compared to the other groups [GB1F $(4, 20) = 20.17$, $P < 0.01$] [GB2F $(4, 20) = 19.01$, $P < 0.01$] (Fig. 7).

Discussion

Research regarding the insula is a new method of understanding the cognitive function of the brain. Studies have shown that the insula is involved in the regulation of pain, formation of addiction, formation of disgust, generation of depression, regulation of cardiac activity, language planning, and empathy [1, 2, 23]. Herpes encephalitis, ischaemic stroke, glioma and other diseases often involve the insula. In addition, neurological and psychiatric disorders, such as temporal lobe epilepsy, schizophrenia, dementia, Alzheimer's disease, anxiety, depression, and autism, are closely related to the insula [24]. Some research on recognition memory has shown that the main structural basis of recognition memory from the perspective of anatomy and function is the highlight network. However, the role and mechanism of the insula, which is the core of the highlight network, is unclear. In addition, there is still considerable controversy regarding the relationship between recollection and familiar memory, its various functional characteristics, the neural basis and other issues [19, 24]. However, GABA, as the most important inhibitory neurotransmitter in the central nervous system, plays an important role in the encoding, sorting and transmission of nerve information [25]. Several studies have shown that GABA is involved in the decision-making process [26] and that the dysfunction of $GABA_B R$ is also associated with a variety of neurological diseases, including epilepsy, anxiety,

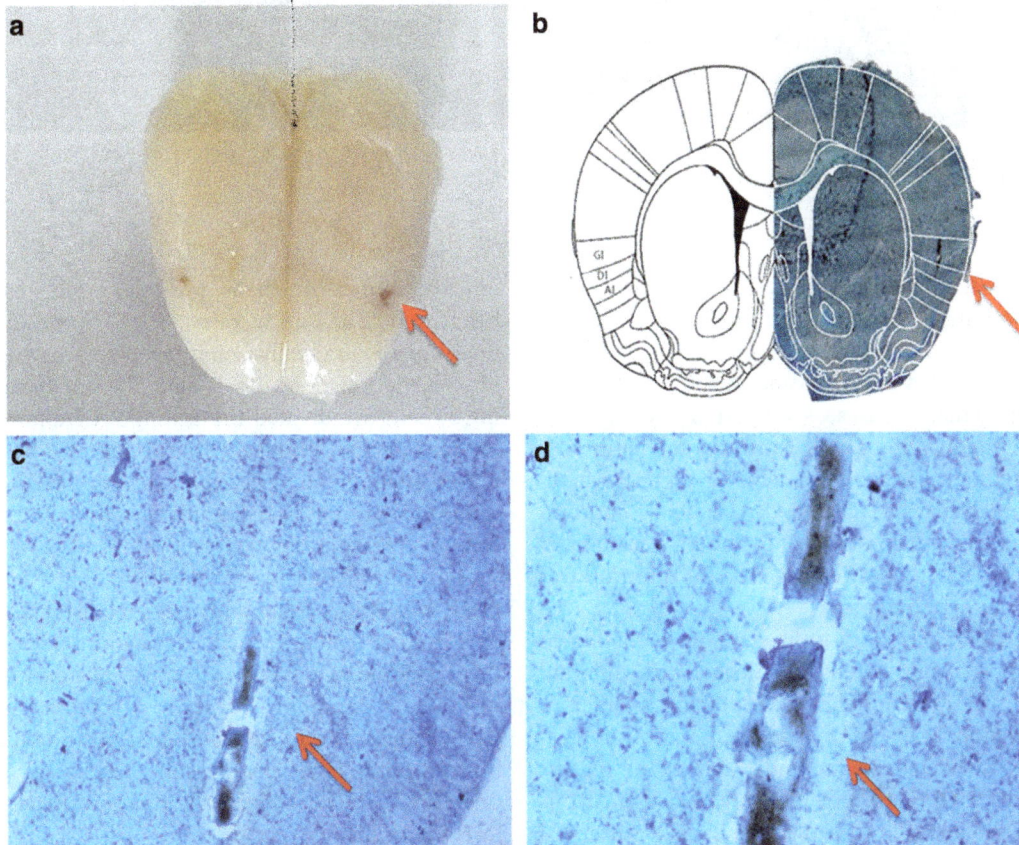

Fig. 4 Nissl (**a**). The appearance of bilateral insular inserts (**b**). Comparison of position and mapping of the left lobes. *Right* a Nissl-stained frozen section of the rat brain (coronal cut, +1.2 mm relative to bregma [39]) was microinjected into the granular insular cortex as detailed in "Methods". *Left* a scheme of the corresponding contralateral hemisphere. *GI* granular insular cortex, *DI* dysgranular insular cortex. **c** ×200 target position of insular, **d** ×400 target position of insular

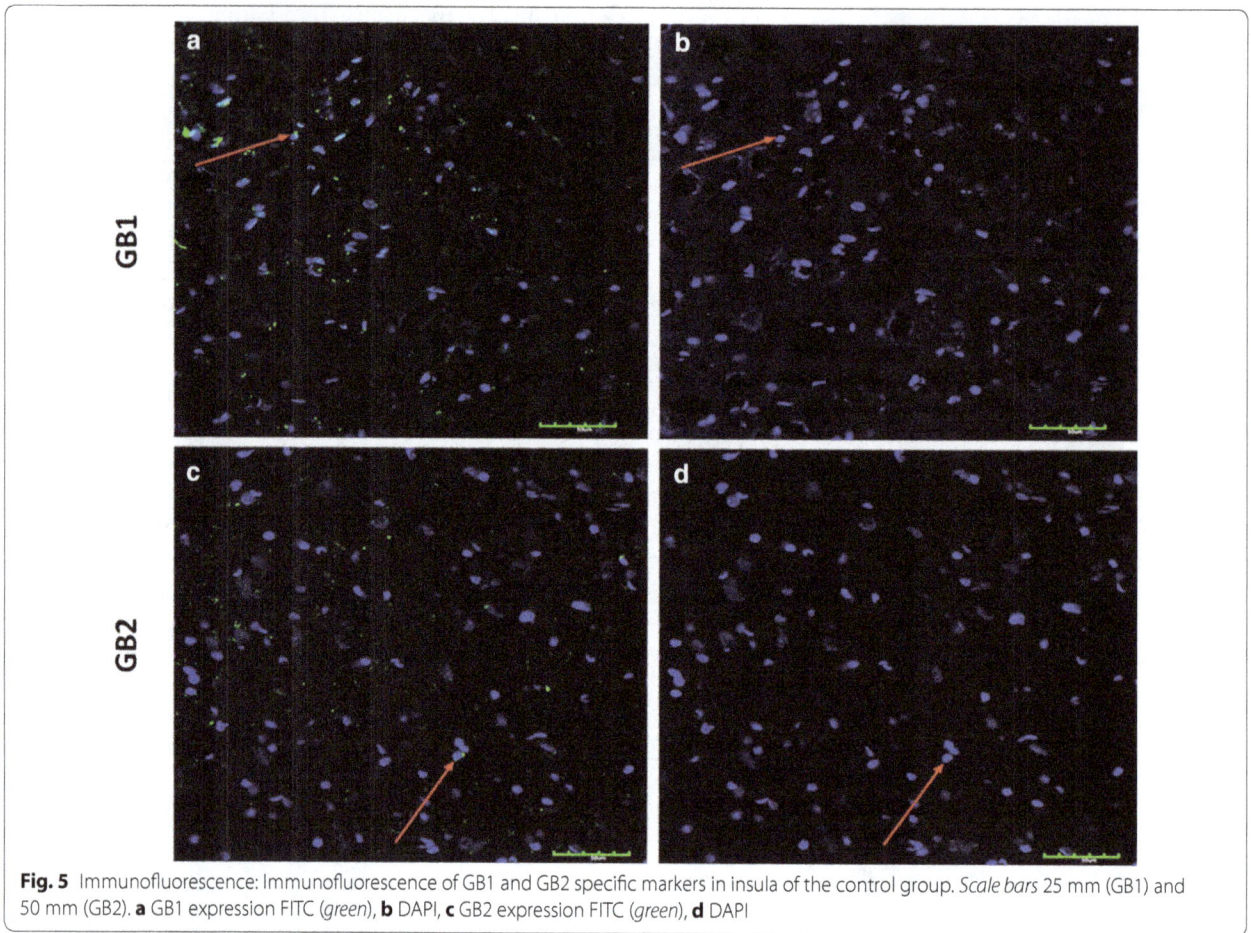

Fig. 5 Immunofluorescence: Immunofluorescence of GB1 and GB2 specific markers in insula of the control group. *Scale bars* 25 mm (GB1) and 50 mm (GB2). **a** GB1 expression FITC (*green*), **b** DAPI, **c** GB2 expression FITC (*green*), **d** DAPI

depression, drug addiction and cognitive disorders [11, 27–29]. To summarize the results of the research regarding GABA and the insula, first, neuropsychiatric diseases are closely associated to the insula and $GABA_BR$. Second, neuropsychiatric diseases are often accompanied by impaired cognitive function. Third, the recognition of cognitive memory is a good indicator of cognitive function. As both the insula and $GABA_BR$ play important roles in recognition memory, we raise some questions of whether there is a link between them. This question was explored in our experiments.

Our behavioural testing utilized a new intelligent behaviour monitoring system, intellicage, with different recognition memory modules. This system is different from the previous water maze, dark test and other classical behavioural detection methods. One of the biggest drawbacks of these classic behavioural experiments is that they are man-made to provide animals a variety of stimuli to observe the animal's learning and memory changes. Alternatively, intellicage is characterized by the location of rats in an environment that closely resembles a natural social environment. This setup avoids human

intervention as much as possible, which can lead to behavioural changes in rats [30, 31]. After years of use, intellicage is gradually being taken seriously in the field of behavioural research. Using the intellicage operating system, we divided the testing programme into four modules, which represent four different types of recognition memory, to verify the effect of $GABA_BR$ expression in the insula on recognition memory. First, we used nosepoke learning to explore the effects of rats' recognition memory (skills learning ability). The second module used position learning and position reversal learning to explore rats' spatial recognition memory changes. In the third module, we explored the use of novel exploration to evaluate the ability of rats to recognize memories of novel things. The fourth module utilized punitive learning and punitive reversal learning to explore a reconsidering memory that reflected spatial positioning and skills learning ability.

Our evidence confirms that after perfusing the $GABA_BR$-selective agonist baclofen and $GABA_BR$-specific antagonist CGP35348 in normal rat insula, the number of corner accesses was reduced in the nosepoke study. This

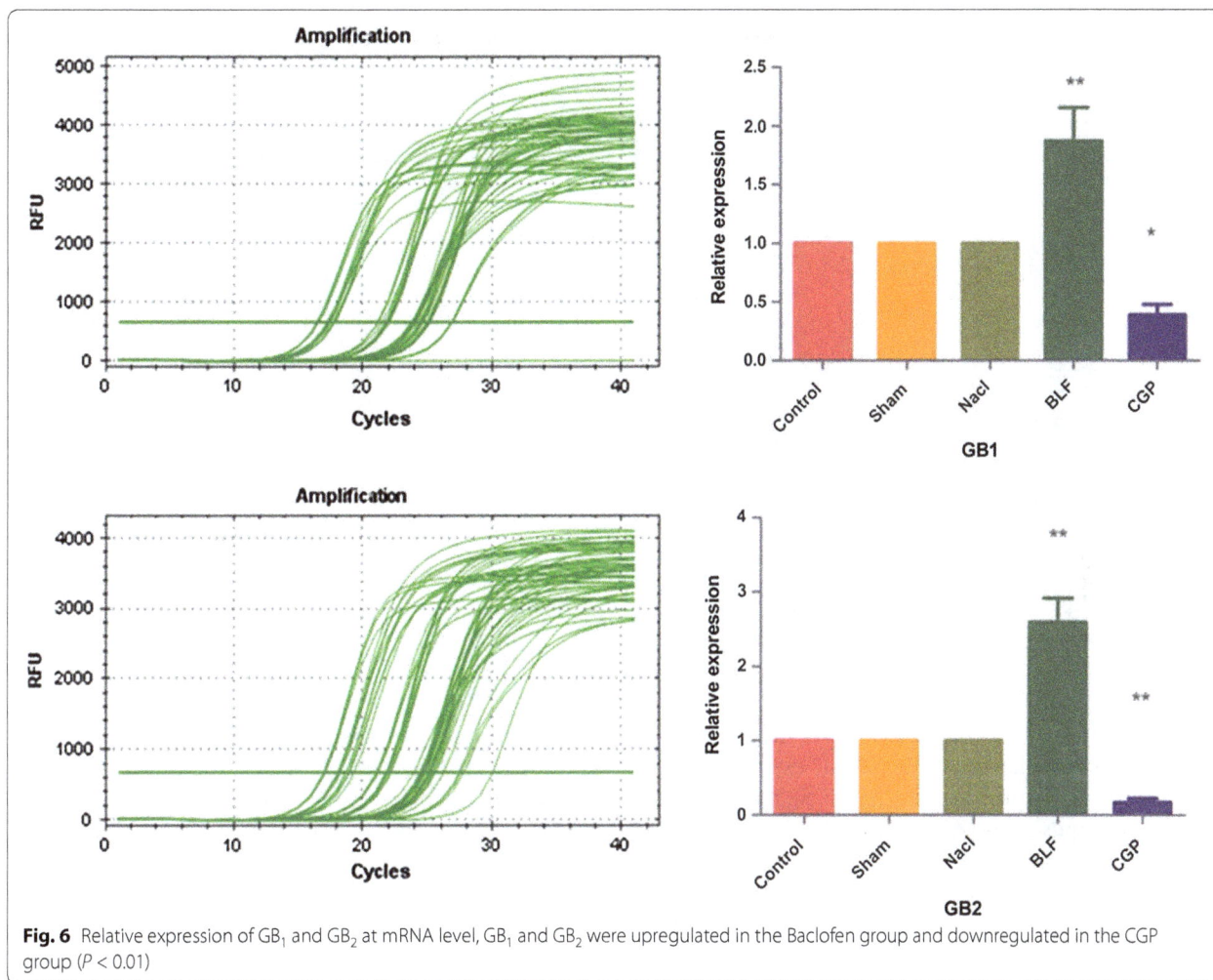

Fig. 6 Relative expression of GB$_1$ and GB$_2$ at mRNA level, GB$_1$ and GB$_2$ were upregulated in the Baclofen group and downregulated in the CGP group ($P < 0.01$)

finding indicated that GABA$_B$R upregulation and down-regulation in the insula resulted in a decrease in the skills learning ability associated with recognition memory. Studies have confirmed that the anterior medial temporal lobes plays a role in food intake [32], and our results confirmed that GABA$_B$R in the insula also affects skills learning as rats learn to drink and remember how to obtain water. In position learning, modulation of rat GABA$_B$R expression also caused a reduction in spatial memory, but the change in GABA$_B$R expression did not affect the spatial recognition memory of the rat in position reversal learning. This finding suggests that upregulation and downregulation of GABA$_B$R in the insula could damage the rat's spatial memory, but it did not affect spatial reversal learning associated with recognition memory. Studies have confirmed that the hippocampus is the node of the memory system [33], but we have determined through experiments that GABA$_B$R in the insula also has such a role. For punitive learning and punitive reversal learning, upregulation and downregulation of GABA$_B$R

expression in the insula of rats could lead to a decrease in the number of correct nosepokes, which indicates that the comprehensive utilization of recognition memory is impaired and interrupted. In recent years, most studies on recognition memory have targeted the hippocampus [34], It has been reported that in the hippocampus, baclofen inhibits GABA$_B$R-induced spatial learning in normal rats by activating the TREK-2K$^+$ channel [15]. CGP35348 inhibits the inhibitory postsynaptic potential (IPSP), enhances GABA$_B$R activation, and improves the memory formation process [35]. However, in our study, up-regulation and down-regulation of GABA$_B$R expression in the insula during the abovementioned test modules affected cognition in normal rats, and GABA$_B$R upregulation in the normal rat insula was more damaging to cognition. Therefore, it cannot be determined whether CGP35348 can improve cognitive function because there are different targets and the roles of the targets are also very different. Thus, increases or decreases in GABA$_B$R expression in the insula will damage memory function.

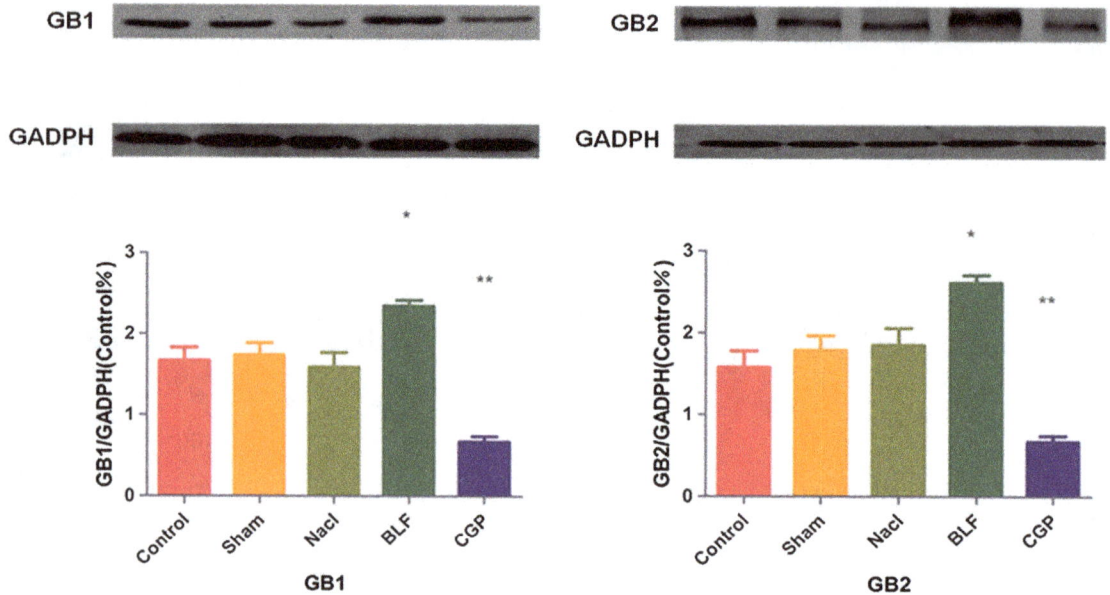

Fig. 7 Western blotting: For the five groups, relative expression of GB1 and GB2. At the protein level expression increased in the Baclofen group but decreased in the CGP group significantly. *$P < 0.05$, **$P < 0.01$

Moreover, with a change in learning pattern, the cognitive changes associated with $GABA_BR$ expression were different. Several studies have confirmed that GABA in the hippocampus plays an important role in novelty recognition and target identification [36, 37], but we found that the change in $GABA_BR$ expression in the insula did not affect the ability of the animals to recognize new things, which indicates that the insula may not be the region involved in novelty recognition.

In this experiment, we also explored the conversion efficiency of rats' recognition memory. In position reversal learning, we found that in the first 5 days, upregulation and downregulation of $GABA_BR$ in the insula resulted in a marked decrease in the recognition memory of rats and that upregulation of $GABA_BR$ expression made this reduction more obvious. However, in the last 5 days of learning, $GABA_BR$ expression in the insula was not associated with a decline in recognition memory capacity. This finding indicates that at the beginning of the first 5 days, upregulation and downregulation of $GABA_BR$ expression in the insula resulted in a reduction in the efficiency of rat spatial recognition of memory transfer, but with an increase in learning time, the efficiency of this conversion was restored in the last 5 days. However, upregulation and downregulation of $GABA_BR$ expression, which occurred both in the first 3 days and in the second 3 days of punitive reversal learning, impaired the conversion efficiency of spatial location recognition memory and the recognition memory of the

skills learning ability, suggesting that changes in $GABA_BR$ expression in the insula influence the efficiency of the transformation of recognition memory. Combining the results of position reversal learning and punitive reversal learning, we conclude that $GABA_BR$ changes in the insula can lead to a reduction in the efficiency of recognition memory, which is a single mode, and this reduction in efficiency will be mitigated with increased learning time; however, for more than one mode of recognition memory, the change in $GABA_BR$ expression in the insula will continue to affect the conversion efficiency of recognition memory.

The insula is located near the temporal lobe. Research has confirmed that the medial temporal lobe and insula are associated with memory consolidation [6] and that temporal lobe lesions, such as temporal lobe epilepsy, can cause patients to have memory damage [38]. It has been found that the relationship between $GABA_BR$ expression in the insula and memory recognition may provide a new target for the treatment of patients with impaired cognitive function. However, in future experiments, we need to study the link between the insula and other brain regions to investigate the behavioural changes of rats in a large sample and to explore the molecular mechanism of $GABA_BR$ expression in insular and recognition memory.

In conclusion, our study demonstrates that $GABA_BR$ plays an important role in the formation of recognition memory and may be become a new target for the study of memory.

Abbreviations
GABA: gamma-aminobutyric acid; PL: position learning; revPL: position reversal learning; NE: novelty of exploration; F5d: five days before; S5d: the second five days; F3d: three days before; S3d: the last three days.

Authors' contributions
NW contributed to the design and planning of the experiment and all the tests, data analyses and writing the manuscript. ZZ and KLW took part in the planning and designing of the experiment and cognitive tests, data analyses and manuscript preparation. FW and TS contributed to the design and planning of the experiment. ZJ contributed to the design and data analyses. TS should be regarded as corresponding author. All authors read and approved the final manuscript.

Author details
[1] Ningxia Key Laboratory of Cerebrocranial Disease, Incubation Base of National Key Laboratory, Ningxia Medical University, Yinchuan, Ningxia, China. [2] Department of Neurosurgery, General Hospital of Ningxia Medical University, Yinchuan, Ningxia, China. [3] Department of Neuroscience, Uppsala University, Uppsala, Sweden.

Competing interests
The authors declare that they have no competing interests.

Funding
This work was supported by the National Natural Science Foundation of China (Nos. 81660226, 81460208) and the Ningxia Science and Technology Support Project.

References
1. Bermudez-Rattoni F. The forgotten insular cortex: its role on recognition memory formation. Neurobiol Learn Mem. 2014;109:207–16.
2. Uddin LQ. Salience processing and insular cortical function and dysfunction. Nat Rev Neurosci. 2015;16(1):55–61.
3. O'Brien LD, Sticht MA, Mitchnick KA, Limebeer CL, Parker LA, Winters BD. CB1 receptor antagonism in the granular insular cortex or somatosensory area facilitates consolidation of object recognition memory. Neurosci Lett. 2014;578:192–6.
4. Blonde GD, Bales MB, Spector AC. Extensive lesions in rat insular cortex significantly disrupt taste sensitivity to NaCl and KCl and slow salt discrimination learning. PLoS ONE. 2015;10(2):e0117515.
5. Fischer DB, Boes AD, Demertzi A, Evrard HC, Laureys S, Edlow BL, Liu H, Saper CB, Pascual-Leone A, Fox MD, et al. A human brain network derived from coma-causing brainstem lesions. Neurology. 2016;87(23):2427–34.
6. Balderas I, Rodriguez-Ortiz CJ, Bermudez-Rattoni F. Consolidation and reconsolidation of object recognition memory. Behav Brain Res. 2015;285:213–22.
7. Warburton EC, Brown MW. Neural circuitry for rat recognition memory. Behav Brain Res. 2015;285:131–9.
8. Rodriguez P, Zhou W, Barrett DW, Altmeyer W, Gutierrez JE, Li J, Lancaster JL, Gonzalez-Lima F, Duong TQ. Multimodal randomized functional MR imaging of the effects of methylene blue in the human brain. Radiology. 2016;281(2):516–26.
9. Padgett CL, Slesinger PA. GABAB receptor coupling to G-proteins and ion channels. Adv Pharmacol. 2010;58:123–47.
10. Craig MT, McBain CJ. The emerging role of GABAB receptors as regulators of network dynamics: fast actions from a 'slow' receptor? Curr Opin Neurobiol. 2014;26:15–21.
11. Lang M, Moradi-Chameh H, Zahid T, Gane J, Wu C, Valiante T, Zhang L. Regulating hippocampal hyperexcitability through GABAB receptors. Physiol Rep. 2014;2(4):e00278.
12. Cullen PK, Dulka BN, Ortiz S, Riccio DC, Jasnow AM. GABA-mediated presynaptic inhibition is required for precision of long-term memory. Learn Mem. 2014;21(4):180–4.
13. Pontes A, Zhang Y, Hu W. Novel functions of GABA signaling in adult neurogenesis. Front Biol. 2013;8(5):496–507.
14. Heaney CF, Kinney JW. Role of GABA(B) receptors in learning and memory and neurological disorders. Neurosci Biobehav Rev. 2016;63:1–28.
15. Deng PY, Xiao Z, Yang C, Rojanathammanee L, Grisanti L, Watt J, Geiger JD, Liu R, Porter JE, Lei S. GABA(B) receptor activation inhibits neuronal excitability and spatial learning in the entorhinal cortex by activating TREK-2K+ channels. Neuron. 2009;63:230–43.
16. Heinrichs SC, Leite-Morris KA, Carey RJ, Kaplan GB. Baclofen enhances extinction of opiate conditioned place preference. Behav Brain Res. 2010;207(2):353–9.
17. Rajalu M, Fritzius T, Adelfinger L, Jacquier V, Besseyrias V, Gassmann M, Bettler B. Pharmacological characterization of GABAB receptor subtypes assembled with auxiliary KCTD subunits. Neuropharmacology. 2015;88:145–54.
18. Balderas I, Rodriguez-Ortiz CJ, Salgado-Tonda P, Chavez-Hurtado J, McGaugh J, Bermudez-Rattoni F. The consolidation of object and context recognition memory involve different regions of the temporal lobe. Learn Mem. 2008;15(9):618–24.
19. Berman DE, Hazvi S, Neduva V, Dudai Y. The role of identified neurotransmitter systems in the response of insular cortex to unfamiliar taste: activation of ERK1-2 and formation of a memory trace. J Neurosci. 2000;20(18):7017–23.
20. St Onge JR, Floresco SB. Prefrontal cortical contribution to risk-based decision making. Cereb Cortex. 2010;20(8):1816–28.
21. Ataie Z, Babri S, Ghahramanian Golzar M, Ebrahimi H, Mirzaie F, Mohaddes G. GABAB receptor blockade prevents antiepileptic action of ghrelin in the rat hippocampus. Adv Pharm Bull. 2013;3(2):353–8.
22. Urbach YK, Raber KA, Canneva F, Plank AC, Andreasson T, Ponten H, Kullingsjo J, Nguyen HP, Riess O, von Horsten S. Automated phenotyping and advanced data mining exemplified in rats transgenic for Huntington's disease. J Neurosci Methods. 2014;234:38–53.
23. Feng Q, Chen X, Sun J, Zhou Y, Sun Y, Ding W, Zhang Y, Zhuang Z, Xu J, Du Y. Voxel-level comparison of arterial spin-labeled perfusion magnetic resonance imaging in adolescents with internet gaming addiction. Behav Brain Funct. 2013;9(1):33.
24. Brown MW, Banks PJ. In search of a recognition memory engram. Neurosci Biobehav Rev. 2015;50:12–28.
25. Gogolla N, Takesian AE, Feng G, Fagiolini M, Hensch TK. Sensory integration in mouse insular cortex reflects GABA circuit maturation. Neuron. 2014;83(4):894–905.
26. Nussbaum D, Honarmand K, Govoni R, Kalahani-Bargis M, Bass S, Ni X, Laforge K, Burden A, Romero K, Basarke S. An eight component decision-making model for problem gambling: a systems approach to stimulate integrative research. J Gambl Stud. 2011;27(4):523–63.
27. Kantamneni S. Cross-talk and regulation between glutamate and GABAB receptors. Front Cell Neurosci. 2015;9:135.
28. Enna SJ, Blackburn TP. GABAB receptor pharmacology—a tribute to Norman Bowery. Preface. Adv Pharmacol. 2010;58:123–47.
29. Fu Z, Yang H, Xiao Y, Zhao G, Huang H. The gamma-aminobutyric acid type B (GABAB) receptor agonist baclofen inhibits morphine sensitization by decreasing the dopamine level in rat nucleus accumbens. Behav Brain Funct. 2012;8:20.
30. Onishchenko N, Tamm C, Vahter M, Hokfelt T, Johnson JA, Johnson DA, Ceccatelli S. Developmental exposure to methylmercury alters learning and induces depression-like behavior in male mice. Toxicol Sci. 2007;97(2):428–37.
31. Krackow S, Vannoni E, Codita A, Mohammed Ah, Cirulli F, Branchi I, Alleva E, Reichelt A, Willuweit A, Voikar V. Consistent behavioral phenotype differences between inbred mouse strains in the IntelliCage. Genes Brain Behav. 2010;9(7):722–31.
32. Coppin G. The anterior medial temporal lobes: their role in food intake and body weight regulation. Physiol Behav. 2016;167:60–70.
33. Eichenbaum H. Memory: organization and control. Annu Rev Psychol. 2017;68:19–45.
34. Lee JQ, Zelinski EL, McDonald RJ, Sutherland RJ. Heterarchic reinstatement of long-term memory: a concept on hippocampal amnesia in rodent memory research. Neurosci Biobehav Rev. 2016;71:154–66.

35. Gillani Q, Iqbal S, Arfa F, Khakwani S, Akbar A, Ullah A, Ali M, Iqbal FA. Effect of GABAB receptor antagonist (CGP35348) on learning and memory in albino mice. Sci World J. 2014;2014:983651.

36. Terunuma M, Revilla-Sanchez R, Quadros IM, Deng Q, Deeb TZ, Lumb M, Sicinski P, Haydon PG, Pangalos MN, Moss SJ. Postsynaptic GABAB receptor activity regulates excitatory neuronal architecture and spatial memory. J Neurosci. 2014;34(3):804–16.

37. Khanegheini A, Nasehi M, Zarrindast MR. The modulatory effect of CA1 GABAb receptors on ketamine-induced spatial and non-spatial novelty detection deficits with respect to Ca(2+). Neuroscience. 2015;305:157–68.

38. Schipper S, Aalbers MW, Rijkers K, Lagiere M, Bogaarts JG, Blokland A, Klinkenberg S, Hoogland G, Vles JS. Accelerated cognitive decline in a rodent model for temporal lobe epilepsy. Epilepsy Behav. 2016;65:33–41.

39. Paxinos G, Watson C. The rat brain in stereotaxic coordinates. San Diego, CA: Academic Press; 1986.

8

Association of tryptophan hydroxylase-2 polymorphisms with oppositional defiant disorder in a Chinese Han population

Chang-Hong Wang[1†], Cong Liu[1†], En-Zhao Cong[1], Gai-Ling Xu[1], Ting-Ting Lv[1], Ying-Li Zhang[1], Qiu-Fen Ning[1], Ji-Kang Wang[1], Hui-Yao Nie[1*‡] and Yan Li[2*‡]

Abstract

Background: Oppositional defiant disorder (ODD) is a behavioral disorder of school-age population. It is well known that 5-HT dysfunction is correlated with impulsivity, which is one of the common characteristics of ODD. The enzyme tryptophan hydroxylase-2 (TPH-2) synthesizes 5-HT in serotonergic neurons of the midbrain raphe. The purposes of this study were to investigate the potential association of *TPH-2* polymorphisms with susceptibility to ODD in a Han Chinese school population.

Methods: Four polymorphisms (rs4570625, rs11178997, rs1386494 and rs7305115) of the TPH-2 gene were analyzed by using polymerase chain reaction and DNA microarray hybridization in a case–control study of 276 Han Chinese individuals (124 ODD and 152 controls).

Results: In single marker analyses,there was a significant difference in the genotype ($x^2 = 4.163$, $P = 0.041$) and allele frequency ($x^2 = 3.930$, $P = 0.047$) of rs1386494 between ODD and control groups. Haplotype analyses revealed higher frequencies of haplotypes TA (rs4570625-rs11178997), TAG (rs4570625-rs11178997-rs1386494), TAA (rs4570625-rs11178997-rs7305115) and TAGA (rs4570625-rs11178997-rs1386494-rs7305115), but lower frequencies of haplotypes GA (rs4570625-rs11178997) and GAG (rs4570625-rs11178997-rs1386494) in ODD compared to control groups.

Conclusions: These findings suggest the role of these *TPH-2* gene variants in susceptibility to ODD. Some haplotypes might be the risk factors for Chinese Han children with ODD, while others might be preventable factors.

Keywords: Oppositional defiant disorder, Tryptophan hydroxylase-2 gene, Single nucleotide polymorphisms

Background

Oppositional defiant disorder (ODD) is a behavioral disorder mainly characterized by resistance, disobedience, provocation or hostility to authority figures during growth and development in children and adolescents [1, 2]. Children and adolescents with ODD may have trouble controlling their temper, showing intense emotional reaction or impulsive actions in response to mild stimulation. Thus, ODD is considered as a disorder of emotional regulation [3]. Children suffering from ODD are at risk for numerous negative outcomes, such as delinquency, unemployment, depression, anxiety and other psychiatric problems [4]. However, the pathological mechanisms of ODD are still unclear.

Based on DSM-IV-TR, the prevalence rate for ODD is 2–16% [5]. Well established in previous research, this disorder exhibits moderate heritability, and is substantially stable over time, particularly through childhood [6], and genetic underpinning is an important factor which can influence children's disruptive behavior, like ODD [7].

*Correspondence: niehuiyao@163.com; liyanzzu2009@126.com
[†]Chang-Hong Wang and Cong Liu contributed equally to this work
[‡]Yan Li and Hui-Yao Nie have contributed equally to this work
[1] Department of Psychiatry, The Second Affiliated Hospital of Xinxiang Medical University (Psychiatric hospital of Henan province, China), Xinxiang 453002, Henan, China
[2] Department of Child and Adolescent, Public Health College, Zhengzhou University, 100 Kexue Road, Zhengzhou 450001, Henan, China

Familial clustering suggests an underlying genetic component, but hereditary connections are variable [1]. ODD has been consistently associated with attention-deficit/hyperactivity disorder (ADHD) [8, 9] and conduct disorder (CD) [10–13]. The estimated heritability of ADHD is approximately 0.76 [14] and 40–60% of ADHD were also diagnosed with ODD [15], suggesting that ODD might share common genetic mechanisms with ADHD [8]. However, the comorbidity of ODD may influence the clinical characteristics, progression and treatment response for ADHD cases [14].

Serotonin (5-HT) is a neurotransmitter involved in various bodily functions, such as aggression, attention, appetite and locomotion. The deficiency of the 5-HT functions is related to depression, anxiety, irregular appetite, aggression, increased pain sensation, and ADHD symptoms [16]. Especially, 5-HT dysfunction is correlated with impulsivity, which is one of the common characteristics of ADHD, ODD, personality disorder [17] and substance abuse [18, 19]. Early studies reported a clear association between low cerebrospinal fluid 5-HT and impulsive aggression [20]. The conversion of tryptophan to 5-hydroxytryptophan is the first and rate limiting step in 5-HT synthesis catalyzed by two subtypes of the enzyme tryptophan hydroxylase (TPH-1 and TPH-2); 5-HT is then formed by decarboxylation of 5-hydroxytryptophan. The studies revealed differential expression of classical TPH-1 synthesizing 5-HT in peripheral tissues, and TPH-2 synthesizing 5-HT mainly in serotonergic neurons of the midbrain raphe [21]. In mice brain stems, the expression of TPH-1 appears to be 150 times lower than TPH-2 [21], suggesting that TPH-2 may play a much more important role in serotonin synthesis in the brain than TPH-1. Thus, the studies have focused on the role of brain-specific TPH-2 in the pathophysiology of various psychiatric disorders, including ADHD [16].

The human TPH-2 gene spans less than 100 kb, consists of 11 exons and is located in the chromosome 12q21.1 region. Several studies have explored the association between TPH-2 gene polymorphisms and ADHD. For example, Sheehan et al. [22] firstly reported the association between TPH2-rs1843809 and ADHD through a family study. A subsequent study reported association between TPH2-rs4570625 or TPH2-rs11178997 and ADHD through a family study [23]. A more recent study showed that a significant correlation between the frequencies of the rs11179027 and rs1843809 of alleles of TPH-2 and ADHD [16]. In addition, the TPH-2 gene polymorphism have been found to be associated with late-onset depression [24], PTSD [25, 26], suicide in patients with alcohol dependence [27, 28] and suicidal behavior [29], as well as with schizophrenia [30, 31] and panic in bipolar disorders [32] in the Chinese Han population.

In view of the possible shared common genes between ADHD and ODD, the important role of TPH-2 in 5-HT synthesis in brain and the possible association between TPH-2 gene polymorphisms and ADHD, as well as the associations of the TPH-2 gene polymorphism with behavioral and psychiatric disorders in previous studies, it would be of interest to examine the association between TPH-2 gene polymorphisms and ODD, which, to our best knowledge, has not been reported. Therefore, the main purpose of the current study was to examine whether the TPH-2 gene polymorphisms was associated with the susceptibility to ODD in a Chinese Han population.

Methods
Subjects
Using the random group sampling method, 2000 Chinese Han students in primary school in Nanyang, Henan Province, China were assessed with Conners Teachers Rating Scale between 2007 and 2009, all four grandparents and both parents of each child were known to be of Han Chinese origin. To confirm the diagnosis of ODD, one or both parents and teachers were interviewed by a chief physician and resident physician on the basis of DSM-IV diagnostic criteria. Inclusion criteria were: (a) aged 6–14 years; (b) had ODD symptoms at least 6 months; (c) intelligence quotient (IQ) ≥ 70 based on Raven's Progressive Matrices; (d) no physical diseases, mental retardation, low body mass index (BMI, <18.5 kg/m^2) or other mental illnesses, or ADHD or CD symptoms. A total of 125 children were confirmed with ODD diagnosis. Among them, 124 subjects were enrolled in the study, including 70 boys (56.5%) and 54 girls (43.5%) with an average age of 10.4 ± 1.9 years.

Data also consisted of 152 control subjects (boy/girl = 78/74), who were recruited from the same primary school. Mean age was 10.5 ± 1.6 years. Inclusion criteria were: (a) aged 6–14 years; (b) no any ODD symptoms; (c) intelligence quotient (IQ) ≥ 70 based on Raven's Progressive Matrices; (d) no physical diseases, mental retardation, low body mass index (BMI, <18.5 kg/m^2) or other mental illnesses, or ADHD or CD symptoms.

There was no significant differences in gender, age and education between ODD and control groups (all $P > 0.05$). This study was approved by the Ethical Committee of the Second Affiliated Hospital, Xinxiang Medical College, Henan Province. Informed consent was obtained from all subjects and their parents.

TPH-2 genotyping
5 ml blood samples were collected from cubital vein between 8:00 and 9:00 a. m. following an overnight fast and placed into the tubes with EDTA anticoagulant. Samples were stored at -70 °C until assayed.

DNA was extracted using a Genomic DNA extraction kit (DP318) (TIANGEN biotechnology company, Beijing, China). The DNA was amplified by polymerase chain reaction (PCR) methods and the primers for the four loci (rs4570625, rs11178997, rs1386494 and rs7305115) were designed by Invitrogen Corporation (Shanghai, China). Oligonucleotide sequences are presented in Table 1.

The total volume of the PCR reaction was 30 µl which contained 0.5 µl whole genome DNA (50 ng/µl), 3 µl $10\times$ PCR buffer solution, 0.5 µl 10 mm L^{-1} dNTPs, 0.5 µl each primer, 0.3 µl Taq polymerase, 1.5 µl 25 mm L^{-1} MgCl$_2$, and 23.7 µl sterile water. Loop parameters for PCR were as follows: initial denaturation at 95 °C for 5 min, amplification at 94 °C for 30 s, annealing at 54/56 °C for 45 s, and extension at 72 °C for 45 s. The process was repeated 34 times, followed by extension at 72 °C for 5 min. PCR products were placed onto glass slides disposed with acrylamide by a Pixsys5500 microarrayer (Cartesian Products, Inc. America) [33]. The PCR products were hybridized with fluorescence-labeled probes at 37 °C for 5–6 h, and the glass slides were scanned with a LuxScan-10k confocal scanner (Capitalbio Corporation, Beijing, China). The genotype of each sample was detected based on the fluorescent signals [34].

Statistical analysis

Differences between genotype groups were analyzed using Chi squared for categorical variables and the Student's t test or one-way analysis of variance (ANOVA) for continuous variables using the PASW Statistics 18.0 software (SPSS Inc., Chicago, IL, USA).

Deviation from the Hardy–Weinberg equilibrium (HWE) was tested separately in cases and controls using Chi square (χ^2) goodness-of-fit test. The difference in the allele and genotype frequencies for TPH-2 polymorphisms between ODD and normal controls was analyzed using the χ^2 test. Pairwise linkage disequilibrium (LD) between four TPH-2 markers was analyzed in cases and normal controls. Haploview 4.2 was used to compute pairwise

LD statistics for markers, haplotype block, haplotype frequency, and haplotype association. We used a 2–4-window fashion analysis. Rare haplotypes found in less than 3% were excluded from the association analysis. A logistic regression analysis was conducted to examine the independent association of each haplotype on the categorical diagnosis of case (0: control, 1: case) after adjusting for the confounders. To control haplotype analyses for multiple testing, 10,000 permutations were performed for the most significant tests to determine the empirical significance.

The power (power defined as the chance that true differences will actually be detected) of the sample was calculated using Quanto Software [35], with known risk allele frequencies and an ODD population prevalence of 0.02–0.16, and we examined log additive, recessive and dominant models.

Results

Single locus analysis

The genotype and allele frequencies of four SNPs located in the TPH-2 gene are summarized in Table 6. No deviation from HWE was detected in the cases or controls (all $P > 0.05$; Tables 2, 3, 4, 5). Significant differences in the genotype and allele frequencies between cases and controls were observed for rs1386494 (genotype $\chi^2 = 4.163$, $P = 0.041$; allele $\chi^2 = 3.930$, $P = 0.047$). The frequency of the Gallele of rs1386494 was higher in patients than in controls. There was no allelic or genotypic association between the other three SNPs and ODD (all $P > 0.05$, Table 6).

Linkage disequilibrium (LD) analysis

LD analyses were performed for all polymorphism pairs in both case and control subjects. All four polymorphisms were in slight to modest LD or without LD with each other in both control (D' = 0.12–0.92; r^2 = 0.02–0.71) and patient groups (D' = 0.10–0.76; r^2 = 0.00–0.16) (Fig. 1).

Haplotype analysis

Two–four SNP sliding window haplotype analyses were performed. Only those haplotypes with a frequency above 3% were included in the analyses. Estimation of haplotype frequencies and comparison of haplotype frequency distributions between cases and controls were conducted using the program Haploview.

We observed significant differences in the frequencies of TA ($P = 0.014$, $OR = 1.951$, 95% CI 1.140–3.341) and GA ($P = 0.012$, $OR = 0.149$, 95% CI 0.027–0.826) haplotypes containing rs4570625-rs11178997 between case and control groups.

Also, we noted significant differences in the frequencies of TAG ($P = 0.02$, $OR = 1.896$, 95% CI 1.099–3.272)

Table 1 Primer sequences of these four loci

SNP ID	Primer sequence (5′–3′)
rs4570625	F: 5′-GAACCCTTACCTTTCCTTTG-3′
	R: 5′Acry-TCCACTCTTCCAGTTATTTT-3′
rs11178997	F: 5′-GTGTTCGGGAGCACAATAAT-3′
	R: 5′ Acry -AAGCCTGCCACTGGAAGTT-3′
rs1386494	F: 5′-TGTTTCTCGCAGGTTGTTGG-3′
	R: 5′ Acry-AGCAAATGAATCACAAAGGG-3′
rs7305115	F: 5′-TAGTTGGTTTTTCTGTTGC-3′
	R: 5′Acry-CCCTTTTCTCTTTAGGTGAG-3′

Sequences of the four primers

Table 2 rs4570625 Hardy–Weinberg Equilibrium test between ODD and control group

Group	Genotype					
	GG	GT	TT	Total	χ^2	P
ODD group					1.474	0.225
Observation (O)	27	51	38	116		
Expectation (E)	23.761	57.478	34.761	116		
Control group					1.301	0.254
Observation (O)	36	83	33	152		
Expectation (E)	39.515	75.970	36.51	152		

df = 1

Table 3 rs11178997 Hardy–Weinberg equilibrium test between ODD and control group

Group	Genotype				χ^2	χ^{2*}	P
	AA	AT	TT	Total			
ODD group						1.292	0.256
Observation (O)	6	33	84	123			
Expectation (E)	4.116*	36.768	82.116	123			
Control group						0.052	0.820
Observation (O)	4	39	109	152			
Expectation (E)	3.633*	39.734	108.63	152			

df = 1, when E is little than 5, we use Yates corrected Chi squared test, χ^{2*}

Table 4 rs1386494 Hardy–Weinberg equilibrium test between ODD and control group

Group	Genotype				χ^2	χ^{2*}	P
	AA	AG	GG	Total			
ODD group						0.138	0.711
Observation (O)	0	8	116	124			
Expectation (E)	0.129*	7.742	116.129	124			
Control group						0.856	0.355
Observation (O)	0	21	128	149			
Expectation (E)	0.740*	19.520	128.740	149			

df = 1* when E is little than 5, we use Yates corrected Chi squared test, χ^{2*}

Table 5 rs7305115 Hardy–Weinberg equilibrium test between ODD and control group

Group	AA	AG	GG	Total	χ^2	P
ODD group					3.389	0.533
Observation (O)	34	56	29	119		
Expectation (E)	32.303	59.395	27.302	119		
Control group					0.844	0.358
Observation (O)	35	64	40	139		
Expectation (E)	2.295	69.410	37.295	139		

df = 1

Table 6　Genotype and allele frequency distribution of the four loci of *THP-2* between two groups

Locus	Genotype (%)			χ^2	P	Allele (%)		χ^2	P
rs4570625	GG	GT	TT	4.525	0.104	G	T	1.729	0.189
ODD	27 (23.3)	51 (44.0)	38 (32.8)			105 (45.3)	127 (54.7)		
Control	36 (23.7)	83 (54.6)	33 (21.7)			155 (51.0)	149 (49.0)		
rs11178997	AA	AT	TT	1.092	0.579	A	T	0.783	0.376
ODD	6 (4.9)	33 (26.8)	84 (68.3)			45 (18.3)	201 (81.7)		
Control	4 (2.6)	39 (25.7)	109 (71.7)			47 (15.5)	257 (84.5)		
rs1386494	AA	AG	GG	4.163	0.041*	A	G	3.930	0.047*
ODD	0	8 (6.5)	116 (93.5)			8 (3.2)	240 (96.8)		
Control	0	21 (14.1)	128 (85.9)			21 (7.0)	277 (93.0)		
rs7305115	AA	AG	GG	0.756	0.685	A	G	0.780	0.377
ODD	34 (28.6)	56 (47.1)	29 (24.4)			124 (52.1)	114 (47.9)		
Control	35 (25.2)	64 (46.0)	40 (28.8)			134 (48.2)	144 (51.8)		

* $P<0.05$

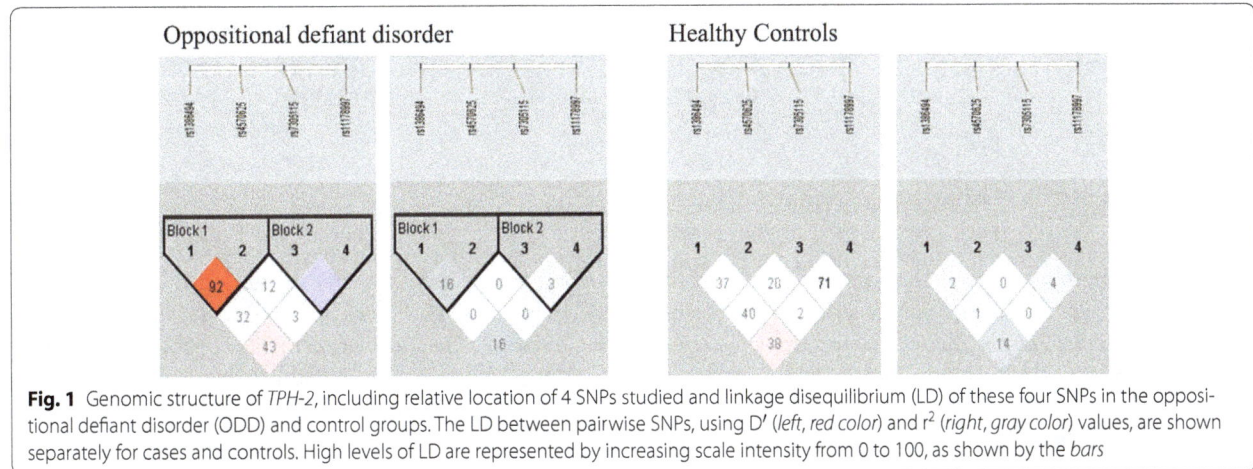

Fig. 1 Genomic structure of *TPH-2*, including relative location of 4 SNPs studied and linkage disequilibrium (LD) of these four SNPs in the opposi-tional defiant disorder (ODD) and control groups. The LD between pairwise SNPs, using D′ (*left, red color*) and r^2 (*right, gray color*) values, are shown separately for cases and controls. High levels of LD are represented by increasing scale intensity from 0 to 100, as shown by the *bars*

and GAG (*P* = 0.013, *OR* = 0.149, 95% *CI* 0.027–0.831) containing rs4570625-rs11178997-rs1386494, as well as TAA (*P* = 0.026, *OR* = 2.315, 95% *CI* 1.088–4.927) con-taining rs4570625-rs11178997-rs7305115 between case and control groups.

Finally, we found significant differences in the frequen-cies of TAGA (*P* = 0.005, *OR* = 3.187, 95% *CI* 1.376–7.382) containing rs4570625-rs11178997-rs1386494-rs7305115 between ODD and control groups (Tables 7, 8).

However, the further analysis by Haploview revealed the nominally significant finding for rs1386494 (χ^2 = 3.846, *P* = 0.0499), and only one haplotypes (TAGA, χ^2 = 4.366, *P* = 0.0367) remained significant. However, the results did not remain statistically sig-nificant after 5000-fold permutation-based analysis incorporating all four SNPs or all the observed hap-lotypes (adjusted both *P* > 0.14). Thus, our study was only considered as preliminary evidence of a possible association.

Power analysis

This total sample had 0.10–0.47 power, 0.31–0.70 power, and 0.36–0.97 power for these four polymorphisms to detect recessive, log additive and dominant polymor-phic inheritance in ODD with an odds ratio (OR) of 2 or greater (alpha = 0.05, two tailed test).

Discussion

To our knowledge, this is the first study to find an association between ODD and the TPH-2 gene poly-morphism rs1386494 or the haplotype formed by this polymorphism and other polymorphisms. While most *TPH-2* association studies have used individual markers, we used polymorphism-based haplotypes and LD analy-sis to show that both ODD and controls shared a homo-geneous LD pattern. This LD suggests that these variants segregate together in a Chinese population.

There is an extensive data consistently showing that decreased functions of the central 5-HT activity are

Table 7 Analysis of genetic linkage disequilibrium of the four loci

SNPs	SNP2		SNP3		SNP4	
	D′	r2	D′	r2	D′	r2
SNP1	0.702	0.090	0.093	0.001	0.405	0.161
SNP2			0.653	0.005	0.001	0.000
SNP3					0.887	0.049

SNP1:rs4570625; SNP2:rs11178997; SNP3:rs1386494; SNP4:rs7305115

Table 8 Haplotype analysis of *TPH-2* between two groups

Haplotype distribution	Case (freq)	Control (freq)	χ^2	Fisher P	OR [95% CI]
SNP1-2					
G-A	1.52 (0.007)	10.57 (0.042)	6.281	0.012233*	0.149 [0.027–0.826]
T-A	40.48 (0.174)	24.43 (0.098)	6.083	0.013679*	1.951 [1.140–3.341]
SNP1-2-3					
G-A-G	1.51 (0.007)	10.51 (0.042)	6.234	0.012562*	0.149 [0.027–0.831]
T-A-G	38.73 (0.167)	24.00 (0.096)	5.409	0.020075*	1.896 [1.099–3.272]
SNP1-2-4					
T-A-A	22.24 (0.096)	10.60 (0.042)	4.981	0.025669*	2.315 [1.088–4.927]
SNP1-2-3-4					
T-A-G-A	21.77 (0.094)	7.79 (0.031)	8.031	0.004617*	3.187 [1.376–7.382]

SNP1:rs4570625; SNP2:rs11178997; SNP3:rs1386494; SNP4:rs7305115 * $P<0.05$

associated with uncontrolled behaviors, including impulsive behavior, aggressiveness, and substance abuse both in humans and in animal models, for example [29, 36, 37]. TPH-2, a rate-limiting enzyme in the biosynthesis of 5-HT, is expressed mainly in brain [38]; thus, it influences the 5-HT level in brain and plays an important role in the development of mental disease [16]. Genetic variation in *TPH-2* activity is likely to represent a critical factor in the pathogenesis of ADHD and impulsivity [16, 23]. Several studies have demonstrated that changes in the 5-HT system were critical in children with ODD [39, 40]. Moreover, the polymorphisms of *TPH-2* have been shown to be associated with ADHD [16, 41, 42], obsessive–compulsive disorder [43], and bipolar affective disorder [44]. Also, *TPH*-2 was found to be associated with major depression [45] and pathogenesis of depression in Chinese females [46] and suicidal behavior [47, 48]. However, there has been no study reporting the relationship between *TPH-2* and ODD.

This study is a case–controlled study in which the frequency of the genotypes and alleles of *TPH-2* polymorphisms were compared between the ODD children and the control group in Chinese Han. The association between the genotypes and alleles of four candidates *TPH-2* SNPs was investigated. Our results showed that there was a significant correlation between the frequencies of the *TPH-2*-rs1386494 and ODD, but not

other three polymorphisms, suggesting that the locus of rs1386494 of *TPH-2* was associated with ODD in Chinese Han children. The association of *TPH-2*-rs1386494 in this study was inconsistent with the result of Walitza et al. [23] study, in which loci of rs4570625 and rs11178997 were found to be associated with ADHD and combined ADHD and ODD, but not rs4565946. There are several reasons to explain the inconsistent results. First, the subjects in Walitza's study included both ADHD and ODD. Second, the linkage disequilibrium analysis in the core family was used in Walitza's study while the case-control association was used in several studies including our current study. Thus, the differential analysis methods and different samples may contribute to discrepant results.

Haplotypes can be more specific risk markers than single alleles, and their use reduces false-positive associations that can occur because common psychiatric disorders are likely to associate with common alleles [49]. Since the four markers analyzed were in the same haplotype block, we performed the two–four SNP sliding window haplotype analysis [50]. We found that the frequencies of the TA and GA haplotypes containing rs4570625-rs11178997, the TAG and GAG haplotypes containing rs4570625-rs11178997-rs1386494, the TAA haplotype containing rs4570625-rs11178997-rs7305115, and the TAGA haplotype containing rs4570625-rs11178997-rs1386494-rs7305115 were significantly different between ODD and controls (all $P < 0.05$). Further, TA, TAG, TAA and TAGA haplotypes might be the risk factors for ODD, while GA and GAG haplotypes might be protective for ODD in Chinese Han children.

Several limitations of this study should be noted. First, the number of subject children was small. The subjects of this study were 124 ODD children and 152 children in the control group. Since our sample size provided only poor statistical power, it is possible that we do see the false-positive results in the present study and our findings need to be considered cautiously. A replication study would be needed to include a large sample size. Second, although we had genotyped four polymorphisms in the present study, the coverage of genetic variation is too limited considering the total *TPH-2* gene variants includes at least 50 polymorphisms. Therefore, it would be much better to use GWAS in larger samples to capture true positive results found in our present study. Third, the samples in our current study were only from local city in Henan province, China. Thus, the findings of this study may not be generalized for the cases of other racial or ethnic groups since the frequency of alleles can vary due to local or racial differences. Fourth, it would be better to use DSM-V as a reference rather than DSM-IV. Unfortunately, we had no DSM-V when our current study was conducted. We will use DSM-V as a reference in our future investigation to remedy this shortcoming.

In summary, we report several convergent findings that implicate an effect of *TPH-2* genotype on increased risk for ODD. We found a potential genetic association of *TPH-2* with risk for ODD, especially the *TPH-2* gene polymorphism rs1386494. Further haplotype analyses showed that TA, TAG, TAA and TAGA haplotypes might be the risk factors for ODD, while GA and GAG haplotypes might be protective for ODD in Chinese Han children. However, the findings in our present study remain preliminary due to the limited sample size and our low statistical power, as well as poor coverage of genetic variations in *THP-2*, which require replication in larger samples of ODD children from different ethnic populations.

Appendix

ODD group

Sex (1=boy; 2=girl)	Age	rs4570625	rs11178997	rs1386494	rs7305115
1	8	GT	AT	GG	AG
2	6	TT	AT	GG	AG
1	7	GT	AT	GG	AG
1	8	TT	AT	GG	AA
2	9	GG	TT	GG	GG

Sex (1=boy; 2=girl)	Age	rs4570625	rs11178997	rs1386494	rs7305115
1	9	GT	TT	GG	AA
2	7	TT	TT	GG	AA
1	10	TT	TT	AG	AA
1	13	TT	AT	GG	AG
1	10	GT	TT	GG	AG
2	10	GT	TT	GG	AG
2	9	TT	AT	GG	AA
2	7	GT	TT	GG	AG
2	9	GG	TT	GG	GG
2	10	GT	TT	AG	AG
2	10	TT	TT	GG	AA
1	9	GT	TT	GG	AG
2	10	GT	TT	GG	GG
1	8	GG	TT	GG	GG
2	9	GG	TT	GG	GG
1	10	GG	TT	GG	GG
2	12	TT	AA	GG	AG
1	10	TT	AT	GG	AA
1	9	GG	TT	GG	AG
2	10	GT	AT	GG	GG
2	10	GT	AT	AG	AA
2	9	TT	AT	GG	AA
1	11	TT	TT	GG	AA
1	14	TT	AT	GG	AG
2	14	TT	AA	AG	AG
1	12	TT	TT	GG	AA
2	14	GT	TT	GG	AG
2	9	GT	AT	GG	AG
1	10	GT	TT	GG	AG
1	11	GG	TT	GG	AG
1	12	GG	TT	AG	AG
1	10	TT	TT	GG	AG
2	12	GT	TT	GG	AG
2	12	GG	TT	GG	AG
2	13	GT	AT	GG	AG
1	11	GT	AT	AG	AG
2	8	GT	AT	GG	GG
2	8	GT	TT	GG	AG
1	8	GT	TT	GG	AG
2	12	GG	TT	GG	GG
1	9	GG	TT	AG	AA
1	11	GT	TT	GG	AG
1	11	GT	TT	GG	AA
1	9	TT	AA	GG	AG
2	10	TT	TT	GG	AA
1	7	TT	TT	GG	AA
2	7	GT	TT	GG	GG
1	11	GT	AT	GG	GG
1	10	GT	TT	GG	AG

Cognitive Neuroscience: Behavioral and Psychological Perspectives

Sex (1=boy; 2=girl)	Age	rs4570625	rs11178997	rs1386494	rs7305115
2	11	GT	TT	GG	AG
1	10	TT	TT	GG	GG
1	11	TT	TT	GG	AA
2	12	GT	TT	GG	AA
2	10	GG	AT	GG	GG
1	12	GT	AT	GG	AG
1	14	TT	TT	GG	GG
1	7	GG	TT	AG	AA
2	8	TT	AA	GG	AA
2	9	GT	TT	GG	AA
2	12	TT	TT	GG	AA
1	9	TT	AT	GG	GG
1	9	GG	TT	GG	AG
2	9	GG	TT	GG	AG
2	12	TT	AT	GG	GG
2	11	TT	TT	GG	AG
1	10	GG	TT	GG	GG
2	11	GG	TT	GG	GG
2	10	GG	TT	GG	AG
1	12	GT	TT	GG	AG
2	11	GT	TT	GG	AG
2	11	GT	TT	GG	AG
1	9	GG	TT	GG	GG
2	8	GT	TT	GG	AG
1	12	GT	AT	GG	AA
1	12	GT	TT	GG	AA
2	7	GT	AT	GG	AG
1	14	TT	TT	GG	AA
1	12	GT	TT	GG	AA
1	10	GT	TT	GG	AG
1	12	TT	TT	GG	AA
2	12	GG	TT	GG	AG
1	11	TT	AT	GG	AA
1	13	TT	TT	GG	AG
1	14	GT	TT	GG	AG
2	8	GG	TT	GG	AG
1	8	GT	TT	GG	AG
2	13	GT	AT	GG	AG
2	10	GG	TT	GG	GG
1	13	GG	TT	GG	GG
2	8	GG	TT	GG	GG
2	9	TT	AA	GG	GG
1	8	GT	TT	GG	AG
2	13	TT	TT	GG	AA
1	13	GT	AT	GG	AG
1	9	TT	AT	GG	GG
2	11	GT	TT	GG	GG
1	13	GG	TT	GG	GG
2	10	GT	TT	GG	AA
1	10	TT	AA	GG	AG
2	10	GT	TT	GG	AG
1	8	GG	TT	GG	AG
1	9	GT	TT	GG	AA
1	9	TT	AT	GG	AA
1	12	GG	TT	GG	GG
2	13	TT	TT	GG	AG
1	9	TT	AT	GG	AG
1	10	GT	TT	GG	AA
1	12	GT	AT	GG	GG
1	13	GT	AT	GG	AA
1	12	GT	AT	GG	GG
1	13	TT	TT	GG	AG
1	11		AT	GG	AA
1	12		AT	GG	AG
1	11		TT	GG	AG
2	12		TT	GG	
1	12		TT	GG	
1	11		TT	GG	
1	12		TT	GG	
1	13			GG	

Control group

Sex (1=boy; 2=girl)	Age	rs4570625	rs11178997	rs1386494	rs7305115
1	8	GG	TT	GG	GG
2	7	TT	TT	GG	AA
1	7	GT	TT	AG	AA
2	9	GT	TT	GG	AG
2	10	GT	TT	GG	AG
1	9	TT	TT	GG	AA
2	8	GT	TT	GG	AG
1	8	GT	TT	AG	AG
1	11	GG	TT	GG	GG
1	9	GG	TT	GG	GG
2	10	TT	AT	AG	AA
2	10	GG	TT	GG	GG
2	13	GT	TT	GG	GG
1	11	TT	TT	GG	AA
1	13	TT	TT	GG	GG
2	7	GT	TT	GG	AG
1	12	GT	TT	GG	AG
1	14	GT	AT	GG	AA
1	10	GG	TT	AG	AA
1	12	GT	TT	GG	GG
2	12	TT	AT	GG	AG
2	11	GG	TT	AG	AG
2	11	GG	TT	GG	GG

Sex (1=boy; 2=girl)	Age	rs4570625	rs11178997	rs1386494	rs7305115
2	9	GG	TT	GG	AA
2	11	GT	TT	GG	AG
2	12	GT	AT	GG	AA
2	10	GT	TT	GG	AA
1	13	GT	TT	GG	AA
1	9	GG	TT	GG	GG
1	9	GT	TT	GG	AG
1	8	GT	TT	GG	AA
2	7	TT	AT	GG	AG
2	10	TT	TT	GG	AA
1	11	GT	TT	AG	AG
1	12	GT	TT	GG	AA
2	10	GG	TT	GG	GG
1	12	TT	AT	GG	AG
2	11	TT	TT	GG	GG
2	11	GG	TT	GG	AG
2	11	GG	TT	GG	AG
1	11	GG	TT	GG	GG
2	12	TT	TT	GG	GG
2	10	GT	AT	GG	AA
1	9	GG	TT	AG	AG
1	11	GT	TT	GG	AG
2	12	GG	AA	GG	AG
1	12	GT	AT	GG	GG
2	12	GT	TT	GG	AG
2	12	GT	TT	GG	AG
2	9	GT	TT	GG	GG
1	9	GT	TT	GG	AG
1	11	TT	AA	GG	AG
2	14	GT	TT	GG	AG
1	12	GG	TT	GG	AG
1	12	GT	AT	GG	AG
1	12	TT	TT	GG	AA
1	11	GG	TT	GG	AG
1	12	GT	TT	GG	AG
1	12	GG	AT	GG	AG
1	12	GT	AT	GG	GG
1	12	TT	TT	GG	AG
1	12	TT	TT	GG	AA
1	12	GG	AT	GG	AG
1	11	GT	AT	GG	AG
1	10	GG	TT	GG	GG
2	11	GT	AT	GG	GG
2	13	GT	TT	GG	AA
2	13	GT	TT	GG	AG
2	12	TT	AT	GG	AG
2	13	TT	TT	GG	GG
2	12	GG	TT	GG	GG
2	11	GT	TT	AG	AA
2	10	GG	TT	GG	GG
1	10	GT	TT	GG	AA
2	10	TT	AT	AG	AA
2	11	GT	TT	AG	AA
2	10	GT	AT	GG	AG
2	10	GT	AT	GG	AG
2	9	GT	TT	GG	AG
2	10	GG	TT	GG	GG
2	9	TT	AT	GG	AA
2	10	GT	AT	GG	GG
2	10	TT	TT	GG	AA
1	8	GT	TT	GG	AG
1	9	TT	TT	AG	AA
2	10	TT	TT	GG	GG
2	9	GT	TT	GG	AG
1	10	GT	AT	AG	AG
1	11	TT	TT	AG	AG
1	12	GT	TT	GG	AG
2	13	GT	TT	GG	AA
2	10	GG	TT	GG	AG
2	11	GT	AT	GG	GG
1	11	GT	TT	AG	AG
2	11	TT	TT	GG	AA
1	11	GT	TT	GG	AG
2	13	GG	TT	GG	AG
1	13	TT	TT	GG	AG
2	13	GT	TT	GG	AG
1	11	TT	AT	GG	AG
2	10	GG	TT	GG	GG
2	8	GT	TT	GG	AG
2	9	GT	TT	GG	AG
1	9	GT	AT	GG	GG
1	10	GT	AT	GG	GG
1	11	GT	TT	GG	AG
1	10	GT	AT	GG	AG
1	11	GT	AT	GG	AG
2	10	GG	TT	GG	GG
1	9	GT	TT	AG	AA
2	12	GT	AA	GG	AG
2	12	GT	TT	GG	AG
1	11	GT	TT	GG	AG
1	7	GT	TT	GG	AG
1	10	TT	TT	· GG	AA
1	8	GG	TT	GG	GG
1	11	GT	TT	GG	AG
2	13	GG	TT	GG	GG
1	12	GG	AT	GG	AA
1	10	GG	TT	GG	AA
1	10	GT	TT	GG	GG

Sex (1=boy; 2=girl)	Age	rs4570625	rs11178997	rs1386494	rs7305115
2	8	GT	TT	GG	AG
2	8	GT	AT	AG	AG
1	12	GG	TT	GG	GG
1	12	GG	TT	GG	GG
2	7	TT	TT	GG	AG
1	7	GT	TT	AG	GG
2	9	GT	AT	GG	GG
2	10	GT	AT	AG	AG
1	9	TT	TT	GG	AA
2	10	GT	AT	GG	GG
1	8	GT	AT	AG	GG
1	11	GG	TT	GG	GG
1	9	GG	AT	GG	AA
2	10	TT	TT	AG	AA
2	10	GT	TT	GG	GG
2	13	GT	TT	GG	AG
1	11	TT	AT	GG	AG
1	11	TT	TT	AG	AA
2	7	GT	TT	GG	
1	12	GT	TT	GG	
1	11	GT	AT	GG	
1	10	GT	TT	GG	
1	12	GT	AT	GG	
1	12	TT	AT	GG	
2	11	GT	AT	GG	
1	11	GT	AT	GG	
2	9	GG	TT	GG	
1	11	GT	TT	GG	
2	12	GT	TT		
2	10	GT	TT		
1	8	GT	AA		

Abbreviations

ODD: oppositional defiant disorder; CD: conduct disorder; ADHD: attention-deficit/hyperactivity disorder; *TPH-2*: the tryptophan hydroxylase-2 gene; 5-HT: serotonin; IQ: intelligence quotient; PCR: polymerase chain reaction; SNP: single nucleotide polymorphisms.

Authors' contributions

C-HW and CL contributed equally for this study and are both considered as first authors, they created the design of the study and the experimental paradigm, managed the acquisition of the data, analyzed and interpreted the data, and wrote the first draft. E-ZC, G-LX and T-TL has been involved in collecting study subjects. Y-LZ did the guidance of laboratory methods in this study, Q-FN managed the acquisition of the data, analyzed and interpreted the data as an assistant, J-KW has been involved in drafting and revising the manuscript. YL and H-YN are the corresponding authors and have contributed equally to this work. All authors read and approved the final manuscript.

Acknowledgements

We warmly thank the children and their parents who kindly took part in this research, as well as the schools and the teachers who agreed to collaborate in this study. We warmly thank Xiang Yang Zhang to help us modify our language errors.

Competing interests

The related authorities and the authors declare that they all have no competing interest. The authors declare that the research was conducted in the absence of any commercial, financial (and non-financial) relationships that could be construed as a potential competing interests.

Funding

This work was supported by grants from the Medical Technology Foundation of Henan Province (142300410025 and 112102310211), Scientific Research Fund of Xinxiang Medical University (2013ZD117) and Ministry of Health research fund projects in China (20090103). Henan Provincial Department of Science and Technology Research Project (102101310400).

References

1. Riley M, Ahmed S, Locke A. Common questions about oppositional defiant disorder. Am Fam Physician. 2016;93(7):586–91.
2. Frick PJ, Nigg JT. Current issues in the diagnosis of attention deficit hyperactivity disorder, oppositional defiant disorder, and conduct disorder. Annu Rev Clin Psychol. 2012;8:77–107. doi:10.1146/annurev-clinpsy-032511-143150.
3. Cavanagh M, Quinn D, Duncan D, Graham T, Balbuena L. Oppositional defiant disorder is better conceptualized as a disorder of emotional regulation. J Atten Disord. 2014;[Epub ahead of print]. doi:10.1177/1087054713520221.
4. Bradshaw CP, Schaeffer CM, Petras H, Ialongo N. Predicting negative life outcomes from early aggressive-disruptive behavior trajectories: gender differences in maladaptation across life domains. J Youth Adolesc. 2010;39(8):953–66. doi:10.1007/s10964-009-9442-8.
5. Gomez R, Hafetz N, Gomez RM. Oppositional defiant disorder: prevalence based on parent and teacher ratings of Malaysian primary school children. Asian J Psychiatry. 2013;6(4):299–302. doi:10.1016/j.ajp.2013.01.008.
6. Pihlakoski L, Sourander A, Aromaa M, Rautava P, Helenius H, Sillanpää M. The continuity of psychopathology from early childhood to preadolescence: a prospective cohort study of 3 to 12-year-old children. Eur Child Adolesc Psychiatry. 2006;15(7):409–17. doi:10.1007/s00787-006-0548-1.
7. Burke JD, Loeber R, Birmaher B. Oppositional defiant disorder and conduct disorder: a review of the past 10 years, part II. J Am Acad Child Adolesc Psychiatry. 2002;41:1275–93. doi:10.1097/01.CHI.0000024839.60748.E8.
8. Tuvblad C, Zheng M, Raine A, Baker LA. A common genetic factor explains the covariation among ADHD ODD and CD symptoms in 9–10 year old boys and girls. J Abnorm Child Psychol. 2009;37(2):153–67. doi:10.1007/s10802-008-9278-9.
9. Gopin CB, Berwid O, Marks DJ, Mlodnicka A, Halperin JM. ADHD preschoolers with and without ODD: do they act differently depending on degree of task engagement/reward? J Atten Disord. 2013;17(7):608–19. doi:10.1177/1087054711432140.
10. Liu L, Cheng J, Li H, Yang L, Qian Q, Wang Y. The possible involvement of genetic variants of NET1 in the etiology of attention-deficit/hyperactivity disorder comorbid with oppositional defiant disorder. J Child Psychol Psychiatry. 2015;56(1):58–66. doi:10.1111/jcpp.12278.
11. Rowe R, Costello EJ, Angold A, Copeland WE, Maughan B. Developmental pathways in oppositional defiant disorder and conduct disorder. J Abnorm Psychol. 2010;119(4):726–38. doi:10.1037/a0020798.
12. Coolidge FL, Thede LL, Young SE. Heritability and the comorbidity of attention deficit hyperactivity disorder with behavioral disorders and executive function deficits: a preliminary investigation. Dev Neuropsychol. 2000;17(3):273–87. doi:10.1207/s15326942dn1703_1.
13. Lahey BB, Waldman ID. Annual research review: phenotypic and causal structure of conduct disorder in the broader context of prevalent forms of psychopathology. J Child Psychol Psychiatry. 2012;53(5):536–57. doi:10.1111/j.1469-7610.2011.02509.x.
14. Faraone SV, Mick E. Molecular genetics of attention deficit hyperactivity disorder. Psychiatr Clin North Am. 2010;33(1):159–80. doi:10.1016/j.psc.2009.12.004.
15. Dittmann RW, Schacht A, Helsberg K, Schneider-Fresenius C, Lehmann M, Lehmkuhl G, Wehmeier PM. Atomoxetine versus placebo in children and adolescents with attention-deficit/hyperactivity disorder and comorbid

oppositional defiant disorder: a double-blind, randomized, multicenter trial in Germany. J Child Adolesc Psychopharmacol. 2011;21(2):97–110. doi:10.1089/cap.2009.0111.

16. Park TW, Park YH, Kwon HJ, Lim MH. Association between *TPH2* gene polymorphisms and attention deficit hyperactivity disorder in Korean children. Genet Test Mol Biomark. 2013;17(4):301–6. doi:10.1089/gtmb.2012.0376.

17. Marazziti D, Baroni S, Masala I, Golia F, Consoli G, Massimetti G, Picchetti M, Catena Dell'osso M, Giannaccini G. Impulsivity, gender, and the platelet serotonin transporter in healthy subjects. Neuropsychiatr Dis Treat. 2010;6:9–15.

18. Brewer JA, Potenza MN. The neurobiology and genetics of impulse control disorders: relationships to drug addictions. Biochem Pharmacol. 2008;75(1):63–75. doi:10.1016/j.bcp.2007.06.043.

19. Coccaro EF, Lee R. Cerebrospinal fluid 5-hydroxyindolacetic acid and homovanillic acid: reciprocal relationships with impulsive aggression in human subjects. J Neural Transm. 2010;117(2):241–8. doi:10.1007/s00702-009-0359-x.

20. Glick A. The role of serotonin in impulsive aggression, suicide, and homicide in adolescents and adults: a literature review. Int J Adolesc Med Health. 2015;27(2):143–50. doi:10.1515/ijamh-2015-5003.

21. Walther DJ, Bader M. A unique central tryptophan hydroxylase isoform. Biochem Pharmacol. 2003;66(9):1673–80. doi:10.1016/S0006-2952(03)00556-2.

22. Sheehan K, Lowe N, Kirley A, Mullins C, Fitzgerald M, Gill M, Hawi Z. Tryptophan hydroxylase 2 (TPH2) gene variants associated with ADHD. Mol Psychiatry. 2005;10(10):944–9. doi:10.1038/sj.mp.4001698.

23. Walitza S, Renner TJ, Dempfle A, Konrad K, Wewetzer Ch, Halbach A, Herpertz-Dahlmann B, Remschmidt H, Smidt J, Linder M, Flierl L, Knölker U, Friedel S, Schäfer H, Gross C, Hebebrand J, Warnke A, Lesch KP. Transmission disequilibrium of polymorphicvariants in the tryptophan hydroxylase-2 gene in attention-deficit/hyperactivity disorder. Mol Psychiatry. 2005;10(12):1126–32. doi:10.1038/sj.mp.4001734.

24. Pereira Pde A, Romano-Silva MA, Bicalho MA, De Marco L, Correa H, de Campos SB, de Moraes EN, Torres KC, de Souza BR, de Miranda DM. Association between tryptophan hydroxylase-2 gene and late-onset depression. Am J Geriatr Psychiatry. 2011;19(9):825–9. doi:10.1097/JGP.0b013e31820eeb21.

25. Goenjian AK, Bailey JN, Walling DP, Steinberg AM, Schmidt D, Dandekar U, Noble EP. Association of TPH1, TPH2, and 5HTTLPR with PTSD and depressive symptoms. J Affect Disord. 2012;140(3):244–52. doi:10.1016/j.jad.2012.02.015.

26. Goenjian AK, Noble EP, Steinberg AM, Walling DP, Stepanyan ST, Dandekar S, Bailey JN. Association of COMT and TPH-2 genes with DSM-5 based PTSD symptoms. J Affect Disord. 2014;172C:472–8. doi:10.1016/j.jad.2014.10.034.

27. Wrzosek M, Łukaszkiewicz J, Wrzosek M, Serafin P, Jakubczyk A, Klimkiewicz A, Matsumoto H, Brower KJ, Wojnar M. Association of polymorphisms in *HTR2A, HTR1A* and *TPH2* genes with suicide attempts in alcohol dependence: a preliminary report. Psychiatry Res. 2011;190(1):149–51. doi:10.1016/j.psychres.2011.04.027.

28. Zupanc T, Pregelj P, Paska AV. Tryptophan hydroxylase 2 (TPH-2) single nucleotide polymorphisms, suicide, and alcohol-related suicide. Psychiatr Danub. 2013;25(Suppl 2):332–6.

29. Perez-Rodriguez MM, Weinstein S, New AS, Bevilacqua L, Yuan Q, Zhou Z, Hodgkinson C, Goodman M, Koenigsberg HW, Goldman D, Siever LJ. Tryptophan-hydroxylase 2 haplotype association with borderline personality disorder and aggression in a sample of patients with personality disorders and healthy controls. J Psychiatr Res. 2010;44(15):1075–81. doi:10.1016/j.jpsychires.

30. Zhang C, Li Z, Shao Y, Xie B, Du Y, Fang Y, Yu S. Association study of tryptophan hydroxylase-2 gene in schizophrenia and its clinical features in Chinese Han population. J Mol Neurosci. 2011;43(3):406–11. doi:10.1007/s12031-010-9458-2.

31. Xu XM, Ding M, Pang H, Wang BJ. TPH2 gene polymorphisms in the regulatory region are associated with paranoid schizophrenia in Northern Han Chinese. Genet Mol Res. 2014;13(1):1497–507. doi:10.4238/2014.March.12.1.

32. Campos SB, Miranda DM, Souza BR, Pereira PA, Neves FS, Tramontina J, Kapczinski F, Romano-Silva MA, Correa H. Association study of tryptophan hydroxylase 2 gene polymorphisms in bipolar disorder patients with panic disorder comorbidity. Psychiatr Genet. 2011;21:106–11. doi:10.1097/YPG.0b013e328341a3a8.

33. Xiao PF, Cheng L, Wan Y, Sun BL, Chen ZZ, Zhang SY, Zhang CZ, Zhou GH, Lu ZH. An improved gel-based DNA microarray method for detecting single nucleotide mismatch. Electrophoresis. 2006;27(19):3904–15. doi:10.1002/elps.200500918.

34. Xiao P, Huang H, Zhou G, Lu Z. Gel immobilization of acrylamide-modified single-stranded DNA template for pyrosequencing. Electrophoresis. 2007;28(12):1903–12. doi:10.1002/elps.200600794.

35. Gauderman WJ. Sample size requirements for association studies of gene-gene interaction. Am J Epidemiol. 2002;155(5):478–84.

36. Silva H, Iturra P, Solari A, Villarroel J, Jerez S, Jiménez M, Galleguillos F, Bustamante ML. Fluoxetine response in impulsive-aggressive behavior and serotonin transporter polymorphism in personality disorder. Psychiatr Genet. 2010;20(1):25–30. doi:10.1097/YPG.0b013e328335125d.

37. Audero E, Mlinar B, Baccini G, Skachokova ZK, Corradetti R, Gross C. Suppression of serotonin neuron firing increases aggression in mice. J Neurosci. 2013;33(20):8678–88. doi:10.1523/JNEUROSCI.2067-12.2013.

38. Chen GL, Miller GM. Advances in tryptophan hydroxylase-2 gene expression regulation: new insights into serotonin-stress interaction and clinical implications. Am J Med Genet B Neuropsychiatr Genet. 2012;159B(2):152–71. doi:10.1002/ajmg.b.32023.

39. Martel MM, Nikolas M, Jernigan K, Friderici K, Nigg JT. Diversity in pathways to common childhood disruptive behavior disorders. J Abnorm Child Psychol. 2012;40(8):1223–36. doi:10.1007/s10802-012-9646-3.

40. Brammer WA, Lee SS. Prosociality and negative emotionality mediate the association of serotonin transporter genotype with childhood ADHD and ODD. J Clin Child Adolesc Psychol. 2013;42(6):809–19. doi:10.1080/15374416.2013.840638.

41. Waider J, Araragi N, Gutknecht L, Lesch KP. Tryptophan hydroxylase-2 (*TPH2*) in disorders of cognitive control and emotion regulation: a perspective. Psychoneuroendocrinology. 2011;36(3):393–405. doi:10.1016/j.psyneuen.

42. Shim SH, Hwangbo Y, Kwon YJ, Jeong HY, Lee BH, Hwang JA, Kim YK. A case-control association study of serotonin 1A receptor gene and tryptophan hydroxylase 2 gene in attention deficit hyperactivity disorder. Prog Neuropsychopharmacol Biol Psychiatry. 2010;34(6):974–9. doi:10.1016/j.pnpbp.

43. Rocha FF, Alvarenga NB, Lage NV, Romano-Silva MA, Marco LA, Corrêa H. Associations between polymorphic variants of the tryptophan hydroxylase 2 gene and obsessive-compulsive disorder. Rev Bras Psiquiatr. 2011;33:176–80.

44. Carkaci-Salli N, Salli U, Tekin I, Hengst JA, Zhao MK, Gilman TL, Andrews AM, Vrana KE. Functional characterization of the S41Y (C2755A) polymorphism of tryptophan hydroxylase 2. J Neurochem. 2014;130(6):748–58. doi:10.1111/jnc.12779.

45. Gao J, Pan Z, Jiao Z, Li F, Zhao G, Wei Q, Pan F, Evangelou E. TPH2 gene polymorphisms and major depression–a meta-analysis. PLoS ONE. 2012;7(5):e36721. doi:10.1371/journal.pone.0036721.

46. Shen X, Wu Y, Qian M, Wang X, Hou Z, Liu Y, Sun J, Zhong H, Yang J, Lin M, Li L, Guan T, Shen Z, Yuan Y. Tryptophan hydroxylase 2 gene is associated with major depressive disorder in a female Chinese population. J Affect Disord. 2011;133(3):619–24. doi:10.1016/j.jad.2011.04.037.

47. Zupanc T, Pregelj P, Tomori M, Komel R, Paska AV. *TPH2* polymorphisms and alcohol-related suicide. Neurosci Lett. 2011;490(1):78–81. doi:10.1016/j.neulet.2010.12.030.

48. Lazary J, Viczena V, Dome P, Chase D, Juhasz G, Bagdy G. Hopelessness, a potential endophenotpye for suicidal behavior, is influenced by *TPH2* gene variants. Prog Neuropsychopharmacol Biol Psychiatry. 2012;36(1):155–60. doi:10.1016/j.pnpbp.2011.09.001.

49. Lohmueller KE, Pearce CL, Pike M, Lander ES, Hirschhorn JN. Meta-analysis of genetic association studies supports a contribution of common variants to susceptibility to common disease. Nat Genet. 2003;33(2):177–82. doi:10.1038/ng1071.

50. Gabriel SB, Schaffner SF, Nguyen H, Moore JM, Roy J, Blumenstiel B, Higgins J, DeFelice M, Lochner A, Faggart M. The structure of haplotype blocks in the human genome. Science. 2002;296(5576):2225–9. doi:10.1126/science.1069424.

9

Cognitive behavioural therapy attenuates the enhanced early facial stimuli processing in social anxiety disorders: an ERP investigation

Jianqin Cao[1], Quanying Liu[2,3], Yang Li[1], Jun Yang[1], Ruolei Gu[4,5], Jin Liang[4,5], Yanyan Qi[4,5], Haiyan Wu[4,5]* and Xun Liu[4,5]

Abstract

Background: Previous studies of patients with social anxiety have demonstrated abnormal early processing of facial stimuli in social contexts. In other words, patients with social anxiety disorder (SAD) tend to exhibit enhanced early facial processing when compared to healthy controls. Few studies have examined the temporal electrophysiological event-related potential (ERP)-indexed profiles when an individual with SAD compares faces to objects in SAD. Systematic comparisons of ERPs to facial/object stimuli before and after therapy are also lacking. We used a passive visual detection paradigm with upright and inverted faces/objects, which are known to elicit early P1 and N170 components, to study abnormal early face processing and subsequent improvements in this measure in patients with SAD.

Methods: Seventeen patients with SAD and 17 matched control participants performed a passive visual detection paradigm task while undergoing EEG. The healthy controls were compared to patients with SAD pre-therapy to test the hypothesis that patients with SAD have early hypervigilance to facial cues. We compared patients with SAD before and after therapy to test the hypothesis that the early hypervigilance to facial cues in patients with SAD can be alleviated.

Results: Compared to healthy control (HC) participants, patients with SAD had more robust P1–N170 slope but no amplitude effects in response to both upright and inverted faces and objects. Interestingly, we found that patients with SAD had reduced P1 responses to all objects and faces after therapy, but had selectively reduced N170 responses to faces, and especially inverted faces. Interestingly, the slope from P1 to N170 in patients with SAD was flatter post-therapy than pre-therapy. Furthermore, the amplitude of N170 evoked by the facial stimuli was correlated with scores on the interaction anxiousness scale (IAS) after therapy.

Conclusions: Our results did not provide electrophysiological support for the early hypervigilance hypothesis in SAD to faces, but confirm that cognitive-behavioural therapy can reduce the early visual processing of faces. These findings have potentially important therapeutic implications in the assessment and treatment of social anxiety.

Trial registration HEBDQ2014021

Keywords: Social anxiety disorder, Cognitive-behavioural therapy, P1, N170, Hyper-vigilance

---

*Correspondence: wuhy@psych.ac.cn
[4] CAS Key Laboratory of Behavioral Science, Institute of Psychology,
Chinese Academy of Sciences, 16 Lincui Road, Chaoyang District,
Beijing 100101, China
Full list of author information is available at the end of the article

Background

Social anxiety disorder (SAD) is a mental disorder characterized by significant fear of negative evaluation and avoidance of interpersonal situations [1, 2]. Over the past decades, an extensive body of research has been devoted to various cognitive symptoms related to SAD, such as attentional biases, negative interpretation biases, and expectancy and memory biases [3–10]. Cognitive models of anxiety [11, 12] have suggested that information processing biases lead patients with social anxiety to view social situations in an excessively negative fashion [13–15]. Due to this interpretation bias, patients with SAD tend to judge ambiguous faces as more angry than happy [16]. However, it is worth mentioning that another study did not report similar interpretation bias [17]. If such interpretation bias exists in SAD for faces, even neutral faces may be viewed as more negative by patients with SAD. Considering that many behavioural and neuroimaging studies have provided convincing evidence that social anxiety is linked to attention bias toward threatening facial stimuli [18–23], there may also be enhanced attention toward neutral faces when compared to those of healthy control subjects.

Compared to other objects, the human face is prominent due to its capacity to convey attractiveness, trustworthiness, or emotions with biological significance in social interactions [24–27]. Studies have indicated that faces with direct eye contact may elicit avoidant and escape responses in individuals with social anxiety disorders [28, 29]. For example, a study using a modified dot-probe task (objects vs. expressions) showed that individuals with social phobia direct their attention away from faces and toward household objects [28]. This suggests that individuals with social anxiety may have impaired processing of faces. Although much effort has been made to examine attention bias or processing abnormalities in response to different emotional expressions in individuals with social anxiety, to our knowledge, no study has directly investigated facial perception abnormalities per se in comparison to object perception in patients with SAD. Therefore, whether SAD is associated with abnormal early processing of facial stimuli remains unclear.

Electrophysiological brain responses may be useful in clarifying whether SAD is associated with enhanced early processing of facial stimuli, as they have high temporal resolution, which may help to differentiate early vs. late attention processes during the processing of facial stimuli. Previous studies have identified different ERP components reflective of different stages of facial perception or attention bias [30–35]. It has been demonstrated that threat-related faces elicit shorter latencies and greater amplitudes of early ERP components (e.g., the P1, N1, and N170) in individuals with high anxiety than in those with low anxiety [30, 36]. An ERP study used the Stroop paradigm with non-emotional stimuli, explicit emotion tasks, and implicit emotion tasks to examine the impact of perceptual and task factors on facial processing in individuals with social anxiety. The authors found that there were enhanced P1 responses during all tasks in individuals with social anxiety, and that this effect was independent of the effects of perceptual or task factors [37]. Such P1 enhancement effects were also found in individuals with sub-clinical SAD in response to happy, angry, fearful, disgusted, and neutral faces. This indicates that there is early attentional capture even by neutral faces in individuals with SAD [38].

Another face-sensitive ERP component is the N170, which is a temporal-parietal negativity associated with facial perceptual coding [39–44]. Prior studies have indicated that N170 is enhanced in response to inverted faces (N170 face inversion effect), but not inverted objects. This supports the idea that N170 is specifically affected by faces [44–46]. The processing of inverted faces typically involves additional early recruitment of visual processing resources when compared to that of upright faces [47]. Social anxiety has been characterized by attentional bias toward threatening or ambiguous faces. However, the manner in which social anxiety affects the processing of inverted faces and whether therapy can alter such processing abnormalities remain unclear.

Cognitive-behavioural therapy (CBT) is a time-limited present-oriented approach to psychotherapy that teaches patients the cognitive and behavioural competencies required to function adaptively in their interpersonal and intrapersonal worlds. CBT is also the most studied non-pharmacologic approach for the treatment of social anxiety disorder [48]. To date, a large number of investigations have demonstrated the efficacy of CBT as a treatment for SAD [49–53]; Scaini et al. [54, 55]. Cognitive-behavioural group therapy (CBGT) has also been reported to be an effective therapeutic approach in reducing the symptoms of anxiety and depression in individuals with anxiety disorders [56–59]. For instance, using an Educational Supportive Group Psychotherapy (ESGP) group as a control, Heimberg et al. [60] examined the effectiveness of CBGT in SAD. They found that the phobic severity rating scale scores of patients undergoing CBGT improved to a great extent after treatment. These patients also reported less anxiety before and during the behavioural test. Interestingly, the 5-year follow-up study (patients who received CBGT or an alternative treatment were contacted 4.5–6.25 years after the initial treatment) also suggested that patients who received CBGT had more lasting improvements than those receiving ESGP treatments [61]. Few studies regarding the treatment of

SAD have investigated neuroimaging data or brain activity changes pre- and post-therapy [62–65].

A handful of studies reported in the literature suggest that therapy leads to global modulations of brain activity, such as attenuated amygdala activity [65]. However, studies of EEG data on therapy effect in patients with SAD are rare. To our knowledge, there are two EEG studies have examined such therapy induced EEG change effect on SAD. One study indicated patients shifted significantly from greater relative right to greater relative left resting frontal EEG activity from pre- to post treatment [66], while another suggested greater coupling between EEG delta and beta oscillations in pre-treatment SAD than control and the coupling EEG normalized after treatment [67]. Compared to these EEG in rest studies, event-related potential(ERP) technique, which permit to investigate behavioural and neural activity(specific ERP components) and relationship between the two with high temporal resolution, may contribute to testing our hypothesis of the underlying early face or object processing mechanism of abnormality in SADs.

Despite these advances, clinical studies have yet to examine whether SAD is associated with abnormal early processing of facial stimuli and whether CBGT can reduce such abnormal neural symptoms. The primary objective of this study was to examine whether social anxiety is associated with abnormalities at the early stages of processing of face-related information, and to investigate neural changes (i.e., P1–N170 effect) after CBGT. The P1–N170 effect, include the P1 effect, the N170 effect and the slope from P1 to N170. Based on the hypervigilance hypothesis of SAD, we expected to observe an enhanced P1–N170 effect in SAD patients. That is, we hypothesized that SAD will show larger P1 and N170 amplitude and larger P1–N170 slope when they processing face-configurational information, especially for inverted faces. Furthermore, we also expect a

treatment effect on theses enhanced early P1/N170 or the P1–N170 slope effect. Specifically, after CBGT, we expected to find decreased P1–N170 responses to faces, which would be reflective of improvements in anxiety symptoms in patients with SAD.

Methods
Participants

The study was carried out in accordance with the Declaration of Helsinki and the experimental protocols used were approved by the institutional review board (IRB) of Harbin Medical University. Eighteen outpatients with SAD were recruited from the Psychology Department of Affiliated Hospital of Harbin Medical University, while 18 healthy control (HC) participants were recruited through advertisements. The patients with SAD (3 men and 15 women, mean age = 33.61 ± 8.84 years) were diagnosed using the validated Chinese translation of the Structured Clinical Interview for Diagnostic and Statistical Manual of Mental Disorders, Fourth Edition (DSM-IV) (SCID-IV) [68], which is the gold standard for assessing SAD in China. Control participants were demographically matched HCs with no history of DSM-IV psychiatric disorders. Specifically, participants' gender, age and education year are being matched and detail information for both groups are shown in Table 1. These individuals were also screened using the SCID. All participants were right-handed and reported no psychoactive substance abuse, no unstable medical illness, and no past or current neurological illness. The subjects' anxiety symptoms were assessed using the brief social phobia scale (BSPS, [69]) and the interaction anxiousness scale (IAS, [70]). All participants provided written informed consent for the experiment. One patient with SAD and the matched HC were excluded because they dropped out from the therapy. We thus carried out the study using a sample of 17 patients with SAD and 17 HC participants.

Table 1 Summary of sociodemographic and self-report measures of mood and symptom severity for participants with social anxiety disorder (SAD) and healthy controls

	SAD group (n = 17)	Healthy controls (n = 17)	T or χ²-test (df = 32)
Age (years)	33.29 (9.01)	33.65 (9.42)	−0.112
Sex (% women)	82%	82%	
Education (years)	13.24 (2.05)	14.29 (2.17)	−1.46
IAS	57.59 (5.23)	34.47 (6.97)	10.932[***]
BSPS	45.12 (11.51)	9.65 (5.43)	11.491[***]
Flower counts	Pre: 60.13; post: 60	Pre: 59.82; post: 59.88	All p > 0.19

Values provided as means (standard deviations)

SAD social anxiety disorder, IAS interaction anxiousness scale, BSPS brief social phobia scale

*** p < 0.001

Demographic data and the self-reported measures of the final 34 participants in the two groups are presented in Table 1. As shown in Table 1, the groups did not differ in demographic characteristics. Compared to those in the HC group, participants in the SAD group reported higher levels of social anxiety.

Stimuli and passive visual detection paradigm

The paradigm was adopted from He et al. [71]. The stimuli used in the study included 60 photographs of unfamiliar young faces, 60 photographs of tables, and 60 photographs of flowers, which were all selected from neutral pictures in the Chinese affective picture system (CAPS). Pictures were all in grey-scale and all were resized to 8 cm × 12 cm, half of the faces were of men and the other half were of women. All face stimuli were trimmed to exclude hair and non-facial contours (Fig. 1). There are five stimulus conditions in the passive visual detection paradigm: upright faces, inverted faces, upright tables, inverted tables, and upright flowers. Sixty trials for each condition were presented in the EEG experiment (total of 300 trials). The stimuli were presented at the centre of a computer screen and were viewed from a distance of 80 cm. All stimuli were presented on a blank background shown on a 17-in. computer screen using a personal computer running E-Prime.

Each trial began with the presentation of a stimulus cross for 1000 ms, followed by a blank screen of 950–1050 ms. All stimuli were presented randomly with 250-ms durations and inter-stimulus intervals randomized to range from 650 ms to 850 ms. Subjects were instructed to pay attention to the presented stimuli and to count the flowers (i.e., targets) in each presentation block. The subjects reported the number of flowers counted upon completion of the viewing of each block. All stimuli were randomized and counterbalanced across participants. Every block comprised of upright faces, upright tables, inverted faces, inverted tables, and targets, 20 trials of each condition in one block. There were 60 trials for each condition presented in three blocks.

Cognitive behavioural group therapy

CBGT was administered by a clinical psychologist and a college psychology teacher. The therapy comprises intensive intervention and consolidation of treatment for 37.5 h over 1 year. The CBGT procedure was conducted following the CBGT treatment guidelines established in Heimberg et al. [72], which includes (1) psychological education, (2) assessment of conceptual ability, (3) cognitive modules, and (4) a behaviour module. The intensive intervention was performed over 12 sessions and lasted 30 h in total (4 sessions/month, lasting 3 months). In the first three sessions, psychological education and

assessment of conceptual ability are conducted to achieve case conceptualization. Patients were taught to understand the normalization and change laws of anxiety, the cognitive model of SAD, factors responsible for the maintenance or an increase in anxiety, and so on. These sessions were designed to enable patients to identify negative cognition ("automatic thoughts" [ATs]), to observe covariation in anxiety, to understand ATs and behavioural responses, to set treatment goals, to master completing homework, etc. The cognitive module and behavioural module are presented in the 4th to 11th sessions. In these sessions, patients are taught to use disputation, coping skills, behavioural experiments, exposure skills, and role-playing to challenge logical errors in their ATs. They are also taught to formulate rational alternatives and behavioural responses. Furthermore, they confront increasingly difficult feared situations (in the session and in real life) while applying cognitive and behavioural skills. When the patients worked on their personal target situations, a standard sequence was followed: identification of ATs and identification of logical errors in ATs, which was followed by disputation of ATs and formulation of rational responses. Thereafter, patients practiced cognitive skills while completing behavioural tasks (e.g., conversing with another group member or giving a speech). Goal attainment and use of cognitive skills were reviewed. Behavioural experiments were used to confront specific reactions to the exposure. Patients were provided with assignments pertinent to exposure to real-life situations across the sessions. In the 12th session, patients were instructed to complete self-administered cognitive restructuring and behavioural skill exercises in real life.

The consolidation treatment is carried out to ensure that the patients implement the self-administered cognitive restructuring and behavioural skill exercises in real life. According to the patient's feedback, the researcher and the intervener provide further guidance for better therapeutic effect. Consolidation treatments were implemented after the 3rd, 6th, and 9th months of the intensive intervention for 7.5 h. The therapy session lasted for about 1 year and the time interval between the two EEG recordings in patients with SAD was 1 year. Patients with SAD performed the passive visual detection paradigm before and after the therapy.

EEG recording and pre-processing

The participants sat comfortably in an electrically shielded room approximately 80 cm from a computer screen. The EEG data were recorded using a 64-channel NeuroScan system (NeuroScan Inc., Herndon, VA). Raw EEG data were sampled at 1000 Hz/channel, with impedances lower than 5 kΩ. Vertical electrooculograms (VEOGs) were recorded supra- and infra-orbitally at the

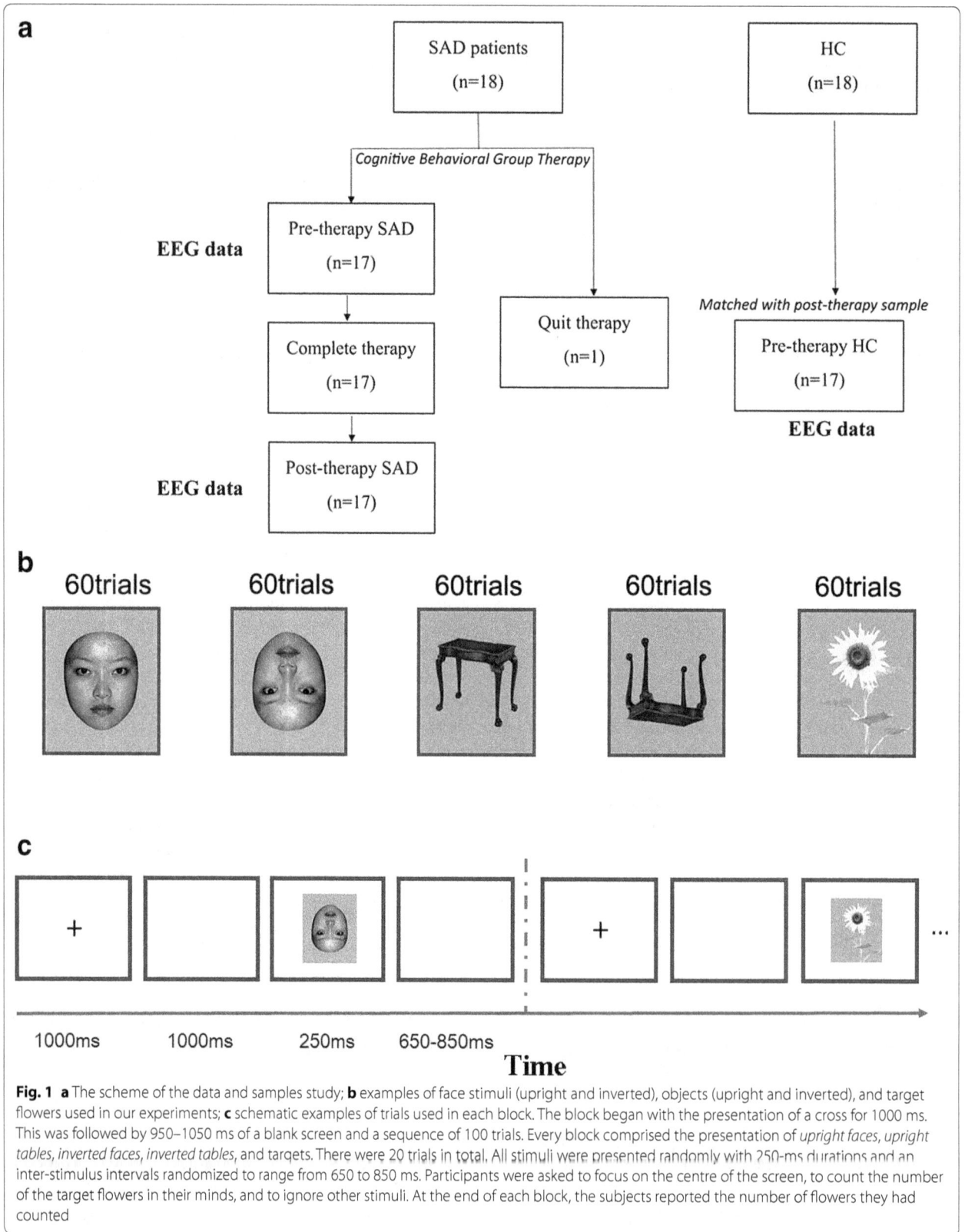

Fig. 1 a The scheme of the data and samples study; **b** examples of face stimuli (upright and inverted), objects (upright and inverted), and target flowers used in our experiments; **c** schematic examples of trials used in each block. The block began with the presentation of a cross for 1000 ms. This was followed by 950–1050 ms of a blank screen and a sequence of 100 trials. Every block comprised the presentation of *upright faces, upright tables, inverted faces, inverted tables,* and *targets.* There were 20 trials in total. All stimuli were presented randomly with 250-ms durations and an inter-stimulus intervals randomized to range from 650 to 850 ms. Participants were asked to focus on the centre of the screen, to count the number of the target flowers in their minds, and to ignore other stimuli. At the end of each block, the subjects reported the number of flowers they had counted

left eye. Horizontal electrooculograms (HEOGs) were recorded by electrodes at the left and right orbital rims. Online recordings were referenced to the nasion. We used a bandpass filter of 0.05–100 Hz.

EEG data were filtered using a low pass of 30 Hz (24 dB/oct) off-line. Epochs were face stimulus-locked and began 200 ms before face onset and ended 600 ms after face onset. Ocular artefacts were removed from EEGs using a regression procedure implemented in Neuroscan software (Scan 4.5). Trials exceeding the threshold of ± 80 µV were excluded from further analysis. As a result, 14.3% of the epochs obtained from all participants were rejected. To test the possible accepted trial numbers difference between group, we run two t-tests of accepted trial numbers for pre-SAD ($M = 51.35$, $SE = 0.99$) vs. HC($M = 52.35$, $SE = 0.55$), and post-SAD ($M = 50.94$, $SE = 1.11$) vs. HC. The results showed no group difference in trial numbers, all $t < 1.009$, all $p > 0.33$. Trials using the four conditions of interest (upright faces, inverted faces, upright tables, and inverted tables) were averaged, and a −200- to 0-ms baseline was used to perform a baseline correction (Fig. 2).

ERP analysis

We first analysed group differences (HC vs. SAD) in ERPs in response to faces and objects before CBGT. The grand-averaged ERPs at PO7/PO8 and the corresponding topography maps of the N170 in the two groups are presented in Fig. 2. Based on previous literature [73] and visual inspection of the grand-averaged ERPs, we analysed the P1 and N170 over P5, P6, P7, P8, PO5, PO6, PO7, and PO8. The P1 amplitude was detected as the peak amplitude in the time window of 70–120 ms, while the N170 amplitude was detected as the peak amplitude in the time window of 120–200 ms. Since existing studies have suggested that the face inversion effect is associated with the slope between the P1 and N170 peaks [74], we also calculated the slope from P1 to N170 using the formula ($P1_{amplitude} - N170_{amplitude}/N170_{latency} - P1_{latency}$). Mean P1/N170 amplitude, peak latencies of P1/N170, and P1–N170 slope values were averaged across selected electrodes, and then entered into three hypothesis-driven testing analyses of variance (ANOVAs). There were 15 total ANOVAs conducted (3 ANOVAs for P1 amplitude, 3 ANOVAS for N170 amplitude, 3 ANOVAs for P1 latency, 3 ANOVAs for N170 latency, 3 ANOVAs for P1–N170 slope). First, a 4 (condition: upright faces vs. inverted faces vs. upright tables vs. inverted tables) × 2 (group: SAD vs. HC) ANOVA was conducted to test assess abnormalities in pre-therapy processing in the SAD and HC groups. An ANOVA was also conducted to examine the therapy effect on SAD for the different conditions, a 4 (condition: upright faces vs. inverted

faces vs. upright tables vs. inverted tables) × 2 (time: pre-therapy SAD vs. post-therapy SAD). Lastly, a 4 (conditions: upright faces vs. inverted faces vs. upright tables vs. inverted tables) × 2 (time: HC pre-therapy vs. SAD post-therapy) ANOVA was conducted to examine whether CBGT "normalized" ERP patterns for the different conditions in patients with SAD post-therapy. Considering the slope test and the P1/N170 component analysis was not independent, we apply multiple comparison correction point of p < 0.025 across measure type (e.g. p < 0.025 for slope analyses for the P1 and N170 components, same for latency analyses, etc.). The reported degrees of freedom of the F-ratio were corrected using the Greenhouse–Geisser method when the sphericity assumption was violated. To investigate relationship between social anxiety symptom ERP component amplitude, we then run correlations between P1/N170 amplitude (P1-pre, N170-pre, P1-post, N170-post) to the anxiety symptoms(IAS-pre, IAS-post). Considering the unique connection is 4 in our initial analysis, the Bonferroni-corrected p value should be $0.05/4_{\text{(total number of comparisons)}} = 0.0125$.

Results
Behavioural results
Overall behavioural performance
There were 60 targets (flowers) in each test, and all participants had equally good accuracy in target monitoring performance. The mean counts were 60.13, 60, 59.82, 59.88 for the SAD pre-therapy, HC, and SAD post-therapy groups, respectively. No differences were found between the HC and SAD pre-therapy groups, or between the SAD pre-therapy and SAD post-therapy groups, $ps > 0.19$.

Anxiety scores and treatment outcomes of CBGT
A t-test on the IAS scores of the SAD and HC groups revealed higher social anxiety in patients with SAD (mean $[M] = 57.58$, standard error $[SE] = 1.27$) than in HCs ($M = 34.47$, $SE = 1.69$) before the therapy, $t_{16} = 8.67$, $p < 0.001$. A t-test on the IAS scores of patients with SAD before and after therapy revealed significantly lower social anxiety after therapy ($M = 38.59$, $SE = 2.29$), $t_{16} = 7.61$, $p < 0.001$. The IAS scores of the patients with SAD post-therapy were not significantly different than those of the healthy controls, $t_{16} = 1.32$, $p = 0.21$.

The SAD group had higher BSPS scores ($M = 45.12$, $SE = 2.79$) than the HC group ($M = 9.65$, $SE = 1.32$) before the therapy, $t_{16} = 10.11$, $p < 0.001$. Changes in the BSPS score also suggested that social anxiety symptoms improved after therapy ($M = 18.24$, $SE = 2.20$), $t_{16} = 10.67$, $p < 0.001$. However, the BSPS score was still higher in patients with SAD post-therapy than in HCs, $t_{16} = 3.31$, $p < 0.01$.

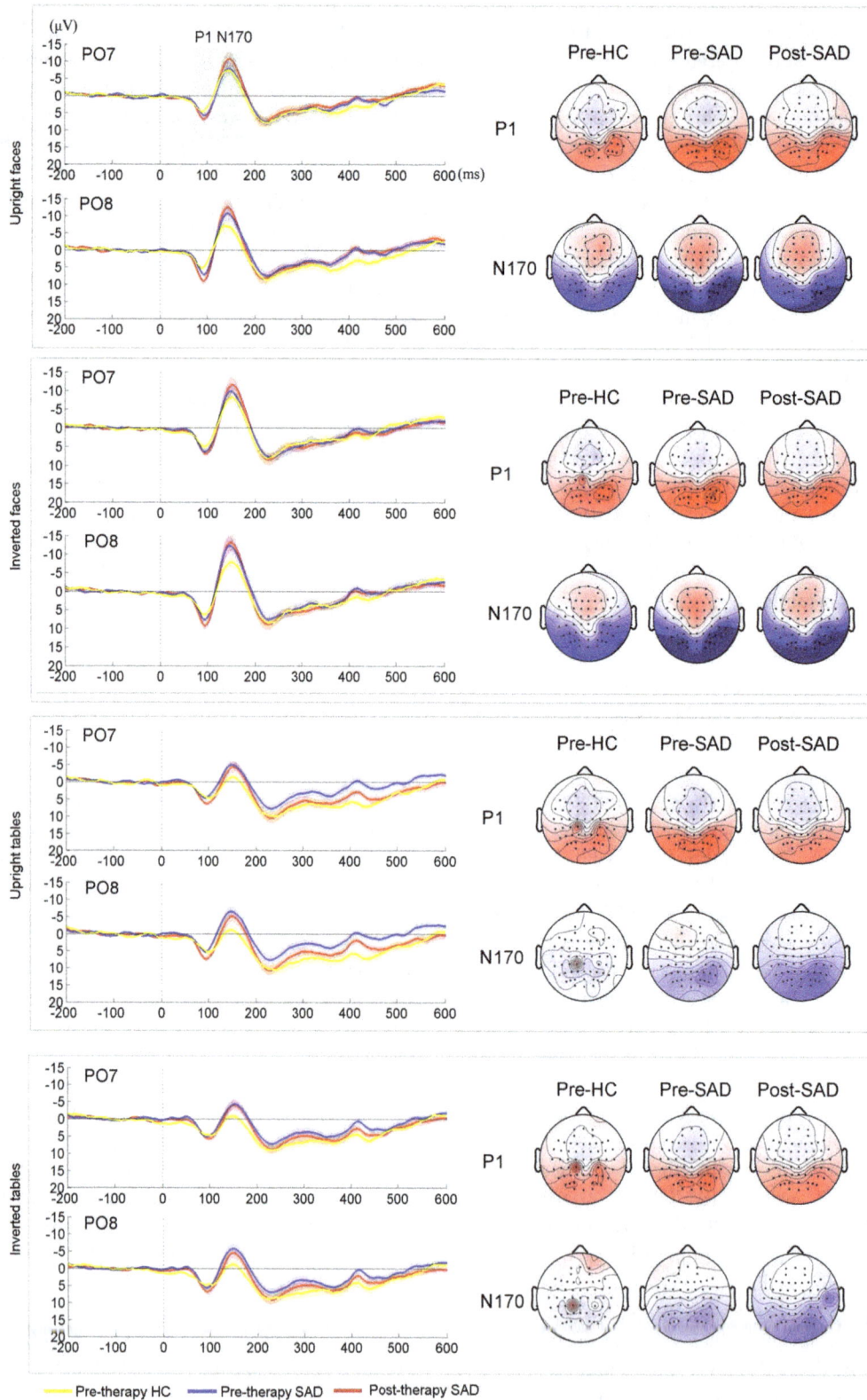

Fig. 2 P1 and N170 analyses for *upright faces*, *inverted faces*, *upright tables*, and *inverted tables*, from *top* to *bottom*. *Left* grand-average ERP time courses according to conditions and groups. The P1 and N170 time periods are marked by *orange* and *green shadows*, respectively. *Middle* scalp topographies of the P1 component over the different conditions and groups. *Right* scalp topographies of the N170 component over different conditions and groups

ERP results

Pre-CBT SAD vs. HC

P1 results We carried out a repeated measures ANOVA on P1 amplitudes of patients with SAD pre-therapy vs. those of HCs. There was no significant group × condition interaction effect ($F_{1, 16} = 1.63$, $p = 0.195$, $\eta_p^2 = 0.092$), the group effect did not reach significance ($F_{1, 16} = 3.58$, $p = 0.062$, $\eta_p^2 = 0.201$). As shown in Fig. 2, the main effect of condition ($F_{3, 14} = 9.82$, $p < 0.001$, $\eta_p^2 = 0.678$) suggested that the inverted faces elicit larger P1 responses ($M = 7.75$ µV, $SE = 0.53$) than upright faces ($M = 6.88$ µV, $SE = 0.49$), upright tables ($M = 6.45$ µV, $SE = 0.48$), or inverted tables ($M = 6.54$ µV, $SE = 0.47$), all $ps < 0.01$ (Fig. 2). The other three conditions were not significant different from each other. An analysis of P1 latency in patients with SAD pre-therapy vs. HCs revealed a main effect of condition ($F_{3, 14} = 12.54$, $p < 0.001$, $\eta_p^2 = 0.729$), with upright faces leading to earlier P1 responses ($M = 93.06$ ms, $SE = 1.85$) than the other three conditions, $ps < 0.05$.

N170 results A repeated measures ANOVA on the N170 amplitude in patients with SAD pre-therapy vs. HCs failed to find significant group effect ($F_{1, 16} = 3.11$, $p = 0.097$, $\eta_p^2 = 0.097$). However, a significant main effect of condition ($F_{3, 14} = 68.00$, $p < 0.001$, $\eta_p^2 = 0.809$) suggested that inverted faces elicit larger N170 responses ($M = -11.29$ µV, $SE = 1.43$) than upright faces ($M = -10.38$ µV, $SE = 1.49$), upright tables ($M = -3.88$ µV, $SE = 1.05$), or inverted tables ($M = -3.42$ µV, $SE = 1.00$), all $ps < 0.05$ (Fig. 2). An analysis of N170 latency in patients with SAD pre-therapy vs. HCs revealed a main effect of condition ($F_{3, 14} = 18.48$, $p < 0.001$, $\eta_p^2 = 0.54$), with upright faces eliciting earlier N170 responses ($M = 145.06$ ms, $SE = 2.18$) than the other three conditions, $ps < 0.001$.

Slope from P1 to N170 To better understand changes in the morphologies of the ERP waveforms, we analysed the slope from P1 to N170 [47]. The SAD group had a steeper change in this slope ($M = 0.32$, $SE = 0.03$) than the HC group ($M = 0.23$, $SE = 0.02$), $F_{1, 16} = 7.02$, $p = 0.017$, $\eta_p^2 = 0.30$. Furthermore, the main effect of condition suggested that the slope is larger in response to faces than to tables, $F_{3, 14} = 16.47$, $p < 0.001$, $\eta_p^2 = 0.779$.

Pre-CBT SAD vs. Post-CBT SAD

P1 results A repeated measures ANOVA of P1 amplitudes in SAD patients pre-therapy vs. post-therapy revealed a significant time effect ($F_{1, 16} = 17.40$, $p < 0.001$, $\eta_p^2 = 0.521$), suggesting that P1 amplitudes are reduced in patients with SAD after therapy ($M = 6.19$ µV, $SE = 0.52$). There was also a significant condition effect ($F_{1, 16} = 12.49$, $p < 0.001$, $\eta_p^2 = 0.438$), suggesting that inverted faces ($M = 7.98$ µV, $SE = 0.68$) and upright faces ($M = 7.57$ µV, $SE = 0.58$) elicit larger P1 responses than upright ($M = 6.09$ µV, $SE = 0.48$) and inverted tables ($M = 6.44$ µV, $SE = 0.58$), $ps < 0.003$ (Fig. 2). However, analysis of P1 latency in patients with SAD pre- vs. post-therapy did not reveal any significant effects, all $Fs < 1.97$, all $ps > 0.18$.

N170 results An ANOVA of N170 amplitude in patients with SAD pre-therapy vs. post-therapy revealed a significant effect of condition ($F_{3, 14} = 45.34$, $p < 0.001$, $\eta_p^2 = 0.739$), suggesting that both inverted ($M = -11.92$ µV, $SE = 1.74$) and upright faces ($M = -10.65$ µV, $SE = 1.69$) elicit larger N170 responses than upright tables ($M = -5.38$ µV, $SE = 1.22$) and inverted tables ($M = -4.93$ µV, $SE = 1.18$), all $ps < 0.05$. Interestingly, we found a significant interaction effect between time and condition, $F_{1, 16} = 6.86$, $p < 0.01$, $\eta_p^2 = 0.30$, suggesting that the reduced N170 effect after therapy only occurs for face stimuli. The simple effect for each condition pre vs. post therapy showed that inverted faces led to a reduction in N170 in SAD post-therapy ($M = -13.11$ µV, $SE = 1.95$) than pre-therapy ($M = -10.79$ µV, $SE = 1.81$), and the significance is approaching the correction point, $p = 0.043$ (Fig. 2). Moreover, the analysis of N170 latency in patients with SAD pre-therapy vs. post-therapy revealed a no significant effects, all $Fs < 3.88$.

Slope from P1 to N170 Interestingly, when we analysed the slope from P1 to N170 in patients with SAD pre-therapy vs. post-therapy, we found a significant interaction between time and condition, $F_{1, 16} = 6.33$, $p = 0.001$, $\eta_p^2 = 0.284$. Further analysis indicated that the slope was generally flattened after therapy, simple effect analyses indicated the pre-post comparison was significant for upright faces (Pre: $M = 0.39$, $SE = 0.05$; Post: $M = 0.33$, $SE = 0.04$) and inverted faces (Pre: $M = 0.39$, $SE = 0.04$; Post: $M = 0.32$, $SE = 0.04$), $ps < 0.013$, but not to objects (Fig. 3).

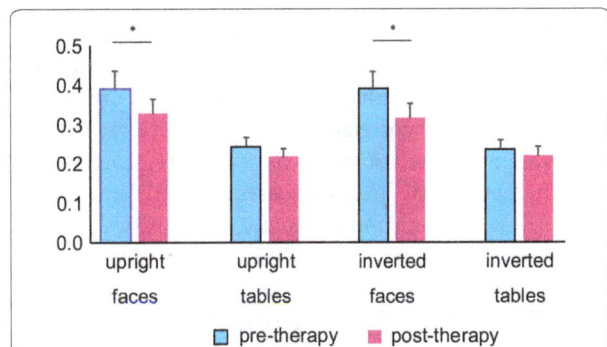

Fig. 3 Slope from P1 to N170 for the *upright faces, upright tables, inverted faces* and *inverted tables*. The slope was calculated for SAD subject's pre-therapy (*blue*) and post-therapy (*red*). Error bars denote standard error. *$p < 0.05$

Post-CBT SAD vs. HC

P1 results ANOVA of P1 amplitudes in HCs pre-therapy vs. patients with SAD post-therapy only revealed a significant condition effect ($F_{1, 16} = 5.84$, $p < 0.01$, $\eta_p^2 = 0.367$), suggesting that inverted faces ($M = 6.79$ μV, $SE = 0.49$) elicit larger P1 responses than upright tables ($M = 5.40$ μV, $SE = 0.42$) and inverted tables ($M = 5.89$ μV, $SE = 0.39$), all ps < 0.008. No other group-related main effect or interaction effect was significant. Analysis of P1 latency in patients with SAD post-therapy compared to HCs showed a pattern that upright faces leading to earlier P1 responses, but was not significant, ps > 0.03 (main effect of condition: $F_{3, 14} = 2.96$, $p = 0.041$, $\eta_p^2 = 0.156$).

N170 results ANOVA of N170 amplitudes in HCs pre-therapy vs. patients with SAD post-therapy only revealed a significant condition effect ($F_{1, 16} = 47.89$, $p < 0.001$, $\eta_p^2 = 0.75$), suggesting that inverted ($M = -10.14$ μV, $SE = 1.35$) and upright faces ($M = -9.38$ μV, $SE = 1.39$) elicit larger N170 responses than upright tables ($M = -4.37$ μV, $SE = 0.88$) and inverted tables ($M = -3.73$ μV, $SE = 0.90$), all ps < 0.025. No other group-related main effect or interaction effect was significant. Analysis of N170 latency in patients with SAD post-therapy compared to HCs only revealed a main effect of condition ($F_{3, 14} = 4.38$, $p < 0.01$, $\eta_p^2 = 0.215$), with upright faces leading to earlier N170 responses ($M = 145.5$ ms, $SE = 2.42$) than the inverted face conditions, $p = 0.001$.

Slope from P1 to N170 ANOVA of the P1–N170 slope in HCs pre-therapy compared to patients with SAD post-therapy only revealed a significant condition effect ($F_{1, 16} = 23.79$, $p < 0.001$, $\eta_p^2 = 0.598$), suggesting that inverted ($M = 0.30$, $SE = 0.03$) and upright faces ($M = 0.31$, $SE = 0.03$) had larger P1–N170 slopes than upright tables ($M = 0.20$, $SE = 0.02$) and inverted tables ($M = 0.19$, $SE = 0.02$), all ps < 0.001. No other group-related main effect or interaction effect was significant.

Correlations between anxiety symptoms and ERP results

To further confirm that higher social anxiety symptoms are correlated with enhanced early face-perception processing, bivariate correlation analyses were performed to examine the relationship between pre-therapy and post-therapy social anxiety scores and P1 and N170, respectively. We only found a significant positive correlation after correction between IAS score in patients with SAD post-therapy and post-therapy N170 amplitude, $r = 0.675$, $p = 0.007$ (Fig. 4). The correlation between pre-therapy social anxiety score and pre-therapy P1/N170 was not significant, ps > 0.23. Correlation analysis of changes in social anxiety scores from pre- to post-treatment and changes in P1/N170 did not reach significance,

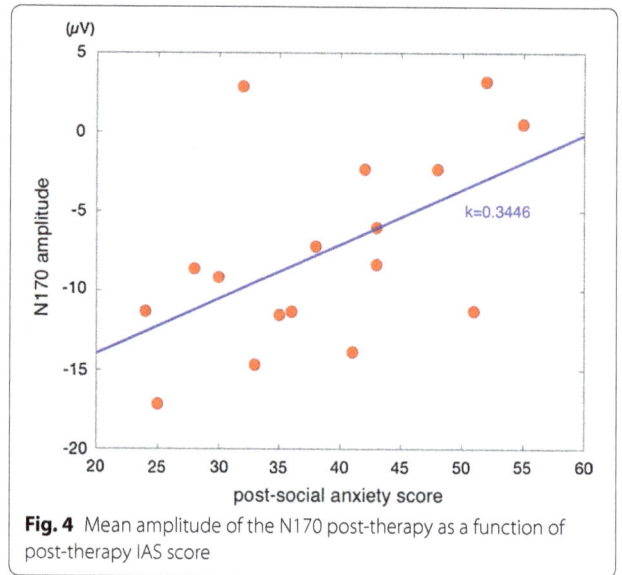

Fig. 4 Mean amplitude of the N170 post-therapy as a function of post-therapy IAS score

all ps > 0.27. No significant correlations were observed for P1.

Discussion

The primary objective of this study was to determine whether social anxiety is associated with enhanced or reduced early neural responses to facial or non-facial stimuli. We also examined whether early perception abnormalities change after CBGT therapy. We assessed behavioural treatment effects on social anxiety symptoms after CBGT therapy using the IAS and the BSPS. Both IAS and BSPS scores were significantly reduced after CBGT. The IAS scores patients with SAD post-therapy were not different than those of HCs. Such results together indicated that social anxiety symptoms were attenuated after CBGT. Although CBGT has been shown to be effective in the treatment of SAD [49–53, 61]; Scaini et al. [54, 55, 75], only few preliminary studies on Chinese samples have been reported [76]. Our results thus provide further evidence for the effectiveness of CBGT for the treatment of SAD.

SAD is a mental disorder characterized by more negative attention to social cues and interpretation of social information. To examine whether individuals with social anxiety pay more early attention to faces than healthy subjects, we first compared data from patients with SAD pre-therapy to data from HCs. Our ERP results revealed a general facial inversion effect in both patients with SAD pre-therapy and HCs, such that inverted faces were associated with larger P1–N170 than other upward faces or non-face objects. Our results are consistent with those of previous studies reporting increased P1 or N170 in response to inverted faces (i.e., facial inversion effect), which mainly reflects the need for configurational processing of faces [31, 44, 77]. The facial inversion effect did not differ between patients with SAD and normal controls in our study, indicating that SAD does not lead to facial stimulus-related specific enhancement processing. However, we found a general trend for increases in the P1–N170 component in response to all stimuli in patients with SAD relative to controls.

The early visual P1 component is an early index of the low-level features of a stimulus and is modulated by emotion or salience [78, 79]. The P1 enhancement effect is also found in response to non-emotional stimuli when the location captures an individual's attention [80] or when there is increased attention to a threat [81]. These findings provide strong evidence for the association between early selective attention and P1. Our results replicated the findings of several previous studies reporting larger P1 for faces than for objects [82, 83]. P1 responses to faces are also faster, which may reflect the early selective attention to social information. We found a trend for larger P1 responses to both faces and tables in individuals with SAD and HCs. This may indicate a common pattern of greater early attention to both faces and objects in individuals with SAD.

The sensitivity of N170 to the inversion of face stimuli has been observed in many previous studies [31, 45]. This reflects a holistic processing mechanism for faces. Our prior ERP study indicated that N170 abnormalities in SAD are associated with response bias [8], and that poor subjective discrimination and recognition ability for faces may stem from abnormal face perception or abnormal attention strategies. However, we did not find significant N170 amplitude group difference in our results.

The above findings seemingly do not support the hypothesis of early hypervigilance to facial stimuli in SAD, as the hypothesis states that socially anxious individuals overtly attend to initial socially relevant cues (e.g., faces) [84]. In other words, the above findings are inconsistent with the hypothesis that selective face processing might be impaired in SAD [8, 28, 85]. At least two interpretations of the lack of a selective attention effect to faces may exist. First, it is possible that previous studies of patients with SAD used different emotional faces [31, 86, 87], see [88], for a review). There is thus no direct evidence that patients with SAD have abnormalities in neutral face processing and not in object processing. An alternative explanation is that the task used in the current study is implicit (task-irrelevant), and that the attention of the participant is focused more on the target stimulus (i.e., flower) in all groups. In this case, both faces and objects are less attended to. If the latter is true, additional studies are required to elucidate the interaction between facial/object attention and social anxiety during explicit attention tasks.

Interestingly, we found a general decrease in the P1–N170 component in patients with SAD after the CBGT therapy sessions. We specifically observed smaller N170 responses in response to face stimuli. Similar changes from pre- to post-treatment change were also partly observed in previous studies of the treatment effects of CBT [66, 67], see [89], for a meta-analysis). For instance, Miskovic et al. [67] have reported frontal alpha EEG asymmetry changes from relatively greater right to relatively greater left frontal alpha EEGs in participants. To our knowledge, this is the first report of a relationship between CBT and ERP responses to faces. As stated above, the early face processing in our task was investigated implicitly (task-irrelevant), as the explicit task was flower-counting. Therefore, CBGT leads to smaller P1–N170 responses to faces even in implicit tests. The current results thus imply that CBGT modulates early face attention and attenuates hypervigilance to social cues even when there is low global attention to the stimuli.

It has been proposed that the facial inversion effect is reflected in the slope between P1 and N170, which combines the peak to peak change in amplitude and the peak to peak change in latency [74, 90]. Although there was no significant group difference on P1 or N170, the SAD abnormal effect occurs in P1–N170 slope. That is, the SAD group showed steeper slope than HC subjects, which may reflect the relative higher early face/object processing sensitivity in SAD. Therefore, it is possible that the P1–N170 slope could serve as a clinical index to determine abnormality in SAD.

Importantly, the CBGT treatment not only weakens anxiety symptoms, but also reduces face-related early components and the P1–N170 slope, especially for face related stimuli. According the cognitive-motivation account of anxiety, anxiety influences the appraisal of stimulus threat value [91]. Compared with objects, facial stimuli are more associated with less threat after the treatment, which could also be changed with the anxiety level [92]. Such treatment effect on face-related early components and the P1–N170 slope in patients with SAD may also be in agreement with our hypothesis that treatment could changes the selective processing in facial stimulus, due to temporal-occipital N170 was more sensitive to holistic processing of faces[93]. Due to the lack of spatial information in the EEG study, further brain imaging studies should be considered to better understand the neural mechanisms underlying such treatment effects in socially anxious individuals.

Although we did not conduct a control therapy procedure in the HCs, the correlation between social anxiety scores after therapy and the corresponding N170 amplitude may provide further support for the relationship between N170 and social anxiety symptoms. In the current study, there was no correlation between symptom improvement and ERP amplitude, which may due to the relatively small sample size. To assess the clinical implications of our work, it would be beneficial to study the possible correlation between clinical social anxiety symptoms and the corresponding ERP amplitude or slope.

Several limitations of this study should be noted. First, the sample size was relatively small due to difficulties with the experimental design (1-year follow-up). Together with the fact that we had a larger proportion of women in our sample, this may have led to reduced statistical power and generalized inference in the current study. Second, our study was limited to neutral face and object conditions in an implicit task. More conditions and tasks should be considered to investigate treatment effects. Another limitation of our study was that we did not carry out control treatment in the HC group due to difficulties with the treatment in HCs (treatment motivation control). It would have been helpful to have a third group in the study that included individuals with SAD who did not complete CBGT to ensure that our findings are in fact related to the intervention and not just familiarity with the stimuli in the task. An additional limitation of the current study is the fact that individuals need to use working memory throughout the task to maintain and manipulate the number of previously viewed flowers. This poses a significant limitation, which may have affected the ERP signal in response to faces in individuals with SAD, as the core element of SAD is fear of negative evaluation [94, 95]. In other words, the subjects with SAD might have been even more motivated to remember the numbers of flowers due to fear of negative evaluation. This would have led to less processing of stimuli in the second viewing task (the post-therapy test), especially for facial stimuli. Further studies with more controls and varied materials should be considered to explore this research question.

Conclusions

In conclusion, data from this study provide support for early enhanced attention and rapid reactions to both faces and objects in patients with SAD. Administration of CBGT can "normalize" this early hyperactivity, especially for facial stimuli in socially anxious individuals who exhibit aberrant P1–N170 responses. Our data provide initial evidence for an implicit processing of faces and objects in individuals with SAD and for brain-based improvements following therapy. It is hoped that the current results encourage further examination of potentially complex conditions and brain imaging methods to carry out brain-based SAD assessments and to predict treatment effects.

Authors' contributions

HW and JC conceived of the study and participated in its design. YL participated in data collection and helped to draft the manuscript. JY and RG participated in diagnostic interviewing of patients with SAD. QL, JL, YQ, and XL participated in data analysis and manuscript discussion. All authors read and approved the final manuscript.

Author details

[1] Department of Nursing, Harbin Medical University, Daqing, Heilongjiang Province, China. [2] Laboratory of Movement Control and Neuroplasticity, KU Leuven, 3001 Louvain, Belgium. [3] Neural Control of Movement Laboratory, ETH Zurich, 8057 Zurich, Switzerland. [4] CAS Key Laboratory of Behavioral Science, Institute of Psychology, Chinese Academy of Sciences, 16 Lincui Road, Chaoyang District, Beijing 100101, China. [5] Department of Psychology, University of Chinese Academy of Sciences, Beijing 100101, China.

Competing interests

The authors declare that they have no competing interests.

Funding

This work was supported by Grants from Heilongjiang Province Social Science Fund Project (15EDB03 and 16EDC03), Ministry of Education of Humanities and Social Science Fund Project (16YJCZH002, 13YJCZH093), and Daqing City Technology Bureau Guidance Project (szdy-2015-04).

References

1. American Psychiatric Association. Diagnostic and statistical manual of mental disorders (DSM-5®). Arlington: American Psychiatric Pub; 2013.
2. Winton EC, Clark DM, Edelmann RJ. Social anxiety, fear of negative evaluation and the detection of negative emotion in others. Behav Res Ther. 1995;33:193–6.
3. Cabeleira CM, Steinman SA, Burgess MM, Bucks RS, MacLeod C, Melo W, Teachman BA. Expectancy bias in anxious samples. Emotion. 2014;14:588–601.
4. Cao J, Gu R, Bi X, Zhu X, Wu H. Unexpected acceptance? Patients with social anxiety disorder manifest their social expectancy in ERPs during social feedback processing. Front Psychol. 2015;6.
5. Huppert JD, Foa EB, Furr JM, Filip JC, Mathews A. Interpretation bias in social anxiety: a dimensional perspective. Cogn Ther Res. 2003;27:569–77.
6. Laposa JM, Cassin SE, Rector NA. Interpretation of positive social events in social phobia: an examination of cognitive correlates and diagnostic distinction. J Anxiety Disord. 2010;24:203–10.
7. Lundh LG, Ost LG. Recognition bias for critical faces in social phobics. Behav Res Ther. 1996;34:787–94.
8. Qi Y, Gu R, Cao J, Bi X, Wu H, Liu X. Response bias-related impairment of early subjective face discrimination in social anxiety disorders: an event-related potential study. J Anxiety Disord. 2017;47:10–20.
9. Stopa L, Clark DM. Social phobia and interpretation of social events. Behav Res Ther. 2000;38:273–83.
10. Wilson JK, Rapee RM. The interpretation of negative social events in social phobia with versus without comorbid mood disorder. J Anxiety Disord. 2005;19:245–74.
11. Clark DM, Wells A. A cognitive model of social phobia. Soc Phobia Diagn Assess Treat. 1995;41:00022–3.
12. Heimberg RG, Brozovich FA, Rapee RM. A cognitive-behavioral model of social anxiety disorder: update and extension. Soc Anxiety Clin Dev Soc Perspect. 2010;2:395–422.
13. Heinrichs N, Hofmann SG. Information processing in social phobia: a critical review. Clin Psychol Rev. 2001;21:751–70.
14. Horley K, Williams LM, Gonsalvez C, Gordon E. Face to face: visual scan-path evidence for abnormal processing of facial expressions in social phobia. Psychiatry Res. 2004;127:43–53.
15. Kashdan TB. Social anxiety spectrum and diminished positive experiences: theoretical synthesis and meta-analysis. Clin Psychol Rev. 2007;27:348–65.

16. Maoz K, Eldar S, Stoddard J, Pine DS, Leibenluft E, Bar-Haim Y. Angry-happy interpretations of ambiguous faces in social anxiety disorder. Psychiatry Res. 2016;241:122–7.

17. Jusyte A, Schonenberg M. Threat processing in generalized social phobia: an investigation of interpretation biases in ambiguous facial affect. Psychiatry Res. 2014;217:100–6.

18. Buckner JD, Maner JK, Schmidt NB. Difficulty disengaging attention from social threat in social anxiety. Cogn Ther Res. 2010;34:99–105.

19. Gilboa-Schechtman E, Foa EB, Amir N. Attentional biases for facial expressions in social phobia: the face-in-the-crowd paradigm. Cogn Emot. 1999;13:305–18.

20. Killgore WD, Yurgelun-Todd DA. Social anxiety predicts amygdala activation in adolescents viewing fearful faces. Neuroreport. 2005;16:1671–5.

21. Mogg K, Bradley BP. Selective orienting of attention to masked threat faces in social anxiety. Behav Res Ther. 2002;40:1403–14.

22. Mogg K, Philippot P, Bradley BP. Selective attention to angry faces in clinical social phobia. J Abnorm Psychol. 2004;113:160–5.

23. Pishyar R, Harris LM, Menzies RG. Attentional bias for words and faces in social anxiety. Anxiety Stress Coping. 2004;17:23–36.

24. Caharel S, Courtay N, Bernard C, Lalonde R, Rebai M. Familiarity and emotional expression influence an early stage of face processing: an electrophysiological study. Brain Cogn. 2005;59:96–100.

25. Green MJ, Phillips ML. Social threat perception and the evolution of paranoia. Neurosci Biobehav Rev. 2004;28:333–42.

26. Lindstrom KM, Guyer AE, Mogg K, Bradley BP, Fox NA, Ernst M, Nelson EE, Leibenluft E, Britton JC, Monk CS, Pine DS, Bar-Haim Y. Normative data on development of neural and behavioral mechanisms underlying attention orienting toward social-emotional stimuli: an exploratory study. Brain Res. 2009;1292:61–70.

27. Nummenmaa L, Calder AJ. Neural mechanisms of social attention. Trends Cogn Sci. 2009;13:135–43.

28. Chen YP, Ehlers A, Clark DM, Mansell W. Patients with generalized social phobia direct their attention away from faces. Behav Res Ther. 2002;40:677–87.

29. Mansell W, Clark DM, Ehlers A, Chen Y-P. Social anxiety and attention away from emotional faces. Cogn Emot. 1999;13:673–90.

30. Bar-Haim Y, Lamy D, Glickman S. Attentional bias in anxiety: a behavioral and ERP study. Brain Cogn. 2005;59:11–22.

31. Bentin S, Allison T, Puce A, Perez E, McCarthy G. Electrophysiological studies of face perception in humans. J Cogn Neurosci. 1996;8:551–65.

32. Huang YX, Luo YJ. Temporal course of emotional negativity bias: an ERP study. Neurosci Lett. 2006;398:91–6.

33. Luo W, Feng W, He W, Wang NY, Luo YJ. Three stages of facial expression processing: ERP study with rapid serial visual presentation. Neuroimage. 2010;49:1857–67.

34. van Hooff JC, Crawford H, van Vugt M. The wandering mind of men: ERP evidence for gender differences in attention bias towards attractive opposite sex faces. Soc Cogn Affect Neurosci. 2011;6:477–85.

35. Vuilleumier P. How brains beware: neural mechanisms of emotional attention. Trends Cogn Sci. 2005;9:585–94.

36. Santesso DL, Meuret AE, Hofmann SG, Mueller EM, Ratner KG, Roesch EB, Pizzagalli DA. Electrophysiological correlates of spatial orienting towards angry faces: a source localization study. Neuropsychologia. 2008;46:1338–48.

37. Peschard V, Philippot P, Joassin F, Rossignol M. The impact of the stimulus features and task instructions on facial processing in social anxiety: an ERP investigation. Biol Psychol. 2013;93:88–96.

38. Rossignol M, Philippot P, Bissot C, Rigoulot S, Campanella S. Electrophysiological correlates of enhanced perceptual processes and attentional capture by emotional faces in social anxiety. Brain Res. 2012;1460:50–62.

39. Batty M, Taylor MJ. Early processing of the six basic facial emotional expressions. Brain Res Cogn Brain Res. 2003;17:613–20.

40. Eimer M, Holmes A. An ERP study on the time course of emotional face processing. Neuroreport. 2002;13:427–31.

41. Henson RN, Goshen-Gottstein Y, Ganel T, Otten LJ, Quayle A, Rugg MD. Electrophysiological and haemodynamic correlates of face perception, recognition and priming. Cereb Cortex. 2003;13:793–805.

42. Itier RJ, Taylor MJ. N170 or N1? Spatiotemporal differences between object and face processing using ERPs. Cereb Cortex. 2004;14:132–42.

43. Jemel B, Schuller AM, Cheref-Khan Y, Goffaux V, Crommelinck M, Bruyer R. Stepwise emergence of the face-sensitive N170 event-related potential component. Neuroreport. 2003;14:2035–9.

44. Rossion B, Gauthier I, Tarr MJ, Despland P, Bruyer R, Linotte S, Crommelinck M. The N170 occipito-temporal component is delayed and enhanced to inverted faces but not to inverted objects: an electrophysiological account of face-specific processes in the human brain. Neuroreport. 2000;11:69–74.

45. Eimer M. The face-specific N170 component reflects late stages in the structural encoding of faces. Neuroreport. 2000;11:2319–24.

46. Kanwisher N. Domain specificity in face perception. Nat Neurosci. 2000;3:759–63.

47. Sadeh B, Yovel G. Why is the N170 enhanced for inverted faces? An ERP competition experiment. Neuroimage. 2010;53:782–9.

48. Heimberg RG. Cognitive-behavioral therapy for social anxiety disorder: current status and future directions. Biol Psychiatry. 2002;51:101–8.

49. Cabral Mululo SC, de Menezes GB, Fontenelle L, Versiani M. Cognitive behavioral-therapies, cognitive therapies and behavioral strategies for the treatment of social anxiety disorder. Revista De Psiquiatria Clinica. 2009;36:221–8.

50. Ciraulo DA, Barlow DH, Gulliver SB, Farchione T, Morissette SB, Kamholz BW, Eisenmenger K, Brown B, Devine E, Brown TA, Knapp CM. The effects of venlafaxine and cognitive behavioral therapy alone and combined in the treatment of co-morbid alcohol use-anxiety disorders. Behav Res Ther. 2013;51:729–35.

51. Hudson JL. Mechanisms of change in cognitive behavioral therapy for anxious youth. Clin Psychol-Sci Pract. 2005;12:161–5.

52. Price M, Anderson PL. The impact of cognitive behavioral therapy on post event processing among those with social anxiety disorder. Behav Res Ther. 2011;49:132–7.

53. Queen AH, Donaldson DL, Luiselli JK. Interpersonal psychotherapy and cognitive-behavioral therapy as an integrated treatment approach for co-occurring bipolar i and social anxiety disorder. Clin Case Stud. 2015;14:434–48.

54. Scaini S, Belotti R, Ogliari A, Battaglia M. A comprehensive meta-analysis of cognitive-behavioral interventions for social anxiety disorder in children and adolescents. J Anxiety Disord. 2016;42:105–12.

55. Wergeland GJH, Fjermestad KW, Marin CE, Haugland BS-M, Bjaastad JF, Oeding K, Bjelland I, Silverman WK, Ost L-G, Havik OE, Heiervang ER. An effectiveness study of individual vs. group cognitive behavioral therapy for anxiety disorders in youth. Behav Res Ther. 2014;57:1–12.

56. Dugas MJ, Ladouceur R, Léger E, Freeston MH, Langolis F, Provencher MD, Boisvert J-M. Group cognitive-behavioral therapy for generalized anxiety disorder: treatment outcome and long-term follow-up. J Consult Clin Psychol. 2003;71:821–5.

57. McEvoy PM, Saulsman LM. Imagery-enhanced cognitive behavioural group therapy for social anxiety disorder: a pilot study. Behav Res Ther. 2014;55:1–6.

58. Mendlowitz SL, Manassis K, Bradley S, Scapillato D, Miezitis S, Shaw BE. Cognitive-behavioral group treatments in childhood anxiety disorders: the role of parental involvement. J Am Acad Child Adolesc Psychiatry. 1999;38:1223–9.

59. Silverman WK, Kurtines WM, Ginsburg GS, Weems CF, Lumpkin PW, Carmichael DH. Treating anxiety disorders in children with group cognitive-behavioral therapy: a randomized clinical trial. J Consult Clin Psychol. 1999;67:995–1003.

60. Heimberg RG, Dodge CS, Hope DA, Kennedy CR, Zollo LJ, Becker RE. Cognitive behavioral group treatment for social phobia: comparison with a credible placebo control. Cogn Ther Res. 1990;14:1–23.

61. Heimberg RG, Salzman DG, Holt CS, Blendell KA. Cognitive—behavioral group treatment for social phobia: effectiveness at five-year followup. Cogn Ther Res. 1993;17:325–39.

62. Doehrmann O, Ghosh SS, Polli FE, Reynolds GO, Horn F, Keshavan A, Triantafyllou C, Saygin ZM, Whitfield-Gabrieli S, Hofmann SG, Pollack M, Gabrieli JD. Predicting treatment response in social anxiety disorder from functional magnetic resonance imaging. JAMA Psychiatry. 2013;70:87–97.

63. Evans KC, Simon NM, Dougherty DD, Hoge EA, Worthington JJ, Chow C, Kaufman RE, Gold AL, Fischman AJ, Pollack MH, Rauch SL. A PET study of

120

Cognitive Neuroscience: Behavioral and Psychological Perspectives

tiagabine treatment implicates ventral medial prefrontal cortex in generalized social anxiety disorder. Neuropsychopharmacology. 2009;34:390–8.

64. Furmark T, Tillfors M, Marteinsdottir I, Fischer H, Pissiota A, Langstrom B, Fredrikson M. Common changes in cerebral blood flow in patients with social phobia treated with citalopram or cognitive-behavioral therapy. Arch Gen Psychiatry. 2002;59:425–33.

65. Mansson KN, Carlbring P, Frick A, Engman J, Olsson CJ, Bodlund O, Furmark T, Andersson G. Altered neural correlates of affective processing after internet-delivered cognitive behavior therapy for social anxiety disorder. Psychiatry Res. 2013;214:229–37.

66. Moscovitch DA, Santesso DL, Miskovic V, McCabe RE, Antony MM, Schmidt LA. Frontal EEG asymmetry and symptom response to cognitive behavioral therapy in patients with social anxiety disorder. Biol Psychol. 2011;87:379–85.

67. Miskovic V, Moscovitch DA, Santesso DL, McCabe RE, Antony MM, Schmidt LA. Changes in EEG cross-frequency coupling during cognitive behavioral therapy for social anxiety disorder. Psychol Sci. 2011;22:507–16.

68. Ruying Z, Yuanhui Z, Bin P. Comparison of three diagnostic criteria for the diagnosis of schizophrenia and mood disorders. Chinese J Psychiatry. 1997;30:45–9.

69. Davidson JR, Miner CM, De Veaugh-Geiss J, Tupler LA, Colket JT, Potts NLS. The brief social phobia scale: a psychometric evaluation. Psychol Med. 1997;27:161–6.

70. Leary MR, Kowalski RM. The Interaction Anxiousness Scale: construct and criterion-related validity. J Pers Assess. 1993;61:136–46.

71. He J-B, Liu C-J, Guo Y-Y, Zhao L. Deficits in early-stage face perception in excessive internet users. Cyberpsychol Behav Soc Netw. 2011;14:303–8.

72. Heimberg RG, Liebowitz MR, Hope DA, Schneier FR, Holt CS, Welkowitz LA, Juster HR, Campeas R, Bruch MA, Cloitre M, Fallon B, Klein DF. Cognitive behavioral group therapy vs phenelzine therapy for social phobia-12-week outcome. Arch Gen Psychiatry. 1998;55:1133–41.

73. de Gelder B, Stekelenburg JJ. Naso-temporal asymmetry of the N170 for processing faces in normal viewers but not in developmental prosopagnosia. Neurosci Lett. 2005;376:40–5.

74. Jacques C, Rossion B. Early electrophysiological responses to multiple face orientations correlate with individual discrimination performance in humans. Neuroimage. 2007;36:863–76.

75. Stangier U, Heidenreich T, Peitz M, Lauterbach W, Clark D. Cognitive therapy for social phobia: individual versus group treatment. Behav Res Ther. 2003;41:991–1007.

76. Wong D, Sun S. A preliminary study of the efficacy of group cognitive-behavioural therapy for people with social anxiety in Hong Kong. Hong Kong J Psychiatry. 2006;16:50.

77. Freire A, Lee K, Symons LA. The face-inversion effect as a deficit in the encoding of configural information: direct evidence. Perception. 2000;29:159–70.

78. Batty M, Taylor MJ. Early processing of the six basic facial emotional expressions. Cogn Brain Res. 2003;17:613–20.

79. Delplanque S, Lavoie ME, Hot P, Silvert L, Sequeira H. Modulation of cognitive processing by emotional valence studied through event-related potentials in humans. Neurosci Lett. 2004;356:1–4.

80. Hillyard SA, Anllo-Vento L. Event-related brain potentials in the study of visual selective attention. Proc Natl Acad Sci. 1998;95:781–7.

81. Pourtois G, Grandjean D, Sander D, Vuilleumier P. Electrophysiological correlates of rapid spatial orienting towards fearful faces. Cereb Cortex. 2004;14:619–33.

82. Gao L, Xu J, Zhang BW, Zhao L, Harel A, Bentin S. Aging effects on early-stage face perception: an ERP study. Psychophysiology. 2009;46:970–83.

83. Itier RJ, Latinus M, Taylor MJ. Face, eye and object early processing: what is the face specificity? Neuroimage. 2006;29:667–76.

84. Amir N, Foa EB, Coles ME. Automatic activation and strategic avoidance of threat-relevant information in social phobia. J Abnorm Psychol. 1998;107:285–90.

85. Horley K, Williams LM, Gonsalvez C, Gordon E. Social phobics do not see eye to eye: a visual scanpath study of emotional expression processing. J Anxiety Disord. 2003;17:33–44.

86. Kolassa I-T, Kolassa S, Bergmann S, Lauche R, Dilger S, Miltner WH, Musial F. Interpretive bias in social phobia: an ERP study with morphed emotional schematic faces. Cogn Emot. 2009;23:69–95.

87. Kolassa I-T, Kolassa S, Musial F, Miltner WH. Event-related potentials to schematic faces in social phobia. Cogn Emot. 2007;21:1721–44.

88. Staugaard SR. Threatening faces and social anxiety: a literature review. Clin Psychol Rev. 2010;30:669–90.

89. Olatunji BO, Cisler JM, Deacon BJ. Efficacy of cognitive behavioral therapy for anxiety disorders: a review of meta-analytic findings. Psychiatr Clin North Am. 2010;33:557–77.

90. Webb SJ, Merkle K, Murias M, Richards T, Aylward E, Dawson G. ERP responses differentiate inverted but not upright face processing in adults with ASD. Soc Cogn Affect Neurosci. 2012;7:578–87.

91. Mogg K, McNamara J, Powys M, Rawlinson H, Seiffer A, Bradley BP. Selective attention to threat: a test of two cognitive models of anxiety. Cogn Emot. 2000;14:375–99.

92. Mathews A, Mackintosh B. A cognitive model of selective processing in anxiety. Cogn Ther Res. 1998;22:539–60.

93. Itier RJ, Batty M. Neural bases of eye and gaze processing: the core of social cognition. Neurosci Biobehav Rev. 2009;33:843–63.

94. Rapee RM, Heimberg RG. A cognitive-behavioral model of anxiety in social phobia. Behav Res Ther. 1997;35:741–56.

95. Weeks JW, Heimberg RG, Fresco DM, Hart TA, Turk CL, Schneier FR, Liebowitz MR. Empirical validation and psychometric evaluation of the brief fear of negative evaluation scale in patients with social anxiety disorder. Psychol Assess. 2005;17:179.

10

Chronic cigarette smoking is linked with structural alterations in brain regions showing acute nicotinic drug-induced functional modulations

Matthew T. Sutherland[1*][iD], Michael C. Riedel[1,2], Jessica S. Flannery[1], Julio A. Yanes[3], Peter T. Fox[4,5,6], Elliot A. Stein[7] and Angela R. Laird[2]

Abstract

Background: Whereas acute nicotine administration alters brain function which may, in turn, contribute to enhanced attention and performance, chronic cigarette smoking is linked with regional brain atrophy and poorer cognition. However, results from structural magnetic resonance imaging (MRI) studies comparing smokers versus nonsmokers have been inconsistent and measures of gray matter possess limited ability to inform functional relations or behavioral implications. The purpose of this study was to address these interpretational challenges through meta-analytic techniques in the service of clarifying the impact of chronic smoking on gray matter integrity and more fully contextualizing such structural alterations.

Methods: We first conducted a coordinate-based meta-analysis of structural MRI studies to identify consistent structural alterations associated with chronic smoking. Subsequently, we conducted two additional meta-analytic assessments to enhance insight into potential functional and behavioral relations. Specifically, we performed a multimodal meta-analytic assessment to test the structural–functional hypothesis that smoking-related structural alterations overlapped those same regions showing acute nicotinic drug-induced functional modulations. Finally, we employed database driven tools to identify pairs of structurally impacted regions that were also functionally related via meta-analytic connectivity modeling, and then delineated behavioral phenomena associated with such functional interactions via behavioral decoding.

Results: Across studies, smoking was associated with convergent structural decreases in the left insula, right cerebellum, parahippocampus, multiple prefrontal cortex (PFC) regions, and the thalamus. Indicating a structural–functional relation, we observed that smoking-related gray matter decreases overlapped with the acute functional effects of nicotinic agonist administration in the left insula, ventromedial PFC, and mediodorsal thalamus. Suggesting structural-behavioral implications, we observed that the left insula's task-based, functional interactions with multiple other structurally impacted regions were linked with pain perception, the right cerebellum's interactions with other regions were associated with overt body movements, interactions between the parahippocampus and thalamus were linked with memory processes, and interactions between medial PFC regions were associated with face processing.

Conclusions: Collectively, these findings emphasize brain regions (e.g., ventromedial PFC, insula, thalamus) critically linked with cigarette smoking, suggest neuroimaging paradigms warranting additional consideration among smokers (e.g., pain processing), and highlight regions in need of further elucidation in addiction (e.g., cerebellum).

*Correspondence: masuther@fiu.edu
[1] Department of Psychology, Florida International University,
AHC-4, RM 312, 11200 S.W. 8th St, Miami, FL 33199, USA
Full list of author information is available at the end of the article

Keywords: Cigarettes, Nicotine, Addiction, Gray matter, Morphometry, Insula, Mediodorsal thalamus, Ventromedial prefrontal cortex, Cerebellum

Background

Over the past two decades, neuroimaging has contributed important insight into the structural and functional brain alterations linked with drug abuse in general [1–3] and nicotine addiction in particular [4–6]. For example, such studies have revealed that nicotine administration alters functional brain activity, inducing enhanced activity in some regions involved with attention and cognition (e.g., thalamus, lateral frontoparietal cortices, anterior cingulate cortex [ACC]) yet reducing activity in other regions involved with task-irrelevant mental operations (e.g., mind wandering; ventromedial prefrontal cortex, posterior cingulate cortex, parahippocampus) [6–8]. These functional brain alterations may, in part, provide a neurobiological account of the well-documented cognitive enhancing properties of acute nicotine administration [9, 10]. On the other hand, chronic cigarette smokers, compared with nonsmokers, exhibit poorer global cognition and impaired performance on specific measures of working memory, cognitive flexibility, visuospatial learning and memory, and processing speed [11–13]. Aligning with such neurocognitive observations, structural magnetic resonance imaging (MRI) studies have detected reduced gray matter integrity among smokers in multiple discrete brain regions including the prefrontal cortex (PFC), ACC, insula, thalamus, and cerebellum [e.g., 14–17]. Such regional atrophy may result from the deleterious impact of cigarette smoking and/or reflect predisposing neurobiological, neurocognitive, or personality factors.

However, structural MRI results among chronic smokers, to some degree, have been inconsistent. For example, gray matter in the insula of smokers has been reported to be decreased [15, 18, 19], increased [20], or comparable to that among nonsmokers [17, 21]. Similarly, whereas some studies have detected smoking-related structural decreases in the ventromedial PFC [17, 19, 22] or thalamus [17, 21, 23], others have not [14, 21, 24]. Heterogeneous findings may be the product of cross-sectional designs with modest-to-moderate sample sizes, between-study variability in participant attributes (e.g., varying age ranges, smoking histories, sex ratios, or other sociodemographic characteristics), and/or methodological differences in MRI acquisition or data analysis parameters (e.g., smoothing, registration techniques, or normalization templates). Such issues constrain interpretations from single studies and necessitate the post hoc integration of results from multiple independently conducted studies to better estimate parameters of interest [25].

Accordingly, neuroimaging meta-analytic techniques have been increasingly adopted to delineate spatially convergent results across studies, including identification of consistently observed gray matter alterations among specific phenotypes [26–28].

Although useful for elucidating potential structural alterations among smokers, measures of gray matter are limited in their ability to inform interpretation of functional relations or behavioral implications. Regarding structural–functional relations, a plausible hypothesis is that brain regions showing chronic smoking-related structural alterations overlap those same regions showing acute nicotinic drug-induced functional modulations. One perspective is that the repeated impact of nicotine exposure within discrete brain regions over an individual's extended smoking history culminates in neuroadaptations that may manifest as gray matter perturbations in those same regions. An alternative perspective is that pre-existing structural alterations may render some individuals more susceptible to acute pharmacologic effects and, in turn, to addiction. Regardless of the causative pathway (or combination thereof), integrating structural and functional neuroimaging results may provide insight into the neurobiological processes potentially contributing to the initiation, escalation, and/or maintenance of cigarette smoking. In other words, a multimodal perspective may allow for enhanced interpretation of structural alterations [29, 30]. Regarding structural-behavioral implications, a frequently posed question not easily answered by considering morphometric outcomes is: what are the behavioral consequences of structural alterations in a particular brain region (or set of regions). As opposed to conjectural discussion of behavioral relevance, empirical approaches to more fully contextualize gray matter alterations are of growing interest [e.g., 31–33]. Such approaches provide an objective means to support behavioral interpretations and/or suggest neuroimaging paradigms warranting additional consideration among a particular phenotype.

In the current study, we aimed to address these interpretational challenges by employing established and emergent meta-analytic techniques to clarify the impact of cigarette smoking on gray matter integrity and to more fully contextualize such morphometic alterations. The specific goals of our study were threefold. First, we sought to identify convergent structural alterations across studies associated with chronic smoking via the well-established, coordinate-based activation likelihood estimation (ALE) meta-analytic framework. We operationalized the effects of chronic smoking as gray matter alterations identified in studies utilizing smoker versus nonsmoker comparisons. Second, we tested the structural–functional hypothesis that chronic smoking-related gray matter alterations overlap those same regions showing acute nicotinic drug-induced functional effects via a multimodal meta-analytic assessment. Whereas we operationalized *chronic effects* as structural alterations identified in smoker versus nonsmoker (i.e., between-subjects) comparisons, we operationalized the *acute effects* of nicotinic acetylcholine receptor (nAChR) agonist administration as functional alterations indentified in pharmacological neuroimaging studies, the vast majority of which employed within-subjects (i.e., drug versus control condition) comparisons. Third, we sought to provide enhanced structural-behavioral insight via emergent database driven meta-analytic tools, which allow for the characterization of typical patterns of task-based co-activation and associated behavioral phenomenon for user-specified seed regions of interest. Specifically, using smoking-related gray matter alterations to define seed regions, we performed meta-analytic connectivity modeling [33] and behavioral decoding assessments [34, 35] on data archived in an extensive neuroimaging repository (http://www.brainmap.org/) to objectively support behavioral interpretations of structural alterations.

Methods

Structural MRI study search and selection

We performed an iterative literature search to compile structural neuroimaging studies interrogating gray matter alterations among chronic cigarette smokers compared with nonsmokers. In the first iteration, we searched the *Web of Science* (http://www.webofknowledge.com) and *PubMed* (http://www.pubmed.gov) databases for peer-reviewed articles with the following logical conjunction of terms: ("voxel-based morphometry" OR "morphometry" OR "gray matter density" OR "gray matter volume") AND ("nicotine" OR "tobacco" OR "cigarette" OR "smok*"). In a second iteration, we consulted the bibliographies of recent review articles [5, 36] and one existing meta-analysis [37] for studies potentially not identified by the database queries. Although a previous meta-analysis has considered the structural impact of chronic smoking, we note that several additional studies have emerged subsequent to that report and highlight our emphasis on structural–functional and structural-behavioral relations as a further distinguishing characteristic. In a final iteration, we tracked the references of and citations to relevant papers, thereby compiling additional studies.

We included studies in this meta-analysis that: (1) assessed gray matter using structural MRI, (2) reported a set of coordinates (i.e., foci) from a between-subjects contrast comparing smokers to matched nonsmoking participants, (3) reported coordinates in a defined stereotaxic space (i.e., Talairach or Montreal Neurological Institute [MNI]), (4) performed a whole-brain analysis, and (5) provided sufficient information regarding characterization of smoking behaviors (e.g., pack-years, Fagerström Test of Nicotine Dependence [FTND] scores, years smoking, number of cigarettes smoked per day), basic demographics of the study samples (e.g., age, sex, N), and data analysis strategies (e.g., smoothing parameters, statistical thresholds).

Accordingly, we identified 15 peer-reviewed articles involving 761 cigarette smokers and 1182 nonsmokers (Additional file 1: Figure S1; Table S1) [14, 15, 17–24, 38–42]. Across these 15 identified studies, the smoker samples were on average 41.8 ± 16.2 (mean ± SD) years of age and were composed of 40.9 ± 25.6 % females. At the time of scanning, smokers reported cigarette use for 22.9 ± 17.0 years, smoked 17 ± 4.0 cigarettes per day, and were moderately nicotine dependent as indicated by FTND scores (4.5 ± 1.3 out of 10). These characteristics were rather consistent across studies and are generally representative of community-based samples of smokers. The nonsmoker samples did not differ from smokers in terms of age (41.1 ± 17.5 years; $t[14] = -0.9$, $p = 0.4$) or sex (41.6 ± 25.0 % female: $t[13]^1 = 0.5$, $p = 0.6$). Most studies mitigated the influence of other drug use by screening via interview and/or urine toxicology on scan days (11 of 15 studies; Additional file 1: Table S2). For each study, we also tabulated information on the type of MRI scanner used and data collection/analysis parameters (Additional file 1: Table S2). All included studies utilized significance thresholds corrected for multiple comparisons or uncorrected thresholds combined with a spatial extent criterion. These studies distinguished gray matter alterations by the nonsmoker > smoker (i.e., smoking-related decreases) and smoker > nonsmoker directions (i.e., smoking-related increases). Of those included, 14 studies (78 foci) reported gray matter decreases among smokers and 5 studies (10 foci) reported increases. Given the limited number of studies and recent arguments that ALE meta-analyses based on less than 10 experiments/studies run the risk of obtaining results driven by a single experiment as opposed to identifying convergence across experiments [43], gray matter increases were not considered further.

---

[1] Paired sample t test. One study did not report the number of females/males.

Structural impact of chronic cigarette smoking: meta-analytic procedures

To identify areas of convergent gray matter decreases across studies, we performed a coordinate-based meta-analysis using the revised version [44, 45] of the activation (in this application, Anatomic) likelihood estimation (ALE) algorithm [26, 46] as implemented in *GingerALE v2.3.4* (http://www.brainmap.org/ale/). ALE is a voxel-wise approach for combining neuroimaging results across a collection of experiments/contrasts and thereby identifying locations of statistically significant spatial convergence. The ALE framework models foci as centers of three-dimensional Gaussian probability distributions, thus accounting for spatial uncertainty due to within- and between-study variability. Foci are weighted by study sample size, where larger samples are associated with narrower distributions and smaller samples with wider distributions. We first linearly transformed foci reported in MNI to Talairach space [47] and then generated modeled maps of each individual contrast using their respective foci (paralleling the modeled activation maps of functional MRI [fMRI] meta-analyses). Next, we calculated a voxel-wise ALE score (i.e., the union of all contrasts' modeled maps) quantifying the spatial convergence of structural alterations across the brain. To identify clusters of statistically significant convergence, we compared these obtained ALE scores with those from an empirical null-distribution derived from a permutation procedure [27]. This comparison resulted in nonparametric p value maps, which we then thresholded at a cluster-corrected level ($p_{corrected} < 0.05$; voxel-level: $p < 0.005$, cluster extent: 344 mm^3) and exported to *MANGO* (http://www.ric.uthscsa.edu/mango/) for visualization on an anatomical (Talairach) template.

Conjoint chronic smoking-related structural effects and acute drug-induced functional effects: multimodal meta-analytic procedures

We leveraged previous meta-analytic outcomes regarding the impact of acute nAChR agonist exposure on brain function to enhance interpretation of structural alterations observed among chronic cigarette smokers. Specifically, in a previous meta-analysis [6] we identified 38 pharmacological fMRI studies that assessed the acute functional effects of nAChR agonist administration (i.e. pharmacologic administration or cigarette smoking) relative to a baseline condition (i.e. placebo administration or smoking abstinence condition) across various cognitive and affective neuroimaging paradigms. The studies meeting selection criteria in that functional meta-analysis involved 796 participants, reported 364 foci from 77 contrasts, and distinguished functional activity modulations by the baseline > drug (i.e., activity decrease) and

drug > baseline (i.e., activity increase) directions. We characterized the impact of nAChR agonists on brain function using the ALE framework (paralleling that described above) and separately identified brain regions showing either convergent activity increases or decreases using a cluster-level corrected threshold ($p_{corrected} < 0.05$).

To test the hypothesis that smoking-related gray matter decreases overlap those same regions showing acute drug-induced effects, we conducted a multimodal meta-analytic assessment. Specifically, we performed a conjunction analysis to identify those brain regions, if any, showing statistically significant convergence when considering both: (1) chronic smoking-related structural effects (smokers versus nonsmokers), and (2) acute drug-induced functional effects (nAChR agonist manipulation versus control condition). Employing a conservative minimum statistic conjunction [48], we identified brain regions showing conjoint structural and functional effects by computing the intersection of the two thresholded meta-analytic maps combined with an additional overlap-cluster extent criterion (100 mm^3).

Behavioral relevance of structurally impacted regions: meta-analytic connectivity modeling and behavioral decoding

As gray matter assessments possess limited ability to inform functional or behavioral interpretations, we subsequently employed emergent meta-analytic tools to more fully contextualize the brain circuit-level and behavioral consequences of structural alterations identified among smokers [28, 49, 50]. Specifically, to determine whether structurally impacted brain regions reflect disruption of functionally interrelated neurocircuits, we utilized *meta-analytic connectivity modeling* (MACM), a validated database driven approach for delineating brain areas that co-activate with a seed region of interest (ROI) across many neuroimaging tasks [33, 51, 52]. This assessment was conducted using the BrainMap database (http://www.brainmap.org/) which is an online repository of over 13,500 neuroimaging contrasts from ~2800 journal articles (as of January, 2016) archived as three-dimensional coordinate-based results (x, y, z) as well as relevant metadata describing the associated experimental design [53–55]. Whereas we utilized the database's archived activation coordinates to characterize the co-activation/connectional profile of structurally-identified ROIs, we utilized the metadata to facilitate behavioral interpretation of smoking-related structural alterations via *meta-analytic behavioral decoding*. Although the data utilized in these assessments were from healthy participants, they nonetheless offer a useful path to enhance interpretation of observed structural alterations among smokers. These analyses attempt to identify within a typical range of function whether pairs of regions interact and, if so, under what behavioral context. If two brain regions are structurally impacted by a certain neuropsychiatric condition and those same regions also appear to interact among healthy participants under a specific behavioral context, one plausible inductive conclusion is that the psychological processes associated with that behavioral context may be disrupted in the neuropsychiatric condition.

Moving beyond isolated regions, we conducted a MACM assessment to characterize the typical pattern of task-based, whole-brain co-activation for each of the structurally-identified ROIs. A MACM assessment aims to identify, across a domain-arching pool of studies interrogating various mental operations and task paradigms, brain areas that simultaneously co-activate with a user-specified seed region. In other words, a MACM assessment identifies brain areas most likely to be activated across all tasks, given activation within a seed. Similar to seed-based resting-state functional connectivity assessments of fMRI data, a MACM identifies those regions that are significantly related to, and presumably interact with the seed. First, we identified experiments in the database that reported one or more activation coordinates within a seed ROI using the *Sleuth* software application (http://www.brainmap.org/sleuth/). The seeds were 8 mm radius spheres centered on the voxels with maximum ALE values within each of the smoking-related gray matter loss regions identified above. We conducted separate searches and computed separate MACMs for each of these ROIs. As practiced in previous MACM assessments to achieve sufficient power [e.g., 56], only those ROIs associated with 30 or more experiments in the database were considered for further analyses. We employed 8 mm radial spheres to equate each ROIs volume and to seek a balance between returning a sufficient number of experiments from the database and minimizing overlap between ROIs that were in close proximity. Next, we extracted the whole-brain coordinates of all foci that co-activated with the seed, constraining this extraction to only activation foci (i.e., no deactivations) reported in studies examining healthy participants (i.e., no intervention or group comparisons). After converting foci reported in MNI to Talairach space [47], we supplied these foci as input to the ALE methodology described above thereby delineating regions of convergent co-activation with the seed when employing a cluster-corrected threshold of $p_{corrected} < 0.05$ (voxel-level: $p < 0.001$). These thresholded MACM maps for each ROI represent the above-chance probability that identified voxels co-activated with the respective seed across many neuroimaging tasks. To determine whether smoking-related gray matter loss regions reflected disruption of functionally

interrelated neurocircuits, we quantified the degree to which one ROI's MACM map intersected with any of the other structurally impacted ROIs. If one ROI's MACM map overlapped at least 50 voxels of any other ROI, those two regions were considered to constitute a circuit-level functional interaction.

In addition to the co-activation coordinates, we also extracted the corresponding BrainMap metadata allowing for the generation of behavioral profiles for each pair of co-activating, and presumably functionally-related, ROIs. The metadata in the database are coded according to a well-defined taxonomy (http://www.brainmap.org/taxonomy/) cataloguing each contributing study's experimental design, stimulus type, behavioral domain (and subcategory), and paradigm class [57, 58]. Under this taxonomy, behavioral domains (BD) represent the mental processes interrogated by the primary study's statistical contrasts and comprise the main categories of *action*, *cognition*, *emotion*, *interoception*, and *perception* as well as BD subcategories (BD-S; e.g., *perception: somesthesis-pain*). Paradigm classes (PC) further categorize the specific task employed (e.g., *pain monitoring/discrimination*, *Go/No-Go*). We used these metadata terms to delineate behavioral phenomena linked with the concurrent activation of those pairs of structurally-identified ROIs considered to constitute circuit-level functional interactions in the above MACM assessments.

Specifically, we created behavioral profiles for circuits of interest by performing forward and reverse inference analyses [34, 35] on the associated distribution of metadata terms [59, 60]. In the forward inference approach, we tested whether the conditional probability of brain activation given a particular behavioral phenomenon (i.e., BD, BD-S, or PC), p(Activation|Phenomenon), was higher than the baseline probability of brain activation, p(Activation). Baseline activation was defined as the probability of finding a random activation from the database in the region(s) of interest. Significance was established with a binomial test ($p_{FDR-corrected} < 0.05$). In the reverse inference approach, we identified the most likely behavioral phenomenon (i.e., BD, BD-S, or PC) given activation in a region. This likelihood, p(Phenomenon|Activation), was derived from p(Activation|Phenomenon) as well as p(Phenomenon) and p(Activation) using Bayes' Rule. Significance was established with a Chi-squared test ($p_{FDR-corrected} < 0.05$). Only BD, BD-S, and PC terms that were significant in both the forward and reverse inference approaches are reported.[2]

---

[2] We note that these analyses represent an attempt to relate behavioral phenomena with identified ROIs as opposed to claiming "a unique role" of those ROIs with respect to behavior [34]. In other words, an association of "*behavioral phenomenon x to brain region y*" obtained from these analyses does not necessarily imply that activity in "*region y is limited to behavioral phenomenon x*".

Results

Structural impact of chronic cigarette smoking

To elucidate structural alterations associated with an extended smoking history, we conducted a meta-analysis identifying consistent gray matter decreases among smokers. This meta-analysis included 78 distinct foci from 14 peer-reviewed studies involving a total of 750 smokers and 1073 nonsmokers (Additional file 1: Table S1). Across these studies, ALE revealed convergent gray matter decreases in 12 distinct clusters, notably in the ventromedial PFC (vmPFC), left insula, and mediodorsal (MD) thalamus, as well as in the medial orbitofrontal cortex (mOFC), ventrolateral PFC (vlPFC), dorsomedial PFC (dmPFC), medial PFC (mPFC), left parahippocampal gyrus, and right cerebellum (Fig. 1; Table 1).

Conjoint chronic smoking-related structural effects and acute drug-induced functional effects

To delineate regions displaying *both* structural alterations linked with chronic smoking *and* functional modulations linked with acute nicotinic agonist administration, we performed a multimodal assessment. Specifically, we conducted a conjunction analysis identifying regions showing both convergent: (1) smoking-related *structural* decreases (Fig. 1), and (2) nAChR agonist-induced *functional* decreases or increases [6]. This multimodal assessment identified overlapping structural and functional effects within the vmPFC, left insula, and MD thalamus (Fig. 2; Table 2). Specifically, whereas gray matter decreases in the vmPFC and insula overlapped with clusters of acute drug-induced functional activity *decreases* (Fig. 2, green; Additional file 1: Figure S2), gray matter decreases in MD thalamus overlapped with drug-induced activity *increases* (Fig. 2, orange; Additional file 1: Figure S3). We arrived at similar outcomes and the same conclusions when performing this multimodal assessment when considering only functional studies involving nicotine administration (i.e., excluding other nAChR agonists; Additional file 1: Figure S4) and when considering only functional results involving cigarette smokers (Additional file 1: Figure S5).

Behavioral relevance of structurally impacted regions: MACM and behavioral decoding

To enhance insight into the circuit-level consequences of smoking-related structural alterations, we first performed a MACM assessment thereby identifying clusters

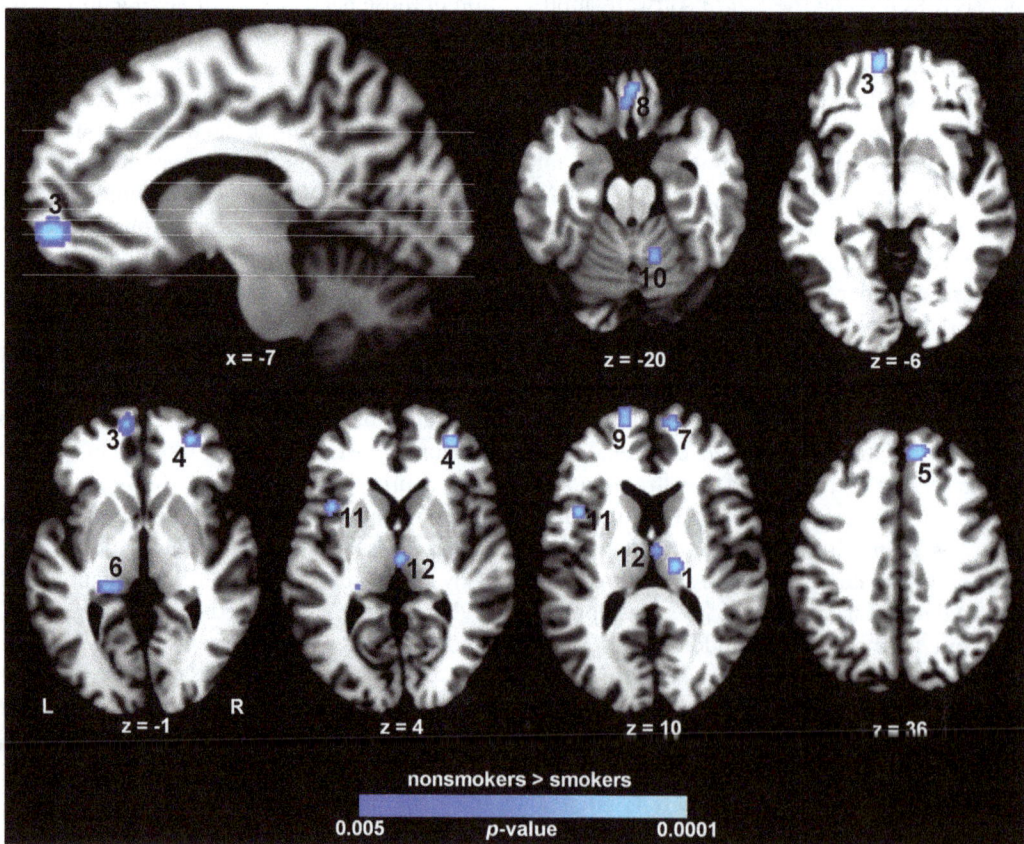

Fig. 1 Structural impact of chronic cigarette smoking. Convergent gray matter decreases among smokers (nonsmokers > smokers) were observed notably in multiple PFC regions, the left insula, thalamus, and cerebellum. *Numbering* corresponds to coordinates listed in Table 1

Table 1 Convergent gray matter decreases associated with chronic smoking: cluster coordinates

Cluster	Region		Volume	X	Y	Z
Nonsmokers > smokers						
1	Thalamus (lateral posterior nucleus)	R	592	16	−22	14
2	dmPFC (BA 6) (superior frontal gyrus)	R	576	16	24	52
3	vmPFC (BA10) (superior frontal gyrus)	L	568	−8	56	−4
4	vlPFC (BA 10) (middle frontal gyrus)	R	480	32	46	4
5	dmPFC (BA 8) (medial frontal gyrus)	R	480	10	40	36
6	Parahippocampal gyrus	L	432	−20	−34	0
7	mPFC (BA10) (medial frontal gyrus)	R	416	12	58	8
8	Medial OFC (BA 11)	B	384	2	34	−20
9	mPFC (BA10) (medial frontal gyrus)	L	376	−14	58	8
10	Cerebellum (dentate)	R	368	14	−58	−20
11	Insula (BA 13)	L	368	−40	8	10
12	Thalamus (medial dorsal nucleus)	B	360	2	−18	4

Numbering corresponds to brain regions shown in Fig. 1. Coordinates (X, Y, Z) of the clusters' peak voxels are reported in Talairach space. Volume is mm^3

B bilateral, *R* right, *L* left, *BA* Brodmann area, *OFC* orbitofrontal cortex, *vmPFC* ventromedial prefrontal cortex, *vlPFC* ventrolateral prefrontal cortex, *dmPFC* dorsomedial prefrontal cortex, *mPFC* medial prefrontal cortex

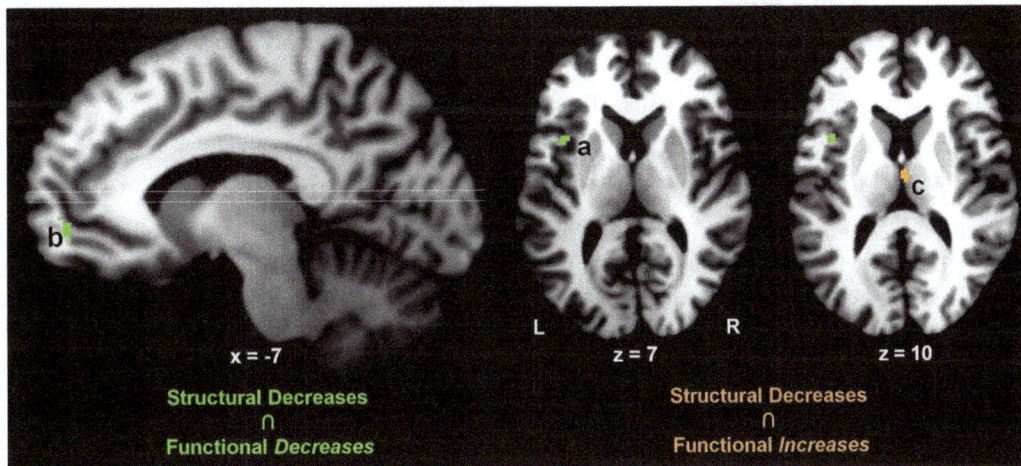

Fig. 2 Conjoint structural and functional effects. Structural alterations (nonsmokers > smokers) overlapped with acute drug-induced activity *decreases* (baseline > drug) in the insula and ventromedial PFC (*green* **a**, **b**). Structural alterations (nonsmokers > smokers) overlapped with acute drug-induced activity *increases* (drug > baseline) in the mediodorsal thalamus (*orange* **c**). Lettering corresponds to coordinates listed in Table 2. See Additional file 1: Figures S2 and S3 for visualization of overlapping and non-overlapping regions from the structural and functional meta-analyses

Table 2 Conjoint chronic smoking-related structural alterations and acute drug-induced functional activity changes: cluster coordinates

Cluster	Region		Volume	X	Y	Z
Gray matter decreases ∩ functional decreases						
a	Insula (BA 13)	L	185	−39	7	9
b	vmPFC (BA10) (superior frontal gyrus)	L	103	−9	50	−3
Gray matter decreases ∩ functional increases						
c	Thalamus (medial dorsal nucleus)	B	142	2	−14	11

Lettering corresponds to brain regions shown in Fig. 2. Coordinates (X, Y, Z) of the clusters' peak voxels are reported in Talairach space. Volume is mm^3

B bilateral, *R* right, *L* left, *BA* Brodmann area, *vmPFC* ventromedial prefrontal cortex

of convergent co-activation for each of the structurally impacted ROIs. One region (mOFC) failed to return a sufficient number of experiments from the BrainMap database and was not considered further (Additional file 1: Table S3). The remaining 11 whole-brain MACM maps represent voxels with an above-chance probability of co-activating with the seed when considering various neuroimaging tasks (Fig. 3; Additional file 1: Table S4). For example, the MACM map for: (1) the *vmPFC* seed (Fig. 3, ROI 3) indentified convergent co-activation within the posterior cingulate cortex, dmPFC, parahippocampus, and inferior frontal gyrus, (2) the *left insula* seed (Fig. 3, ROI 11) displayed notable co-activation with the right insula, posterior medial prefrontal cortex (encompassing the ACC and supplemental motor area), the thalamus, parietal cortex, and cerebellum, and (3) the *MD thalamus* seed (Fig. 3, ROI 12) encompassed the posterior medial PFC, bilateral insula, parietal cortex, and cerebellar regions. These and similarly-derived MACM maps delineating networks of task-based co-activation resemble networks identified when considering task-independent resting-state fMRI data [28, 61–64].

We then further assessed these co-activation maps to determine whether structurally impacted regions reflected functionally interrelated neurocircuits. Those structurally impacted ROIs that also appeared to be functionally related are summarized in Fig. 4a. In this representation, the paths between regions indicate the observation of one ROI intersecting with another ROI's MACM map. For example, the left insula's MACM map (Fig. 4a, ROI 11) overlapped the lateral posterior thalamus (ROI 1), cerebellum (ROI 10), and the MD thalamus (ROI 12) and vice versa (represented by double-headed arrows), whereas the left insula ROI was overlapped by the MACM map derived for the vlPFC seed (ROI 4, single-headed arrow). For the 11 ROIs, 12 unique paths were identified (out of 55; Additional file 1: Figure S6) representing pairs of regions with an above-chance probability of co-activation.

To characterize behavioral phenomena linked with these pairs of functionally-related ROIs, we performed behavioral decoding via forward and reverse inference techniques on the associated BrainMap metadata terms (BD, BD-S, and PC). Those behavioral phenomena significantly associated with co-activation of ROI pairs are represented in Fig. 4b. We highlight four observations from this assessment. First, the left insula's co-activation with multiple other ROIs was linked with aspects of pain processing. Specifically, insula and vlPFC co-activation (Fig. 4b, path: ROI 4–11) was significantly associated with the BD *perception* (purple), the BD-S *somesthesis-pain*, and the PC *pain monitoring/discrimination*. Similarly, concurrent activation of the insula and MD thalamus

(Fig. 4b, path: ROI 11–12) was linked with *perception*, *somesthesis-pain*, and *pain monitoring/discrimination* in addition to the PC *recitation/repetition (overt)*. Insula and lateral posterior thalamus co-activation (Fig. 4b, path: ROI 11–1) was associated with *perception* and *somesthesis-pain*. Second, the right cerebellum's co-activation with multiple other ROIs was related to aspects of overt body movements. Specifically, cerebellum and insula co-activation (Fig. 4b, path: ROI 10–11) was associated with the BD *action* (red), the BD-S *execution-speech*, and the PC *recitation/repetition*. Similarly, concurrent activation of the cerebellum and MD thalamus (Fig. 4b, path: ROI 10–12) was related to *action*, *execution* (non-speech), *execution-speech*, and *recitation/repetition* in addition to the PCs of *flexion/extension* and *Go/No-Go* (i.e., inhibiting an overt body movement). Co-activation of the cerebellum and lateral posterior thalamus (Fig. 4b, path: ROI 10–1) was linked with the BD *action*, BD-S *execution* (non-speech), and PC *finger tapping/button press*. Third, co-activation of the parahippocampus and MD thalamus (Fig. 4b, path: ROI 6–11) was related to the BD *cognition* (green), the BD-S *memory-explicit*, and the PCs *cued-explicit* and *recognition/recall*. Lastly, concurrent activation of the vmPFC and mPFC (Fig. 4b, path: ROI 3–9) was associated with the PC *face monitoring/discrimination*.

Discussion

We compiled structural MRI results to clarify the impact of cigarette smoking on gray matter integrity. Our meta-analytic results revealed convergent gray matter decreases among smokers in multiple regions including the prefrontal cortex, insula, thalamus, and cerebellum. Given that such structural measures provide limited insight into functional or behavioral implications, we subsequently performed two additional meta-analytic assessments to more fully contextualize these gray matter decreases. Indicative of a structural–functional relation, we observed via a multimodal assessment that chronic smoking-related structural effects overlapped with the acute functional effects of nAChR agonist administration in the vmPFC, left insula, and MD thalamus. Suggestive of structural-behavioral implications, we then identified pairs of structurally impacted regions that tended to co-activate across various tasks and delineated behavioral phenomena linked with such co-activation via MACM and behavioral decoding, respectively. These assessments linked the left insula's co-activation with multiple other brain regions to pain perception, the right cerebellum's co-activation with other regions to overt body movement, co-activation of the parahippocampus and MD thalamus with memory processes, and co-activation of medial PFC regions with face processing.

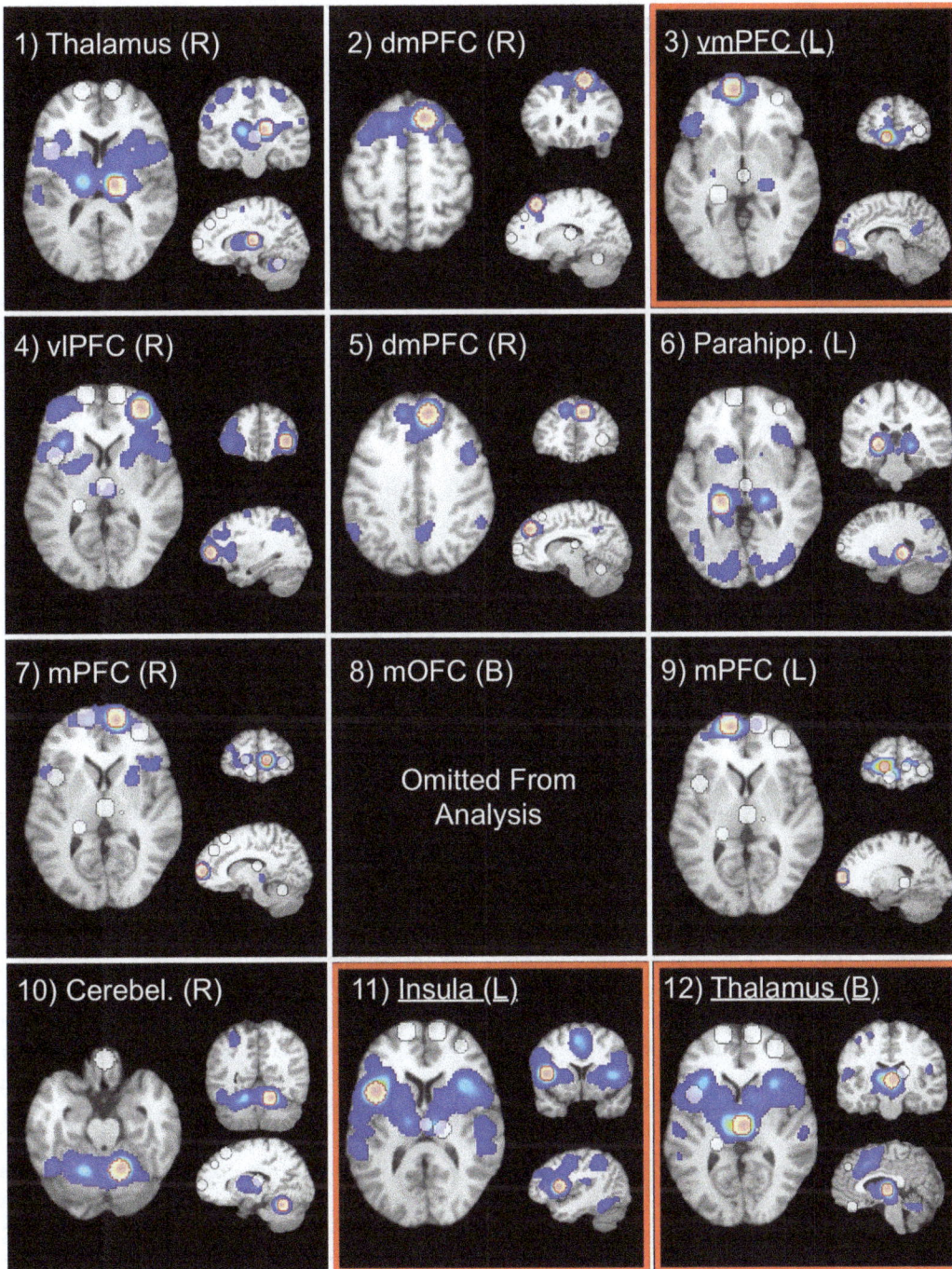

Fig. 3 Meta-analytic connectivity modeling (MACM) maps of task-related co-activation for each structurally impacted ROI. These thresholded MACM maps ($p_{corrected} < 0.05$) represent voxels with an above-chance probability of co-activating with the respective seed regions (8 mm radius *spheres* centered on the voxels with maximum ALE values within each smoking-related gray matter loss region). One region (ROI 8; mOFC) failed to return a sufficient number of contrasts from the database and was omitted from further analyses. *Numbering* corresponds to that in Table 1. The seed ROI of each MACM map is outlined in *red*. MACM maps for ROIs *boxed* in *red* are discussed in the main text. See Additional file 1: Table S4 for each seed ROI's co-activation coordinates

Across studies, we observed convergent smoking-related structural decreases in discrete brain regions notably in the PFC (i.e., ventromedial, ventrolateral, dorsomedial, orbitofrontal), insula, thalamus, and cerebellum. Although we can only speculate on the pathogenesis of such decreases, structural differences between

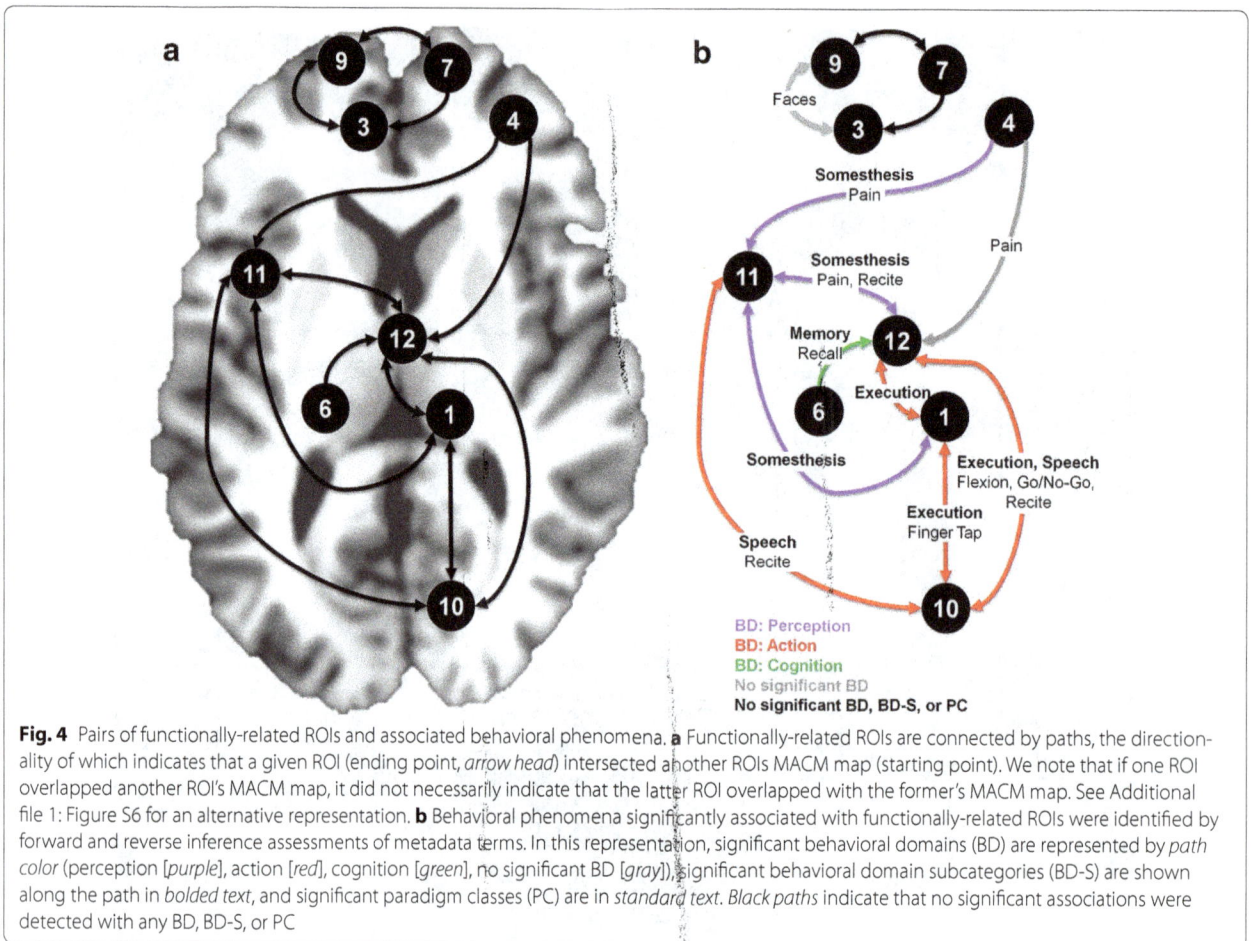

Fig. 4 Pairs of functionally-related ROIs and associated behavioral phenomena. **a** Functionally-related ROIs are connected by paths, the direction-ality of which indicates that a given ROI (ending point, *arrow head*) intersected another ROIs MACM map (starting point). We note that if one ROI overlapped another ROI's MACM map, it did not necessarily indicate that the latter ROI overlapped with the former's MACM map. See Additional file 1: Figure S6 for an alternative representation. **b** Behavioral phenomena significantly associated with functionally-related ROIs were identified by forward and reverse inference assessments of metadata terms. In this representation, significant behavioral domains (BD) are represented by *path color* (perception [*purple*], action [*red*], cognition [*green*], no significant BD [*gray*]), significant behavioral domain subcategories (BD-S) are shown along the path in *bolded text*, and significant paradigm classes (PC) are in *standard text*. *Black paths* indicate that no significant associations were detected with any BD, BD-S, or PC

smokers and nonsmokers could be products of predis-posing neurobiological risk factors [65], the deleterious impact of cigarette smoking on microvascular function-ing [66], neurotoxic events (e.g., oxidative stress, inflam-mation) associated with many of the >4000 compounds present in tobacco smoke [67], and/or be mediated directly or indirectly by nicotine itself. Focusing on the last possibility, nAChRs are ubiquitous throughout the human brain with particularly high densities in the thala-mus, insula, and vmPFC [68, 69]. Widespread upregula-tion of nAChRs, likely related to receptor desensitization from nicotine exposure, has been observed among smok-ers [70, 71] and, conversely, smoking cessation associ-ated with decreases in regional nAChR densities [72]. Evidence from preclinical models suggests neurotoxic events and protracted consequences on cholinergic neurotransmission following nicotine exposure particu-larly during adolescence [73–75]. As such, one plausible mechanistic account is that repeated stimulation of high densities of nAChRs by nicotine may contribute to neu-rotoxicity within discrete regions and/or increase the vul-nerability of those regions to other volatile compounds

in tobacco smoke [19] which ultimately manifest as gray matter decreases.

Speaking to such an account, we conducted a mul-timodal meta-analytic assessment to determine if smoking-related structural decreases overlapped with nicotinic agonist-induced functional modulations and observed conjoint effects in the vmPFC, insula, and MD thalamus. In addition to possessing relatively high nAChR densities, these regions also are critically impli-cated in addiction-related psychological processes. For example, the vmPFC, in concert with other regions such as the OFC and striatum, is thought to play a role in rep-resenting subjective value information, behavioral choice selection, and evaluating outcomes and alterative rewards [76–78]. The insula, a functionally heterogeneous region, is involved with monitoring the physiological state of the body, appears causally related to the initiation, mainte-nance, and adjustment of attentional control, and likely plays a role in maladaptive decision-making among drug addicts [79–82]. Dysfunction of the MD thalamus, a primary node within a thalamic-PFC-basal ganglia net-work involved in associative learning, is implicated in the transition from goal-directed action (e.g., recreational drug use) to habitual forms of responding (e.g., dysregulated drug seeking) [83, 84]. Consistent with the notion that structural alterations in these regions are a product of prolonged nicotine/tobacco exposure, group differences between smokers and nonsmokers within, for example, the insula were not detected among an adolescent/young adult participant sample with relatively lower exposure levels (0.9 ± 0.7 pack-years on average) [85] but were observed among similarly aged individuals with relatively higher exposure levels (4.0 ± 1.8 pack-years) [86]. Furthermore, multiple studies have provided evidence for dose-dependent exposure effects on gray matter integrity within the insula [18, 85] and vmPFC [19, 22, 86] as well as within the lateral PFC [14, 20] and cerebellum [23]. Widespread dose-dependent negative relations between pack-years and cortical thickness were recently corroborated in a large sample of older adults ($N > 500$) with particularly robust effects in the medial and lateral PFC [87]. Interestingly, positive relations between number of years since last cigarette and cortical thickness, suggesting potential recovery with smoking cessation, were also detected in medial PFC and posterior insula regions, amongst others [87]. Our multimodal meta-analytic outcomes add to a growing literature implicating the vmPFC, insula, and thalamus as contributors to the initiation, escalation, maintenance, and/or cessation of cigarette smoking.

Representing one objective approach for providing insight into the behavioral relevance of convergent gray matter decreases among smokers, we utilized emergent meta-analytic tools to delineate structurally impacted ROIs that tended to co-activate and their associated behavioral phenomena. Similar approaches have been used to quantitatively aid interpretation of regions identified via structural assessments or networks commonly observed via resting-state fMRI (i.e., assessments inherently lacking direct behavioral insight) [28, 33]. Although we adopted a quantitative approach to infer behavioral relevance of structural alterations, we note that our interpretations remain largely speculative until experimentally verified. We observed that co-activation of the left insula with thalamic and lateral PFC regions were generally linked with pain perception. Dysregulated pain processing is increasingly recognized as a potential barrier to smoking cessation [88, 89] and emerging evidence suggests bidirectional relations between pain and smoking behaviors [90, 91]. In laboratory assessments (e.g., cold pressor test), minimally-deprived or abstinent smokers, compared with nonsmokers, exhibit lower pain tolerance and report greater subjective experiences of pain where such pain reports positively correlate with nicotine withdrawal severity [92–94]. As such, nicotine abstinence

may contribute to enhanced pain sensitivity that could maintain cigarette smoking via negative reinforcement mechanisms similar to other withdrawal symptoms [95]. Although the insula's role in interoceptive monitoring has been well characterized [80] and higher nAChR availability in the thalamus, PFC, and cerebellum has been positively correlated with increased pain sensitivity among abstinent smokers [96], relatively little neuroimaging work has focused on the neurobiological processes that may contribute to smoking- or withdrawal-related pain dysregulation. Our meta-analytic outcomes suggest that neuroimaging investigations of pain perception among smokers, with emphasis on the putative functional interactions between the insula and MD thalamus, may be a productive avenue for future research.

We also observed that co-activation of the right cerebellum with insula and thalamic regions were generally linked with overt body movements. Acutely administered, nicotine augments performance in simple motor tasks [9] and increases cerebellar vermis activity during externally paced finger tapping [97]. On the other hand, chronic cigarette smokers perform worse than nonsmokers on neurocognitive measures of fine motor skills and postural stability [11]. Smoking-related decreases in right cerebellum gray matter, identified via an ROI-based approach [16] (i.e., a study not meeting inclusion criteria for the current meta-analysis), further corroborate our observation of convergent decreases in this region. Whereas our outcomes are consistent with the cerebellum's critical role in motor coordination, they also align with contemporary views emphasizing the region's contribution to cognitive processes [98, 99] and relevance to drug addiction [100, 101]. For example, we observed that co-activation of the cerebellum and MD thalamus was significantly associated with Go/No-Go paradigms that require inhibitory control. Although current neurobiological models of addiction have yet to provide an integrative account of this region's contribution, altered cerebellar structure and function appears to be a common characteristic across drugs of abuse [100]. Our meta-analytic outcomes serve to further draw attention to the cerebellum in the context of addiction in general and cigarette smoking in particular.

Lastly, co-activation of the parahippocampus and MD thalamus was linked with memory processes and co-activation of medial PFC regions linked with face processing. Regarding the former observation, neurocognitive assessments have consistently identified visuospatial learning and memory deficits among older (>60 years) as well as middle-aged smokers (30–60 years) relative to nonsmokers [11, 12]. Regarding the latter observation, as face processing paradigms often directly or indirectly involve affective components, a plausible interpretation is that smoking-related structural effects in medial PFC regions may relate to disrupted emotional processing and/or regulation [102, 103]. Indeed, smokers tend to report elevated negative mood and a reduced ability to self-regulate such states when compared with nonsmokers [104, 105].

Our findings should be considered in light of remaining issues. First, the ALE framework is a coordinate-based meta-analytic approach that does not incorporate the size of identified clusters from the primary studies, which leads to less precise representations relative to image-based approaches [106], which, on the other hand, are themselves often less feasible. Second, we only considered gray matter decreases among smokers owing to a small number of reported experiments/foci in the literature with respect to increases. Nonetheless, neuroimaging studies have documented smoking-related volumetric increases in the caudate and putamen [17, 86], positive correlations between putamen volume and lifetime nicotine/tobacco exposure [107], and positive correlations between greater striatal volume and more intense cue-induced tobacco craving [108]. Third, we followed previous recommendations that at least 10-15 experiments should be included in an ALE meta-analysis and note that the meta-analysis identifying gray matter decreases among smokers involved 14 studies. Based on recent data simulations [43], closer to ~20 experiments has been prescribed to achieve sufficient power to detect moderately sized effects. Fourth, meta-analytic results are limited by the methodology commonly employed by the included studies. With respect to the use of T1-weighted MRIs to assess gray matter, we note recent commentaries regarding the potential for drug-induced cerebral blood flow alterations to complicate interpretation of structural outcomes [109, 110]. Given that many studies included in this meta-analysis did not report the time elapsed between last cigarette smoked and MRI data collection (Additional file 1: Table S2), this potential confounding factor cannot be ruled out. Fifth, our behavioral decoding outcomes are limited by the studies archived in the BrainMap database at the time of analysis as well as its associated taxonomy. Sixth, although some studies have begun to characterize the impact of smoking on gray matter in young adult/adolescent smokers [85, 86], the concurrent influence of marijuana [111] or alcohol use [112], and sex differences among smokers [17], as more studies accumulate regarding the influence of these and other important factors on gray matter alterations, it will become possible to better characterize the specificity of the meta-analytic effects identified herein. Lastly, it remains for future work, perhaps through multi-site longitudinal investigations, to determine whether regional

structural alterations are a cause or consequence of cigarette smoking (or a combination thereof) and the extent to which such alterations recover following cessation.

In sum, cigarette smoking was associated with convergent structural decreases across studies in the PFC, insula, thalamus, and cerebellum. Some of these chronic smoking-related structural effects overlapped with regions showing acute nicotinic drug-induced functional effects. This study highlights the utility of using neuroimaging meta-analytic techniques to compile, synthesize, and inform neuroimaging investigations aiming to elucidate the neurobiological factors underlying the initiation, escalation, maintenance, and/or cessation of cigarette smoking. Collectively, our findings emphasize brain regions (e.g., vmPFC, insula, thalamus) and circuits (e.g., insula-thalamus) linked with chronic smoking, suggest neuroimaging paradigms warranting additional consideration among smokers (e.g., pain processing), and point to regions in need of further elucidation in addiction (e.g., cerebellum).

Authors' contributions

MTS and ARL conceived and designed the study. MTS, MCR, JF, JAY contributed to the acquisition, analysis, and visualization of the meta-analytic data. PTF and ARL contributed data analysis tools and technical support. MTS, EAS, ARL contributed to the interpretation of study results. MTS and ARL supervised the study. MTS, PTF, and ARL obtained funding. MTS and ARL supervised the study. MTS drafted the manuscript. All authors critically reviewed the manuscript for important intellectual content. All authors read and approved the final manuscript.

Author details
[1] Department of Psychology, Florida International University, AHC-4, RM 312, 11200 S.W. 8th St, Miami, FL 33199, USA. [2] Department of Physics, Florida International University, Miami, FL, USA. [3] Department of Psychology, Auburn University, Auburn, AL, USA. [4] Research Imaging Institute, University of Texas Health Science Center, San Antonio, TX, USA. [5] South Texas Veterans Health Care System, San Antonio, TX, USA. [6] State Key Laboratory for Brain and Cognitive Sciences, University of Hong Kong, Hong Kong, China. [7] Neuroimaging Research Branch, National Institute on Drug Abuse, Intramural Research Program, NIH/DHHS, Baltimore, MD, USA.

Acknowledgements
This work was supported by the National Institute on Drug Abuse (K01-DA037819, MTS) and the National Institute of Mental Health (R01-MH074457 and R56-MH097870, ARL and PTF) of the NIH. EAS is supported by the Intramural Research Program of the National Institute on Drug Abuse. The content is solely the responsibility of the authors and does not necessarily represent the official views of the NIH.

Competing interests
The authors declare that they have no competing interests.

References

1. Koob GF, Volkow ND. Neurocircuitry of addiction. Neuropsychopharm. 2010;35:217–38.
2. Droutman V, Read SJ, Bechara A. Revisiting the role of the insula in addiction. Trends Cogn Sci. 2015;19:414–20.
3. Konova AB, Goldstein RZ. Role of the value circuit in addiction and addiction treatment. In: Wilson SJ, editor. The Wiley-Blackwell handbook on the neuroscience of addiction. Hoboken: Wiley-Blackwell; 2015. p. 109–27.
4. Fedota JR, Stein EA. Resting-state functional connectivity and nicotine addiction: prospects for biomarker development. Ann NY Acad Sci. 2015;1349:64–82.
5. Jasinska AJ, Zorick T, Brody AL, Stein EA. Dual role of nicotine in addiction and cognition: a review of neuroimaging studies in humans. Neuropharmacology. 2014;84:111–22.
6. Sutherland MT, Ray KL, Riedel MC, Yanes JA, Stein EA, Laird AR. Neurobiological impact of nicotinic acetylcholine receptor agonists: an activation likelihood estimation meta-analysis of pharmacologic neuroimaging studies. Biol Psychiatry. 2015;78:711–20.
7. Menossi HS, Goudriaan AE, de Azevedo-Marques Perico C, Nicastri S, de Andrade AG, D'Elia G, Li CS, Castaldelli-Maia JM. Neural bases of pharmacological treatment of nicotine dependence—insights from functional brain imaging: a systematic review. CNS drugs. 2013;27:921–41.
8. Bentley P, Driver J, Dolan RJ. Cholinergic modulation of cognition: insights from human pharmacological functional neuroimaging. Prog Neurobiol. 2011;94:360–88.
9. Heishman SJ, Kleykamp BA, Singleton EG. Meta-analysis of the acute effects of nicotine and smoking on human performance. Psychopharmacology. 2010;210:453–69.
10. Newhouse PA, Potter AS, Dumas JA, Thiel CM. Functional brain imaging of nicotinic effects on higher cognitive processes. Biochem Pharmacol. 2011;82:943–51.
11. Durazzo TC, Meyerhoff DJ, Nixon SJ. A comprehensive assessment of neurocognition in middle-aged chronic cigarette smokers. Drug Alcohol Depend. 2012;122:105–11.
12. Durazzo TC, Meyerhoff DJ, Nixon SJ. Chronic cigarette smoking: implications for neurocognition and brain neurobiology. Int J Environ Res Public Health. 2010;7:3760–91.
13. Corley J, Gow AJ, Starr JM, Deary IJ. Smoking, childhood IQ, and cognitive function in old age. J Psychosom Res. 2012;73:132–8.
14. Brody AL, Mandelkern MA, Jarvik ME, Lee GS, Smith EC, Huang JC, Bota RG, Bartzokis G, London ED. Differences between smokers and non-smokers in regional gray matter volumes and densities. Biol Psychiatry. 2004;55:77–84.
15. Fritz HC, Wittfeld K, Schmidt CO, Domin M, Grabe HJ, Hegenscheid K, Hosten N, Lotze M. Current smoking and reduced gray matter volume-a voxel-based morphometry study. Neuropsychopharmacology. 2014;39:2594–600.
16. Kuhn S, Romanowski A, Schilling C, Mobascher A, Warbrick T, Winterer G, Gallinat J. Brain grey matter deficits in smokers: focus on the cerebellum. Brain Struct Funct. 2012;217:517–22.
17. Franklin TR, Wetherill RR, Jagannathan K, Johnson B, Mumma J, Hager N, Rao H, Childress AR. The effects of chronic cigarette smoking on gray matter volume: influence of sex. PLoS ONE. 2014;9:e104102.
18. Stoeckel LE, Chai XJ, Zhang J, Whitfield-Gabrieli S, Evins AE. Lower gray matter density and functional connectivity in the anterior insula in smokers compared with never smokers. Addict Biol. 2015. doi:10.1111/adb.12262.
19. Hanlon CA, Owens MM, Joseph JE, Zhu X, George MS, Brady KT, Hartwell KJ. Lower subcortical gray matter volume in both younger smokers and established smokers relative to non-smokers. Addict Biol. 2016;21(1):185–95.
20. Zhang X, Salmeron BJ, Ross TJ, Geng X, Yang Y, Stein EA. Factors underlying prefrontal and insula structural alterations in smokers. Neuroimage. 2011;54:42–8.
21. Liao Y, Tang J, Liu T, Chen X, Hao W. Differences between smokers and non-smokers in regional gray matter volumes: a voxel-based morphometry study. Addict Biol. 2012;17:977–80.
22. Kuhn S, Schubert F, Gallinat J. Reduced thickness of medial orbitofrontal cortex in smokers. Biol Psychiatry. 2010;68:1061–5.
23. Gallinat J, Meisenzahl E, Jacobsen LK, Kalus P, Bierbrauer J, Kienast T, Witthaus H, Leopold K, Seifert F, Schubert F, Staedtgen M. Smoking and structural brain deficits: a volumetric MR investigation. Eur J Neurosci. 2006;24:1744–50.
24. Yu R, Zhao L, Lu L. Regional grey and white matter changes in heavy male smokers. PLoS ONE. 2011;6:e27440.
25. Fox PT, Laird AR, Lancaster JL. Coordinate-based voxel-wise meta-analysis: dividends of spatial normalization. Report of a virtual workshop. Hum Brain Mapp. 2005;25:1–5.
26. Laird AR, Fox PM, Price CJ, Glahn DC, Uecker AM, Lancaster JL, Turkeltaub PE, Kochunov P, Fox PT. ALE meta-analysis: controlling the false discovery rate and performing statistical contrasts. Hum Brain Mapp. 2005;25:155–64.
27. Eickhoff SB, Bzdok D, Laird AR, Kurth F, Fox PT. Activation likelihood estimation meta-analysis revisited. Neuroimage. 2012;59:2349–61.
28. Goodkind M, Eickhoff SB, Oathes DJ, Jiang Y, Chang A, Jones-Hagata LB, Ortega BN, Zaiko YV, Roach EL, Korgaonkar MS, et al. Identification of a common neurobiological substrate for mental illness. JAMA Psychiatry. 2015;72:305–15.
29. Radua J, Borgwardt S, Crescini A, Mataix-Cols D, Meyer-Lindenberg A, McGuire PK, Fusar-Poli P. Multimodal meta-analysis of structural and functional brain changes in first episode psychosis and the effects of antipsychotic medication. Neurosci Biobehav Rev. 2012;36:2325–33.
30. Cooper D, Barker V, Radua J, Fusar-Poli P, Lawrie SM. Multimodal voxel-based meta-analysis of structural and functional magnetic resonance imaging studies in those at elevated genetic risk of developing schizophrenia. Psychiatry Res. 2014;221:69–77.
31. Nickl-Jockschat T, Kleiman A, Schulz JB, Schneider F, Laird AR, Fox PT, Eickhoff SB, Reetz K. Neuroanatomic changes and their association with cognitive decline in mild cognitive impairment: a meta-analysis. Brain Struct Funct. 2012;217:115–25.
32. Nickl-Jockschat T, Schneider F, Pagel AD, Laird AR, Fox PT, Eickhoff SB. Progressive pathology is functionally linked to the domains of language and emotion: meta-analysis of brain structure changes in schizophrenia patients. Eur Arch Psychiatry Clin Neurosci. 2011;261(Suppl 2):S166–71.
33. Laird AR, Eickhoff SB, Li K, Robin DA, Glahn DC, Fox PT. Investigating the functional heterogeneity of the default mode network using coordinate-based meta-analytic modeling. J Neurosci. 2009;29:14496–505.
34. Poldrack RA. Can cognitive processes be inferred from neuroimaging data? Trends Cogn Sci. 2006;10:59–63.
35. Yarkoni T, Poldrack RA, Nichols TE, Van Essen DC, Wager TD. Large-scale automated synthesis of human functional neuroimaging data. Nat Methods. 2011;8:665–70.
36. Wang C, Xu X, Qian W, Shen Z, Zhang M. Altered human brain anatomy in chronic smokers: a review of magnetic resonance imaging studies. Neurol Sci. 2015;36:497–504.
37. Pan P, Shi H, Zhong J, Xiao P, Shen Y, Wu L, Song Y, He G. Chronic smoking and brain gray matter changes: evidence from meta-analysis of voxel-based morphometry studies. Neurol Sci. 2013;34:813–7.
38. Wang K, Yang J, Zhang S, Wei D, Hao X, Tu S, Qiu J. The neural mechanisms underlying the acute effect of cigarette smoking on chronic smokers. PLoS ONE. 2014;9:e102828.
39. Morales AM, Lee B, Hellemann G, O'Neill J, London ED. Gray-matter volume in methamphetamine dependence: cigarette smoking and changes with abstinence from methamphetamine. Drug Alcohol Depend. 2012;125:230–8.
40. Almeida OP, Garrido GJ, Alfonso H, Hulse G, Lautenschlager NT, Hankey GJ, Flicker L. 24-month effect of smoking cessation on cognitive function and brain structure in later life. Neuroimage. 2011;55:1480–9.
41. Almeida OP, Garrido GJ, Lautenschlager NT, Hulse GK, Jamrozik K, Flicker L. Smoking is associated with reduced cortical regional gray matter density in brain regions associated with incipient Alzheimer disease. Am J Geriatr Psychiatry. 2008;16:92–8.
42. Chen X, Wen W, Anstey KJ, Sachdev PS. Effects of cerebrovascular risk factors on gray matter volume in adults aged 60–64 years: a voxel-based morphometric study. Psychiatry Res. 2006;147:105–14.
43. Eickhoff SB, Nichols TE, Laird AR, Hoffstaedter F, Amunts K, Fox PT, Bzdok D, Eickhoff CR. Behavior, sensitivity, and power of activation likelihood estimation characterized by massive empirical simulation. Neuroimage. in press.
44. Eickhoff SB, Laird AR, Grefkes C, Wang LE, Zilles K, Fox PT. Coordinate-based activation likelihood estimation meta-analysis of neuroimaging

data: a random-effects approach based on empirical estimates of spatial uncertainty. Hum Brain Mapp. 2009;30:2907–26.

45. Turkeltaub PE, Eickhoff SB, Laird AR, Fox M, Wiener M, Fox P. Minimizing within-experiment and within-group effects in Activation Likelihood Estimation meta-analyses. Hum Brain Mapp. 2012;33:1–13.

46. Turkeltaub PE, Eden GF, Jones KM, Zeffiro TA. Meta-analysis of the functional neuroanatomy of single-word reading: method and validation. Neuroimage. 2002;16:765–80.

47. Lancaster JL, Tordesillas-Gutierrez D, Martinez M, Salinas F, Evans A, Zilles K, Mazziotta JC, Fox PT. Bias between MNI and Talairach coordinates analyzed using the ICBM-152 brain template. Hum Brain Mapp. 2007;28:1194–205.

48. Nichols T, Brett M, Andersson J, Wager T, Poline JB. Valid conjunction inference with the minimum statistic. Neuroimage. 2005;25:653–60.

49. Laird AR, Fox PM, Eickhoff SB, Turner JA, Ray KL, McKay DR, Glahn DC, Beckmann CF, Smith SM, Fox PT. Behavioral interpretations of intrinsic connectivity networks. J Cogn Neurosci. 2011;23:4022–37.

50. Reetz K, Dogan I, Rolfs A, Binkofski F, Schulz JB, Laird AR, Fox PT, Eickhoff SB. Investigating function and connectivity of morphometric findings–exemplified on cerebellar atrophy in spinocerebellar ataxia 17 (SCA17). Neuroimage. 2012;62:1354–66.

51. Eickhoff SB, Jbabdi S, Caspers S, Laird AR, Fox PT, Zilles K, Behrens TE. Anatomical and functional connectivity of cytoarchitectonic areas within the human parietal operculum. J Neurosci. 2010;30:6409–21.

52. Robinson JL, Laird AR, Glahn DC, Lovallo WR, Fox PT. Metaanalytic connectivity modeling: delineating the functional connectivity of the human amygdala. Hum Brain Mapp. 2010;31:173–84.

53. Laird AR, Eickhoff SB, Fox PM, Uecker AM, Ray KL, Saenz JJ Jr, McKay DR, Bzdok D, Laird RW, Robinson JL, et al. The BrainMap strategy for standardization, sharing, and meta-analysis of neuroimaging data. BMC Res Notes. 2011;4:349.

54. Laird AR, Eickhoff SB, Kurth F, Fox PM, Uecker AM, Turner JA, Robinson JL, Lancaster JL, Fox PT. ALE meta-analysis workflows via the BrainMap database: progress towards a probabilistic functional brain atlas. Front Neuroinform. 2009;3:23.

55. Fox PT, Lancaster JL. Opinion: mapping context and content: the Brain-Map model. Nat Rev Neurosci. 2002;3:319–21.

56. Riedel MC, Ray KL, Dick AS, Sutherland MT, Hernandez Z, Fox PM, Eickhoff SB, Fox PT, Laird AR. Meta-analytic connectivity and behavioral parcellation of the human cerebellum. Neuroimage. 2015;117:327–42.

57. Fox PT, Laird AR, Fox SP, Fox PM, Uecker AM, Crank M, Koenig SF, Lancaster JL. BrainMap taxonomy of experimental design: description and evaluation. Hum Brain Mapp. 2005;25:185–98.

58. Turner JA, Laird AR. The cognitive paradigm ontology: design and application. Neuroinformatics. 2012;10:57–66.

59. Nickl-Jockschat T, Rottschy C, Thommes J, Schneider F, Laird AR, Fox PT, Eickhoff SB. Neural networks related to dysfunctional face processing in autism spectrum disorder. Brain Struct Funct. 2015;220:2355–71.

60. Cieslik EC, Zilles K, Caspers S, Roski C, Kellermann TS, Jakobs O, Langner R, Laird AR, Fox PT, Eickhoff SB. Is there "one" DLPFC in cognitive action control? Evidence for heterogeneity from co-activation-based parcellation. Cereb Cortex. 2013;23:2677–89.

61. Bzdok D, Heeger A, Langner R, Laird AR, Fox PT, Palomero-Gallagher N, Vogt BA, Zilles K, Eickhoff SB. Subspecialization in the human posterior medial cortex. Neuroimage. 2015;106:55–71.

62. Raichle ME, MacLeod AM, Snyder AZ, Powers WJ, Gusnard DA, Shulman GL. A default mode of brain function. PNAS. 2001;98:676–82.

63. Seeley WW, Menon V, Schatzberg AF, Keller J, Glover GH, Kenna H, Reiss AL, Greicius MD. Dissociable intrinsic connectivity networks for salience processing and executive control. J Neurosci. 2007;27:2349–56.

64. Gu H, Salmeron BJ, Ross TJ, Geng X, Zhan W, Stein EA, Yang Y. Mesocorticolimbic circuits are impaired in chronic cocaine users as demonstrated by resting-state functional connectivity. Neuroimage. 2010;53:593–601.

65. Peters J, Bromberg U, Schneider S, Brassen S, Menz M, Banaschewski T, Conrod PJ, Flor H, Gallinat J, Garavan H, et al. Lower ventral striatal activation during reward anticipation in adolescent smokers. Am J Psychiatry. 2011;168:540–9.

66. Rossi M, Pistelli F, Pesce M, Aquilini F, Franzoni F, Santoro G, Carrozzi L. Impact of long-term exposure to cigarette smoking on skin microvascular function. Microvasc Res. 2014;93:46–51.

67. Swan GE, Lessov-Schlaggar CN. The effects of tobacco smoke and nicotine on cognition and the brain. Neuropsychol Rev. 2007;17:259–73.

68. Picard F, Sadaghiani S, Leroy C, Courvoisier DS, Maroy R, Bottlaender M. High density of nicotinic receptors in the cingulo-insular network. Neuroimage. 2013;79:42–51.

69. Paterson D, Nordberg A. Neuronal nicotinic receptors in the human brain. Prog Neurobiol. 2000;61:75–111.

70. Staley JK, Krishnan-Sarin S, Cosgrove KP, Krantzler E, Frohlich E, Perry E, Dubin JA, Estok K, Brenner E, Baldwin RM, et al. Human tobacco smokers in early abstinence have higher levels of beta2* nicotinic acetylcholine receptors than nonsmokers. J Neurosci. 2006;26:8707–14.

71. Esterlis I, Ranganathan M, Bois F, Pittman B, Picciotto MR, Shearer L, Anticevic A, Carlson J, Niciu MJ, Cosgrove KP, D'Souza DC. In vivo evidence for beta2 nicotinic acetylcholine receptor subunit upregulation in smokers as compared with nonsmokers with schizophrenia. Biol Psychiatry. 2014;76:495–502.

72. Brody AL, Mukhin AG, Stephanie S, Mamoun MS, Kozman M, Phuong J, Neary M, Luu T, Mandelkern MA. Treatment for tobacco dependence: effect on brain nicotinic acetylcholine receptor density. Neuropsychopharmacology. 2013;38:1548–56.

73. Abreu-Villaca Y, Seidler FJ, Tate CA, Slotkin TA. Nicotine is a neurotoxin in the adolescent brain: critical periods, patterns of exposure, regional selectivity, and dose thresholds for macromolecular alterations. Brain Res. 2003;979:114–28.

74. Slotkin TA, Ryde IT, Seidler FJ. Separate or sequential exposure to nicotine prenatally and in adulthood: persistent effects on acetylcholine systems in rat brain regions. Brain Res Bull. 2007;74:91–103.

75. Jain A, Flora SJ. Dose related effects of nicotine on oxidative injury in young, adult and old rats. J Environ Biol. 2012;33:233–8.

76. Bartra O, McGuire JT, Kable JW. The valuation system: a coordinate-based meta-analysis of BOLD fMRI experiments examining neural correlates of subjective value. Neuroimage. 2013;76:412–27.

77. Levy DJ, Glimcher PW. The root of all value: a neural common currency for choice. Curr Opin Neurobiol. 2012;22:1027–38.

78. Hare TA, Camerer CF, Rangel A. Self-control in decision-making involves modulation of the vmPFC valuation system. Science. 2009;324:646–8.

79. Dosenbach NUF, Visscher KM, Palmer ED, Miezin FM, Wenger KK, Kang HSC, Burgund ED, Grimes AL, Schlaggar BL, Petersen SE. A core system for the implementation of task sets. Neuron. 2006;50:799–812.

80. Craig AD. How do you feel—now? The anterior insula and human awareness. Nature Rev Neurosci. 2009;10:59–70.

81. Naqvi NH, Bechara A. The insula and drug addiction: an interoceptive view of pleasure, urges, and decision-making. Brain Struct Funct. 2010;214:435–50.

82. Paulus MP. Decision-making dysfunctions in psychiatry—altered homeostatic processing? Science. 2007;318:602–6.

83. Balleine BW, Morris RW, Leung BK. Thalamocortical integration of instrumental learning and performance and their disintegration in addiction. Brain Res. 2015;1628:104–16.

84. Hogarth L, Balleine BW, Corbit LH, Killcross S. Associative learning mechanisms underpinning the transition from recreational drug use to addiction. Ann NY Acad Sci. 2013;1282:12–24.

85. Morales AM, Ghahremani D, Kohno M, Hellemann GS, London ED. Cigarette exposure, dependence, and craving are related to insula thickness in young adult smokers. Neuropsychopharmacology. 2014;39:1816.

86. Li Y, Yuan K, Cai C, Feng D, Yin J, Bi Y, Shi S, Yu D, Jin C, von Deneen KM, et al. Reduced frontal cortical thickness and increased caudate volume within fronto-striatal circuits in young adult smokers. Drug Alcohol Depend. 2015;151:211–9.

87. Karama S, Ducharme S, Corley J, Chouinard-Decorte F, Starr JM, Wardlaw JM, Bastin ME, Deary IJ. Cigarette smoking and thinning of the brain's cortex. Mol Psychiatry. 2015;20:778–85.

88. Zale EL, Ditre JW, Dorfman ML, Heckman BW, Brandon TH. Smokers in pain report lower confidence and greater difficulty quitting. Nicotine Tob Res. 2014;16:1272–6.

89. Ditre JW, Kosiba JD, Zale EL, Zvolensky MJ, Maisto SA. Chronic pain status, nicotine withdrawal, and expectancies for smoking cessation among lighter smokers. Ann Behav Med. 2016;50:427.

90. Ditre JW, Brandon TH, Zale EL, Meagher MM. Pain, nicotine, and smoking: research findings and mechanistic considerations. Psychol Bull. 2011;137:1065–93.

91. Parkerson HA, Zvolensky MJ, Asmundson GJ. Understanding the relationship between smoking and pain. Expert Rev Neurother. 2013;13:1407–14.

92. Nakajima M, Al'Absi M. Nicotine withdrawal and stress-induced changes in pain sensitivity: a cross-sectional investigation between abstinent smokers and nonsmokers. Psychophysiology. 2014;51:1015–22.

93. Al'Absi M, Lemieux A, Nakajima M, Hatsukami DK, Allen S. Circulating leptin and pain perception among tobacco-dependent individuals. Biol Psychol. 2015;107:10–5.

94. Pulvers K, Hood A, Limas EF, Thomas MD. Female smokers show lower pain tolerance in a physical distress task. Addict Behav. 2012;37:1167–70.

95. Baker TB, Piper ME, McCarthy DE, Majeskie MR, Fiore MC. Addiction motivation reformulated: an affective processing model of negative reinforcement. Psychol Rev. 2004;111:33–51.

96. Cosgrove KP, Esterlis I, McKee S, Bois F, Alagille D, Tamagnan GD, Seibyl JP, Krishnan-Sarin S, Staley JK. Beta2* nicotinic acetylcholine receptors modulate pain sensitivity in acutely abstinent tobacco smokers. Nicotine Tob Res. 2010;12:535–9.

97. Wylie KP, Tanabe J, Martin LF, Wongngamnit N, Tregellas JR. Nicotine increases cerebellar activity during finger tapping. PLoS ONE. 2013;8:e84581.

98. Ramnani N. Frontal lobe and posterior parietal contributions to the cortico-cerebellar system. Cerebellum. 2012;11:366–83.

99. Stoodley CJ. The cerebellum and cognition: evidence from functional imaging studies. Cerebellum. 2012;11:352–65.

100. Moulton EA, Elman I, Becerra LR, Goldstein RZ, Borsook D. The cerebellum and addiction: insights gained from neuroimaging research. Addict Biol. 2014;19:317–31.

101. Miquel M, Vazquez-Sanroman D, Carbo-Gas M, Gil-Miravet I, Sanchis-Segura C, Carulli D, Manzo J, Coria-Avila GA. Have we been ignoring the elephant in the room? Seven arguments for considering the cerebellum as part of addiction circuitry. Neurosci Biobehav Rev. 2016;60:1–11.

102. Lindquist KA, Wager TD, Kober H, Bliss-Moreau E, Barrett LF. The brain basis of emotion: a meta-analytic review. Behav Brain Sci. 2012;35:121–43.

103. Foland-Ross LC, Altshuler LL, Bookheimer SY, Lieberman MD, Townsend J, Penfold C, Moody T, Ahlf K, Shen JK, Madsen SK, et al. Amygdala reactivity in healthy adults is correlated with prefrontal cortical thickness. J Neurosci. 2010;30:16673–8.

104. Lyvers M, Carlopio C, Vicole Bothma H, Edwards MS. Mood, mood regulation, and frontal systems functioning in current smokers, long-term abstinent ex-smokers, and never-smokers. J Psychoact Drugs. 2014;46:133–9.

105. Lyvers M, Carlopio C, Bothma V, Edwards MS. Mood, mood regulation expectancies and frontal systems functioning in current smokers versus never-smokers in China and Australia. Addict Behav. 2013;38:2741–50.

106. Salimi-Khorshidi G, Smith SM, Keltner JR, Wager TD, Nichols TE. Meta-analysis of neuroimaging data: a comparison of image-based and coordinate-based pooling of studies. Neuroimage. 2009;45:810–23.

107. Das D, Cherbuin N, Anstey KJ, Sachdev PS, Easteal S. Lifetime cigarette smoking is associated with striatal volume measures. Addict Biol. 2012;17:817–25.

108. Janes AC, Park MT, Farmer S, Chakravarty MM. Striatal morphology is associated with tobacco cigarette craving. Neuropsychopharmacology. 2015;40:406–11.

109. Franklin TR, Wang Z, Shin J, Jagannathan K, Suh JJ, Detre JA, O'Brien CP, Childress AR. A VBM study demonstrating 'apparent' effects of a single dose of medication on T1-weighted MRIs. Brain Struct Funct. 2013;218:97–104.

110. Franklin TR, Wetherill RR, Jagannathan K, Hager N, O'Brien CP, Childress AR. Limitations of the use of the MP-RAGE to identify neural changes in the brain: recent cigarette smoking alters gray matter indices in the striatum. Front Hum Neurosci. 1052;2014:8.

111. Wetherill RR, Jagannathan K, Hager N, Childress AR, Rao H, Franklin TR. Cannabis, cigarettes, and their co-occurring use: disentangling differences in gray matter volume. Int J Neuropsychopharmacol. 2015;18:pyv061.

112. Luhar RB, Sawyer KS, Gravitz Z, Ruiz SM, Oscar-Berman M. Brain volumes and neuropsychological performance are related to current smoking and alcoholism history. Neuropsychiatric Dis Treat. 2013;9:1767–84.

11

Effect of parsley (*Petroselinum crispum*, Apiaceae) juice against cadmium neurotoxicity in albino mice (*Mus Musculus*)

Saleh N. Maodaa[1], Ahmed A. Allam[1,2*], Jamaan Ajarem[1], Mostafa A. Abdel-Maksoud[1], Gadah I. Al-Basher[1] and Zun Yao Wang[3*]

Abstract

Background: Parsley was employed as an experimental probe to prevent the behavioral, biochemical and morphological changes in the brain tissue of the albino mice following chronic cadmium (Cd) administration.

Methods: Non-anesthetized adult male mice were given parsley juice (*Petroselinum crispum*, Apiaceae) daily by gastric intubation at doses of 10 and 20 g/kg/day. The animals were divided into six groups: Group A, mice were exposed to saline; Groups B and C, were given low and high doses of parsley juice, respectively; Group D, mice were exposed to Cd; Groups E and F, were exposed to Cd and concomitantly given low and high doses of parsley, respectively.

Results: Cd intoxication can cause behavioral abnormalities, biochemical and histopathological disturbances in treated mice. Parsley juice has significantly improved the Cd-associated behavioral changes, reduced the elevation of lipid peroxidation and normalized the Cd effect on reduced glutathione and peroxidase activities in the brain of treated mice. Histological data have supported these foundations whereas Cd treatment has induced neuronal degeneration, chromatolysis and pyknosis in the cerebrum, cerebellum and medulla oblongata.

Conclusion: The low dose (5 g/kg/day) of parsley exhibited beneficial effects in reducing the deleterious changes associated with Cd treatment on the behavior, neurotransmitters level, oxidative stress and brain neurons of the Cd-treated mice.

Keywords: Heavy metal, Cerebellum, Cerebrum, Medulla oblongata, Neurotransmitter

Background

Cadmium (Cd) is among the most hazardous heavy metals that is not chemically degraded in the environment and can enter into the food chain [1]. Both natural and anthropogenic sources of this heavy metal, including industrial emissions and the application of fertilizer and sewage sludge to farm land, may lead to the contamination of soils and the increased Cd uptake by crops and vegetables grown for human consumption [2]. Some important sources of Cd exposure for humans can be the emissions from industries of petroleum mining, batteries, metal plating, pigments, plastics, toys and alloy, cigarette smoking and through dietary consumption [3]. Total human intake of Cd from food has been estimated by Järup [4] as 2.8–4.2 µg/kg body weight/week, which equates to approximately 40–60 % of the current provisional tolerable weekly intake of 7 µg/kg body weight/week.

Cd has no essential biochemical roles, but can exert diverse and severe toxicity in multiple body systems as it can bind to tissues, trigger oxidative stress, affect endocrine function, block aquaporins, and interfere with functions of essential cations such as magnesium and zinc [5]. Cd can pose some particular risks to the young,

*Correspondence: aallam@ksu.edu.sa; allam1081981@yahoo.com; wangzun315cn@163.com
[1] Department of Zoology, College of Science, King Saud University, Riyadh 11451, Saudi Arabia
[3] State Key Laboratory of Pollution Control and Resources Reuse, School of the Environment, Nanjing University, Nanjing 210023, Jiangsu, People's Republic of China
Full list of author information is available at the end of the article

as exposures in early life can compromise development, with lifelong physical, intellectual, and behavioral impairments [6]. The International Agency for Research on Cancer classified cadmium as a well-known carcinogen [7]. Cd represented one of the most toxic and carcinogenic heavy metals [8]. It is considered as a serious health hazard to humans and other animals [9]. Exposure to Cd may cause lesions in many organs such as brain, liver, kidney and testis [10], thus leading to cerebral, hepatic, renal and testicular dysfunction [11]. It has been reported that Cd exposure produced long-term impairments of neurobehavioral status such as alterations in attention and memory as well as in the psychomotor and visuomotor functioning and speed in workers [12, 13]. Clinical data have shown aggressive elevation and anxiety-like behaviors, impaired learning and memory processes, and changes in the development of the visual system [14]. Previous studies on Cd toxicity have reported behavioral impairments in both animal models and humans after exposure to Cd [15]. Acetylcholine esterase is an important enzyme that hydrolyses the neurotransmitter acetylcholine in the synaptic cleft of cholinergic synapses and neuromuscular junctions [16]. Alterations in the acetylcholine activity in various diseases and poisonings suggested that this enzyme could be an important physiological and pathological biomarker [17, 18].

Additionally, Cd can increase blood–brain barrier permeability, thus penetrating and accumulating in brain tissue of animals [17] and leading to brain intracellular accumulation, cellular dysfunction, and cerebral edema. Also, it can affect the degree and balance of excitation–inhibition in synaptic neurotransmission as well as the antioxidant levels in animal's brain [19, 20]. Cd toxicity is partly due to oxidative DNA damage associated with the increased production of reactive oxygen species (ROS), such as superoxide ion, hydroxyl radicals and hydrogen peroxide [21]. Previous studies have indicated that Cd can decrease antioxidant enzyme levels [21]. Free radicals cause the oxidation of biomolecules (e.g., protein, amino acids, lipid and DNA), which leads to cell injury and death [22]. For example, ROS markedly alter the physical, chemical, and immunological properties of superoxide dismutase (SOD), which further exacerbates oxidative damage in cells. This has raised the possibility that antioxidants could acts as prophylactic agents against many pathological conditions. It has long been recognized that naturally occurring substances in higher plants have antioxidant activities. Many culinary herbs (e.g., parsley) have been shown to function as natural antioxidants [23].

Parsley (*Petroselinum crispum*, Apiaceae) is an annual herb, which is important dietary source of vitamins and essential metals. It's usage at sufficient levels whether cooked or not cooked can promote the levels of vitamins

and essential metals in human body, which in turn can decrease the risks of Cd toxicity [24]. Phytochemical screening of parsley has revealed the presence of some compounds such as flavonoids [25], carotenoids [26], ascorbic acid [27] and tocopherol [28]. These components of fresh parsley leaf can scavenge superoxide anion in vitro and hydroxyl radical in addition to protecting against ascorbic acid-induced membrane oxidation [25]. Supplementation of diets with fresh parsley leaf can increase antioxidant capacity of rat plasma and decrease oxidative stress in humans [29]. Similarly, aqueous and ethanol extracts of fresh parsley leaf strongly inhibit linoleic acid oxidation and lipid oxidation [30]. Biological mobility, tissue concentrations, and excretion of Cd are determined by oxidation state, solubility, a complex set of equilibria between complexing sites, as well as active transport through membranes [31]. Chelation is central to natural detoxification of heavy metals, via formation of complexes, particularly with glutathione and other small molecules and their excretion [7]. Essential oil extracted from parsley possessed a certain degree of antioxidant activities in terms of β-carotene bleaching capacity and free radical scavenging activity [32]. Therefore, parsley was also reported as a possible source of antioxidants which may prevent Cd toxicity.

Also, parsley is one of the most used medicinal plants to treat arterial hypertension [33]; diabetes, cardiac [33] and renal diseases [34]. Moreover, in experimental studies, it has been reported that this herb has strong diuretic [35], anti-hyperglycemic, anti-hyperlipidemic, anticoagulant [36], anti-oxidant [32], anti-microbial [37] and laxative activities [38]. It has been reported that parsley alcoholic extract has a protective effect against toxicity induced by sodium valproate in male rats [39]. Parsley leaves were used for treatment of constipation, jaundice, colic, flatulence edema, rheumatism. It was used to treat eczema, knee, ache, impotence and bleeding [40]. However, according to our knowledge, the reported literatures on the protective effect of parsley against Cd neurotoxicity are still limited.

In the present work, we investigated the hypothesis that parsley juice may protect against Cd-induced pathological changes in albino mice.

Methods
Chemicals
Cadmium chloride ($CdCl_2$) was of analytical grade and purchased from Sigma Chemical Company (St Louis, MO, USA).

Parsley juice preparation
petroselinum crispum (*mill.*) *nymex a.w. hill* from the family Apiaceae (alt. Umbelliferae) is commonly known

as parsley. The origin of parsley is from Mediterranean region, but today is cultivated wherever of the world. Botanic identification was performed by taxonomist in the Department of botany and microbiology, Faculty of Sciences, King Saud University (Riyadh, Saudi Arabia) where a voucher specimen has been deposited (collection number AL 1021). The plain leaf parsley type daily collected from vegetable market in Riyadh (Saudi Arabia) was carefully washed under tap water. The fresh parsley juice was prepared daily using a vegetable juicer. Two concentrations of the juice were prepared: the first is 10 % juice, i.e., 10 g parsley squash in 100 ml drinking water. The second is 5 % juice, i.e., 5 g parsley squash in 100 ml drinking water. The prepared juice has been filtered using a filter paper after preparation and before drinking by the animals to remove fibers and other insoluble components.

Ethics statement

All the experimental protocols and investigations were approved and complied with the *Guide for Care and Use of Laboratory Animals* published by the US National Institutes of Health (NIH Publication No. 85–23, revised 1996) and was approved by the Ethics Committee for Animal Experimentation at King Saud University (Permit Number: PT 983).

Animals and dosing schedule

A total of 48 adult male albino mice (*Mus musculus*) weighing 30–35 g were obtained from College of Pharmacy, King Saud University, Saudi Arabia and housed in stainless steel wire cages (5 animals/cage) under specific pathogen-free conditions. The animals were maintained at 22–25 °C on a 12:12 h light/dark cycle and provided with food and water ad libitum. Parsley juice was orally administered daily to non-anesthetized parsley treated groups by gastric intubation at two doses of 10 and 20 g/kg/day for 28 days (D). Totally, 30 mg/kg of $CdCl_2$ dissolved in saline was intraperitoneally injected to partially anesthetized Cd treated groups by three exposure times D1, D7 and D15 (10 mg/kg every time). The animals were labeled into six groups as follows:

Group A: mice were given with tab water orally and saline intraperitoneally (*Control group*).
Group B: mice were given with 5 % Parsley juice orally and saline intraperitoneally (5 % *Parsley group*).
Group C: mice were given with 10 % Parsley juice orally and saline intraperitoneally (10 % *Parsley group*).
Group D: mice were given with tab water orally and Cd doses intraperitoneally (*Cd intoxicated group*).
Group E: mice were given with 5 % Parsley juice orally and Cd doses intraperitoneally (5 % *Parsley-Cd group*).

Group F: mice were given with 10 % Parsley juice orally and Cd doses intraperitoneally (10 % *Parsley-Cd group*).

Cd estimation assay
Instrumentation
The analytical determination of Cd in mice brain was carried out by ICP-MS (inductively coupled plasma mass spectrometer): ELAN 9000 (Perkin Elmer Sciex Instrumento, Concord, Ontario, Canada).

Reagents
Nitric acid (69 % v/v), super purity grade was supplied from Romil, England. Hydrochloric acid (37 % v/v) and hydrofluoric acid (40 % v/v) were supplied from Merck (Germany). High purity water obtained from Millipore Milli-Q water purification system was used throughout the work.

Calibration
The ICP-MS calibration was carried out by external calibration with the blank solution and three working standard solutions (20, 40 and 60 ppm), starting from 1000 mg/l single standard solutions for ICP-MS (A ristar grade, BDH laboratory supplies, England for Cd).

Sample collection and preparation
Samples were prepared by accurately weighing 200 mg of longitudinal section of brain into a dry and clean Teflon digestion beaker, 6 ml of HNO_3, 2 ml HCl and 2 ml HF were added to the Teflon beaker. Samples were digested on the hot plate at 120–150 °C for approximately 40 min. The resulting digest was not clear, so it was filtered through whatman filtered paper No. 42. The filtered digest was transferred to a 50 ml plastic volumetric flask and made up to mark using deionized water. A blank digest was carried out in the same way.

Behavioral assays
8 male mice from each group were used in the present study at the beginning of the 5th week (D28–30) after finishing the dosing period. The animals were used only in one test of the present tests per day. For the tests, the animals were brought in a room (25 °C) of dim red light reserved for that purpose. All tests were conducted blindly by the same experimenter [41].

T-maze conducting assay
The six groups of animals were prevented from food all the night before this examination. The elevated T-maze consisted of three closed arms to be T like structure. The main arm (100 × 10 × 20 cm) and two lateral arms (40 × 10 × 20 cm) at an elevation of 20 cm above the

floor. Arms of the maze form T like structure. The rodent food was placed at the end of the right lateral arm. The maze was cleaned with a 20 % ethanol after each test. The hungry animals were placed in the terminal end of the main arm of the elevated T-maze facing the passage to the two lateral arms. The mice left to explore the maze for 1 min, then the animal removed from the maze and kept in its cage for 2 h. The mice replaced in the same position in the main arm and the behavior analyzed for 5 min by an experimenter who is blind for the experimental protocol. The frequency and duration in food and main arm visits (under red illumination) were recorded. The time spent exploring the arms to reach food (seconds), and the time spent in food arm in seconds, were determined. The frequency and time of entering the food lateral arm not the other lateral arm was considered to be memory reflector according to Leret [42].

Cage activity assay

The Ugo Basile 47420-Activity Cage was used to record spontaneous co-ordinate activity of mice and variation of this activity in time either horizontal or vertical movements. This test was performed for 3 min/animal.

Grip-strength meter assay

The Ugo Basile 47200-Grip-Strength Meter suitable for mice automatically measures grip-strength (i.e. peak force and time resistance) of forelimbs in mice. The aim was to assess forelimbs muscle strength. Each animal was tested for three times and the peak force of each mouse was recorded. The mean of three values of each mouse was recorded.

Rota-rod assay

The Ugo Basile rota-rod instrument was used in this test, the mouse is placed on a horizontally oriented and mechanically rotating at 15 rpm rod. The rod is suspended above a cage floor, which is low enough not to injure the animal, but high enough to induce avoidance of fall. Mice naturally try to stay on the rotating rod, or rota-rods, and avoid falling to the ground. The length of time that a given animal stays on this rotating rod is a measurement of their balance, coordination, physical condition, and motor-activity.

Biochemical assays

8 animals of each group were anesthetized by light ether and sacrificed at D30. Brain was dissected and 0.5 g tissue was homogenized in 5 ml of cold 0.1 M $HClO_4$ containing 0.05 % EDTA. The homogenate was centrifuged at 10,000 rpm for 10 min at 4 °C and the clear supernatant collected in a microfuge tube (0.5 ml each) and stored at −40 °C until assays.

Dopamine and serotonin determination

The level of neurotransmitters 5-hydroxytryptamine or serotonin and dopamine was estimated in the brain. The monoamines dopamine and serotonin was estimated using the modified method of Patrick [43]. A 10 % homogenate of the brain has been re-centrifuged at 17,000 rpm at 4 °C for 5 min. The supernatants were filtered using 0.45 μm pore filters and analyzed by high performance liquid chromatography. The mobile phase consisted of 32 mM citric acid monohydrate, 12.5 mM disodium hydrogen orthophosphate, 7 % methanol, 1 mM octane sulfonic acid and 0.05 mM EDTA. The mobile phase was filtered through 0.22 μm filter and degassed under vacuum before use. Bondpak C_{18} column was used at a flow rate of 1.2 ml/min and the injection volume of the sample was 20 μl. The levels of dopamine and serotonin were calculated using a calibration curve and the results were expressed as ng/mg tissue weight.

Determination of acetylcholine

The method has been described previously which didn't use acetylcholine esterase inhibitor [44]. Inbrief, dialysate samples were directly injected into the liquid chromatography/electrochemistry system assisted by a chromatography manager (Millennium; Waters, Milford, MA) and analyzed for acetylcholine. Acetylcholine was separated on a coiled cation exchanger acetylcholine column (analytical column) (Sepstik 530 × 1.0 mm I.D., packed with polymetric strong exchanger, 10 μm in diameter; BAS, West Lafayette, IN), followed by the post-immobilized enzyme reactor which consisted of choline oxidase/acetylcholine esterase. Acetylcholine was hydrolyzed by acetylcholine esterase to form acetate and choline in the post-immobilized enzyme reactor, and then choline was oxidized by choline oxidase to produce betaine and hydrogen peroxide (H_2O_2). H_2O_2 is detected via oxidation of horseradish peroxidase, which in turn oxidized Os (bpy) entrapped in the redox polymer coated on the surface of the glassy carbon electrode (MF-9080; BAS), set at +100 mV (LC-4C; BAS) versus Ag/AgCl reference electrode. This reduction was analyzed with the detector (LC-4C; BAS) as a signal indicating acetylcholine on the chromatogram.

Lipid peroxidation assay (TBARS)

Lipid peroxidation was determined by assaying thiobarbituric acid-reactive substances (TBARS) according to the method of Preuss [45]. Briefly, 1.0 ml supernatant was precipitated with 2 ml 7.5 % trichloroacetic acid and centrifuged at 1000g for 10 min. Clear supernatant was mixed with 1 ml 0.70 % thiobarbituric acid, incubated at 80 °C and the absorbance measured at 532 nm. Tetramethoxypropane was used as the standard.

Glutathione (GSH) assay

Glutathione content was determined according to the procedure of Beutler [46] with some modifications. Briefly, 0.20 ml of tissue supernatant was mixed with 1.5 ml precipitating solution containing 1.67 % glacial metaphosphoric acid, 0.20 % Na-EDTA and 30 % NaCl. The mixture was allowed to stand for 5 min at room temperature and centrifuged at $1000g$ for 5 min. One ml clear supernatant was mixed with 4 ml 0.30 M Na_2HPO_4 and 0.50 ml DTNB reagent (40 mg 5, 5′ dithiobis-(2-nitrobenzoic acid dissolved in 1 % sodium citrate). A blank was similarly prepared in which 0.20 ml water was used instead of the brain supernatant. The absorbance of the color was measured at 412 nm in a spectrophotometer.

Peroxidase activity determination

Peroxidase activity was determined according to the method of Kar and Mishra [47]. Briefly, 1.0 ml supernatant was mixed with 3.0 ml of 0.01 M phosphate- buffered saline (pH 6.8), 315 μl of 2 % pyrogallol, 154 μl H_2O_2 and incubated for 15 min at 25 °C. The reaction was stopped by the addition of 0.50 ml of 5 % H_2SO_4 and the absorbance was recorded at 420 nm. Peroxidase activity was expressed as the amount of purpurogallin formed per unit absorbance.

Histological preparations

For the histological preparations, left loop of cerebellum, cerebral cortex and medulla oblongata of three sacrificed animals were immediately fixed in 20 % formalin saline for 24 h. The tissues were washed to remove the excessive fixative and then dehydrated in ascending grades (70, 80, 90 and 95 %) of ethyl alcohol for 45 min each, then in two changes of absolute ethyl alcohol for 30 min each. This was followed by two changes of xylene for 30 min each. The tissues were then impregnated with paraplast plus (three changes) at 60 °C for 3 h and then embedded in paraplast plus. Sections (4–5 μm) were prepared with a microtome, de-waxed, hydrated and stained in Mayer's haemalum solution for 3 min. The sections were stained in Eosin for one min, washed in tap water and dehydrated in ethanol as described above. Hematoxylin and eosin (H&E) stained sections were prepared according to the method of Mallory [48].

Statistical analysis

The Statistical Package for the Social Sciences (SPSS for windows version 11.0; SPSS Inc, Chicago) was used for the statistical analyses. Comparative analyses were conducted by using the general linear models procedure (SPSS, Inc). Also, the data were analyzed using one-way and two-way analysis of variance (ANOVA) followed by LSD computations to compare various groups with each other. Results were expressed as mean ± S.D. The level of significance was expressed as significant at $P < 0.05$, highly significant at $P < 0.01$ and very highly significant at $P < 0.001$.

Results
Cd bioaccumulation

Cd concentrations in the brain tissues of exposed mice were estimated. As shown in Fig. 1, Cd bioaccumulation in the brain of both parsley groups (Groups B and C) was significantly ($P < 0.05$) reduced in comparison to the control group. On the other hand, a highly significant ($P < 0.001$) increase in the level of Cd in Cd-intoxicated

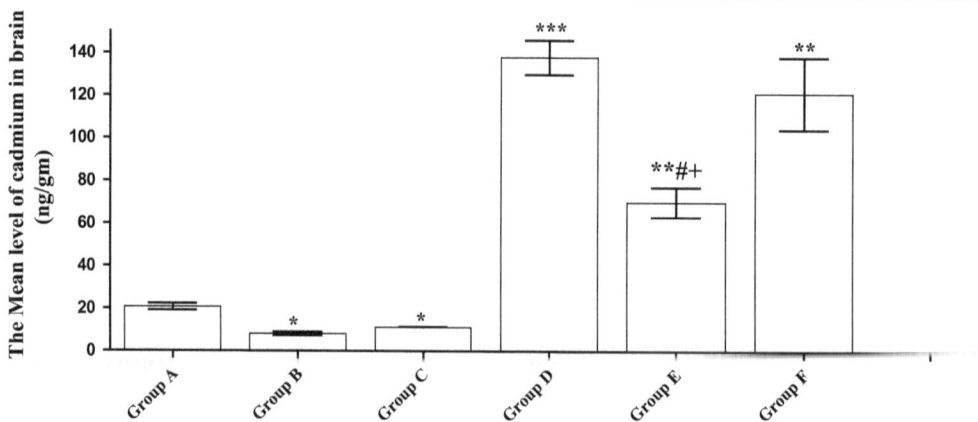

Fig. 1 The mean concentration of Cd in the brain tissue of Cd-treated animals in comparison to control groups. Data are expressed as mean ± SEM (N = 8) (F = 28.446). *P < 0.05 for parsley (Groups B and C), Cd (Group D) and parsley + Cd treated groups (Groups E and F) versus control (Group A); #P < 0.05 for parsley + Cd treated groups versus cadmium group; +P < 0.05 for low dose parsley treated group versus high dose parsley treated group. (**P < 0.01; ***P < 0.001)

group (Group D) in comparison to the control group, was monitored. Meanwhile, parsley treatment has an obvious ameliorating effect on Cd-intoxication. Both the low (5 %) and the high (10 %) doses of parsley have clearly decreased the Cd level in the brain tissues of Cd-parsley groups in comparison to the Cd-group (Group D) with the more reducing effect being associated with the low parsley dose (Group E).

Effect of parsley treatment on the body weight change in Cd- treated mice

Toxicological studies have illustrated that many toxicants are usually associated with weight loss in exposed animals. In the current study, we have investigated the dampening effect of Cd toxicity on the body weight increase in treated mice and the possible restoring capacity of parsley on this effect. Table 1 illustrates that both parsley groups (B and C) have exhibited a similar pattern of body weight change in comparison to the control group (A) during the experiment time. Conversely, Cd-intoxicated group (D) has showed a significant decrease in the body weight in comparison to the control group. Parsley treatment has restored to some extent, the normal pattern of body weight change seen in the control groups.

Behavioral investigations

The behavior of animals in the T-maze showed that the Cd treated animals have bad memory and low smell ability. This was elucidated by the decreased number of entrances to the main arm (Fig. 2a) and to the food arm (Fig. 2c) concomitant with the long time consumed by the Cd-treated animals to reach to the food (Fig. 2b) and to the food arm (Fig. 2d) in comparison to the control animals. Parsley treatment has showed an ameliorating effect that was clearer in the low dose parsley group in comparison to the high dose one. In the activity cage,

Table 1 Effect of parsley treatment on the animal's body weight change

	Initial weight	Final weight
Group A	32.21 ± 3.818	35.8 ± 4.131
Group B	32.87 ± 4.079	35.122 ± 5.638
Group C	32.81 ± 5.178	33.72 ± 5.5
Group D	33.7 ± 6.549	32.9 ± 7.1*
Group E	31.2 ± 4.589	33.97 ± 4.095#
Group F	31.8 ± 4.131	32.2 ± 6.71#

Initial and final body weights were estimated for all the five groups of animals. Data are expressed as mean ± SEM (N = 8). *P < 0.05, **P < 0.01, ***P < 0.001, for parsley (Groups B and C), Cd (Group D) and parsley + Cd treated groups (Groups E and F) versus control (Group A); # P < 0.05 for parsley + Cd treated groups versus cadmium group; +P < 0.05 for low dose parsley treated group versus high dose parsley treated group

the animals of Cd-intoxicated group showed a significant elevation in the vertical and horizontal movements as compared to the control group. On the contrary of the vertical movement, the animals of both parsley groups (Groups B and C) showed significant increases in the values of horizontal movements. After parsley treatment, the animals of Groups E and F displayed values of vertical and horizontal movements that were near to that of the control group animals (Fig. 3a, b).

The fore-limb muscles of mice in Groups A, B and C recorded relatively similar beaks in the grip strength examination scores. The recorded beaks of Group D animals appeared significantly lower in comparison to the control, the beaks achieved by the animals of Groups E and F showed significant improvements (Fig. 3c).

In rota-rod test and in comparison to the control group, the latency to fall by the Cd-intoxicated group on the rod was significantly reduced. Parsley treatment has resulted in increasing the staying times of the animals of Groups E and F on the rod to become near to that of the control group (Fig. 3d).

Biochemical studies
Neurotransmitters

Dopamine is an important neurotransmitter and its concentration is usually linked with the functioning of the nervous system and the behavior of living organisms. In both of the control and the parsley groups (A, B and C), the dopamine level in mice brain appeared nearly similar with little elevation in Group C. In comparison to the control group, a highly significant depletion of dopamine concentration has been detected in Cd-intoxicated group (P < 0.001). Parsley treatment has slightly ameliorated this effect but still, a significant reduction in Groups E and F (P < 0.01) was recorded (Fig. 4a). Serotonin level, another important neurotransmitter, was investigated in all the experimental groups. Both parsley groups (B and C) have showed no significant difference in the brain level of serotonin in comparison to the control group. A significant reduction in the level of serotonin was detected in Cd-intoxicated group (D). Following parsley treatment with two different doses, the level of serotonin was significantly reduced in the low dose parsley group (E) while the high dose one (F) has showed no significant reduction as compared to the control (Fig. 4b).

The present acetylcholine concentrations showed similar results to dopamine. In Groups A, B and C, its concentration did not show any significant difference, while it displayed a highly significant (P < 0.01) depletion in Cd-intoxicated group. In Groups E and F, a significant (P < 0.05) reduction in serotonin level was also monitored but still, parsley treatment has an obvious lowering effect on the Cd-induced pathology (Fig. 4c).

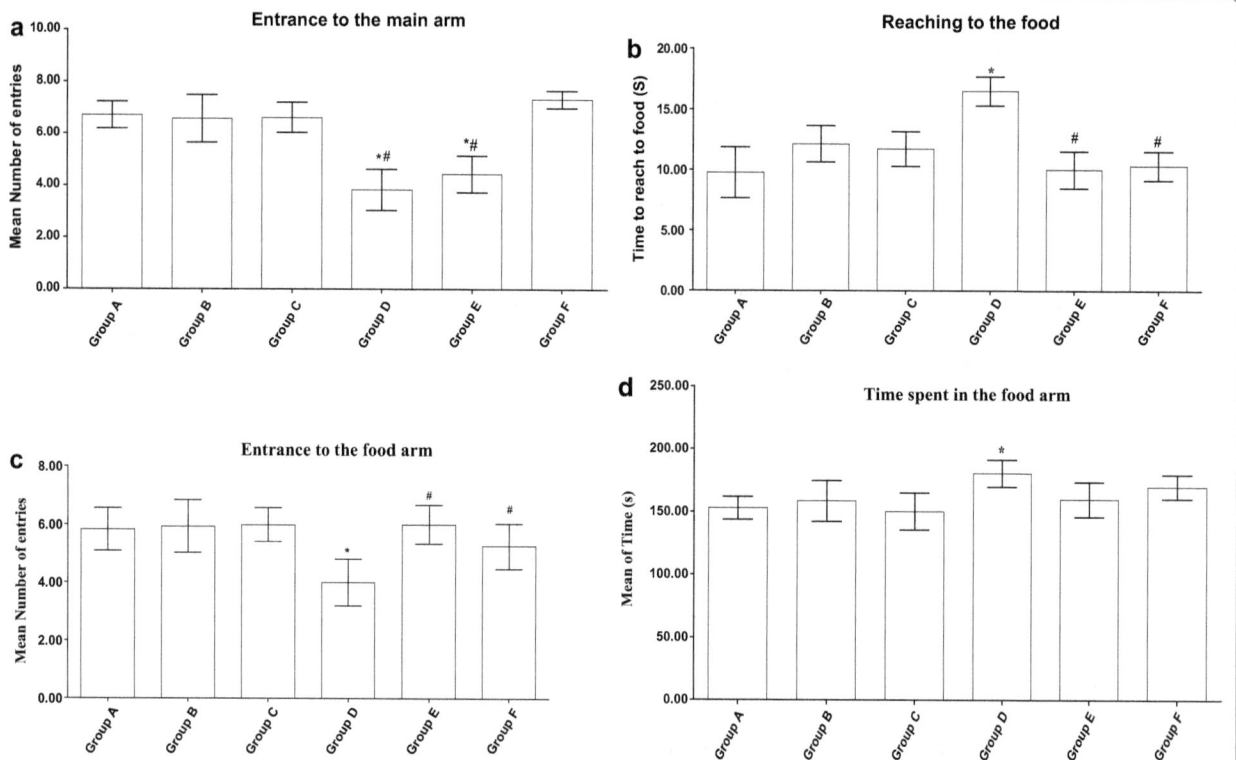

Fig. 2 Parsley treatment can affect animal's behavior. Animal's behavior in T-maze. **a** The number of entrances of main arm (F = 3.448). **b** The time consumed to reach to the food (F = 8.076). **c** The number of entrances to the food arm (F = 3.471). **d** The time spent in the food arm (F = 8.780). Data are expressed as mean ± SEM (N = 8). *P < 0.05 for parsley (Groups B and C), Cd (Group D) and parsley + Cd treated groups (Groups E and F) versus control (Group A); #P < 0.05 for parsley + Cd treated groups versus cadmium group; +P < 0.05 for low dose parsley treated group versus high dose parsley treated group

Oxidative stress

As illustrated in Fig. 5a, the change in brain lipid peroxidation in parsley groups was not significant in comparison to the control group. Conversely, a significant (P < 0.01) elevation in TBARS level was detected in Cd-intoxicated group. However, after parsley treatment the TBARS level was significantly lowered in both Cd-parsley groups (Groups E and F) in comparison to Cd group (Group D).

In addition to the increased level of TBARS, Cd treatment has also produced a significant (P < 0.001) decrease in GSH content in Cd-intoxicated group. Parsley has exerted a positive impact and improvement was observed in both of parsley-Cd groups as indicated from the significant increase in Groups E and F in comparison to the Cd group (D) (Fig. 5b).

Peroxidase activity was also monitored as an important indicator for oxidative stress. While both parsley groups have a similar level of peroxidase in comparison to the control, Cd-intoxicated group has showed a significant elevation in the peroxidase activity as compared to the

control (Fig. 5c). After parsley treatment, both parsley-Cd groups have showed decreased level of peroxidase as compared to the Cd group.

Brain histopathological changes

The normal pyramidal neurons exhibited their general characteristic shape. The nuclei of these cells were rounded, large and centrally located (Fig. 6). The normal cells of the cerebral cortex had spherical or pyramidal perikaryon, whose nuclei were large; also the neurons were arranged in a regular pattern (Fig. 6a–c). The cerebral neurons appeared more developed toward the white matter. In Cd-treated group, chromatolysis and pyknosis have been observed in the pyramidal neurons. In Groups E and F, parsley juice showed significant neuronal protection through reducing the rate of chromatolysis and pyknosis (Fig. 6d–f).

In the cerebellum, the fold layers (molecular, Purkinje cells and internal granular) became completely mature and the external granular layer disappeared completely (Fig. 7). The neuronal density in the molecular layer

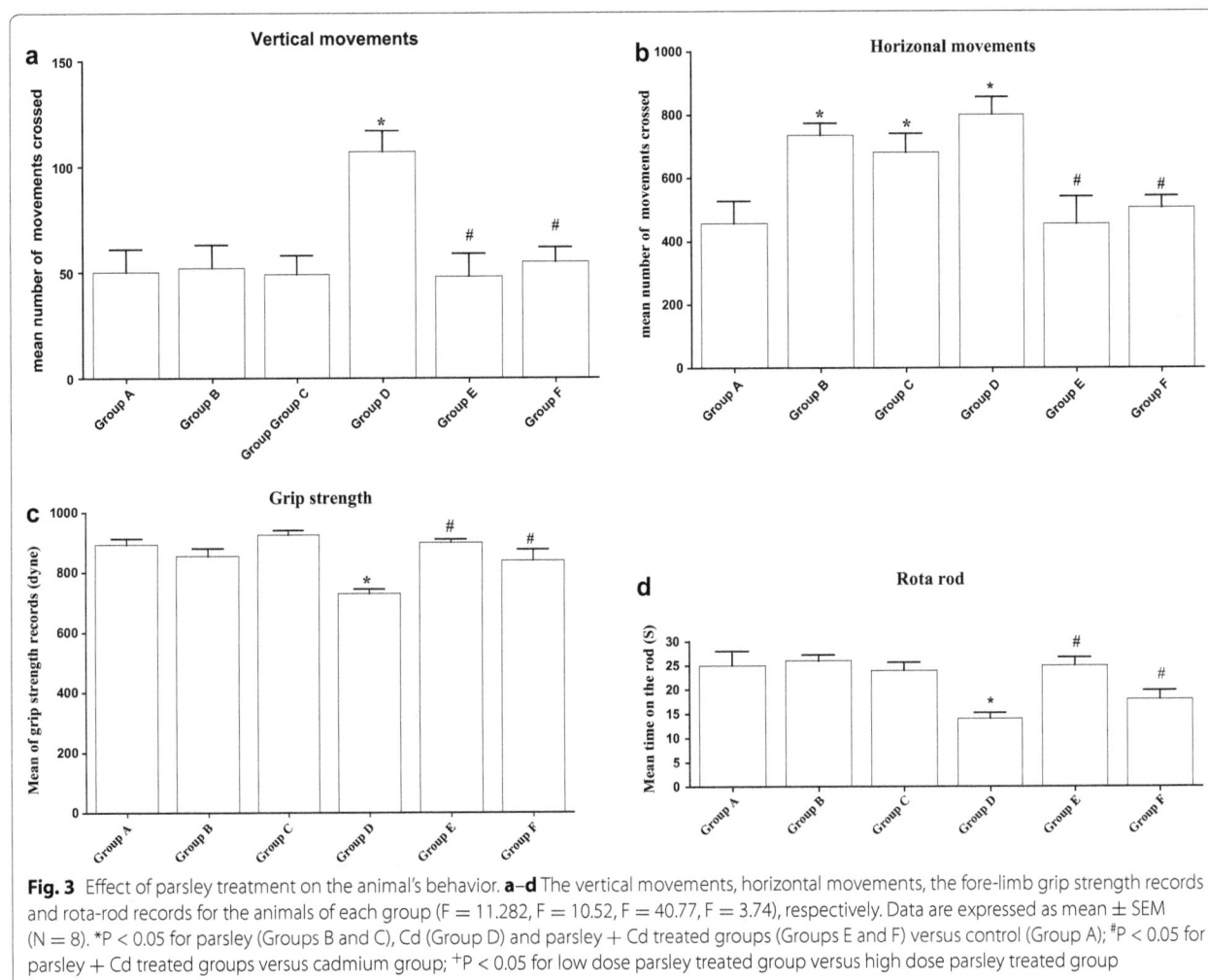

Fig. 3 Effect of parsley treatment on the animal's behavior. **a–d** The vertical movements, horizontal movements, the fore-limb grip strength records and rota-rod records for the animals of each group (F = 11.282, F = 10.52, F = 40.77, F = 3.74), respectively. Data are expressed as mean ± SEM (N = 8). *P < 0.05 for parsley (Groups B and C), Cd (Group D) and parsley + Cd treated groups (Groups E and F) versus control (Group A); #P < 0.05 for parsley + Cd treated groups versus cadmium group; +P < 0.05 for low dose parsley treated group versus high dose parsley treated group

of both the control and the parsley treated groups was the highest as compared to Cd-treated groups. The normal Purkinje cells were arranged in a single row of large neurons with pear-shaped perikaryon and large nucleus. The lateral processes were disappeared and the apical processes formed the permanent dendritic tree (Fig. 7). In Cd-treated groups, some degenerated and pyknotic Purkinje cells were detected. Of which, some were more spindle-shaped and small. These numbers of degenerated Purkinje neurons were reduced in Cd-parsley groups (Groups E and F) (Fig. 7d–f). Variations have been observed in the folds size of the groups, where small folds appeared in Group D.

The normal medulla neurons appeared large in size, polygonal, varied in shape and had round nuclei (Fig. 8a–c). In Cd-treated group, most medulla neurons appeared small and pyknotic (Fig. 8d). In Cd-parsley treated groups, the medulla neurons showed improvement (Fig. 8e, f).

Discussion

The present study was designed to investigate the protective role of parsley juice against Cd neurotoxicity in albino mice. The obtained results suggested that intake of parsley may partly improve the malformations induced by exposure of adult mice to Cd. The effects of daily supplementation of two different doses of parsley on the deleterious changes of Cd on animal's behavioral activities, neurotransmitters level, oxidative stress parameters and histopathology of brain were investigated in the current study. The high concentration of Cd in brain tissues of Cd-treated groups may be due to the Cd bioaccumulation. The current results of Groups E and F showed that parsley juice has an observable protective effect against Cd accumulation especially at the low dose. This may be due to the significant effect of parsley in the excretion of heavy metals from body, an effect that was documented before [35]. In fact the dose dependence of parsley has been illustrated before [49] and it seems in the current study that the low parsley dose is considered as a therapeutic dose while the high dose

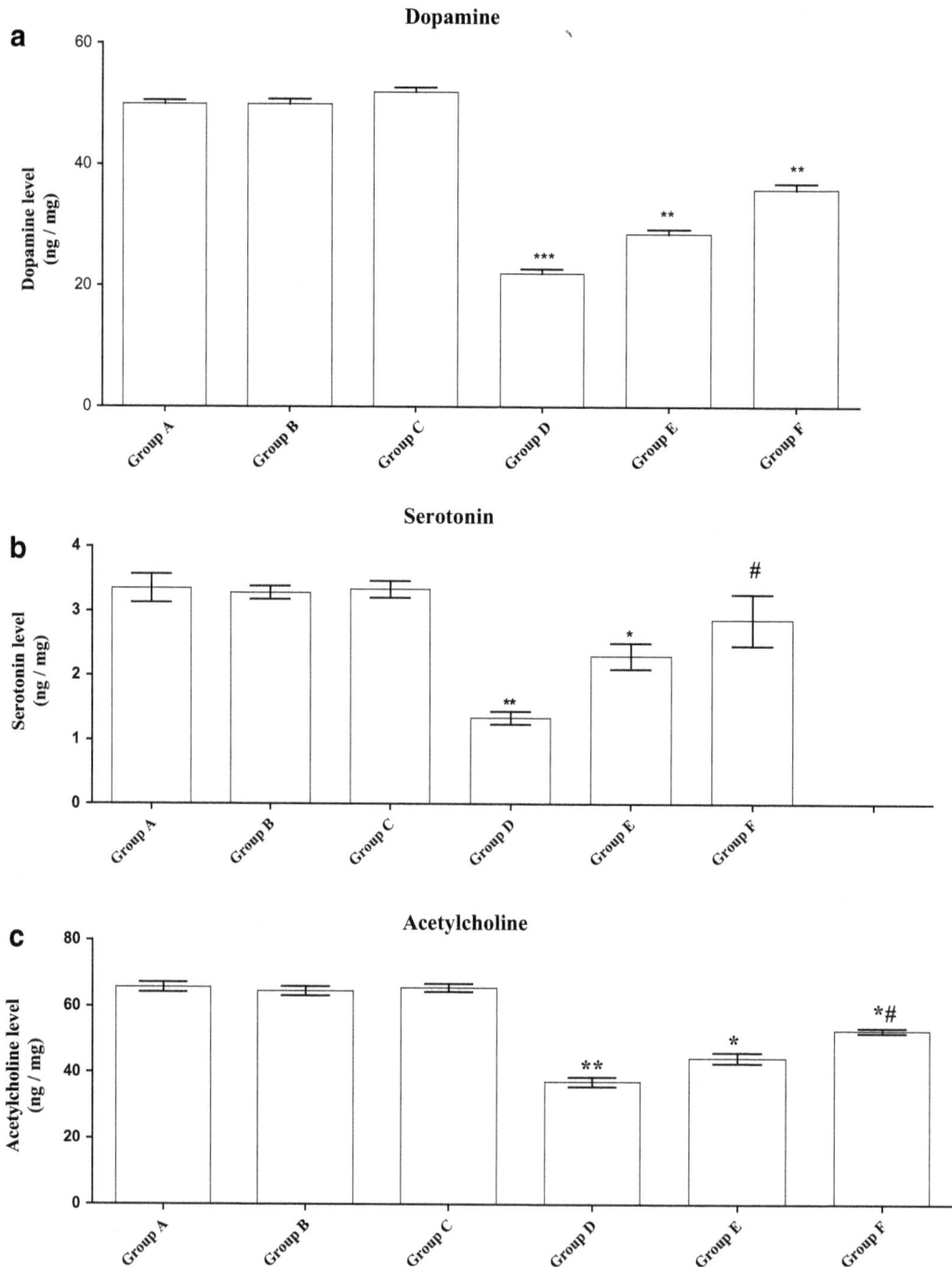

Fig. 4 Effect of parsley treatment on the brain level of neurotransmitters. **a–c** The mean concentration of extra cellular dopamine, serotonin and acetylcholine in the animals brain tissues of each group (F = 249.63, F = 31.24, F = 169.79), respectively. Data are expressed as mean ± SEM (N = 8). *P < 0.05, **P < 0.01,***P < 0.001, for parsley (Groups B and C), Cd (Group D) and parsley + Cd treated groups (Groups E and F) versus control (Group A); #P < 0.05 for parsley + Cd treated groups versus cadmium group; +P < 0.05 for low dose parsley treated group versus high dose parsley treated group

one is considered as overdose. Previously, animal's body weight was known to be one of the most sensitive indicators of toxicity [49]. In a recent study of Gonçalves [17], the rodents exposed to Cd were reported to display a lowered body weight. Our data supports these previous foundations in Cd-intoxicated group. However, in Cd-parsley groups,

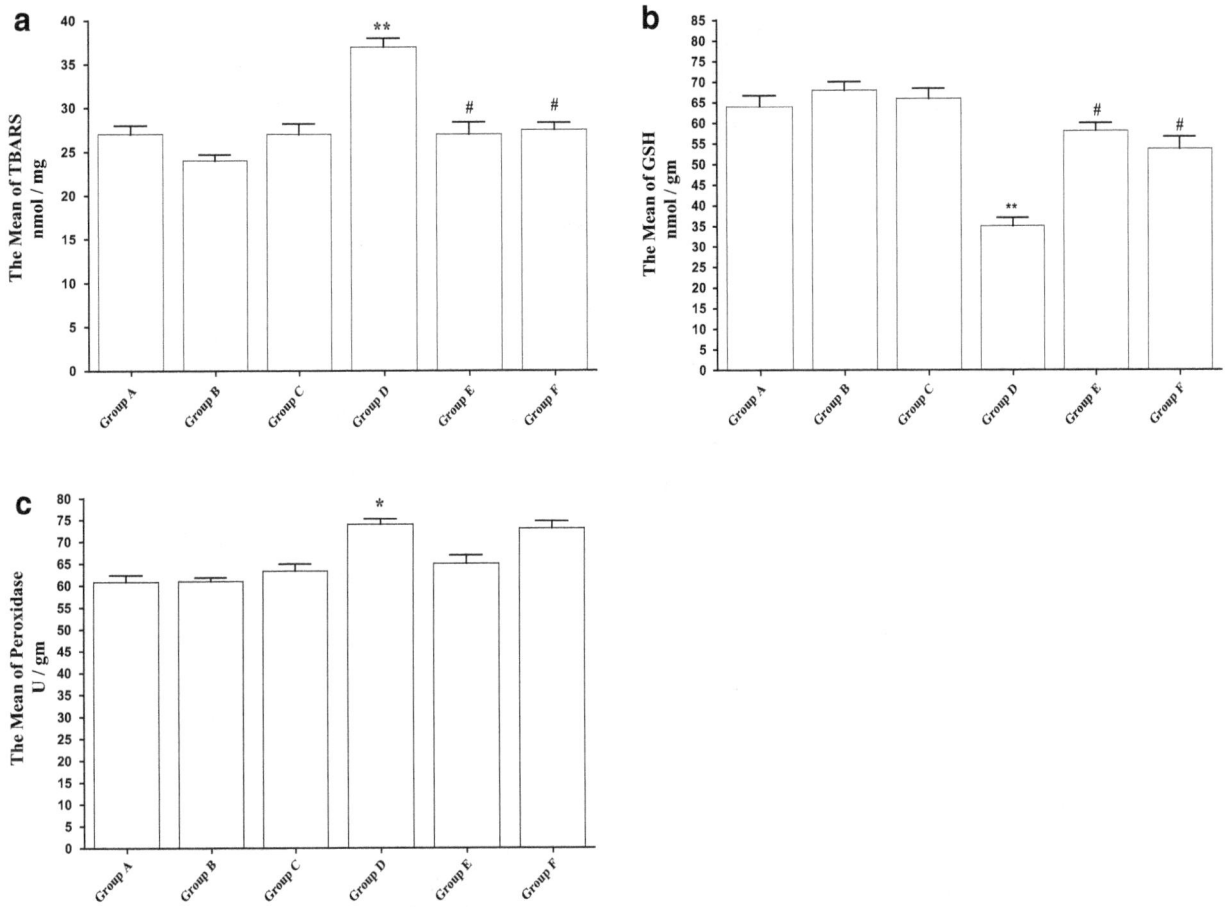

Fig. 5 Effect of parsley treatment on Cd-induced oxidative stress. **a–c** The mean concentration of TBARS, GSH and peroxidase in the brain tissues of each group (F = 124.53, F = 189.94, F = 154.65), respectively. Data are expressed as mean ± SEM (N = 8). *P < 0.05, **P < 0.01, ***P < 0.001, for parsley (Groups B and C), Cd (Group D) and parsley + Cd treated groups versus control (Groups E and F); #P < 0.05 for parsley + Cd treated groups versus cadmium group; +P < 0.05 for low dose parsley treated group versus high dose parsley treated group

parsley could improve this effect and this may be attributed, in part, to the beneficial actions that parsley exerts on the gastrointestinal tract [51].

The results of the present study showed that the brain levels of neurotransmitters were significantly depleted by Cd treatment in Cd-exposed mice. It was reported previously that neurotransmitter depletion is nutritionally based. Neurotransmitters are made from amino acids that are required for its creation. Consequently, if the diet is deficient, neurotransmitter deficiency develops [52]. Here, Cd-intoxication may have been resulted in anorexia and consequently diet deficiency. There is an evidence of an inhibitory role of dopamine and serotonin mediated receptors in depressing the hyperexcitability of brain neurons as appeared by the poor performance of the treated animals in the current behavioral examinations [8]. Recently, many research groups have focused on the participation of serotonin in the neurochemical mechanisms of cognition, especially of learning and

memory. Potential toxic mechanisms of action for Cd may include the disruption in serotonergic neurotransmission through disturbed levels of neurotransmitters in mice brain [50]. It was reported before that Cd toxicity has resulted in disrupted acetylcholine esterase activity [15]. Cd-intoxicated group of animals showed greater oxidative stress and a marked depletion of the antioxidants, than Groups E and F animals that were exposed to Cd and parsley juice. The results presented in the current study showing higher increase of the lipid peroxidation in Group D which is in accordance with the results obtained by Méndez-Armenta and Ríos [19] that reported an enhanced lipid peroxidation and increased TBARS after acute Cd exposure. Glutathione is one of the essential compounds for maintenance of cell integrity and participation in cellular metabolism [51]. Alterations in the ratio of reduced (GSH) and oxidized (GSSG) glutathione are well accepted as one of the indicators of oxidative stress in humans and experimental animals [52, 53].

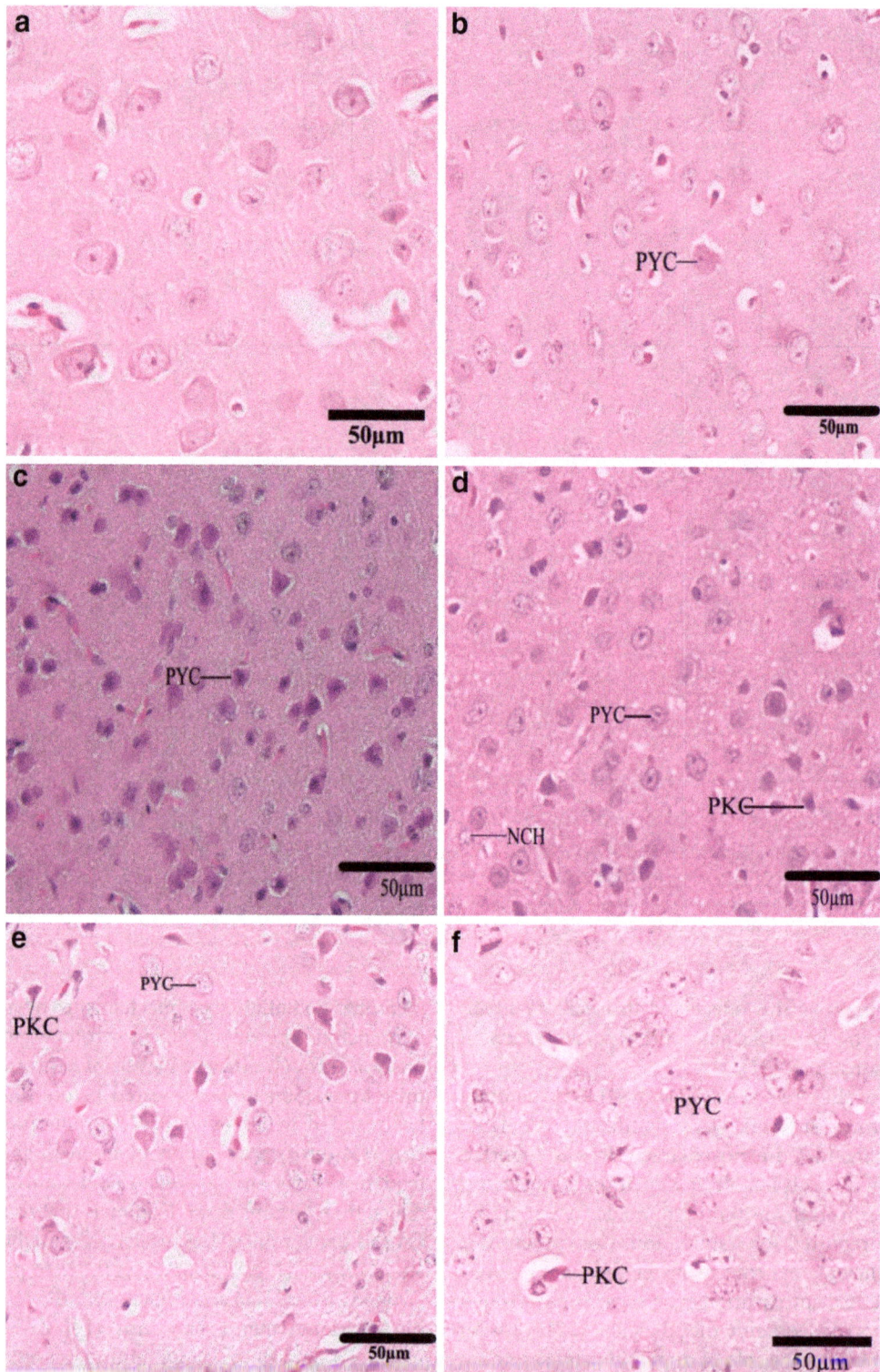

Fig. 6 Effect of parsley treatment on the histology of cerebral cortex. Photographs of the cerebral cortex of the newborns at D30 showing pyramidal neurons (PYC) degenerated pyramidal cells (PKC), neurocytechromatolysis (NCH). **a** Control group, **b** Parsley 5 % group (Group B), **c** Parsley 10 % group (Group C), **d** Cd-group (Group D), **e** Cd + 5 % parsley group (Group E) and **f** Cd + 10 % parsley group (Group F) (H & E stain)

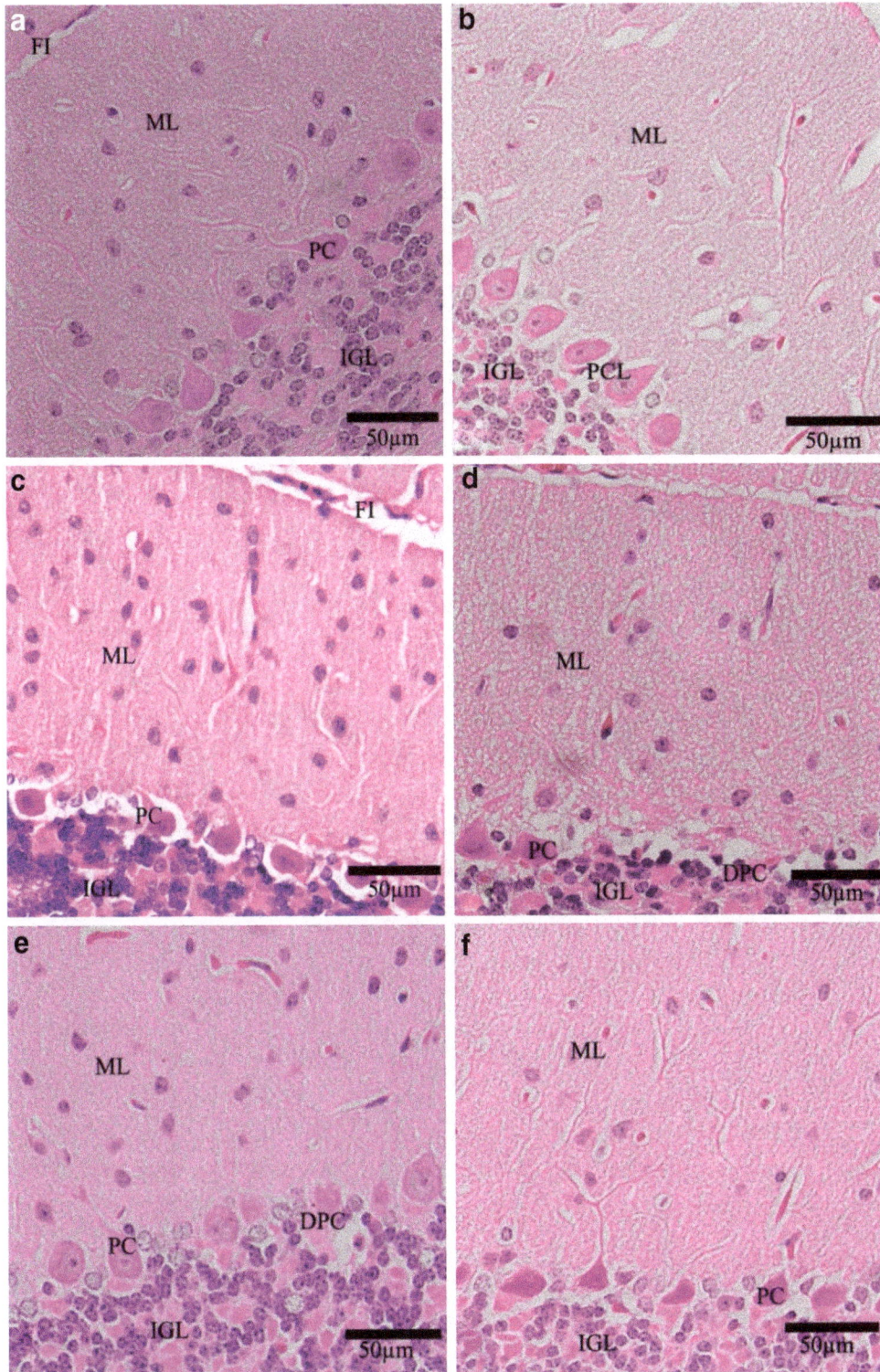

Fig. 7 Effect of parsley treatment on the histology of cerebellar cortex. Photographs of the cerebellar cortex of the newborns at D30 showing Purkinje cell (PC),Purkinje cell layer (PCL), degenerated Purkinje cell (DPC), fissure (FI), hemorrhage (H), internal granular layer (IGL), molecular layer (ML) and white matter (WM). **a** Control group, **b** parsley 5 % group (Group B), **c** parsley 10 % group (Group C), **d** Cd-group (Group D), **e** Cd + 5 % parsley group (Group E) and **f** Cd + 10 % parsley group (Group F) (H & E stain)

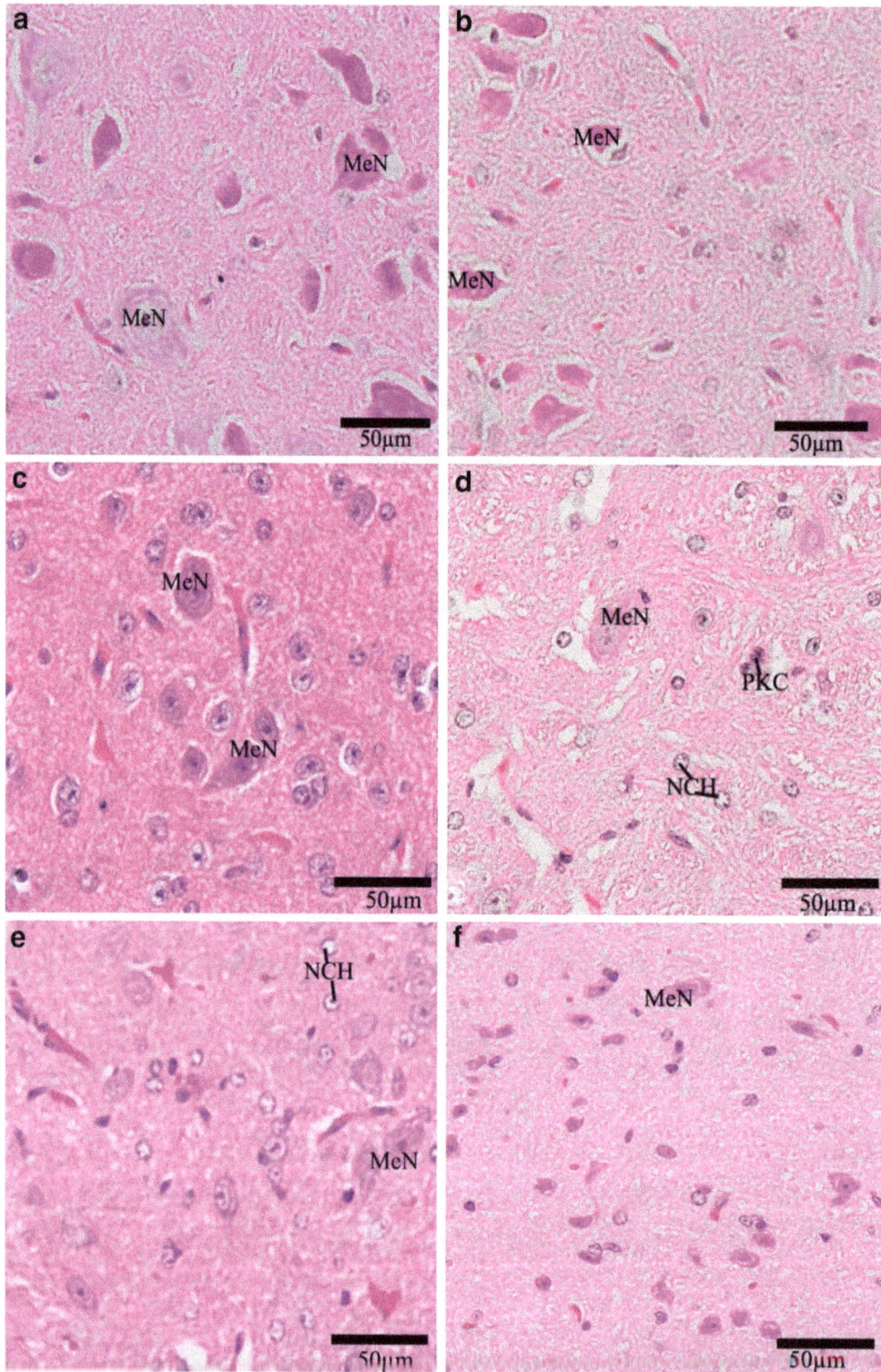

Fig. 8 Effect of parsley treatment on the histology of medulla oblongata. Photographs of the medulla oblongata of the newborns at D30 showing medulla neurons (MeN), degenerated medullary cells (PKC), neurocytechromatolysis (NCH). **a** Control group, **b** parsley 5 % group (Group B), **c** parsley 10 % group (Group C), **d** Cd-group (Group D), **e** Cd + 5 % parsley group (Group E) and **f** Cd + 10 % parsley group (Group F) (H & E stain)

The depletion of GSH may lead to lipid peroxidation. Therefore, GSH is considered as an important biomarker of oxidative stress [54]. The level of GSH is regulated by NADPH dependent enzyme, glutathione reductase (GR), and therefore an inhibition of GR may adversely affect GSH levels [54]. Furthermore, conjugation of heavy metals metabolites, with GSH forms glutathione-S-conjugates, which ultimately forms mercapturic acids [55]. This may further deplete GSH in the cell. Abu-Taweel [8] reported that Cd depleted GSH content and increased peroxidase enzymes activities in mice. Increased peroxidase activity might be due to generation of free radicals [56]. The antioxidant enzymes (e.g. peroxidases) constituted a mutually supportive team of defense against ROS [54].

Several mechanisms can contribute to the increased oxidative stress in toxicity induced by heavy metals, especially chronic exposure to Cd. Accumulated evidence pointed out that Cd inhalation can lead to elevated ROS and reactive nitrogen species (RNS) production by the mitochondrial respiratory system, antioxidant enzyme inactivation and an imbalance of glutathione redox status [13]. Cd toxicity can promote an important oxidative imbalance, favoring the production of free radicals and the reduction of antioxidant defenses. At high concentrations, ROS/RNS can damage the major components of the cellular structure, including nucleic acids, proteins, amino acids, and lipids [57]. Such oxidative modifications would affect several cell functions, metabolism, and gene expression, which in turn can cause some other pathological conditions [58]. The oxidative stress leads to neuronal damage in several brain regions [54–59]. For example, neuronal loss in the cerebrum can impair animal's memory [60] while, neuronal loss in the cerebellum can have some adverse effects on balance and coordination [55]. In addition, neuronal loss in the medulla oblongata and the spinal cord can affect physical activity of mice [61]. Supplementation with parsley juice for 28 days alleviated somewhat the Cd-induced toxicity, which showed significant improvement in the physical balance, memory, coordination, motor activities, muscles strength and brain neurotransmitters levels in Cd-treated animals. Parsley supplementation also restored GSH balance and decreased lipid peroxidation and peroxidase activity. Overall, this study demonstrated that the low dose (10 g/kg/day) of parsley supplementation could improve the pathological alterations in mice and this is in accordance with the results reported by Zhang [32]. Parsley has also been found to significantly suppress hydroperoxide and ROS levels in brain and other tissues in mice by stimulating production of glutathione synthesis and thereby boosting cellular antioxidant defenses [32]. Taken together, our data demonstrates that parsley may be an important therapeutic tool to combat Cd toxicity-associated effects. This parsley ameliorating effect may be due to its ability to neutralize free radicals and thereby prevent neuronal damage caused by oxidative stress.

Conclusion
Parsley has protective effects against Cd neurotoxicity in albino mice. Parsley juice supplementation improves the abnormal behavior of Cd intoxicated mice and reduces neuronal aberrations in the brain.

Abbreviations
D: day; EDTA: ethylene diamine tetraacetic Acid; ICP-MS: inductively coupled plasma mass spectrometer; GSH: reduced glutathione; ROS: reactive oxygen species; RNS: reactive nitrogen species; TBARS: thiobarbituric acid-reactive substances.

Authors' contributions
AA and SM carried out the experiments, participated in the design of the study, performed the statistical analysis and drafted the manuscript. JA and ZW provided expertise in the HPLC–MS analysis and participated in the design and coordination of the study. MA revised the whole Ms, performed statistical revision and performed the body weight change follow up and data analysis. GA revised the discipline of the statistical work and whole manuscript. All authors read and approved the final manuscript.

Author details
[1] Department of Zoology, College of Science, King Saud University, Riyadh 11451, Saudi Arabia. [2] Department of Zoology, Faculty of Science, Beni-Suef University, Beni-Suef, Egypt. [3] State Key Laboratory of Pollution Control and Resources Reuse, School of the Environment, Nanjing University, Nanjing 210023, Jiangsu, People's Republic of China.

Acknowledgements
The authors would like to extend their sincere appreciation to the Deanship of Scientific Research at King Saud University for its funding of this research through the Research Group Project no RGP- VPP- 240.

Competing interests
The authors declare that they have no competing interests.

References
1. ATSDR. Agency for toxic substance and disease registry. Atlanta: U.S. Toxicological Profile for Cadmium, Department of Health and Humans Services, Public Health Service, Centers for Disease Control; 2005.
2. Järup L, Akesson A. Current status of cadmium as an environmental health problem. Toxicol Appl Pharmacol. 2009;238:201–8.
3. de Souza PF, Diamante MA, Dolder H. Testis response to low doses of cadmium in Wistar rats. Int J Exp Pathol. 2010;91(2):125–31.
4. Järup L, Berglund M, Elinder CG, Nordberg G, Vahter M. Health effects of cadmium exposure—a review of the literature and a risk estimate. Scan J Work Environ Health. 1998;42:1–52.
5. Fowler BA. Monitoring of human populations for early markers of cadmium toxicity: a review. Toxicol Appl Pharmacol. 2009;238(3):294–300.
6. Sears ME. Chelation: harnessing and enhancing heavy metal detoxification—a review. ScientificWorldJournal. 2013;2013:1–13.
7. Matovic VA, Bulat ZB, Cosi D. Cadmium toxicity revisited: focus on oxidative stress induction and interactions with zinc and magnesium. Arch Ind Hyg Toxicol. 2011;62:65–76.

8. Abu-Taweel GM, Ajarem JS, Ahmad M. Protective effect of curcumin on anxiety, learning behavior, neuromuscular activities, brain neurotransmitters and oxidative stress enzymes in cadmium intoxicated mice. J Behav Brain Sci. 2013;3:74–84.

9. Brzoska MM, Majewska K, Kupraszewicz E. Effects of low, moderate and relatively high chronic exposure to cadmium on long bones susceptibility to fractures in male rats. Environ Toxicol Pharmacol. 2010;29(3):235–45.

10. Xu LC, Sun H, Wang SY, Song L, Chang HC, Wang XR. The roles of metallothionein on cadmium induced testes damages in Sprague dawley rats. 2005.

11. Ognjanovic BI, Markovic SD, Ethordevic NZ, Trbojevic IS, Stajn AS, Saicic ZS. Cadmium induced lipid peroxidation and changes in antioxidant defense system in the rat testes: protective role of coenzyme Q(10) and vitamin E. Reprod Toxicol. 2010;29(2):191–7.

12. Viaene MK, Masschelein R, Leeders J, De Groof M, Swerts LJVC, Roels HA. Neurobehavioural effects of occupational exposure to cadmium: a cross sectional epidemiological study. Occup Environ Med. 2000;57:19–27.

13. Haider S, Anis L, Batool Z, Sajid I, Naqvi F, Khaliq S, Ahmed S. Short term cadmium administration dose dependently elicits immediate biochemical, neurochemical and neurobehavioral dysfunction in male rats. Metab Brain Dis. 2015;30(1):83–92.

14. Terçariol SG, Almeida AA, Godinho AF. Cadmium and exposure to stress increase aggressive behavior. Environ Toxicol Pharmacol. 2011;32:40–5.

15. Gonçalves JF, Fiorenza AM, Spanevello RM, Mazzanti CM, Bochi GV, Antes FG, Stefanello N, Rubin MA, Dressler VL, Morsch VM, Schetinger MRC. N-Acetylcysteine prevents memory deficits, the decrease in acetylcholinesterase activity and oxidative stress in rats exposed to cadmium. Chem Biol Interact. 2010;186:53–60.

16. Soreq H, Seidman S. Acetylcholinesterase—new roles for an old actor. Nat Rev Neurosci. 2001;2:294–302.

17. Gonçalves JF, Fernando T, da Costa NP, Farias GJ, et al. Behavior and brain enzymatic changes after long-term intoxication with cadmium salt or contaminated potatoes. Food Chem Toxicol. 2012;50:3709–18.

18. Schmatz R, Mazzanti CM, Spanevello R, Stefanello N, Gutierres J, Corrêa M, Rosa MM, Rubin MA, Schetinger MRC, Morsch VM. Resveratrol prevents memory deficits and the increase in acetylcholinesterase activity in streptozotocin-induced diabetic rats. Eur J Pharmacol. 2009;610:42–8.

19. Méndez-Armenta M, Ríos C. Cadmium neurotoxicity. Environ Toxicol Appl Pharmacol. 2007;23:350–8.

20. Ji LY, Zhang WW, Yu D, Cao YR, Xu H. Effect of heavy metal-solubilizing microorganisms on zinc and cadmium extractions from heavy metal contaminated soil with Tricholomalobynsis. World J Microbiol Biotechnol. 2012;28(1):293–301.

21. Stohs SJ, Bagchi D, Hassoun E, Bagchi M. Oxidative mechanism in the toxicity of chromium and cadmium ions. J Environ Pathol Toxicol Oncol. 2000;19:201–13.

22. Paniagua-Castro N, Escalona-Cardoso G, Madrigal-Bujaidar E, Martínez-Galero E, Chamorro-Cevallos G. Protection against cadmium-induced teratogenicity in vitro by glycine. Toxicol In Vitro. 2008;22(1):75–9.

23. Jaswir I, Che Man YB, Kitts DD. Synergistic effect of rosemary, sage and citric acid on retention of fatty acids fromre fined, bleached and deodorized palm olein during repeated deepfat frying. J Am Oil Chem Soc. 2000;77:527–33.

24. Zhai Q, Narbad A, Chen W. Dietary strategies for the treatment of cadmium and lead toxicity. Nutrients. 2015;7:552–71.

25. Fejes S, Blazovics A, Lemberkovics E, Petri G, Szöke E, Kery A. Free radical scavenging and membrane protective effects of methanol extracts from Anthriscuscerefolium L. (Hoffm.) and Petroselinum crispum (Mill.) nym. ex A.W. Hill. Phytother Res. 2000;14:362–5.

26. Francis GW, Isaksen M. Droplet counter current chromatography of the carotenoids of parsley: Petroselinum crispum. Chromatographia. 1989;27:549–51.

27. Davey MW, Bauw G, Montagu MV. Analysis of ascorbate in plant tissues by high-performance capillary zone electrophoresis. Anal Biochem. 1996;239:8–19.

28. Fiad S, El Hamidi M. Vitamin E and trace elements. SeifenOeleFetteWasche. 1993;119:25–6.

29. Nielsen SE, Young JF, Daneshvar B, Lauridsen ST, Knuthsen P, Sandstrom B, et al. Effect of parsley (Petroselinumcrispum) intake on urinary apigenin excretion, blood antioxidant enzymes and biomarkers for oxidative stress in human subjects. Br J Nutr. 1999;81:447–55.

30. Wong PY, Kitts DD. Studies on the dual antioxidant and antibacterial properties of parsley (Petroselinumcrispum) and cilantro (Coriandrumsativum) extracts. Food Chem. 2006;97:505–15.

31. Nordberg GF, Nogawa K, Nordberg M, Friberg LT. Foreword metals–a new old environmental problem and chapter 23: cadmium. In: Nordberg GF, Fowler BA, Nordberg M, Friberg LT, editors. Handbook on the toxicology of metals. 3rd ed. Academic Press: Academic Press; 2011. p. vii–446–451, 463–470, 600–609.

32. Zhang H, Chen F, Wang Xi, Yao HY. Evaluation of antioxidant activity of parsley (Petroselinumcrispum) essential oil and identification of its antioxidant constituents. Food Res Int. 2006;39:833–9.

33. Eddouks M, Maghrani M, Lemhadri A, Ouahidi ML, Jouad H. Ethnopharmacological survey of medicinal plants used for the treatment of diabetes mellitus, hypertension and cardiac diseases in the south-east region of Morocco (Tafilalet). J Ethnopharmacol. 2002;82:97–103.

34. Jouad H, Haloui M, Rhiouani H, El Hilaly J, Eddouks M. Ethnobotanical survey of medicinal plants used for the treatment of diabetes, cardiac and renal diseases in the North centre region of Morocco (Fez-Boulemane). J Ethnopharmacol. 2001;77:175–82.

35. Darias V, Martin-Herrera D, Abdalla S, Fuente D. Plant used in urinary pathologies in the Canary island. Pharm Biol. 2001;39:170–80.

36. Yazicioglu A, Tuzlaci E. Folkmedicinal plants of Trabzon (Turkey). Fitoterapia. 1996;67:307–18.

37. Ojala T, Remes S, Haansuu P, Vuorela H, Hiltunen R, Haahtela K, Vuorela P. Antimicrobial activity of some coumarin containing herbal plants growing in Finland. J Ethnopharmacol. 2000;73:299–305.

38. Kreydiyyeh SI, Usta J, Kaouk I, Al-Sadi R. The mechanism underlying the laxative properties of parsley extract. Phytomedicine. 2001;8:382–8.

39. Jassim AM. Protective Effect of Petroselinumcrispum (parsley)extract on histopathological changes in liver, kidney and pancreas induced by sodium valproate-in male rats. Kufa J Vet Med Sci. 2013;4(1):20–7.

40. Manderfeld MM, Schafer HW, Davidson PM, Zottola EA. Isolation and identification of antimicrobial furocoumarins from parsley. J Food Prot. 1997;60:72–7.

41. Ajarem JS, Ahmad M. Behavioral and biochemical consequences of perinatal exposure of mice to instant coffee: a correlative evaluation. Pharmacol Biochem Behav. 1991;40(4):847–52.

42. Leret ML, San Millán JA, Antonio MT. Perinatal exposure to lead and cadmium affects anxiety-like behavior. Toxicology. 2003;186:125–30.

43. Patrick OE, Hirohisa M, Masahira K, Koreaki M. Central nervous system bioaminergic responses to mechanic trauma. Surg Neurol. 1991;35(4):273–9.

44. Ichikawa J, Li Z, Dai J, Meltzer HY. Atypical antipsychotic drugs, quetiapine, iloperidone, and melperone, preferentially increase dopamine and acetylcholine release in rat medial prefrontal cortex: role of 5-HT1A receptor agonism. Brain Res. 2002;956(2):349–57.

45. Preuss HG, Jarrel ST, Scheckenbach R, Lieberman S, Anderson RA. Comparative effects of chromium, vanadium and Gymnema sylvestre on sugar-induced blood pressure elevations in SHR. J Am Coll Nutr. 1998;17(2):116–23.

46. Beutler E, Duron O, Kelly BM. Improved method for determination of blood glutathione. J Lab Clin Med. 1963;61:882–8.

47. Kar M, Mishra D. Catalase, peroxidase and polyphenoloxidase activities during rice leaf senescence. Plant Physiol. 1976;57:315–9.

48. Mallory FB. Pathological techénique. Philadelphia: Saunders; 1988.

49. Yousofi A, Daneshmandi S, Soleimani N, Bagheri K, Karimi MH. Immunomodulatory effect of parsley (Petroselinumcrispum) essential oil on immune cells: mitogen-activated splenocytes and peritoneal macrophages. Immunopharmacol Immunotoxicol. 2012;34(2):303–8.

50. Wise LD, Gordon LR, Soper KA, Duchai DM, Morrissey RE. Developmental neurotoxicity evaluation of acrylamide in Sprague-Dawley rats. Neurotoxicol Teratol. 1995;17:189–98.

51. Moazedi AA, Mirzaie DN, Seyyednejad SM, Zadkarami MR, Amirzargar A. Spasmolytic effect of Petroselinumcrispum (Parsley) on rat's ileum at different calcium chloride concentrations. Pak J Biol Sci. 2007;10(22):4036–42.

52. Rao TS, Asha MR, Ramesh BN, Rao KS. Understanding nutrition, depression and mental illnesses. Indian J Psychiatry. 2008;50(2):77–82.

53. Richter-Levin G, Segal M. The effects of serotonin depletion and raphe grafts on hippocampal electrophysiology and behavior. J Neurosci. 1991;11(6):1585–96.

54. Conklin KA. Dietary antioxidants during cancer chemotherapy: impact on chemotherapeutic effectiveness and development of side effects. Nutr Cancer. 2000;37(1):1–18.

55. Gohil K, Viguie C, Stanley WC, Brooks GA, Packer L. Blood glutathione oxidation during human exercise. J Appl Physiol. 1988;64(1):115–9.

56. Ajarem J, Allam AA, Ebaid H, Maodaa SN, Al-Sobeai SM, Rady AM, Met-walli A, Altoom NG, Ibrahim KE, Sabri MI. Neurochemical, structural and neurobehavioral evidence of neuronal protection by whey proteins in diabetic albino mice. Behav Brain Funct. 2015;11:7.

57. Allam AA, El-Ghareeb AA, Abdul-Hamid M, Gad MA, Sabri I. Effect Of prenatal and perinatal acrylamide on the biochemical and morphological changes in liver of developing albino rat. Arch Toxicol. 2010;84(2):129–41.

58. Allam AA, El-Ghareeb AA, Abdul-Hamid M, Bkry A, Sabri I. Prenatal and perinatal acrylamide disrupts the development of cerebellum in rat: biochemical and morphological studies. Toxicol Ind Health. 2011;27(4):291–306.

59. Allam AA, Ajarem J, Abdul-Hamid M, Bakry A. Acrylamide disrupts the development of medulla oblongata in albino rat: biochemical and mor-phological studies. Afr J Pharm Pharmacol. 2013;7(20):1320–31.

60. Valko M, Leibfritz D, Moncol J, Cronin MTD, Mazur M, Telser J. Free radicals and antioxidants in normal physiological functions and human disease. Int J Biochem Cell Biol. 2007;39(1):44–84.

61. Young IS, Woodside JV. Antioxidants in health and disease. J Clin Pathol. 2001;54(3):176–86.

12

Mitochondrial dysfunction and autism: comprehensive genetic analyses of children with autism and mtDNA deletion

Noémi Ágnes Varga[1], Klára Pentelényi[1], Péter Balicza[1], András Gézsi[1,2], Viktória Reményi[1], Vivien Hársfalvi[1], Renáta Bencsik[1], Anett Illés[1], Csilla Prekop[3] and Mária Judit Molnár[1*]

Abstract

Background: The etiology of autism spectrum disorders (ASD) is very heterogeneous. Mitochondrial dysfunction has been described in ASD; however, primary mitochondrial disease has been genetically proven in a small subset of patients. The main goal of the present study was to investigate correlations between mitochondrial DNA (mtDNA) changes and alterations of genes associated with mtDNA maintenance or ASD.

Methods: Sixty patients with ASD and sixty healthy individuals were screened for common mtDNA mutations. Next generation sequencing was performed on patients with major mtDNA deletions (mtdel-ASD) using two gene panels to investigate nuclear genes that are associated with ASD or are responsible for mtDNA maintenance. Cohorts of healthy controls, ASD patients without mtDNA alterations, and patients with mitochondrial disorders (non-ASD) harbouring mtDNA deletions served as comparison groups.

Results: MtDNA deletions were confirmed in 16.6% (10/60) of patients with ASD (mtdel-ASD). In 90% of this mtdel-ASD children we found rare SNVs in ASD-associated genes (one of those was pathogenic). In the intergenomic panel of this cohort one likely pathogenic variant was present. In patients with mitochondrial disease in genes responsible for mtDNA maintenance pathogenic mutations and variants of uncertain significance (VUS) were detected more frequently than those found in patients from the mtdel-ASD or other comparison groups. In healthy controls and in patients without a mtDNA deletion, only VUS were detected in both panel.

Conclusions: MtDNA alterations are more common in patients with ASD than in control individuals. MtDNA deletions are not isolated genetic alterations found in ASD; they coexist either with other ASD-associated genetic risk factors or with alterations in genes responsible for intergenomic communication. These findings indicate that mitochondrial dysfunction is not rare in ASD. The occurring mtDNA deletions in ASD may be mostly a consequence of the alterations of the causative culprit genes for autism or genes responsible for mtDNA maintenance, or because of the harmful effect of environmental factors.

Keywords: Autism, Mitochondrial dysfunction, mtDNA deletion, ASD associated genetic alterations, Intergenomic communication

Background

In recent years, the number of patients diagnosed with autism spectrum disorders (ASD) has increased with current studies reporting a prevalence of 1% [1]. ASD shows extreme clinical heterogeneity; however, the diagnosis of ASD according to the Diagnostic and Statistical Manual of Mental Disorders (5th edition) is based on deficits in two areas—social communication and restricted, repetitive behaviour or interests. The patient must have deficits in both areas, and symptoms must be present from early childhood [2]. The genetic architecture of ASD

*Correspondence: molnar.mariajudit@med.semmelweis-univ.hu
[1] Institute of Genomic Medicine and Rare Disorders, Semmelweis University, Tömő Str. 25-29, Budapest 1083, Hungary
Full list of author information is available at the end of the article

is very diverse consisting of a variety of genetic alterations, such as chromosomal abnormalities, copy number variations, rare single nucleotide variants (SNVs), common polymorphic variations, and epigenetic modifications; however, only 6–15% of children with ASD have well-defined genetic syndromes [3]. Because of the development of high-throughput sequencing methods, many highly penetrant genetic causes of ASD have been identified, but the underlying genetic background of 70% of cases remains unexplained [4].

Mitochondrial disease (MD) is presently one of the most recognized metabolic diseases caused by the failure of both nuclear and/or mitochondrial DNA (mtDNA). The prevalence of mtDNA mutations responsible for MD is 1 in 5000, whereas that of nuclear mutations is 2.9 per 100,000 cases [5]. Although MD frequently results in a spectrum of disorders with multisystemic presentations, neurological symptoms are common because tissues with high-energy demands, such as neural tissue, are often the most strongly affected by mitochondrial dysfunction. Even though the diagnosis of MD is increasing and becoming more frequent, the exact genetic background in many cases remains unconfirmed. Mitochondrial dysfunction can be caused by either primary MD or secondary mitochondrial damage [6]. Primary MD is because of genetic defects in mtDNA or a defect in a nuclear gene that is important for mitochondrial function. These mutations usually affect proteins involved in reactions of oxidative phosphorylation (OXPHOS). However, many disorders show similar effects in terms of mitochondrial dysfunction, but are elicited by mutations in other genes not related directly to normal mitochondrial function [7]. In other cases environmental factors, associated disorders or ageing are resulting in secondary alterations.

Several authors have proposed that mitochondrial dysfunction may be one of the most common medical conditions associated with autism [8, 9]. Lombard et al. [10] proposed that ASD may be a condition with abnormal mitochondrial function. Clinical and biochemical studies have uncovered an emerging link between mitochondrial dysfunction and neurodevelopmental disorders, including intellectual disability [11], childhood epilepsy, and ASD [9]. Furthermore, mitochondrial dysfunction has been associated with some forms of syndromic ASD [8, 11]. In many of these studies, biochemical changes, such as elevated levels of creatine kinase, lactate, pyruvate, carnitine, ammonia, and alanine were detected in the serum of patients with ASD [11–14]. In other studies, altered respiratory chain enzyme activities [15] or decreased expression of OXPHOS genes were detected in autistic brain [16], findings which indicate abnormal or altered mitochondrial function.

Damage to the OXPHOS system was found in individuals with ASD by Napoli et al. [17] and reviewed by Valenti et al. [11]. Oliveira et al. [14] found that 7% (7/100) of children with ASD, who were clinically indistinguishable from other affected children with ASD, exhibited a mitochondrial respiratory chain disorder. Weissman et al. [18] proposed that defective mitochondrial OXPHOS may be an additional underlying pathogenic mechanism in a subset of individuals with autism.

Despite evidence of altered mitochondrial function in some individuals with ASD, it is not known whether mitochondrial dysfunction is a cause or an effect of ASD. Although a mitochondrial subgroup in ASD could be identified [19], findings from review articles, such as those of Palmieri and Persico [19] and Rossignol and Frye [9], found that even in this subgroup the causative genetic factor could be identified in a proportion of cases (23%). In cases of non-syndromic ASD, mitochondrial dysfunction without mtDNA alterations has been frequently observed [8, 9]. In a systematic review and meta-analysis, Rossignol reported that MD was present in 5% of children with ASD [9], and in this ASD/MD subgroup, mtDNA abnormalities were found in 23% of patients [9]. These findings demonstrate that primary MD may be present in a subgroup of children with ASD.

Some studies have reported mtDNA deletions in individuals with ASD [12, 20–22]. Single mtDNA deletions have a role in different paediatric and adult onset primary MDs such as Kearns–Sayre syndrome, Pearson syndrome, and progressive ophthalmoplegia externa [23]. Multiple mtDNA deletions occur mostly because of pathogenic mutations in genes responsible for intergenomic communication; however, they are often related to ageing or harmful environmental factors as well because mtDNA has a poor DNA repair system [6, 24].

The aim of the present study was to investigate the presence of the most common pathogenic mtDNA alterations in patients with ASD and to elucidate the etiology of these mtDNA alterations by analysing their co-occurrence with both known ASD-associated genes and genes responsible for mtDNA maintenance and by comparison the targeted NGS data (ASD associated genes and genes responsible for mtDNA maintenance) of cases with and without mtdel-ASD, patients with primary mitochondrial disorders and healthy controls.

Methods

Patients

Detailed clinical examinations consisting of a general medical examination and neurological assessment were performed. A diagnosis of ASD was made using the ADI-R (autism diagnostic interview—revised) and ADOS (autism diagnostic observation schedule). Patients were screened for minor physical abnormalities, which were selected based on the Méhes Scale [25]. Family history and detailed environmental/societal data were collected from the first degree relatives of each patient. Any disorders present in the parents as well as environmental factors were registered. Written informed consent was obtained from the parents of the patient. This study was performed in accordance with the Helsinki Declaration of 1975 and was approved by the Hungarian Research Ethics Committee (44599-2/2013/EKU). The diagnosis of ASD was based on the standardized ADI-R in Hungarian, which was published by the Autism Foundation (Kapocs Publisher), according to the following scores: A $\geq$ 10 (social interaction), B $\geq$ 7 (communication), C $\geq$ 3 (repetitive stereotype manner), D $\geq$ 1 (abnormal development under 36 months). Sixty children with ASD [6 females and 54 males, median age = 7 years, interquartile range (IQR) = 7.25] were included in our study. Before patient selection our ASD patients were screened for Fragile X syndrome and only negative cases were included in our cohort. Of our 60 patients with ASD, 58 are of European descent and 2 are Roma. Our control group for mtDNA screening consisted of 60 European adults (26 females and 34 males, median age = 28 years, IQR = 13.75) selected from our biobank [26]. All controls were healthy individuals under 45 years of age and free from addiction (alcohol, smoking, and drugs). For the interpretation of our next generation sequencing (NGS) results, we compared data from the following cohorts: patients with ASD and without mtDNA deletion, labelled non-mtdel-ASD, (6 males and 1 female, median age = 8 years, IQR = 5.5), patients with MD and mtDNA deletion, without ASD (4 males and 3 females, median age = 18 years, IQR = 19), and healthy control individuals (1 male and 5 females, median age = 27 years, IQR = 2.25). The investigated patients and controls were not related. All patients without a mtDNA deletion were considered to have non-syndromic ASD. The study design is illustrated in Table 1.

Genetic analysis

DNA was isolated from peripheral blood samples from all participants using the QIAamp DNA blood kit (Qiagen, Hilden, Germany) according to manufacturer's instructions. To identify single and multiple mtDNA deletions, long range PCR was performed as described by Remenyi et al. [27]. MtDNA single and multiple deletions were screened with long PCR in 20 µl volume: 20 pmol primers Fw 5′-TAAAAATCTTTGAAATAGGGC-3′ and Rev 5′-CGGATACAGTTCACTTTAGCT-3′, 0.2 µl Phusion DNA Polymerase (Finnzymes, Vantaa, Finland), 4 µl Phusion GC Reaction Buffer (Finnzymes, Vantaa, Finland), 0.4 µl dNTP and 12.4 µl water (qPCR grade water, AMBION). PCR program was the following: 98 °C 30 s, 30 cycles: 98 °C 10 s, 63 °C 10 s, 72 °C 3/8 min, then the last synthesis at 72 °C 7 min. Amplicates were visualised by ethidium-bromide (2% agarose) and determined with QuantityOne Software (Bio-Rad Corp. Hertfordshire, UK). The three most-frequent pathogenic mtDNA point mutations were screened by PCR–RFLP using a GeneAmp PCR System 9700 (Applied Biosystems, MA, USA) [20]. The most well-known ASD-associated genes [28] and 51 genes responsible for intergenomic communication (Additional file 1: Table S1) were investigated using NGS, which was performed on a MiSeq (Illumina, CA, USA) using the TruSight Autism Rapid Capture Kit (Illumina, CA, USA) and the SureSelect QXT Kit (Agilent Technologies, CA, USA) according to the manufacturer's instructions. In the intergenomic panel, 16/32 samples were multiplexed in one sequencing run, whereas in the autism panel 24 samples were multiplexed in a single run using the MiSeq reagent kit v2 and 300 cycles (Illumina, CA, USA). The mean read depth was 152 × in the intergenomic gene panel and 135 × in the ASD-associated gene panel. In both panels, 20 × coverage was achieved in a minimum of 90% of target regions. Pathogenic and likely pathogenic mutations from NGS data were validated by Sanger sequencing, and segregation analysis was performed within individual families.

Table 1 The design of the study

Cohorts	M.3243 A > G, m.8993 T > C/G, m.8344 A > G	mtDNA deletion	IG NGS (51 genes)	ASD NGS (101 genes)
ASD cases (n = 60)	✓	✓	✓a	✓a
Healthy controls (n = 60)	✓	✓	✓b	✓b
mtdel-MD (n = 7)	✓	✓	✓	–

The investigated cohorts and the performed genetic analysis are shown in the Table 1. NGS testing for intergenomic panel and ASD panel has been performed in the cohort of the 10 mtdel ASD cases and in subgroup of 7 non-mtdel ASD cases and a subgroup of healthy controls (N = 6). Patients with primary mitochondrial disease (N = 7) served as further control group. All investigated person were Caucasian except 2 non-mtdel ASD cases

ASD autism spectrum disorder, *MD* mitochondrial disease, *mtDNA* mitochondrial DNA, *IG NGS* next generation sequencing for genes responsible for intergenomic communication, *ASD NGS* next generation sequencing for autism associated genes

a The 10 mtdel-ASD cases and 7 non-mtdel ASD were investigated

b 6 cases were investigated

Statistical and bioinformatics analysis

Chi square test with Yates correction/Fisher exact test were used to determine significant differences between patient and control groups [29]. Raw sequences were filtered with Picard tools (version 2.1.0) [30] and quality filtered reads were aligned to the hg19 reference genome with BWA-mem [31] using default parameters. Variant calling was performed using GATK HaplotypeCaller (version 3.3-0) [32] and VCF files were annotated with SnpEff (version 4.1) [33]. We analysed only those variants that were found in the canonical transcript of the gene. To identify potentially causal genetic variations, we used VariantAnalyzer, which is an in-house software developed by András Gézsi from the Budapest University of Technology and Economics [34]. This software application annotates SNPs and short indels with several types of annotations, such as their predicted function on genes using SnpEff, observed allele frequencies in several genomic projects including the 1000 Genomes Project and the ESP6500 Project, conservation scores based on PhyloP or PhastCons, predicted function of non-synonymous SNPs using dbNSFP, and disease associations with HGMD and ClinVar. By creating filter cascades based on these annotations and other information (e.g., genotypes and variant quality annotations), the software can easily be used to filter the variants through a user-friendly graphical interface. Analysis and variant calling of SureSelect libraries was performed with SureCall software (Agilent, CA, USA). First, we filtered for variants known to be disease-causing, using human gene mutation database (HGMD) Professional 2015.1 edition [35]. Second, we filtered for rare variants based on the minor allele frequency and frequency of the mutation in our NGS data repository. Since large-scale genomic data of the Hungarian population is not available, a mutation with a low minor allele frequency may also be population-specific. We labelled a variant as a rare mutation if it was present in one or two samples within our cohort and the minor allele frequency in Europeans from the 1000 Genomes and ExAC databases was less than 0.5%. It is important to note that a limitation of this method is that it may exclude identification of founder mutations and disease-associated polymorphisms. Finally, mutations were prioritized based on their predicted effects. Exonic frameshift and stop mutations were considered always damaging, whereas the effects of missense mutations were predicted using Polyphen2, SIFT (Sort Intolerant From Tolerant), or MutationTaster (MT).

Results

Sixty children with ASD (6 females and 54 males, median age = 7 years, IQR = 7.25) were investigated. In our analysed cohort of 60 patients, 29 patients were sporadic (from simplex families) and their family histories were negative for other neurodevelopmental disorders and major psychiatric or neurological disorders. The distribution of the relevant symptoms for mitochondrial disorders in mtdel-ASD and idiopathic ASD group are shown in Fig. 1. There were some differences between ASD cases with and without mtDNA deletion regarding the clinical phenotype. Developmental regression, muscle hypotonia, and additional neurological signs were most common in the mtdel-ASD cases. Multisystemic abnormality appeared also more frequently. Referring to seizures no major differences has been observed between these two groups. Family history was not available in two cases because these children were not living with their biological parents. A positive family history was found in 48% of cases, of which 20 cases (33.3%) had a family history for psychiatric disorders (bipolar disorder, depression, and schizophrenia). In four cases (6.7%), visual and hearing impairments, ataxia, complex endocrine disorders, or a combination of these factors was noted. The co-occurrence of these symptoms is an indicator for MD according to mitochondrial disease criteria (MDC) [36]. In five cases (8%), we found a positive family history for psychiatric disorders and some MDC-related symptoms were also noted.

Minor physical anomalies were identified in 44 children. All children were diagnosed with ASD based on ADI-R, and in most cases, with ADOS as well. We found that serum lactate levels and/or the lactate:pyruvate ratio supported the presence of mitochondrial dysfunction in four patients.

Genetic investigation—mtDNA mutation screening

Mitochondrial deletions were identified in 16.6% (10/60) of our patients with ASD. Two children had multiple deletions, whereas a single major deletion was detected in the range of 2.4–7.9 kb in eight children. Detailed clinical and family history data as well as associated phenotype of the patients harbouring mtDNA deletions are shown in Table 2. An evaluation of clinical phenotype, family history, and laboratory data suggested MD in seven cases with mtDNA deletion. None of the investigated families had a previous diagnosis of primary MD. In all cases, the rate of heteroplasmy (HP) was > 20% in blood samples (Table 2). In the 60 healthy control individuals, a mtDNA deletion was found in two cases. Based on our statistical analysis, there was a significant difference in the frequency of mtDNA deletions between our ASD and control cohorts (χ^2 with Yates correction = 4.5; p = 0.03; odds ratio = 5.8; 95% CI 1.21–27.72). Further analysis of mtDNA mutational "hotspot" regions (m.3243 A > G, m.8993 T > C/G, and m.8344 A > G) did not detect any alterations in our ASD cohort.

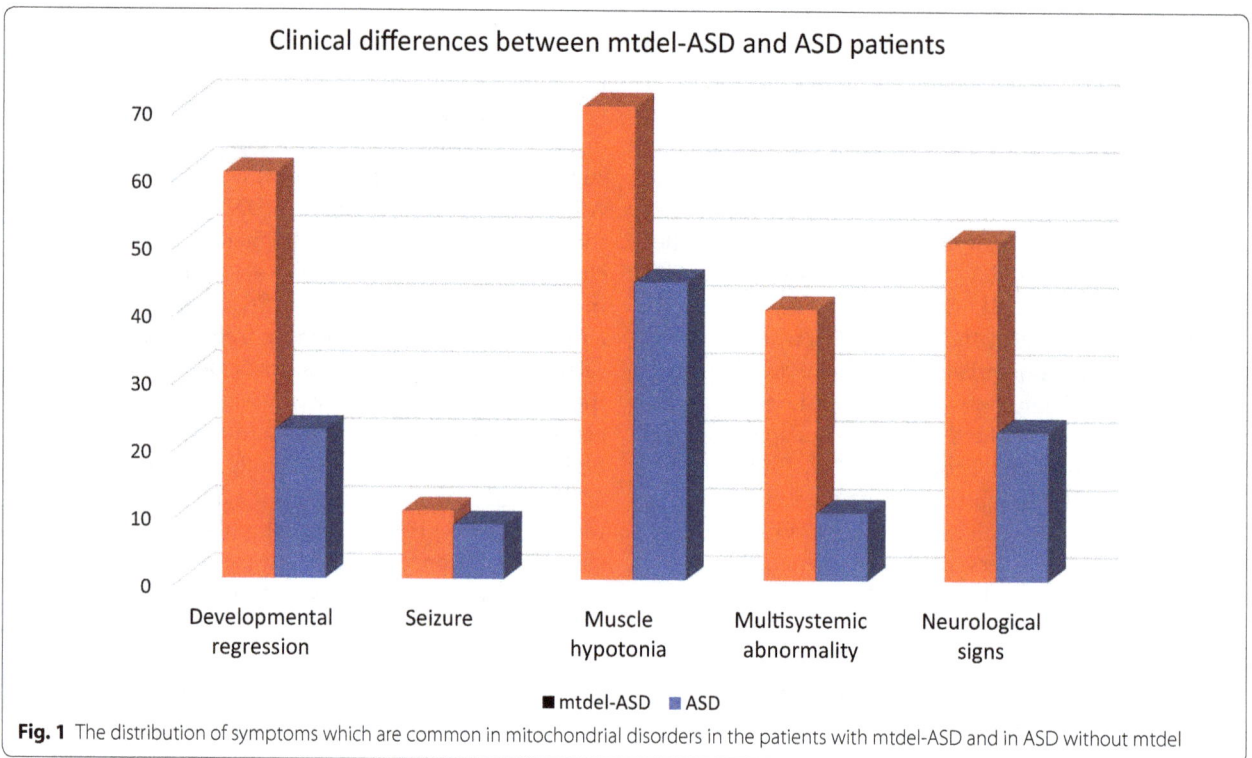

Fig. 1 The distribution of symptoms which are common in mitochondrial disorders in the patients with mtdel-ASD and in ASD without mtdel

Genetic investigation—nuclear DNA mutation screening of genes responsible for intergenomic communication

Next, we focused on those patients with mtDNA deletions (mtdel-ASD) and performed nuclear DNA (nDNA) mutation screening to investigate genes involved in intergenomic communication. In this subgroup, we found one rare likely pathogenic variant and one variant with uncertain significance (VUS). The rare variants identified in two patients were both present in only one allele, however the mode of inheritance of these disorders is autosomal recessive (Table 3). In *Patient 5* (P5), the likely pathogenic heterozygous T265I mutation in the mitochondrial genome maintenance exonuclease 1 (*MGME1*) is responsible for mtDNA integrity [37]. In *Patient 9* (P9), we found a de novo VUS mutation (Clin-Var ID203970) in succinate-CoA ligase alpha subunit (*SUCLG1*) in a heterozygous form.

In our cohort of seven patients with MD (without ASD) harbouring mtDNA deletions, we found a pathogenic rare variants in two case, and rare VUS in five further cases (Table 2). In one patient the compound heterozygous state of one pathogenic and one VUS in *C10orf2* gene were detected. In cohorts without MD (patients with ASD lacking mtDNA deletion and healthy individuals) we found two–two rare VUS in genes responsible for intergenomic communications (Table 3).

Comparing the intergenomic NGS panel results for our different cohorts, we found no significant difference between mtdel-ASD cases and healthy controls with one tailed Fisher exact test (p: 0.4890 odds: 0.5, CI 0.05–4.97); and mtdel-ASD and ASD without mtDNA deletion groups (p:0.55882, Odds: 0625 CI 0.06–5.96). Likely pathogenic variant and VUS were identified in higher number in MD patients with mtDNA deletion and without ASD (p = 0.013, Odds: 0.04 CI 0.003–0.5743), in a heterozygous form (Table 3).

Genetic investigation—nDNA mutation screening of ASD-associated genes

Using the TruSight Autism NGS panel, we detected rare SNVs in 90% (9/10) of our affected children with mtDNA deletion. Syndromic ASD was identified in a single case, *Patient 3* (P3), from our mtdel-ASD cohort. A heterozygous pathogenic mutation in chromodomain helicase DNA-binding protein 7 (*CHD7*) was found in this patient as well as a heterozygous mutation of uncertain significance in tuberin (*TSC2*). The *CHD7* rare variant regarding the ACMG guideline, fulfils the PVS1 and one PS2 criteria [38] and based on this we evaluated it as pathogenic. The patient's phenotype and the family segregation pattern indicated this *CHD7* mutation as a de novo mutation resulting in CHARGE syndrome (OMIM 214800) [39].

Table 2 Mitochondrial DNA deletion status and clinical data of children with ASD and mtDNA deletion

Family history	Associated diseases	Minor anomalies	Symptoms beside ASD	Laboratory results	mtDNA (HP)
MS + FS: intellectual disability, epilepsy	Chronic otitis	+	Hypoacusis, orofacial dyspraxia, intellectual disability, limb ataxia, tremor	Lactate level: 3.6 mmol/l (norm: ≤ 1.6 mmol/l), low testosterone levels, high LDH level, normal CK	Multiple (> 20%)
MS: autoimmune hypothyreosis	Gluten sensitivity	+	Attention deficit, intellectual disability, Slight macrocephaly, constipation	Lactate level: 0.6 mmol/l (norm: ≤ 1.6 mmol/l), elevated lactate/pyruvate ratio, normal CK and LDH levels	Major deletion (80%)
MS: epilepsy FS: anxiety	Tooth problems	+	Multiple congenital anomalies, coloboma, visual problems, hypotonic muscles, truncal ataxia, breathing difficulties	Lactate level: 1.9 mmol/l (norm: ≤ 1.6 mmol/l). elevated progesterone level, high LDH levels, low insulin levels	Major deletion (20%)
Mother: panic syndrome	Gastro-oesophageal reflux	+	Postnatal growth deficiency, failure to thrive, intellectual disability	Lactate level: 1.3 mmol/l (norm: ≤ 1.6 mmol/l)	Major deletion (65%)
Negative	Atopic dermatitis	−	No	Lactate levelel: 0.9 mmol/l (norm: ≤ 1.6 mmol/l)	Major deletion (35%)
Previous foetus: aborted, FS: hydrocephalus, anal atresia, MS: depression, anxiety, ptosis, OCD, carcinoma	Neonatal jaundice, strabismus	+	Microcephaly, visual problems, hypotonic muscles	Lactate level: 2.3 mmol/l (norm: ≤ 1.6 mmol/l), elevated LDH levels, normal CK level	Major deletion (20%)
Negative	No	+	Mild truncal ataxia	Lactate level: 1.2 mmol/l (norm: ≤ 1.6 mmol/l)	Major deletion (85%)
MS: bipolar disorder (3 relatives), suspected thyroid problems	Atopic dermatitis, CMV, hepatitis	+	Sensorineural hearing loss, mild myopathy, ptosis	Lactate level: 1.5 mmol/l (norm: ≤ 1.6 mmol/l), elevated LDH, norm CK level. High anti-CMV antibody titer after birth, elevated liver enzymes	Major deletion (85%)
MS + FS: PD, AD, intellectual disability; FS: suspicion of ASD	No	+	Mild truncal ataxia, calf hypertrophy	Lactate level: 1.5 mmol/l (norm: ≤ 1.6 mmol/l). Elevated lactate/pyruvate ratio, normal CK and LDH level	Major deletion (90%)
Negative	No	+	No	Lactate level: 1.2 mmol/l (norm: ≤ 1.6 mmol/l)	Multiple (> 20%)

The detected mtDNA deletion, family history, clinical data as well as associated phenotype of the ASD patients harbouring mtDNA deletions are shown in Table 2

MS maternal side of the family, *FS* paternal side of the family, *OCD* obsessive–compulsive disorder, *PD* Parkinson's diseases, *AD* Alzheimer's disease, *LDH* lactate dehydrogenase, *CK* creatine kinase, *CMV* cytomegalovirus, *mtDNA* mitochondrial DNA, *HP* ratio of heteroplasmy

Table 3 Results of the intergenomic NGS panel

Patient ID	Gene	Mutation	Zygosity	Inheritance	Clinical relevance	Polyphen2	SIFT	MT	dbSNP	ExAC	1000 Genomes/EUR AF
Patients with ASD and mtDNA deletion (N = 10)											
P5	MGME1	T265I	HET	AR	Likely pathogenic [37]	0.95	0.25	D	rs76599088	0.007875	0.0044/0.0139
P9	SUCLG1	G79D	HET	AR	Uncertain significance	0.99	0	D	n/d	n/d	n/d
Patients with ASD and without mtDNA deletion (N = 7)											
C-ASD1	MTO	K321E	HET	AR	Uncertain significance	1	0.001	D	rs148667065	0.0000908	n/d
C-ASD2	EARS2	R99Q	HET	AR	Uncertain significance	n/d	1	D	n/d	n/d	n/d
Patients with MD and mtDNA deletion, without ASD (N = 7)											
C-MD1	WARS2	H151R	HET	AD/AR	Uncertain significance	0.1	0.02	D	rs150022801	0.001779	0.0008/0.003
C-MD2	APEX	R202P	HET	n/d	Uncertain significance	0.6	0.01	P	n/d	0.000008242	n/d
C-MD3	ATP5F1	I173V	HET	AR	Uncertain significance	0.02	0.1	D	n/d	n/d	n/d
C-MD4	MTO1	V517M	HET	AR	Uncertain significance	0.03	0.1	D	n/d	n/d	n/d
C-MD5	C10orf2	N399S	HET	AR	Pathogenic [38]	0.896	0.09	D	n/d	n/d	n/d
	C10orf2	A453Q	HET	AR	Uncertain significance	0.053	0.27	D	n/d	n/d	n/d
C-MD6	MRPL3	S75N	HET	AR	Pathogenic [56]	0.8	0.34	D	rs151331067	0.001606	0.0008/n/d
Healthy controls without mtDNA deletion (N = 6)											
C-H3	EARS2	S482N	HET	AR	Uncertain significance	n/d	0.28	D	n/d	n/d	n/d
C-H4	SLC25I3	V219F	HET	AD	Uncertain significance	0.62	0.001	D	n/d	n/d	n/d

Pathogenic, likely pathogenic, and rare variants of uncertain significance detected in the 10 mtdel-ASD cases and different comparison groups are presented (benign variations are not shown)

P mtdel-ASD patient, *non-mtdel-ASD* ASD patient without mtDNA deletion, *MD* patient with mitochondrial disease, *H* healthy control individual, *HET* heterozygous, *AR* autosomal recessive, *AD* autosomal dominant, *n/d* no data, *SIFT* sorting intolerant from tolerant prediction database, *MT* mutation t@ster prediction database, *D* disease causing according to mutation t@ster prediction, *P* polymorphism according to mutation t@ster prediction, *ExAC* allele frequency data from exome aggregation consortium, *1000 Genomes* allele frequency data from 1000 Genomes project, *EUR AF* allele frequency in the European Super Population of the 1000 Genomes project

In *Patient 8* (P8), we found a pathogenic nonsense mutation in 7-dehydrocholesterol reductase (*DHCR7*), which was present in only one allele.

In Patient 2 (P2) a rare mutation was detected in autism susceptibility candidate 2 (*AUTS2*), which previously was associated with syndromic ASD form. The significance of the missense mutation identified in our study is uncertain; during segregation analysis the same mutation was present in the healthy mother, however we do not know exactly the penetrance of the genetic defects of *AUTS2*. This rare *AUTS2* variant coexisted with a rare variant in retinoic acid induced gene 1 (*RAI1*) (Table 4).

Using in silico analysis, alterations of uncertain significance were detected in ASD-associated genes in 60% (6/10) of the mtdel-ASD cases and 71% (5/7) of non-mtdel-ASD cases (Table 4). In the six control individuals only four rare VUS were detected in genes associated with ASD. The rare variant in zinc finger protein 804A (*ZNF804A*) was found in two healthy controls, indicating a variant that is likely population-specific (Table 4).

Detailed phenotype of a patient with mtDNA deletion and CHARGE syndrome (*CHD7* mutation)

An 11-year-old male patient (P3) had multiple congenital anomalies, such as coloboma of the eyes, oxycephaly, epicanthus, convergent strabismus, mild bifid nose/broad nasal tip, low settled cup ears, mild facial asymmetry, dental dysgenesis, asymmetric chest, macroglossia, cryptorchidism, testicular hypoplasia, and atrial septal defect. He began walking at 3 years of age and suffers from obsessive hand movements, erratic behavior, and sleep disturbance. Aside from his developmental abnormalities, neurological investigation detected pes varus, severe visual impairment, bilateral ptosis, chewing difficulties, mild atrophy and weakness in the distal muscles of the extremities, and truncal ataxia. High lactate levels were detected in both serum and cerebrospinal fluid, and decreased levels of serum melatonin, calcium, and vitamin D3 were measured. A brain MRI detected hypoplastic vermis and transverse sinus on the right side. An EEG found generalized irritative signs, and VEP found an increased P100 on the left side. Brainstem auditory evoked potentials was normal. Family history identified arrhythmia, diabetes mellitus, and colon polypomatosis on the maternal side, and diabetes mellitus, arrhythmia, and dementia on the paternal side.

Detailed phenotype of a patient with congenital cytomegalovirus infection and mtDNA deletion

The 5-year-old female patient (P8) was born at a gestational age of 39 weeks by Caesarean section with a birth weight of 3000 g. The pregnancy was complicated with a partial placental abruption at 11 weeks. Evidence of prolonged neonatal jaundice, highly elevated liver enzymes, low prothrombin level, and high IgM and IgG type anti-cytomegalovirus (CMV) antibodies led to the diagnosis of a congenital CMV infection-induced hepatic lesion. She had congenital sensorineural hearing loss, mild myopathic facies, mild ptosis, and atopic facial dermatitis. A brain MRI identified several T2 hyperintense supratentorial lesions (5–10 mm in size), which were suggested to have an infectious etiology. A heterozygous nonsense mutation in *DHCR7* and a major large single deletion in mtDNA were found. The healthy mother also harbours the detected heterozygous mutation. Cholesterol and 7-dehydrocholesterol levels of the child are in the normal range. Homozygous or compound heterozygous mutations in *DHCR7* result in Smith–Lemli–Opitz (SLOS) syndrome, which is an autosomal recessive disease. However, human CMV infection may lead to altered mitochondrial biogenesis [40]. We believe that this case demonstrates a direct interaction between genetic and environmental risk factors in some forms of ASD.

Discussion

In this study, we provide for the first time a comprehensive genetic analysis of patients with ASD that investigates co-occurrence of the most frequent mtDNA alterations, intergenomic communication disturbances (51 genes), and 101 genes previously associated with ASD. We found co-occurrence of mtDNA deletions with ASD-associated genetic alterations, which supports the previous observation that mitochondrial alterations are frequently associated with ASD. In one patient with ASD (P3), we found a mtDNA deletion with CHARGE syndrome caused by a de novo mutation in *CHD7*. These genetic alterations in P3 were also accompanied by a *TSC2* mutation of uncertain significance. Autistic symptoms are present in approximately 30% of patients with CHARGE syndrome [39], and lactic acidosis is a rare alteration. Based on the phenotype, we conclude that the driving genetic alteration in this patient is the *CHD7* mutation, and the mitochondrial gene defect may not be the true causative factor in the etiology of the disease; however, CHD7 function is strongly ATP-dependent [41]. In addition, the associated heterozygous *TSC2* mutation is likely a modifying gene. *CHD7* is a member of the chromo-domain helicase DNA-binding (CHD) protein family and plays a role in transcription regulation through chromatin remodelling. Mutations in *TSC2* are known to cause one syndromic form of ASD; however, our patient did not develop the classic symptoms of tuberous sclerosis until recently. *TSC2* mutations may induce activation of mTORC1 leading to increased mtDNA expression and mitochondrial density. mTOR is a Ser/Thr kinase that forms complexes with numerous

Cognitive Neuroscience: Behavioral and Psychological Perspectives

Table 4 Results of the ASD-NGS panel

Patient ID	Gene	Mutation	Zygosity	Inheritance	Clinical relevance	Polyphen2
Patients with ASD and mtDNA deletion (N = 10)						
P1	FOXP2	A280T	HET	AD	Uncertain significance	0.99
P2	RAI1	V1565M	HET	AD	Uncertain significance	0.845
	AUTS2	L433P	HET	AD	Uncertain significance	1
P3	TSC2	K22N	HET	AD	Uncertain significance	1
	CHD7	Fs	HET	AD	Pathogenic [38]	n/d
P4	RELN	L496P	HET	AD/AR	Uncertain significance	0.98
	KATNAL2	R1382S	HET	AR/AD	Uncertain significance	0.99
P6	ZNF804A	A1108T	HET	n/d	Uncertain significance	1
P7	RAI1	G1070R	HET	AD	Uncertain significance	0.99
P8	DHCR7	W119*	HET	AR	Pathogenic	n/d
	NHS	R409Q	HET	XLD	Uncertain significance	1
P10	PDE10A	P477A	HOM	AR/AD	Uncertain significance	0.99
Patients with ASD and without mtDNA deletion (N = 7)						
C-ASD1	SHANK2	A1129P	HET	n/d	Uncertain significance	0.86
C-ASD2	PON3	S820N	HET	n/d	Uncertain significance	1
	NRXN1	S820N	HET	AR	Uncertain significance	0
	CNTNAP2	Y716C	HET	n/d	Uncertain significance	0.9
C-ASD3	SCN2A	L577I	HET	AD	Uncertain significance	0
C-ASD4	NLGN4X	Q89H	HET	XLD	Uncertain significance	0.99
C-ASD6	GNA14	Y287C	HET	n/d	Uncertain significance	1
Healthy controls (N = 6)						
C-H1	ZNF804A	A1108T	HET	n/d	Uncertain significance	1
	NIPBL	R765K	HET	AD	Uncertain significance	0.001
C-H2	ZNF804A	A1108T	HET	n/d	Uncertain significance	1
C-H3	RELN	A150V	HET	AD/AR	Uncertain significance	0.974

Patient ID	SIFT	MT	dbSNP	ExAC	1000 Genome/ EUR AF
Patients with ASD and mtDNA deletion (N = 10)					
P1	0.23	D	n/d	0.000008278	n/d
P2	0.02	P	rs368106957	0.0001819	0.0002/0
	n/d	D	n/d	0.0002025	n/d
P3	0.42	P	n/d	n/d	n/d
	n/d	D	n/d	n/d	n/d
P4	0.02	D	n/d	n/d	n/d
	0.14	P	rs148791504	0.0009651	0.0016/n/d
P6	0.16	P	rs112183442	0.02529	0.0158/0.0457

Table 4 continued

Patient ID	SIFT	MT	dbSNP	ExAC	1000 Genome/ EUR AF
P7	0.01	D	rs370633684	0.0004679	0.0004/0.00077
P8	0.12	P	rs11555217	0.0007	n/d
	0.31	P	n/d	0.00002282	n/d
P10	1	P	rs61733392	0.004515	0.0024/0.006
Patients with ASD and without mtDNA deletion (N = 7)					
C-ASD1	0.29	D	rs377255888	0.00004137	n/d
C-ASD2	0	D	rs139856535	0.002787	0.0016/n/d
	0.33	D	rs80293130	0.0002235	0.0002/n/d
	0.18	D	n/d	0.00008303	n/d
C-ASD3	0.91	D	n/d	n/d	n/d
C-ASD4	0.1	D	n/d	n/d	n/d
C-ASD6	1	D	rs61755085	0.001506	0.0014/0.004
Healthy controls (N = 6)					
C-H1	0.16	P	rs112183442	0.02529	0.0158/0.0457
	0.64	D	rs185678374	0.0005529	0.0004/n/d
C-H2	0.16	P	rs112183442	0.02529	0.0158/0.0457
C-H3	0.01	n/d	n/d	0.000008245	n/d

The detected rare variants of the 10 mtdel-ASD cases, in ASD patients without a mtDNA deletion, and in healthy controls are presented (only pathogenic, likely pathogenic variations and variations with uncertain significance variations are shown)

P mtdel-ASD patient, *non-mtdel-ASD* ASD patient without mtDNA deletion, *MD* patient with mitochondrial disease, *H* healthy control individual, *HET* heterozygous, *AR* autosomal recessive, *AD* autosomal dominant, *n/d* no data, *SIFT* sorting intolerant from tolerant prediction database, *D* disease causing according to mutation t@ster prediction, *P* polymorphism according to mutation t@ster prediction, *MT* mutation t@ster prediction database, *1000 Genomes* allele frequency data from 1000 Genomes project, *EUR AF* allele frequency in the European Super Population of the 1000 Genomes project, *ExAC* allele frequency data from exome aggregation consortium, *1000 Genomes* allele frequency data from 1000 Genomes project

*The symbol of the non sense mutation in protein level

protein partners to regulate cell growth, mitochondrial membrane potential, and ATP synthetic capacity [42].

In *Patient 8*, we found that the mtDNA deletion was accompanied by a heterozygous pathogenic *DHCR7* mutation and a rare variant of uncertain significance in NHS actin remodelling activator (*NHS*). DHCR7 catalyses cholesterol production from 7-dehydrocholesterol, and defects in this protein cause SLOS. Furthermore, a high 7-dehydrocholesterol level results in mitochondrial dysfunction [43]. However, the significance of a heterozygous mutation in this gene is not known. We hypothesize that in the case presented here the co-occurrence of the *DHCR7* heterozygous mutation and CMV infection may play a role in changes of mitochondrial biogenesis and in the pathogenesis of autistic features. The patient was tested for SLOS; both serum cholesterol and 7-dehydrocholesterol levels were normal, which rules out the presence of typical SLOS.

Evidence of mitochondrial dysfunction in ASD was first described 19 years ago [10]. Currently, it is the most common metabolic abnormality known in ASD with a prevalence of 7.2% [14]. In a subgroup of the CHARGE (Childhood Autism Risk from Genes and Environment) study, decreased NADH activity was found in lymphocytes in 8 of 10 cases. In this cohort, only 2 of the 10 patients had mtDNA deletions and 5 patients had altered mtDNA copy numbers [12]. However, the genetic background was not clarified in 79% of the patients with ASD-MD [9]. Therefore, the possibility of secondary damage to mitochondria cannot be excluded. A small pilot study examining 12 patients with ASD described 8 mitochondrial deletions [21], which could be the result of intergenomic communication disturbances, environmental factors, or other gene–gene interactions. As is the case for many other disorders, it is still not clear whether the detected mitochondrial dysfunction in ASD is a primary or secondary event either having a key role in disease pathogenesis or is simply a downstream effect.

In our study, mtDNA deletions were identified in 16.6% of evaluated patients with ASD. During mtDNA hotspot screening and NGS analysis, no concomitant primary MD was detected. To examine whether mtDNA deletion is a primary or secondary event in ASD in our cohort, we used different comparison groups to screen the nDNA background of the mtDNA deletion. Pathogenic or likely pathogenic variants were detected in both mtdel-ASD and MD without ASD cases, all in heterozygous form. A high number of VUS in intergenomic communication genes were detected in the MD without ASD cohort (4/6), and a few rare variants were identified in patients with ASD that lacked mtDNA deletion and in healthy controls (Table 3). Homozygous or compound heterozygous mutations in *MGME1* and *SUCLG1* have been previously correlated with severe early-onset mitochondrial

disorders (OMIM 615084, OMIM 245400) [44]. The importance of the presence of heterozygous mutations is not well understood. It is known in some genes responsible for intergenomic communications heterozygous mutations may result in a less severe phenotype than that found with the homozygous form [45].

The question has also been raised whether patients with MD and ASD symptoms have special characteristics. In a study by Rossignol and Frye [9], a cohort of ASD/MD children were compared to two comparison groups: children with general ASD and children with general MD. In the ASD/MD group, increased lactate and pyruvate levels, seizures, motor delays, and gastrointestinal abnormalities were significantly more prevalent compared to children with general ASD. A more balanced male:female ratio was also detected in the ASD/MD group [9]. Our results confirm the observations by Rossignol and Frye; however, in our ASD cohort with mtDNA deletion, elevated lactate levels and/or an elevated lactate:pyruvate ratio were found in only four cases, whereas most of our ASD patients with mtDNA deletion had symptoms common to MD, such as hypoacusis, muscle weakness, hypotonia, delayed motor development, and movement disorder (Fig. 1). Significant difference between mtdel-ASD and non-mtdel-ASD group was found regarding clinical phenotypes (developmental regression, muscle hypotonia, additional neurological signs and multisystemic alterations were more common in cases mt-delASD). Interestingly, the phenotypes of classic mitochondrial deletion syndromes, such as Pearson syndrome, progressive ophthalmoplegia externa, and Kearns–Sayre syndrome, were not detected in any of our patients. The family histories of mtdel-ASD children in our cohort differed from the family histories of the ASD cohort without a mtDNA deletion, since various psychiatric disorders were common among family members of mtdel-ASD cases both on maternal and paternal side. However none of the parents reached the MDC scoring cut-off value for definitive MD, which could not be independently verified because none of the family members agreed to perform muscle biopsy. MtDNA disorders are usually inherited maternally, however single mtDNA deletions are considered sporadic events with low inheritance risk, whereas multiple mtDNA deletions are the result of primary nuclear defects in genes responsible for mtDNA maintenance or nucleoside metabolism and follow Mendelian inheritance patterns [46].

Mitochondrial haplogroups were also investigated in association with ASD. Chalkia et al. found that individuals with European haplogroups designated I, J, K, X, T and U (55% of the European population) had significantly higher risks of ASD compared to the most common European haplogroup, HHV. Asian and Native American haplogroups A and M also were at increased risk of ASD

[47]. In Hungary it is not rare that a person has ancient European haplotype such as T, K, and U haplotype, and rarely Asian haplotype such as B can occur as well. In some Hungarian patients the mtDNA deletion was coexisting with ancient haplotype [48].

In 90% (9/10) of children from the mtdel-ASD cohort, we found rare SNVs in ASD-associated genes (Table 4). A rare mutation was detected in *AUTS2* in which deletions are inherited in an autosomal dominant manner and are associated with neurological symptoms including intellectual disability and developmental delay [49]. In a modest study of 13 cases of ASD associated with *AUTS2* alterations, only one patient had a nonsense mutation; all the other patients had a deletion [49]. The significance of the missense mutation identified in our study is uncertain (her mother harbours the mutation as well); however, clinical symptoms of the patient correlate with the phenotype of previously published *AUTS2* mutations. This rare *AUTS2* variant coexisted with a rare variant in retinoic acid induced gene 1 (*RAI1*). The gene–gene interaction of these two alterations are hypothesized.

In addition, we found that patients had mutations of uncertain significance in forkhead box P2 (*FOXP2*), *RAI1*, phosphodiesterase 10A (*PDE10A*), katanin catalytic subunit A1 like 2 (*KATNAL2*), and reelin (*RELN*). Most of these genes play a role in cell regulation, signal transduction, and various signalling pathways, which could influence mitochondrial function. *FOXP2* is an evolutionarily conserved transcription factor that regulates the expression of a variety of genes. Mutations in this gene cause speech-language disorder 1 (OMIM 602081), which is also known as autosomal dominant speech and language disorder with orofacial dyspraxia [50]. *RAI1* acts as a transcriptional regulator of chromatin remodelling by interacting with basic transcriptional machinery [51]. *RAI1* deletion is associated with Smith–Magenis syndrome, whereas duplications are associated with Potocki–Lupski syndrome [52]. Several heterozygous mutations are also associated with Smith–Magenis syndrome [53]. In our case, we found that the typical symptoms of Smith–Magenis syndrome were not present. Mutations in *PDE10A* can affect cyclic nucleotide concentrations. This phosphodiesterase selectively catalyzes the hydrolysis of 3′ cyclic phosphate bonds in cAMP and/or cGMP. The phosphodiesterase family of proteins regulates cellular levels, localization, and duration of action of these second messengers by controlling the rate of their degradation. In addition, phosphodiesterases are involved in many signal transduction pathways and are implicated in the pathogenesis of bipolar disorder [54].

Mitochondrial dysfunction may be associated with several forms of syndromic ASD, but is also frequently related to non-syndromic cases [8, 9]. During our comprehensive analysis, we found examples of both but in most cases we did not find the causative genetic mutation that accounts for the mitochondrial dysfunction. In the examined children from the general ASD cohort (without mtDNA deletion), we found several VUS, most of which were identified in genes without previous correlation to mitochondrial dysfunction. Based on our findings, we conclude that the detected mitochondrial DNA deletions in patients with ASD in our cohort are a secondary effect. By investigating the most common mtDNA alterations and the most common nuclear genes responsible for intergenomic communications, we did not identify the clear genetic etiology in most of our cases. Therefore, further investigation and characterization is warranted.

Limitations

We identified certain limitations in our study. We focused our investigation to analyse mutational hotspots and large mtDNA deletions and did not sequence the entire mitochondrial genome. The mtDNA mutations were analysed from blood samples; postmitotic tissue was not available. The used long PCR method detects deletions in the mtDNA with high sensitivity and low specificity. Deletions under 10% of heteroplasmy could be missed due to technical barrier, overestimation of the HP ratio is not expected. The detection of mtDNA deletion from NGS data will be in the future a new perspective, but today it is not in the everyday praxis. We used targeted NGS panels comprised of the most important genes associated with intergenomic communication and ASD. However, these panels do not include all currently associated genes and the number of these genes is continuously increasing. Finally, our healthy control group was older than our ASD cohort and had different gender ratios. However, we felt that ethically it was not appropriate to obtain biomaterial from healthy children for genetic testing. Since somatic mtDNA deletion may occur in association with ageing, and we detected the mtDNA deletion less frequently in the control group it had no impact on our data. Mitobreak Database [55] supports or presumption since deletion were present mostly only aged healthy controls, otherwise they were associated or to sporadic primary mitochondrial disorders (single deletion) or to disorders due to intergenomial gene alterations (multiple deletions).

Conclusions

The aim of our study was to gain a better understanding of mitochondrial dysfunction in autism. We found that mtDNA alterations were more common among our cohort of patients with ASD than in control individuals. In addition, we found that the mtDNA deletion was usually not the single genetic alteration identified in ASD, but co-occurred in both syndromic and non-syndromic forms of ASD with either ASD-associated genetic risk factors and/or alterations in genes responsible for intergenomic communication. Our findings indicate a very complex pathophysiology of ASD in which mitochondrial dysfunction is not rare and can be caused by mtDNA deletion, which may be considered as de novo mutations or the consequence of the alterations of the causative culprit genes for autism or genes responsible for mtDNA maintenance.

Abbreviations

ACMG: American College Medical Genetics; AD: autosomal dominant inheritance; AD: Alzheimer's disease; ADI-R: autism diagnostic interview—revised; ADOS: autism diagnostic observation schedule; AR: autosomal recessive inheritance; ASD: autism spectrum disorder; ASD NGS: next generation sequencing for autism associated genes; ATP: adenosine-triphosphate; BWA: Burrows–Wheeler alignment tool; C-ASD: control ASD patient; C-H: healthy control individual; CHARGE: coloboma, heart defect, atresia choanae, retarded growth and development, genital-, ear abnormality; CHARGE: childhood autism risk from genes and environment; CHD: chromo-domain helicase DNA-binding; CK: creatine kinase; C-MD: control patient with MD; CMV: cytomegalovirus; D: disease-causing according to mutation t@ster prediction; dbNSFP: database for nonsynonymous SNPs' functional predictions; DNA: deoxyribonucleic acid; EEG: electroencephalography; ESP6500: NHLBI GO exome sequencing project; EUR AF: Allele frequency in the European super population of the 1000 Genomes project; ExAC: exome aggregation consortium; FS: on father's side; Fs: frameshift mutation; FS: father's side of the family; HET: heterozygous; HGMD: human gene mutation database; HOM: homozygous; HP: heteroplasmy; IG NGS: next generation sequencing for genes responsible for intergenomic communication; IQR: interquartile range; LDH: lactate dehydrogenase; MD: mitochondrial disease; MDC: mitochondrial disease criteria; MRI: magnetic resonance imaging; MS: on mother's side; MS: mother's side of the family; MT: mutation taster prediction; mtdel-ASD: ASD patients with mitochondrial deletion; mtDNA: mitochondrial deoxyribonucleic acid; mTORC: mechanistic target of rapamycin complex; n/d: no data; NADH: nicotinamide adenine dinucleotide; nDNA: nuclear deoxyribonucleic acid; NGS: next generation sequencing; OCD: obsessive-compulsive disease; OXPHOS: oxidative phosphorylation; P: polymorphism according to mutation t@ster prediction; P1-10: mtdel-ASD patient 1-10; PCR: polymerase chain reaction; PD: Parkinson's disease; PS2: pathogenic criterion is weighted as strong; PVS1: pathogenic criterion is weighted as very strong; RFLP: restriction fragment length polymorphism; SIFT: sort intolerant from tolerant amino acid substitution prediction software; SLOS: Smith–Lemli–Opitz syndrome; SNV: single nucleotide variant; VCF: variant call format; VEP: visual evoked potential; VUS: variant of uncertain significance; XLD: X-linked dominant inheritance.

Authors' contributions

MMJ, NÁV and KP designed the study. NÁV and PB performed data collection, physical examination of the patients. KP and VH performed the library preparation for NGS panels, NÁV analyzed the NGS data of the autism panel, and control groups, KP analyzed the NGS data of the intergenomic panel, and participated in mtDNA mutation screening and manuscript drafting. AG provided the bioinformatical platform to analyze the NGS data, VR participated in mtDNA deletion screening, VH preformed NGS sequencing. RB made the validation by Sanger sequencing and the segregation analysis of the family members. AI revised the manuscript. CsP performed the neuropsychological testing of the patients, NÁV wrote the manuscript and performed the statistical analyses. MJM designed the study, coordinated the research team, leaded the manuscript preparation, revised and corrected the manuscript. All authors read and approved the final manuscript.

Author details

[1] Institute of Genomic Medicine and Rare Disorders, Semmelweis University, Tömő Str. 25-29, Budapest 1083, Hungary. [2] Department of Genetics, Cell- and Immunobiology, Semmelweis University, Nagyvárad tér 4, Budapest 1089, Hungary. [3] Vadaskert Foundation for Children's Mental Health, Lipótmezei Str. 1-5, Budapest 1021, Hungary.

Acknowledgements

The authors thank Margit Kovács, Mariann Markó, and Mónika Sáry for their technical assistance, Lisa Hubers for language corrections, and the Metabolic Laboratory of the I. Department of Pediatrics for performing the biochemical investigation.

Competing interests

The authors declare that they have no competing interests.

Funding

This study was supported from Research and Technology Innovation Fund BIOKLIMA KTIA_AIK_12-1-2013-0017 and Hungarian National Brain Research Program KTIA_NAP_13_1-2013-0001.

References

1. Lai MC, Lombardo MV, Baron-Cohen S. Autism. Lancet. 2014;383(9920):896–910.
2. American Psychiatric Association. Diagnostic and statistical manual of mental disorders: DSM-5-. 5th ed. Washington, DC: American Psychiatric Association; 2013. p. 50.
3. Schaefer GB, Mendelsohn NJ. Genetics evaluation for the etiologic diagnosis of autism spectrum disorders. Genet Med. 2008;10(1):4–12.
4. Schaaf CP, Zoghbi HY. Solving the autism puzzle a few pieces at a time. Neuron. 2011;70(5):806–8.
5. Gorman GS, Schaefer AM, Ng Y, Gomez N, Blakely EL, Alston CL, et al. Prevalence of nuclear and mitochondrial DNA mutations related to adult mitochondrial disease. Ann Neurol. 2015;7(5):753–9.
6. Niyazov DM, Kahler SG, Frye RE. Primary mitochondrial disease and secondary mitochondrial dysfunction: importance of distinction for diagnosis and treatment. Mol Syndromol. 2016;7(3):122–37.
7. Martikainen MH, Chinnery PF. Mitochondrial disease: mimics and chameleons. Pract Neurol. 2015;15(6):424–35.
8. Frye RE, Rossignol DA. Mitochondrial dysfunction can connect the diverse medical symptoms associated with autism spectrum disorders. Pediatr Res. 2011;69:41–7.
9. Rossignol DA, Frye RE. Mitochondrial dysfunction in autism spectrum disorders: a systematic review and meta-analysis. Mol Psychiatry. 2012;17:290–314.
10. Lombard J. Autism: a mitochondrial disorder? Med Hypotheses. 1998;50:497–500.
11. Valenti D, de Bari L, De Filippis B, Henrion-Caude A, Vacca RA. Mitochondrial dysfunction as a central act or in intellectual disability-related diseases: an overview of Down syndrome, autism, Fragile X and Rett syndrome. Neurosci Behav Rev. 2014;46:202–17.
12. Giulivi C, Zhang YF, Omanska-Klusek A, Ross-Inta C, Wong S, Hertz-Picciotto I, et al. Mitochondrial dysfunction in autism. JAMA. 2010;304:2389–96.
13. Frye RE. Biomarkers of abnormal energy metabolism in children with autism spectrum disorder. NA J Med Sci. 2012;5:141–7.
14. Oliveira G, Diogo L, Grazina M, Garcia P, Ataíde A, Marques C, et al. Mitochondrial dysfunction in autism spectrum disorders: a population-based study. Dev Med Child Neurol. 2005;47:185–9.
15. Goldenthal MJ, Damle S, Sheth S, Shah N, Melvin J, Jethva R, et al. Mitochondrial enzyme dysfunction in autism spectrum disorders; a novel biomarker revealed from buccal swab analysis. Biomark Med. 2015;9(10):957–65.

16. Parikshak NN, Gandal MJ, Geschwind DH. Systems biology and gene networks in neurodevelopmental and neurodegenerative disorders. Nat Rev Genet. 2015;16(8):441–58.

17. Napoli E, Wong S, Hertz-Picciotto I, Giulivi C. Deficits in bioenergetics and impaired immune response in granulocytes from children with autism. Pediatrics. 2014;133(5):e1405–10.

18. Weissman JR, Kelley RI, Bauman ML, Cohen BH, Murray KF, Mitchell RL, et al. Mitochondrial disease in autism spectrum disorder patients: a cohort analysis. PLoS ONE. 2008;3(11):e3815.

19. Palmieri L, Persico AM. Mitochondrial dysfunction in autism spectrum disorders: cause or effect? Biochim Biophys Acta. 2010;1797(6–7):1130–7.

20. Fillano JJ, Goldenthal MJ, Rhodes CH, Marín-García J. Mitochondrial dysfunction in patients with hypotonia, epilepsy, autism, and developmental delay: HEADD syndrome. J Child Neurol. 2002;17(6):435–9.

21. Smith M, Spence MA, Flodman P. Nuclear and mitochondrial genome defects in autism. Ann NY Acad Sci. 2009;1151:102–32.

22. Gu F, Chauhan V, Kaur K, Brown WT, LaFauci G, Wegiel J, et al. Alterations in mitochondrial DNA copy number and the activities of electron transport chain complexes and pyruvate dehydrogenase in the frontal cortex from subjects with autism. Transl Psychiatry. 2013;3:e299.

23. Pitceathly RD, Rahman S, Hanna MG. Single deletions in mitochondrial DNA–molecular mechanisms and disease phenotypes in clinical practice. Neuromuscul Disord. 2012;22(7):577–86.

24. Haas RH, Parikh S, Falk MJ, Saneto RP, Wolf NI, Darin N, et al. Mitochondrial disease: a practical approach for primary care physicians. Pediatrics. 2007;120:1326–33.

25. Méhes K. Informative morphogenetic variants (minor congenital anomalies). Orv Hetil. 1986;127(49):3001–3.

26. NEPSYBANK. Magyar Klinikai Neurogenetikai Társaság, Budapest. http://molneur.webdoktor.hu. Accessed 03 April 2016.

27. Remenyi V, Inczedy-Farkas G, Komlosi K, Horvath R, Maasz A, Janicsek I, et al. Retrospective assessment of the most common mitochondrial DNA mutations in a large Hungarian cohort of suspect mitochondrial cases. Mitochondrial DNA. 2015;26(4):572–8.

28. Betancur C. Etiological heterogeneity in autism spectrum disorders: more than 100 genetic and genomic disorders and still counting. Brain Res. 2011;1380:42–77.

29. Chi square, Fisher exact test. http://vassarstats.net/odds2x2.html. Accessed 20 Jul 2017.

30. Picard Tools–By Broad Institute. http://broadinstitute.github.io/picard/. Accessed 02 Jun 2017.

31. Li H, Durbin R. Fast and accurate short read alignment with Burrows–Wheeler transform. Bioinformatics. 2009;25(14):754–60.

32. DePristo MA, Banks E, Poplin R, Garimella KV, Maguire JR, Hartl C, et al. A framework for variation discovery and genotyping using next-generation DNA sequencing data. Nat Genet. 2011;43(5):491–8.

33. Cingolani P, Platts A, le Wang L, Coon M, Nguyen T, Wang L, et al. A program for annotating and predicting the effects of single nucleotide polymorphisms, SnpEff: SNPs in the genome of Drosophila melanogaster strain w1118; iso-2; iso-3. Fly. 2012;6(2):80–92.

34. Balicza P, Grosz Z, Gonzalez MA, Bencsik R, Pentelenyi K, Gal A, et al. Genetic background of the hereditary spastic paraplegia phenotypes in Hungary—an analysis of 58 probands. J Neurol Sci. 2016;364:116–21.

35. Cooper DN, Ball EV, Krawczak M. The human gene mutation database. Nucleic Acids Res. 1998;26(1):285–7.

36. Morava E, van den Heuvel L, Hol F, de Vries MC, Hogeveen M, Rodenburg RJ, et al. Mitochondrial disease criteria: diagnostic applications in children. Neurology. 2006;67(10):1823–6.

37. Taylor RW, Pyle A, Griffin H, Blakely EL, Duff J, He L, et al. Use of whole-exome sequencing to determine the genetic basis of multiple mitochondrial respiratory chain complex deficiencies. JAMA. 2014;312(1):68–77.

38. Richards S, Aziz N, Bale S, Bick D, Das S, Gastier-Foster J, et al. Standards and guidelines for the interpretation of sequence variants: a joint consensus recommendation of the American College of Medical Genetics and Genomics and the Association for molecular pathology. Genet Med. 2015;17(5):405–24.

39. Aramaki M, Udaka T, Kosaki R, Makita Y, Okamoto N, Yoshihashi H, et al. Phenotypic spectrum of CHARGE syndrome with CHD7 mutations. J Pediatr. 2006;148:410–4.

40. Karniely S, Weekes MP, Antrobus R, Rorbach J, vanHaute L, Umrania Y, et al. Human cytomegalovirus infection upregulates the mitochondrial transcription and translation machineries. Mbio. 2016;7(2):e00029.

41. Basson MA, van Ravenswaaij-Arts C. Functional insights into chromatin remodelling from studies on CHARGE syndrome. Trends Genet. 2015;31(10):600–11.

42. Koyanagi M, Asahara S, Matsuda T, Hashimoto N, Shingeyama Y, Shibutani Y, et al. Ablation of TSC2 enhances insulin secretion by increasing the number of mitochondria through activation of mTORC1. PLoS ONE. 2011;6:e23238.

43. Chang S, Ren G, Steiner RD, Merkens LS, Roullet JB, Korade Z. Elevated autophagy and mitochondrial dysfunction in the Smith–Lemli–Opitz syndrome. Mol Genet Metabol Rep. 2014;1:431–42.

44. Kornblum C, Nicholls TJ, Haack TB, Schöler S, Peeva V, Danhauser K, et al. Loss-of-function mutations in MGME1 impair mtDNA replication and cause multisystemic mitochondrial disease. Nat Genet. 2013;45:214–9.

45. Tyynismaa H, Ylikallio E, Patel M, Molnar MJ, Haller RG, Suomalainen A. A heterozygous truncating mutation in RRM2B causes autosomal-dominant progressive external ophthalmoplegia with multiple mtDNA deletions. Am J Hum Genet. 2009;5(2):290–5.

46. Suomalianen A, Kaukonen J. Disease caused by nuclear genes affecting mtDNA stability. Am J Meg Genet. 2001;106:53–61.

47. Chalkia D, Singh LN, Leipzig J, Lvova M, Derbeneva O, Lakatos A, et al. Association between mitochondrial DNA Haplogroup variation and autism spectrum disorders. JAMA Psychiatry. 2017;74(11):1161–8.

48. Pentelenyi K, Remenyi V, Gal A, Milley GM, Csosz A, Mende BG, et al. Asian-specific mitochondrial genome polymorphism (9-bp deletion) in Hungarian patients with mitochondrial disease. Mitochondrial DNA A. 2016;27(3):1697–700.

49. Beunders G, van de Kamp J, Vasudevan P, Morton J, Smets K, Kleefstra T, et al. A detailed clinical analysis of 13 patients with AUTS2 syndrome further delineates the phenotypic spectrum and underscores the behavioural phenotype. J Med Genet. 2016;53(8):523–32.

50. Bartlett CW, Flax JF, Logue MW, Vieland VJ, Bassett AS, Tallal P, et al. A major susceptibility locus for specific language impairment is located on 13q21. Am J Hum Genet. 2002;71:45–55.

51. Bi W, Ohyama T, Nakamura H, Yan J, Visvanathan J, Justice MJ, et al. Inactivation of Rai1 in mice recapitulates phenotypes observed in chromosome engineered mouse models for Smith–Magenis syndrome. Hum Mol Genet. 2005;14:983–95.

52. Zhang F, Potocki L, Sampson JB, Liu P, Sanchez-Valle A, Robbins-Furman P, et al. Identification of uncommon recurrent Potocki–Lupski syndrome-associated duplications and the distribution of rearrangement types and mechanisms in PTLS. Am J Hum Genet. 2010;86:462–70.

53. Girirajan S, Elsas LJ, Devriendt K, Elsea SH. RAI1 variations in Smith–Magenis syndrome patients without 17p11.2 deletions. J Med Genet. 2005;42:820–8.

54. McDonald ML, MacMullen C, Liu DJ, Leal SM, Davis RL. Genetic association of cyclic AMP signaling genes with bipolar disorder. Transl Psychiatry. 2012;2(10):e169.

55. MitoBreak. http://mitobreak.portugene.com. Accessed 27 Nov 2017.

56. Guo Y, Deng X, Zhang J, Su L, Xu H, Luo Z, et al. Analysis of the MRPL3, DNAJC13 and OFCC1 variants in Chinese Han patients with TS-CTD. Neurosci Lett. 2012;517(1):18–20.

13

Developmental stress elicits preference for methamphetamine in the spontaneously hypertensive rat model of attention-deficit/hyperactivity disorder

Jacqueline S. Womersley[1]*, Bafokeng Mpeta[1], Jacqueline J. Dimatelis[1], Lauriston A. Kellaway[1], Dan J. Stein[2] and Vivienne A. Russell[1]

Abstract

Background: Developmental stress has been hypothesised to interact with genetic predisposition to increase the risk of developing substance use disorders. Here we have investigated the effects of maternal separation-induced developmental stress using a behavioural proxy of methamphetamine preference in an animal model of attention-deficit/hyperactivity disorder, the spontaneously hypertensive rat, versus Wistar Kyoto and Sprague–Dawley comparator strains.

Results: Analysis of results obtained using a conditioned place preference paradigm revealed a significant strain × stress interaction with maternal separation inducing preference for the methamphetamine-associated compartment in spontaneously hypertensive rats. Maternal separation increased behavioural sensitization to the locomotor-stimulatory effects of methamphetamine in both spontaneously hypertensive and Sprague–Dawley strains but not in Wistar Kyoto rats.

Conclusions: Our findings indicate that developmental stress in a genetic rat model of attention-deficit/hyperactivity disorder may foster a vulnerability to the development of substance use disorders.

Keywords: Addiction, Attention-deficit/hyperactivity disorder, Conditioned place preference, Developmental stress, Methamphetamine, Spontaneously hypertensive rat

Background

Over recent years a substantial and compelling body of literature has emerged to suggest the importance of gene × environment interactions in the development of psychopathology. Genetic inheritance and environmental factors each account for approximately 50 % of the risk of developing a substance use disorder (SUD) [1]. More specifically, both human and animal studies have identified early life stress and a diagnosis of attention-deficit/hyperactivity disorder (ADHD) as individual risk factors

for the development of SUDs [2, 3]. Specific mechanisms involved in such vulnerability have begun to be delineated in humans. A [11C]raclopride positron emission tomography study found that a history of childhood adversity increased amphetamine-induced dopamine release in the ventral striatum [4] while data from a functional magnetic resonance imaging (fMRI) study revealed increased limbic area activity after childhood maltreatment in abstinent methamphetamine-dependent individuals [5]. A further fMRI study examining reward-related brain areas found increased activity in the putamen in individuals who had experienced early life adversity whilst activity in the right insula was associated with ADHD symptomology [6]. Specific animal models may be useful in further investigating such mechanisms. Neonatal

*Correspondence: jacqueline.womersley@gmail.com
[1] Department of Human Biology, Faculty of Health Sciences, University of Cape Town, Anzio Road, Observatory, Cape Town 7925, South Africa
Full list of author information is available at the end of the article

isolation-induced developmental stress in rats was found to increase cocaine self-administration [7]. In a separate study, developmentally stressed rats displayed a reduced threshold for intracranial self-stimulation of the lateral hypothalamus following amphetamine administration, an indication that the reward-enhancing effect of amphetamine was higher than in controls [8]. Combined these results suggest that early life stress and ADHD may render individuals hyper-sensitive to psychostimulants.

Though the shared pathophysiology underlying developmental stress, ADHD and SUDs is not yet clear, altered dopaminergic transmission affects all three processes and thus has emerged as a likely mechanism. Developmental stress induces long-term changes in the dopaminergic system, reducing dopamine type 2 receptor levels in the nucleus accumbens, which is in turn associated with compulsive drug use and impulsivity [9–11]. Altered striatal concentrations and functional polymorphisms of the dopamine transporter (DAT), the presynaptic transporter responsible for the rapid reuptake of synaptic dopamine and therefore of critical importance in dopaminergic homeostasis, have both been implicated in ADHD [12, 13]. Furthermore, the most widely prescribed medications for the treatment of ADHD are psychostimulants, which exert their effects at dopaminergic synapses [14]. DAT is the molecular target for the psychostimulant drug of abuse, methamphetamine, which binds to DAT and reverses its action essentially causing dopamine to be released into, rather than taken up from, synapses [15]. The subsequent supraphysiological levels of dopamine are responsible for the rewarding properties of drugs and in turn influence a number of dopamine-dependent behavioural processes, which are comorbid with the development of SUDs, such as altered motivation, motor output, impulsivity and reward processing [10, 16].

To further probe the common mechanism underlying developmental stress, ADHD and SUDs, we previously used in vivo chronoamperometry to examine the effect of developmental stress, via maternal separation (MS), on striatal dopamine clearance in an animal model of ADHD. The spontaneously hypertensive rat (SHR), in comparison to its normotensive progenitor strain the Wistar Kyoto rat (WKY), is a well-validated animal model of ADHD [17–19]. Our preliminary results indicated that MS delayed the clearance of ejected dopamine in SHR suggesting reduced DAT efficiency [20]. A further study examining the effect of cocaine, a psychostimulant and potent DAT inhibitor, in this model found that the cocaine-induced delay in dopamine uptake was exacerbated by MS in SHR resulting in a prolonged elevated dopamine concentration [21]. Given these results, we hypothesise that the observed decrease in DAT efficiency in MS SHR will translate into an increased preference for

the psychostimulant methamphetamine, a drug with a high potential for dependence and abuse [22]. We examined this proposal using SHR, WKY and an additional comparator strain, Sprague Dawley (SD), to control for the putative depressive/anxious phenotype of WKY, which might influence our results [23, 24]. This study used adolescent rats, an age associated with the onset of drug use and prior to the full development of elevated blood pressure in SHR [25, 26]. We employed the conditioned place preference (CPP) test, a classical conditioning paradigm that pairs drug exposure with one of two visually and tactilely distinct compartments to determine whether drug administration can overcome an innate initial preference. Successful pairing of a drug with the non-preferred compartment and a change in location preference is used as a proxy for the rewarding properties of the drug [27].

Methods
Animals
SHR (Charles River Laboratories, Wilmington, MA, USA), WKY (Harlan Laboratories, Bicester, UK) and SD (Charles River Laboratories, Wilmington, MA, USA) rats were obtained from strains maintained at the University of Cape Town Research Animal Facility. The decision to source WKY from Harlan, UK, rather than Charles River Laboratories, was based on research suggesting that they are the most appropriate behavioural and genetic control [24]. Rats had ad libitum access to water and standard rat chow and were housed in clear Perspex cages with wood chip bedding in a facility maintained at 21–23 °C with a 12/12 h light/dark cycle (lights on at 06h00). All experiments were authorised by the University of Cape Town Faculty of Health Sciences Animal Ethics Committee under application 011/047 and conformed to local and international standards set out for the care and use of animals for scientific purposes [28, 29].

Maternal separation
The MS paradigm was performed as previously described [30]. Briefly, male and female rats were pair bred in the University of Cape Town Human Biology satellite animal facility and the day of birth of the resulting litters was designated as postnatal day 0 (P0). On P2, the dam was removed from the cage and the number and sex of the pups was determined. In order to maintain uniformity of care, litters were culled to 8 pups with males preferentially selected for. However, a minimum of 2 female pups were retained in each litter to control for possible altered maternal behaviour and subsequent anxiety in offspring due to varying litter gender composition [31, 32]. Dams of non-separated (nMS) litters were subsequently returned to the home cage and remained with

the litter in the animal facility until weaning. Conversely, on P2 MS litters were removed from the dam to a separate room maintained at 31–33 °C with infrared heating lamps. Three hours later the litters were returned to the animal facility and the dam returned to the home cage. This separation paradigm occurred between 09h00 and 13h00 over 13 days from P2 to P14. Cleaning of cages and the initial handling of pups on P2 was consistent across MS and nMS groups to ensure that potential differences would be due to the effect of the separation paradigm. On P21 litters were weaned and male rats we co-housed (2–4 rats/cage) for the remainder of the project. No more than 2 rats from any one litter were assigned to an experimental group so as to avoid potential confounding litter effects.

Conditioned place preference

The CPP paradigm was performed over the course of 7 days (P54–P60) in male adolescent rats, thereby corresponding with the most common age of onset for SUDs in humans [33]. This compressed protocol consisted of 3 preconditioning, 3 conditioning and 1 probe trial day. Briefly, a square black Perspex box (43 cm length × 50 cm height) was equally divided by a central partition to produce one chamber with a grid floor and thin vertical white stripes on the walls and a second chamber with unadorned walls and a smooth floor. Rats were allowed to freely explore the apparatus for 30 min during preconditioning, which was performed over the course of 3 days to compensate for the increased exploratory drive and preference for novelty in SHR as well as potential anxiety in WKY [34]. The compartment in which rats spent the most time on the 3rd day of testing was designated as the preferred compartment. The conditioning period was composed of 2 × 1-h trials per day with a vehicle (0.9 % saline administered via intraperitoneal injection at 1 ml/kg volume) injection paired with the preferred compartment, and a methamphetamine (Sigma-Aldrich, St Louis, MO, USA) injection (1.5 mg/kg in 0.9 % saline administered via intraperitoneal injection at 1 ml/kg) paired with the non-preferred compartment. These 2 trials were separated by at least 3 h to allow sufficient time for memory formation with the non-drug pairing conducted first to prevent the association of potential withdrawal effects with the subsequent trial [27]. The selected dose of methamphetamine (1.5 mg/kg calculated as a free base) was based on 3 factors: successful CPP in SHR following conditioning with a 1.25 mg/kg dose; the failure to find an effect of MS on place preference in SD rats administered a 1.0 mg/kg dose; and the need to avoid potential neurotoxic side effects associated with a higher dose, which might reduce locomotor activity due to depressive effects [35–38]. As caudate putamen methamphetamine

concentrations peak between 30 and 60 min post intraperitoneal injection, rats were injected 10 min prior to the onset of conditioning trials to ensure that peak cerebral concentrations of methamphetamine were reached within the 1 h conditioning trial [39]. On the final day of testing, P60, rats were exposed to a 30 min probe trial during which they were allowed to freely explore the apparatus. Behaviour was recorded using a Soni Handicam DCR-SX 83E and time spent in each compartment as well as locomotor activity were analysed using Noldus Ethovision XT 7.0 (Noldus Information Technology, Wageningen, Netherlands). This experimental design produced 6 final groups: nMS SHR (n = 13), MS SHR (n = 11), nMS WKY (n = 10), MS WKY (n = 13), nMS SD (n = 13) and MS SD (n = 10).

Statistical analyses

All data were tested for normal distribution using a Shapiro–Wilk W test. Baseline activity data over the course of the 3 preconditioning days was analysed to check for strain and stress effects. The time spent highly mobile (defined as the period of time during which the area detected as the animal changes by at least 60 % per second) was non-parametrically distributed and therefore tested for potential strain × stress effects using a Kruskal–Wallis test with multiple comparisons of mean ranks with Bonferroni adjustment as a post hoc test. To check for differences in the initial strength of compartment preference, the duration spent in the non-preferred compartment on the third day of preconditioning was subjected to a factorial ANOVA with strain and stress as categorical predictors. Significant differences were further investigated using a Tukey post hoc test. Methamphetamine preference scores were calculated by subtracting the time spent in the non-preferred compartment on the third day of preconditioning from the time spent in the same compartment during the probe trial. Therefore a positive value, i.e. increased time spent in the non-preferred compartment following methamphetamine conditioning, was taken as an indication of increased preference for the drug-paired compartment. Preference scores were normally distributed and thus analysed using a factorial ANOVA with strain and stress as categorical factors. Significant differences between groups were probed using a Tukey post hoc test. To determine which groups displayed behavioural sensitisation to methamphetamine, the total distance covered and the time spent highly mobile on the first and third days of conditioning were compared. As these data were non-parametrically distributed, they were analysed with a Wilcoxon Matched Pairs Test. To check for strain × stress effects on sensitisation, we subjected the mobility data to an aligned rank transform for nonparametric factorial analyses [40]. This preprocessing allows common ANOVA procedures to be used to investigate interaction effects in repeated measures non-parametrically distributed data. All statistical analyses were performed using Statistica 13 (Statsoft, Dell Software, Tulsa, OK, USA) and an α value of 0.05 was used to determine significance. Graphs were generated using GraphPad Prism 6.0 (GraphPad, La Jolla, CA, USA).

Results

The time spent highly mobile was recorded over the 3 preconditioning days and analysed to check for differences in baseline locomotor activity. Kruskal–Wallis tests revealed significant strain × stress effects on the time spent highly mobile on each of the 3 days [day 1 H(5,N = 70) = 23.47, p < 0.001; day 2 H(5,N = 70) = 22.43, p < 0.001; and day 3 H(5,N = 70) = 26.27, p < 0.001] (Fig. 1). Post hoc analysis revealed that MS WKY spent less time highly mobile than MS SHR across all 3 days (day 1 p = 0.022, day 2 p = 0.020, and day 3 p = 0.013). MS WKY also spent less time highly mobile than MS SD on the third day of preconditioning (p = 0.009). Further differences between SHR and WKY rats were also found on days 2 and 3 of preconditioning where nMS SHR spent more time highly mobile than nMS WKY (p = 0.020 and p = 0.039 respectively).

The change in time spent in the non-preferred compartment following methamphetamine administration was analysed by factorial ANOVA and revealed a significant strain x stress interaction (F$_{(2,64)}$ = 6.45, p = 0.003). A post hoc test indicated that MS SHR spent a longer period in the methamphetamine-paired compartment compared to both nMS SHR and MS SD (p = 0.049 and p = 0.029 respectively) (Fig. 2). MS did not alter

preference for the methamphetamine-paired compartment in either WKY or SD and no strain difference was found within the nMS group. The strength of initial compartment preference was analysed by factorial ANOVA and revealed a significant strain effect (F$_{(2,64)}$ = 10.36, p < 0.001). A Tukey post hoc test indicated that WKY spent more time in the preferred compartment initially than both SHR and SD (p < 0.001 and p = 0.002 respectively) (Fig. 2).

Potential sensitisation to methamphetamine was determined by comparing locomotor activity data obtained on the first and third days of methamphetamine conditioning. A Wilcoxon matched pairs test indicated an increase in time spent highly mobile on the third day of conditioning for all groups (T$_{(n=70)}$ = 619.5, p < 0.001). This difference was significant in nMS SHR (T$_{(n=13)}$ = 8.0, p = 0.009), MS SHR (T$_{(n=11)}$ = 2.0, p = 0.006) and MS SD (T$_{(n=10)}$ = 4.0, p = 0.028) (Fig. 3). A further Wilcoxon matched pairs test revealed a significant effect of methamphetamine on total distance covered in all groups (T$_{(n=70)}$ = 640.0, p < 0.001), which was due to MS SHR and MS SD covering significantly greater distances on the third day of conditioning (T$_{(n=11)}$ = 8.0, p = 0.026, and T$_{(n=10)}$ = 6.0, p = 0.028 respectively) (Fig. 4). Repeated measures ANOVAs of aligned rank transformed data revealed no significant strain × stress effects for either the duration highly mobile or the total distance covered.

Discussion

In this study we sought to investigate whether our earlier observation of delayed dopamine reuptake in MS SHR translates into increased preference for the psychostimulant methamphetamine measured using a CPP paradigm. Consistent with our hypothesis, MS SHR displayed increased preference for the methamphetamine-paired compartment compared to both nMS SHR and MS SD. The failure of MS in SD rats to increase methamphetamine preference is consistent with a previous study, in which nMS and MS male SD rats were exposed to 2 conditioning stages (P33–36 and P39–42) with methamphetamine (administered at 1 mg/kg) yet did not differ in their preference for methamphetamine at P37, P43 or P50 [35]. The finding that WKY did not develop methamphetamine CPP is also in keeping with a previous study that showed that rats with high anxiety exhibit less 50 kHz ultrasonic vocalizations—a marker of positive affect [41]. We also investigated whether there were any differences in the initial magnitude of compartment preference and determined that WKY showed a more robust preference for the saline-paired compartment during preconditioning than both SHR and SD rats. Perhaps more importantly for the current results, there was no difference in the strength of compartment preference

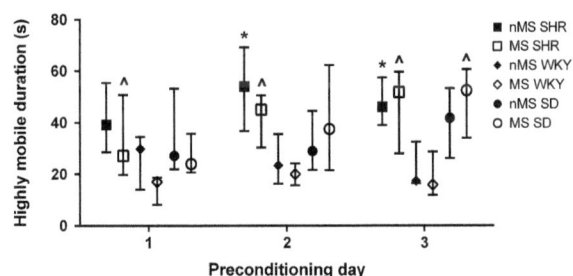

Fig. 1 SHR and WKY rats exhibit baseline differences in the time spent highly mobile during preconditioning. ^MS WKY spent less time highly mobile compared to MS SHR on days 1 through 3 of preconditioning and compared to MS SD on the third day of preconditioning (p < 0.05, Bonferroni post hoc test). *nMS WKY spent less time highly mobile than nMS SHR during the second and third days of preconditioning (p < 0.05, 613 Bonferroni post hoc test). Data are displayed as median and interquartile range

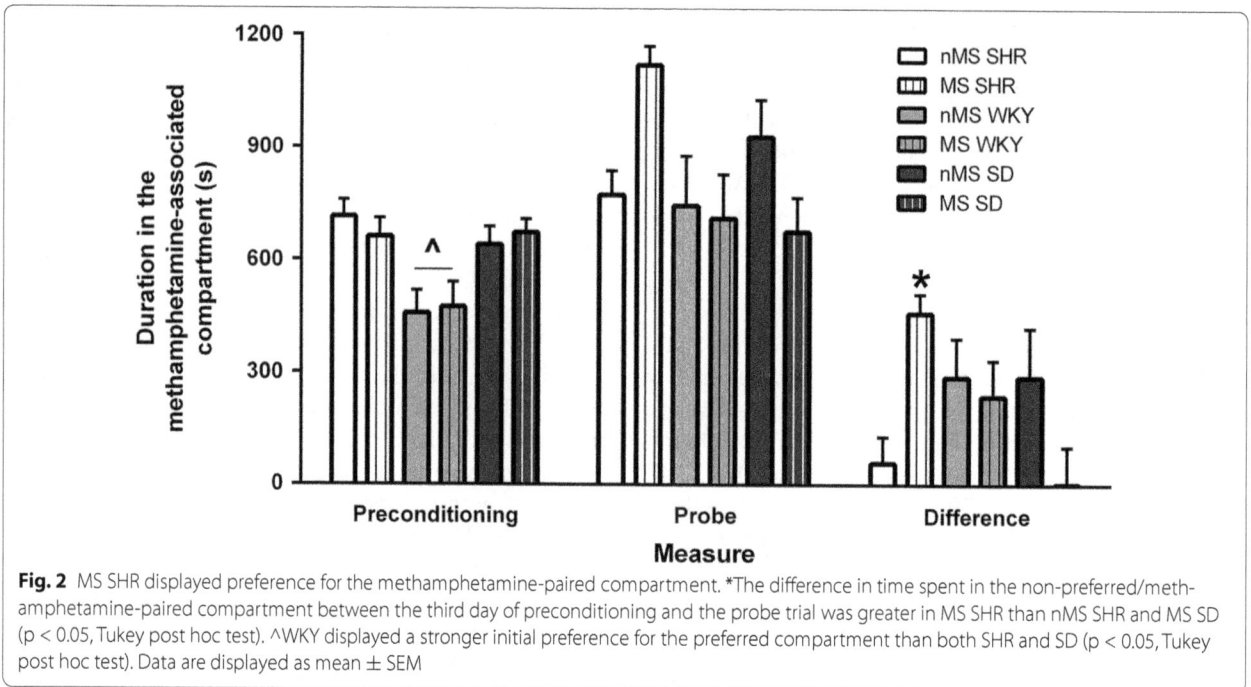

Fig. 2 MS SHR displayed preference for the methamphetamine-paired compartment. *The difference in time spent in the non-preferred/methamphetamine-paired compartment between the third day of preconditioning and the probe trial was greater in MS SHR than nMS SHR and MS SD (p < 0.05, Tukey post hoc test). ^WKY displayed a stronger initial preference for the preferred compartment than both SHR and SD (p < 0.05, Tukey post hoc test). Data are displayed as mean ± SEM

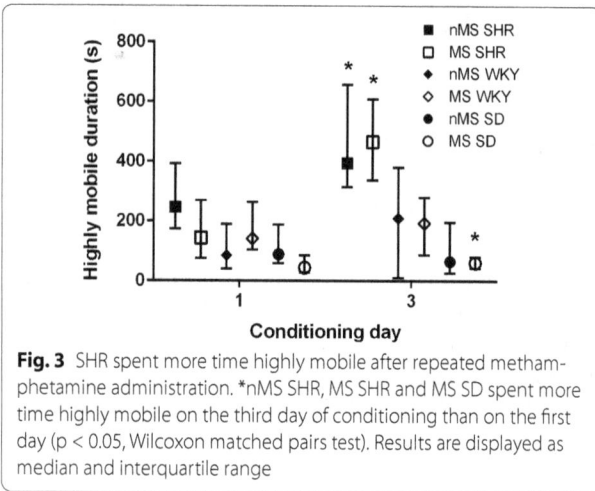

Fig. 3 SHR spent more time highly mobile after repeated methamphetamine administration. *nMS SHR, MS SHR and MS SD spent more time highly mobile on the third day of conditioning than on the first day (p < 0.05, Wilcoxon matched pairs test). Results are displayed as median and interquartile range

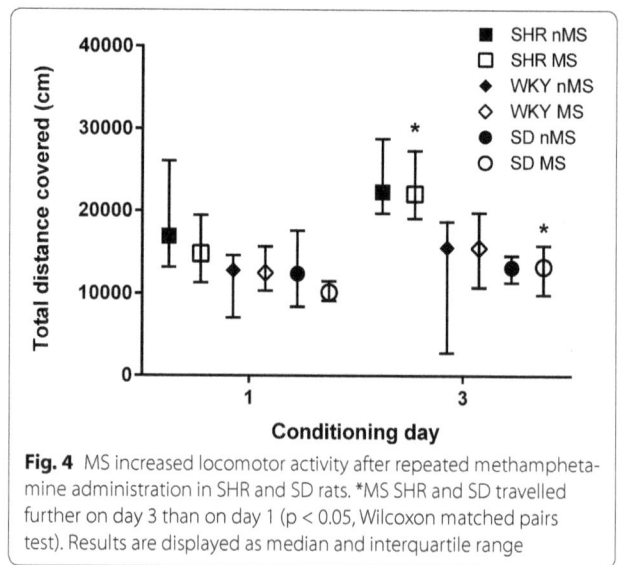

Fig. 4 MS increased locomotor activity after repeated methamphetamine administration in SHR and SD rats. *MS SHR and SD travelled further on day 3 than on day 1 (p < 0.05, Wilcoxon matched pairs test). Results are displayed as median and interquartile range

between nMS and MS SHR. Combined these results suggest that the influence of developmental stress on drug preference is dependent on genetic predisposition.

The failure of nMS SHR to show a robust preference for the methamphetamine-associated compartment is perhaps surprising given the association between ADHD and drug abuse [42]. However, we maintain that previous studies which found that SHR exhibit a preference for psychostimulants differ from our own in several important methodological aspects including the source of the SHR used and the age at testing. For example,

several studies in SHR have found positive preference for methamphetamine (1.25 and 5.0 mg/kg) as well as the psychostimulants amphetamine (5 mg/kg) and methylphenidate (1.25, 5.0 and 20 mg/kg) [37, 38, 43, 44]. Importantly, these studies made use of SHR obtained from Charles River Japan as opposed to the current study which sourced SHR from Charles River USA, a noteworthy distinction given evidence that suggests that SHR from different vendors may display different behavioural characteristics [24]. Furthermore, in the aforementioned studies, the age of the rats at the time of behavioural testing differed by at least a week compared to our protocol. Though a small difference, age has previously been suggested to influence the response to psychostimulants in SHR [45, 46]. A further possible reason for the failure to find methamphetamine CPP in nMS SHR in the current study lies in the behaviour of the strain. Previous research has indicated that, congruent with the hyperactive phenotype, SHR continue to display increased locomotor activity in familiar environments [47]. Indeed, an analysis of preconditioning baseline activity revealed that SHR were more active than their WKY counterparts. It is therefore possible that the rewarding effects of methamphetamine were insufficient to prevent nMS SHR from exploring both chambers of the apparatus during the probe trial.

A repeated measures analysis of the locomotor activity on the first and third days of conditioning found no significant strain × stress effects on the magnitude of sensitisation. However, a matched pairs comparison of locomotor activity on the first and third days of conditioning indicated that nMS SHR, MS SHR and MS SD spent more time highly mobile after repeated methamphetamine administration, which translated into an increased total distance covered in the latter two experimental groups. As these results measure the change in locomotor activity due to methamphetamine, they are not influenced by the higher baseline activity levels of SHR. This suggests that SHR, and in particular MS SHR, display an increased sensitisation to methamphetamine i.e. repeated exposure produces an increased stimulant drug response that is associated with increased motivation to consume the drug [48]. The current study made use of ambulatory activity to measure locomotor sensitisation. However, repeated exposure to psychostimulants may also lead to the development of repetitive motor behaviours or stereotypies such as repeated sniffing, rearing, and head and mouth movements [49]. Previous research using Lewis and Fischer 344 rats has indicated that the developmental time course of stereotyped behaviour in response to methamphetamine may differ between strains [50]. Furthermore, a study comparing the behavioural responses of 6 week old SHR and WKY to d-amphetamine found strain differences in the types of stereotypic movement produced [51]. It is therefore possible that an analysis of stereotyped behaviour in the current study may have revealed further strain and/or stress effects, including sensitisation to methamphetamine in WKY.

Comparison of the methamphetamine preference and sensitisation results reveal a conflict insofar as methamphetamine elicited preference in MS SHR whilst

increasing sensitisation in nMS SHR, MS SHR and MS SD. This apparent contradiction between psychomotor and reward responses to psychostimulants has also been found in previous studies. One such investigation examined the effect of self-administration duration on drug-primed reinstatement and behavioural sensitisation [52]. Rats that advanced from short to extended access durations (1 vs. 6 h) escalated their cocaine consumption during the first hour of their trials such that they infused more cocaine in that period than their short access (1 h only) counterparts [52]. However, this group that displayed increased drug self-administration, a measure of drug preference, did not differ in locomotor sensitisation to the drug. Further, in a study that assessed locomotor activation, sensitisation and place preference in response to cocaine in 6 mouse strains, the authors failed to find locomotor sensitisation in certain strains that displayed drug CPP [53]. This led the authors to hypothesise that the psychomotor and rewarding effects of drugs may be served by distinct mechanisms. Extending this hypothesis to our own results, it is possible that developmental stress may exert different effects on these mechanisms within the strains we tested. Support for this explanation is provided by previous research suggesting that the time course of dopaminergic development differs between SHR and comparator strains. In an in vitro autoradiography study assessing striatal dopaminergic development in pre- and post-hypertensive (2 and 15 week old respectively) SHR and WKY, DAT was elevated in the caudate putamen of SHR at both developmental stages [54]. In addition, SHR putamen followed a lateral-to-medial DAT gradient during early development and displayed elevated dopamine type 1 receptor concentrations compared to WKY by 15 weeks [54]. A further study examining [3H] dopamine uptake into synaptosomes prepared from WKY and SHR (at 1, 2, 3, 6, 8 and 10 weeks of age) found that the rate of dopamine uptake in the prefrontal cortex was persistently lower in SHR from 2 weeks onwards and transiently lower in the striatum at the 6 week time point [55]. Though we were unable to find reports evaluating dopaminergic development in SHR and SD strains, the comparisons between SHR and WKY suggest possible strain differences in the developmental course of multiple dopaminergic pathways. It is therefore possible that the effects of MS may be region specific in different strains, based on the developmental stage of a particular brain area. In this way, MS may affect brain areas responsible for both locomotor activity and reward in SHR, whilst having a more anatomically restricted effect in influencing only locomotor activity in SD.

The potential of early life stress to exert long term changes on neurophysiology is well-recognised [56]. Of relevance to our MS model, immunohistochemical studies have indicated that development of the striatal dopaminergic system continues postnatally with an increase in axospinous connections and a decrease in axodendritic and axosomatic synapses [57]. The overall reduction in total dopaminergic synaptic density bears a closer resemblance to the adult profile [57]. Disruption during this critical window may produce psychopathology associated with dopaminergic dysfunction including ADHD and SUDs [58–60].

Both increased locomotor activity in response to methamphetamine and successful place preference are dependent on dopamine and as such these two measures can be used as a proxy of increased extracellular dopamine concentration [16, 61]. Given the preference for and sensitisation to methamphetamine displayed by MS SHR, it is likely that developmental stress in SHR increased the extracellular dopamine concentration in the brain areas serving these functions. This would also be in keeping with our previous in vivo chronoamperometric studies where the DAT-mediated clearance of dopamine was delayed by MS in SHR [20, 21]. We hypothesise that the dose of methamphetamine used in the study (1.5 mg/kg) was non-saturating i.e. the number of DATs unimpeded by methamphetamine was reduced in MS SHR compared to controls. This scenario could result in a similar dopamine release between groups but prolonged elevated synaptic dopamine in MS SHR due to reduced DAT-mediated clearance. This is consistent with evidence for altered DAT function and responsiveness to psychostimulants in ADHD as found by Stein et al., where children diagnosed with ADHD and possessing the 9/9 repeat DAT allele were less sensitive to the effects of the therapeutic psychostimulants on measures of hyperactivity and impulsivity [62]. However, further experiments measuring methamphetamine-induced dopamine release and DAT-mediated reuptake would be required to either support or refute this proposed mechanism. This hypothesis would also be further refined by an experiment that examines whether MS affects DAT expression differently in SHR compared to WKY and SD.

Conclusions

Our finding of preference for the methamphetamine-associated compartment in MS SHR strongly supports our previous chronoamperometric findings of reduced DAT-mediated dopamine clearance in MS SHR. Given the high cost of SUDs to individuals and society, such mechanistic insights are important in understanding how a diagnosis of ADHD and a history of developmental stress may increase the risk of developing SUDs. Furthermore, these results again reinforce the importance of gene × environment interactions in influencing psychopathology.

Abbreviations

ADHD: attention-deficit/hyperactivity disorder; CPP: conditioned place preference; DAT: dopamine transporter; fMRI: functional magnetic resonance imaging; MS: maternally separated; nMS: non-maternally separated; P: postnatal day; SD: Sprague–Dawley; SHR: spontaneously hypertensive rat; SUD: substance use disorder; WKY: Wistar Kyoto.

Authors' contributions

JW, JD, LK, DS and VR conceived and designed the study. JW and BM conducted the experiments and analysed the data. JD, LK, DS and VR supervised the study. JW drafted the manuscript. All authors critically reviewed the manuscript and gave final approval for the version to be published. This work formed part of the BSc (Honours) project of BM and part of the Ph.D. thesis of JW. All authors read and approved the final manuscript.

Author details

[1] Department of Human Biology, Faculty of Health Sciences, University of Cape Town, Anzio Road, Observatory, Cape Town 7925, South Africa. [2] Department of Psychiatry and Mental Health, Faculty of Health Sciences, University of Cape Town, Groote Schuur Hospital, Observatory, Cape Town 7925, South Africa.

Acknowledgements

Nuraan Ismail and AK Samuels are gratefully acknowledged for animal husbandry and care.

Competing interests

The authors declare that they have no competing interests.

Funding

This work was based on research supported by the South African National Research Foundation and the South African Medical Research Council. Any opinion, finding and conclusion or recommendation expressed in this material is that of the author and the NRF does not accept any liability in this regard. Thanks are also due to the Faculty of Health Sciences Research Committee of the University of Cape Town for their support and the Postgraduate Publication Incentive Award.

References

1. Maze I, Nestler E. The epigenetic landscape of addiction. Ann NY Acad Sci. 2011;1216:99–113.
2. Harstad E, Levy S. Attention-deficit/hyperactivity disorder and substance abuse. Pediatrics. 2014;134:e293–301.
3. Meade CS, Watt MH, Sikkema KJ, Deng LX, Ranby KW, Skinner D, Pieterse D, Kalichmann SC. Methamphetamine use is associated with childhood sexual abuse and HIV sexual risk behaviors among patrons of alcohol-serving venues in Cape Town, South Africa. Drug Alcohol Depend. 2012;126:232–9.
4. Oswald LM, Wand GS, Kuwabara H, Wong DF, Zhu S, Brasic JR. History of childhood adversity is positively associated with ventral striatal dopamine responses to amphetamine. Psychopharmacology. 2014;231:2417–33.
5. Dean AC, Kohno M, Hellemann G, London ED. Childhood maltreatment and amygdala connectivity in methamphetamine dependence: a pilot study. Brain Behav. 2014;4:867–76.

6. Boecker R, Holz N, Buchmann A, Blomeyer D, Plichta M, Wolf I, Baumeister S, Meyer-Lindenberg A, Banaschewski T, Brandeis D, Laucht M. Impact of early life adversity on reward processing in young adults: EEG-fMRI results from a prospective study over 25 years. PLoS ONE. 2014;9:e104185.

7. Kosten T, Miserendino M, Kehoe P. Enhanced acquisition of cocaine self-administration in adult rats with neonatal isolation stress experience. Brain Res. 2000;875:44–50.

8. Der-Avakian A, Markou A. Neonatal maternal separation exacerbates the reward-enhancing effect of acute amphetamine administration and the anhedonic effect of repeated social defeat in adult rats. Neuroscience. 2010;170:1189–98.

9. Li M, Xue X, Shao S, Shao F, Wang W. Cognitive, emotional and neuro-chemical effects of repeated maternal separation in adolescent rats. Brain Res. 2013;1518:82–90.

10. Volkow ND, Koob G, Baler R. Biomarkers in substance use disorders. ACS Chem Neurosci. 2015;6:522–5.

11. Dalley JW, Fryer TD, Brichard L, Robinson ES, Theobald DE, Lääne K, Peña Y, Murphy ER, Shah Y, Probst K, et al. Nucleus accumbens D2/3 receptors predict trait impulsivity and cocaine reinforcement. Science. 2007;315:1267–70.

12. Cook EH, Stein MA, Krasowski MD, Cox NJ, Olkon DM, Kieffer JE, Leventhal BL. Association of attention-deficit disorder and the dopamine trans-porter gene. Am J Hum Genet. 1995;56:993–8.

13. Barr CL, Xu C, Kroft J, Feng Y, Wigg K, Zai G, Tannock R, Schachar R, Malone M, Roberts W, et al. Haplotype study of three polymorphisms at the dopa-mine transporter locus confirm linkage to attention-deficit/hyperactivity disorder. Biol Psychiatry. 2001;49:333–9.

14. Pasini A, Sinibaldi L, Paloscia C, Douzgou S, Pitzianti M, Romeo E, Curatolo P, Pizzuti A. Neurocognitive effects of methylphenidate on ADHD children with different DAT genotypes: a longitudinal open label trial. Eur J Paedi-atr Neurol. 2013;17:407–14.

15. Riddle E, Fleckenstein A, Hanson G. Mechanisms of methamphetamine-induced dopaminergic neurotoxicity. AAPS J. 2006;8:E413–8.

16. Tobler PN. Behavioral Functions of Dopamine Neurons. In: Iversen L, Iversen S, Dunnett S, Bjorklund A, editors. Dopamine Handbook. 1st ed. New York: Oxford University Press; 2010. p. 316–30.

17. Sagvolden T. Behavioral validation of the spontaneously hypertensive rat (SHR) as an animal model of attention-deficit/hyperactivity disorder (AD/HD). Neurosci Biobehav Rev. 2000;24:31–9.

18. Sagvolden T, Russell V, Aase H, Johansen E, Farshbaf M. Rodent models of attention-deficit/hyperactivity disorder. Biol Psychiatry. 2005;57:1239–47.

19. Russell V. Neurobiology of animal models of attention-deficit hyperactiv-ity disorder. J Neurosci Methods. 2007;161:185–98.

20. Womersley JS, Hsieh JH, Kellaway LA, Gerhardt GA, Russell VA. Maternal separation affects dopamine transporter function in the spontaneously hypertensive rat: an in vivo electrochemical study. Behav Brain Funct. 2011;7:49.

21. Womersley JS, Kellaway LA, Stein DJ, Gerhardt GA, Russell VA. Effect of cocaine on striatal dopamine clearance in a rat model of developmental stress and attention-deficit/hyperactivity disorder. Stress. 2016;19:78–82.

22. Barr AM, Panenka WJ, MacEwan GW, Thornton AE, Lang DJ, Honer WG, Lecomte T. The need for speed: an update on methamphetamine addic-tion. J Psychiatry Neurosci. 2006;31:301–13.

23. Garza RDL, Mahoney J. A distinct neurochemical profile in WKY rats at baseline and in response to acute stress: implications for animal models of anxiety and depression. Brain Res. 2004;1021:209–18.

24. Sagvolden T, Johansen EB, Wøien G, Walaas SI, Storm-Mathisen J, Berger-sen LH, Hvalby O, Jensen V, Aase H, Russell VA, et al. The spontaneously hypertensive rat model of ADHD-the importance of selecting the appro-priate reference strain. Neuropharmacology. 2009;57:619–26.

25. Kandel D, Logan J. Patterns of drug use from adolescence to young adult-hood: I. Periods of risk for initiation, continued use, and discontinuation. Am J Public Health. 1984;74:660–6.

26. Okamoto K, Aoki K. Development of a strain of spontaneously hyperten-sive rats. Jpn Circ J. 1963;27:282–93.

27. Carlezon WA. Place conditioning to study drug reward and aversion. Methods Mol Med. 2003;84:243–9.

28. SABS: South African National Standard. The Care and Use of Animals for Scientific Purposes (SANS 10386:2008). 1st edn. Pretoria: South African Bureau of Standards, Standards Division; 2008.

29. Mohr B. The current status of laboratory animal ethics in South Africa. ATLA. 2013;41:48–51.

30. Daniels WM, Pietersen CY, Carstens ME, Stein DJ. Maternal separation in rats leads to anxiety-like behavior and a blunted ACTH response and altered neurotransmitter levels in response to a subsequent stressor. Metab Brain Dis. 2004;19:3–14.

31. Kosten TA, Huang W, Nielsen DA. Sex and litter effects on anxiety and DNA methylation levels of stress and neurotrophin genes in adolescent rats. Dev Psychobiol. 2014;56:392–406.

32. Kosten TA, Nielsen DA. Litter and sex effects on maternal behavior and DNA methylation of the Nr3c1 exon 17 promoter gene in hippocampus and cerebellum. Int J Dev Neurosci. 2014;36:5–12.

33. Volkow ND. What do we know about drug addiction? Am J Psychiatry. 2005;162:1401–2.

34. Wultz B, Sagvolden T, Moser E, Moser M. The spontaneously hyperten-sive rat as an animal model of attention-deficit hyperactivity disorder: effects of methylphenidate on exploratory behavior. Behav Neural Biol. 1990;53:88–102.

35. Faure J, Stein D, Daniels W. Maternal separation fails to render animals more susceptible to methamphetamine-induced conditioned place preference. Metab Brain Dis. 2009;24:541–59.

36. Silva CD, Neves AF, Dias AI, Freitas HJ, Mendes SM, Pita I, Viana SD, Oliveira PAD, Cunha RA, Ribeiro CAF. A single neurotoxic dose of methamphet-amine induces a long-lasting depressive-like behaviour in mice. Neurotox Res. 2014;25:295–304.

37. dela Peña I, Ahn H, Choi J, Shin C, Ryu J, Cheong J. Reinforcing effects of methamphetamine in an animal model of attention-deficit/hyperactiv-ity disorder- the spontaneously hypertensive rat. Behav Brain Funct. 2010;6:72.

38. dela Peña I, Lee JC, Lee HL, Woo TS, Lee HC, Sohn AR, Cheong JH. Dif-ferential behavioral responses of the spontaneously hypertensive rat to methylphenidate and methamphetamine: lack of a rewarding effect of repeated methylphenidate treatment. Neurosci Lett. 2012;514:189–93.

39. Zhang Y, Loonam T, Noailles P, Angulo J. Comparison of cocaine- and methamphetamine-evoked dopamine and glutamate overflow in somatodendritic and terminal field regions of the rat brain during acute, chronic, and early withdrawal conditions. Ann NY Acad Sci. 2001;937:93–120.

40. Wobbrock J, Findlater L, Gergle D, Higgins J. The aligned rank transform for nonparametric factorial analyses using only ANOVA procedures In Proceedings of the ACM Conference on Human Factors in Computing Systems (CHI'11). New York: ACM Press; 2011. p. 143–6.

41. Lehner MH, Taracha E, Kaniuga E, Wisłowska-Stanek A, Wróbel J, Sobolewska A, Turzyńska D, Skórzewska A, Płaźnik A. High-anxiety rats are less sensitive to the rewarding affects of amphetamine on 50 kHz USV. Behav Brain Res. 2014;275:234–42.

42. Roberts W, Peters J, Adams Z, Lynam D, Milich R. Identifying the facets of impulsivity that explain the relation between ADHD symptoms and substance use in a nonclinical sample. Addict Behav. 2014;39:1272–7.

43. dela Peña I, Ahn H, Choi J, Shin C, Ryu J, Cheong J. Methylphenidate self-administration and conditioned place preference in an animal model of attention-deficit hyperactivity disorder: the spontaneously hypertensive rat. Behav Pharmacol. 2011;22:31–9.

44. dela Peña I, de la Peña J, Kim B, Han D, Noh M, Cheong J. Gene expression profiling in the striatum of amphetamine-treated spontaneously hyper-tensive rats which showed amphetamine conditioned place preference and self-administration. Arch Pharm Res. 2015;38:865–75.

45. Yang P, Cuellar D III, Swann A, Dafny N. Age and genetic strain differences in response to chronic methylphenidate administration. Behav Brain Res. 2011;218:206–17.

46. Yang P, Swann A, Dafny N. Acute and chronic methylphenidate dose-response assessment on three adolescent male rat strains. Brain Res Bull. 2006;71:301–10.

47. Langen B, Dost R. Comparison of SHR, WKY and Wistar rats in different behavioural animal models: effect of dopamine D1 and alpha2 agonists. Atten Defic Hyperact Disord. 2011;3:1–12.

48. Everitt BJ, Robbins TW. From the ventral to the dorsal striatum: devolv-ing views of their roles in drug addiction. Neurosci Biobehav Rev. 2013;37:1946–54.

49. Kelley A. Measurement of rodent stereotyped behavior. Curr Protoc Neurosci. 2001;4:8.8.1–8.13.

50. Camp D, Browman K, Robinson T. The effects of methamphetamine and cocaine on motor behavior and extracellular dopamine in the ventral striatum of Lewis versus Fischer 344 rats. Brain Res. 1994;668:180–93.

51. McCarty R, Chiueh C, Kopin I. Differential behavioral responses of spontaneously hypertensive (SHR) and normotensive (WKY) rats to d-amphetamine. Pharmacol Biochem Behav. 1980;12:53–9.

52. Knackstedt L, Kalivas P. Extended access to cocaine self-administration enhances drug-primed reinstatement but not behavioral sensitization. J Pharmacol Exp Ther. 2007;322:1103–9.

53. Eisener-Dorman AF, Grabowski-Boase L, Tarantino LM. Cocaine locomotor activation, sensitization and place preference in six inbred strains of mice. Behav Brain Funct. 2011;7:29.

54. Watanabe Y, Fujita M, Ito Y, Okada T, Kusuoka H, Nishimura T. Brain dopamine transporter in spontaneously hypertensive rats. J Nucl Med. 1997;38:470–4.

55. Myers M, Whittemore S, Hendley E. Changes in catecholamine neuronal uptake and receptor binding in the brains of spontaneously hypertensive rats (SHR). Brain Res. 1981;220:325–38.

56. Provençal N, Binder E. The effects of early life stress on the epigenome: from the womb to adulthood and even before. Exp Neurol. 2015;268:10–20.

57. Antonopoulos J, Dori I, Dinopoulos A, Chiotelli M, Parnavelas J. Postnatal development of the dopaminergic system of the striatum in the rat. Neuroscience. 2002;110:245–56.

58. Marco EM, Macrì S, Laviola G. Critical age windows for neurodevelopmental psychiatric disorders: evidence from animal models. Neurotox Res. 2011;19:286–307.

59. Money K, Stanwood G. Developmental origins of brain disorders: roles for dopamine. Front Cell Neurosci. 2013;7:260.

60. Martin LJ, Spicer DM, Lewis MH, Gluck JP, Cork LC. Social deprivation of infant rhesus monkeys alters the chemoarchitecture of the brain: I, subcortical regions. J Neurosci. 1991;11:3344–58.

61. Cagniard B, Sotnikova T, Gainetdinov R, Zhuang X. The dopamine transporter expression level differentially affects responses to cocaine and amphetamine. J Neurogenet. 2014;28:112–21.

62. Stein MA, Waldman I, Newcorn J, Bishop J, Kittles R, Cook EH. Dopamine transporter genotype and stimulant dose-response in youth with attention-deficit/hyperactivity disorder. J Child Adolesc Psychopharmacol. 2014;24:238–44.

63. Womersley JS, Mpeta B, Dimatelis JJ, Kellaway LA, Stein DJ, Russell VA. Developmental stress elicits preference for methamphetamine in the spontaneously hypertensive rat model of attention-deficit/hyperactivity disorder. Zenodo. 2016. doi:10.5281/zenodo.52569.

14

Neuropsychological and neurophysiological benefits from white noise in children with and without ADHD

Simon Baijot[1,2,3*], Hichem Slama[1,2,5,6], Göran Söderlund[7], Bernard Dan[3,8], Paul Deltenre[4], Cécile Colin[1,2,4†] and Nicolas Deconinck[3†]

Abstract

Background: Optimal stimulation theory and moderate brain arousal (MBA) model hypothesize that extra-task stimulation (e.g. white noise) could improve cognitive functions of children with attention-deficit/hyperactivity disorder (ADHD). We investigate benefits of white noise on attention and inhibition in children with and without ADHD (7–12 years old), both at behavioral and at neurophysiological levels.

Methods: Thirty children with and without ADHD performed a visual cued Go/Nogo task in two conditions (white noise or no-noise exposure), in which behavioral and P300 (mean amplitudes) data were analyzed. Spontaneous eye-blink rates were also recorded and participants went through neuropsychological assessment. Two separate analyses were conducted with each child separately assigned into two groups (1) ADHD or typically developing children (TDC), and (2) noise beneficiaries or non-beneficiaries according to the observed performance during the experiment. This latest categorization, based on a new index we called "Noise Benefits Index" (NBI), was proposed to determine a neuropsychological profile positively sensitive to noise.

Results: Noise exposure reduced omission rate in children with ADHD, who were no longer different from TDC. Eye-blink rate was higher in children with ADHD but was not modulated by white noise. NBI indicated a significant relationship between ADHD and noise benefit. Strong correlations were observed between noise benefit and neuropsychological weaknesses in vigilance and inhibition. Participants who benefited from noise had an increased Go P300 in the noise condition.

Conclusion: The improvement of children with ADHD with white noise supports both optimal stimulation theory and MBA model. However, eye-blink rate results question the dopaminergic hypothesis in the latter. The NBI evidenced a profile positively sensitive to noise, related with ADHD, and associated with weaker cognitive control.

Keywords: ADHD, White noise, ERP (P300), Dopamine, Optimal stimulation

Background

Attention-deficit/hyperactivity disorder (ADHD) is a highly prevalent developmental disorder that affects about 5 % of school-aged children and adolescents [1–4]. These children typically exhibit pervasive behavioral symptoms of hyperactivity, inattention and impulsivity [1], which substantially affect their quality of life (for a review, see [5]). Moreover, these symptoms are associated with adverse educational [6], interpersonal [7], and occupational outcomes [8]. Furthermore, deficits in attention, cognitive and executive functioning are considered as core behavioral symptoms in ADHD and are concerned in most contemporary ADHD models [9]. The most prominent deficits seen in ADHD are response inhibition [10], inattention (vigilance), working memory,

*Correspondence: sbaijot@ulb.ac.be
†Cécile Colin and Nicolas Deconinck contributed equally to this work
[1] Center for Research in Cognition and Neurosciences (CRCN), Université Libre de Bruxelles (ULB), Campus du Solbosch CP 191, Avenue F.D. Roosevelt 50, CP 151, 1050 Brussels, Belgium
Full list of author information is available at the end of the article

planning [11] and reaction time (RT), particularly RT variability [12].

While stimulant medication has been shown to improve behavioral symptoms [13] and school performance in ADHD [14], adverse effects from such medication have also been reported [15–19]. The immediate environment, which is the main concern of the present study, is also known to have a significant impact on the expression of certain ADHD symptoms such as hyperactivity, impulsivity or inattention [20–26].

Several models, including the optimal stimulation theory [20], the cognitive-energetic model [27], the stochastic resonance (SR) effect [28] and the moderate brain arousal (MBA) model [29], have tentatively incorporated an improvement of cognitive functioning related to environmental stimulation. The optimal stimulation theory is based on a homeostatic model, suggesting that each individual has its own biologically determined optimal level of arousal enabling him/her to reach the best level of cognitive functioning [20, 30]. Zentall, Zentall [30] hypothesized that children with ADHD suffer from under-arousal, which lowers their level of performance under "normal" conditions. They interpreted the restless and inattentive behavior of ADHD children as self-stimulation in order to raise their arousal level and, consequently, performance. Zentall, Zentall [30] suggest that the motor activity of children with ADHD increases more when they are exposed to a stimulus-poor environment in order to reach their high-stimulation threshold. The optimal stimulation theory was first proposed as a theoretical model but was later supported by empirical behavioral evidence from improvement in children with ADHD when extra-task stimulation was added, such as background linguistic noise during a reading/arithmetic task [31], pictures during a continuous performance test (CPT) auditory task [32], colored items during a CPT task [33, 34] and background music during arithmetic tasks [35]. Thus, apparent distraction might have a positive effect on performance and is therefore not always detrimental. In line with the optimal stimulation theory, the cognitive-energetic model postulates that ADHD symptoms and deficits occur because of problems with regulating energetic factors [27]. Sergeant et al. [27] suggest that performance is not only influenced by cognitive capacity but also by environmentally determined levels of arousal and activation as well as the extent to which variations in these energetic factors can be managed to ensure optimal performance.

One possible explanation for why adding stimulation might be beneficial lies in the stochastic resonance (SR) phenomenon [36]. SR is a phenomenon in which an optimal amount of random noise (e.g. white noise[1]), may be

beneficial for cognitive performance under certain circumstances [36]. Jepma et al. [37] showed, for example, that task-irrelevant auditory white noise can speed up responses to stimuli in the visual modality.

The MBA model [38] is a neurocomputational model related to the concept of SR but has been developed in the framework of ADHD research. MBA model posits that random noise in the environment introduces, through the perceptual system, internal noise into the neural system. This noise is assumed to compensate for the reduced background neural activity in ADHD related to their hypofunctioning dopaminergic system [38, 39]. Soderlund et al. [22] propose that the required level of extra-task stimulation (noise) depends on dopamine functioning so that participants with low dopamine levels (such as children with ADHD) require more noise to reach optimal cognitive performance in comparison with typically developing children (TDC).

MBA model is corroborated by three studies using a long-term memory task [22, 26, 40], which indicate that an optimal level of noise for inattentive children has detrimental consequences for TDC. Helps et al. [26] also showed benefits from white noise in a Go/Nogo task in children who were considered as "sub-attentive" by their teachers, while performance in "super-attentive" children worsened. The benefits concerned omission errors, which were significantly reduced in the sub-attentive group (in the white noise exposure condition), while there was no effect on commission errors for any group. However, a direct link between dopaminergic functioning and the beneficial effect of white noise on cognition has not yet been clearly demonstrated [26, 38]. In a study with a rat model of ADHD [41], white noise exposure did not increase dopamine levels, and noise benefit could be found even in dopamine-lesioned rats. In humans, spontaneous eye-blink rate, a marker of dopamine functioning in the striatum [42, 43], might help to further investigate this relationship.

To our knowledge, the potential effect of a white noise exposure on a visual Go/Nogo task has not been previously examined in children with ADHD, nor at behavioral or at neurophysiological levels. The P300 is an event-related potential (ERP) component that allows different processes (see below) to be studied and is often used as an interest marker in ADHD [44–47]. ERP studies in ADHD using Go/Nogo tasks have generally shown reductions in P300 amplitudes at centro-parietal sites in children with ADHD when compared to TDC (in Woltering et al. [48]), though this may not always be the case (see [49, 50]). This attenuation of P300 amplitudes in individuals with ADHD may suggest that less attentional resources are allocated to inhibitory control and related evaluative processes [48].

---

[1] White noise is a continuous random signal-sound from 20 to 20,000 Hz [23].

In this study, the first objective was to compare noise benefit between children with ADHD and TDC in a visual cued Go/Nogo task using both behavioral and neurophysiological measures. This task, in which a non-informative cue precedes each Go or Nogo trial, enables the separate examination of P300 evoked by: (1) preparation (Cue P300); (2) inhibition (Nogo P300); (3) attention and orienting processes (Go P300; [51]). The Cued Go/Nogo was chosen because the high target/non-target ratio in this task is adapted to rapidly obtain the minimum of 36 artifact-free trials (by condition) required for measuring a P300 [52]. Moreover, white noise was already found to be beneficial in a study using Go/Nogo in children considered "sub-attentive" but without an ADHD diagnosis [26]. The Go/Nogo task is also one of the most frequent inhibition tasks used in ADHD [53]. The second objective was to investigate potential correlations between noise benefit and individual neuropsychological profiles. For that purpose, we proposed a new marker of performance, the "Noise Benefit Index" (NBI), which allowed us to consider whether or not participants had benefited from noise (present during the task), regardless of their group categorization (ADHD or TDC). The third objective was to investigate whether this NBI has a neurophysiological impact, i.e. whether differences in the P300 component can be observed between "noise-beneficiaries" (subjects who benefit from noise) and "noise non-beneficiaries" (subjects who do not). Finally, the fourth objective, was to measure spontaneous eye-blink rates to test the MBA model assumption that white noise would increase arousal through dopaminergic system modulation [38]. We hypothesized that (1) neuropsychological and neurophysiological differences would be observed between children with ADHD and TDC submitted to the visual cued Go/Nogo paradigm. We expected to observe more omissions, more impulsive errors, and slower and more variable RTs in the ADHD group but only in the no noise condition. In electrophysiological data, we expected to observe attenuated P300 amplitudes in children with ADHD compared to TDC in the no-noise condition. (2) We expected to observe increased P300 mean amplitude in the noise condition for noise beneficiaries and correlations between noise benefit and neuropsychological (and clinical) markers of attention and inhibition. (3) We expected a significant relationship between ADHD categorization and noise benefit categorization. (4) We hypothesized that children with ADHD would exhibit different eye-blink rates than TDC (in a no-noise condition) but that this difference would be reduced during white noise exposure.

Methods

Participants

Children with ADHD were recruited and assessed according to DSM IV-TR criteria [54] by a multidisciplinary team including pediatric neurologists and neuropsychologists in local university hospitals. If the child was regularly treated by methylphenidate, medication was stopped 48 h before testing. Exclusion criteria were a seizure disorder, IQ below 80, being in a specialized school, psychiatric comorbidities (assessed through the CBCL questionnaire; listed in Table 1), non-corrected sensory deficits and pharmacological treatment (other than methylphenidate) that could interfere with behavioral performance and/or with neurophysiological results. Children who have had otitis or other ear problems had an audiometry to ensure they had normal hearing.

At first, 36 children (7–12 years old) were recruited for the study. Three children were excluded because of a too poor signal-to-noise ratio after EEG qualitative observation. Two children were excluded because their estimated IQ was below 80, and one child asked to stop the experiment because it was too long for him. The two groups (ADHD and TDC) consisted then of 13 children with ADHD (5 girls; mean age = 9.2; SD = 1.3) and 17 TDC (9 girls; mean age = 8.5; SD = 1.2). TDC were recruited from primary schools.

In addition to the neuropsychological assessment (see 2.1.1.), each child performed subtests of the Wechsler Intelligence Scale for Children (WISC-IV: Wechsler, 2005). Estimated IQ was computed based on two perceptual processing subtests (picture concepts, matrix reasoning) and two verbal comprehension subtests (similarities, vocabulary) of the WISC-IV. Intellectual assessment was aimed at excluding children who presented an intellectual weakness but was not used for group comparison as it is known to be influenced by attentional and executive factors [55, 56]. Parents were asked to fill in the Child Behavior Checklist–CBCL [57]. Results from CBCL and IQ testing are shown in Table 1. As gender influences symptom expression and cognitive profile in ADHD [58], we performed a *Chi* square test of independence to assess whether the gender ratio was different between the groups. It showed that the gender ratio was not statistically different between the groups [*Chi* square $(1) = 1.23$, $p = .27$].

Informed consents were obtained from all subjects and from their parents with the prior approval of the Ethics Committee of the Queen Fabiola Children's University Hospital (ULB, Belgium), of the Erasme Hospital (ULB, Belgium) and of the Faculty of Psychology and Education (ULB, Belgium).

Table 1 Means, standard deviations and group comparison for estimated IQ, age and parent-rated CBCL T-scores

Measure	Group				t test and ANOVA	
	TDCN = 17		ADHDN = 13		t	p
	Mean	SD	Mean	SD		
Estimated IQ	111.2	6.8	102.9	9.9	−2.72	.01*
Age	9.2	1.3	8.5	1.2	−1.66	.11
CBCL[a]						p[b]
Affective problems[a]	56.3	6.8	62.8	7.0	2.39	.14
Anxiety problems[a]	58.1	7.1	59.6	7.9	.53	.99
Somatic problems[a]	56.8	5.6	55.9	6.9	−0.36	1
ADHD problems[a]	53.2	5.5	64.8	7.6	4.51	<.01*
Oppositional defiant problems[a]	56.9	7.7	60.3	9.5	1.00	.99
Conduct problems[a]	58.4	8.9	62.7	9.5	1.18	.95

* p value indicating significant difference between groups; overall α = .05

[a] Child behavior checklist; T-scores

[b] p values below are corrected for multiple comparisons (Bonferroni correction)

Material and procedure
Data was acquired during two separate sessions: a neuropsychological assessment and an experimental session.

Neuropsychological assessment
During this session, we used the computerized TAP battery [59, 60] and a Counting Stroop task [61] to assess different components of attention and executive functions. The TAP battery allows assessing several attentional and executive processes and is well normed (n > 500), both for children (from 6 years old) and adults, which allows using the same battery in children and adult studies. It has been shown to be an effective instrument to investigate both cognitive functions in ADHD (in children and adults) [60] and treatment efficacy in ADHD [62]. Attentional abilities were assessed using the Alertness subtest of the TAP. Alertness included a simple reaction time (tonic alertness) and an auditory-cued reaction time task (phasic alertness). The tonic condition represents a good measure of intrinsic alertness and the phasic alertness is used to evaluate the effect of a warning cue during attention tasks. Inhibition was evaluated using the Go/Nogo subtest of the TAP and a Counting Stroop task [61, 63]. The Go/Nogo task requires either a button press response (Go) or the inhibition of a response (Nogo), depending on the stimuli presented (the "go" is represented by an "×" and the "nogo" by a "+"). The Counting Stroop task included three conditions: counting, reading and interference. Items were presented on a computer screen in 10 lines, presented one at time, with 10 stimuli per line (squares with numbers or dots). In the counting condition, children had to report as fast as possible the number of dots within each square. In the reading condition, they

had to read the number written within each square. In the interference condition, they had to report how many numbers were written within each square, while avoiding reading the number itself.

IQ testing as well as the completion of the CBCL questionnaire and the informed consent was performed during this session.

Experimental session
In the visual cued Go/Nogo task, the child was submitted to three kinds of 3 × 3 cm stimuli briefly displayed (150 ms), in black, one by one on a grey background. A square (the warning stimulus hereafter called the cue) always preceded Go ("×") or Nogo ("+") stimuli. Go and Nogo stimuli each had a 50 % of probability of following a cue and were pseudo-randomly displayed (see Fig. 1). The inter-stimulus interval (ISI) between the cue and the following stimulus was varied randomly (1–2 s, mean = 1.5 s) while the ISI between Go or Nogo stimuli and the following cue was constant (2.5 s). The task was divided into two different blocks, each lasting 4 min 20 s. In each block, 60 cues were presented, 30 Go and 30 Nogo stimuli. Subjects had to perform each block twice, once with and once without white noise. There were thus altogether four blocks per participant. The order of the blocks and conditions (noise or no-noise exposure) was counterbalanced. Noise was delivered binaurally at 77 dB SPL with Etymotic earphones (model ER-3A) connected through a 25 cm long silicon tube ending in a hollowed foam cylinder inserted into the entrance of the ear canals.

The children were asked to press a button as fast as possible each time a Go stimulus was displayed and had to inhibit pressing when a Nogo was presented. We

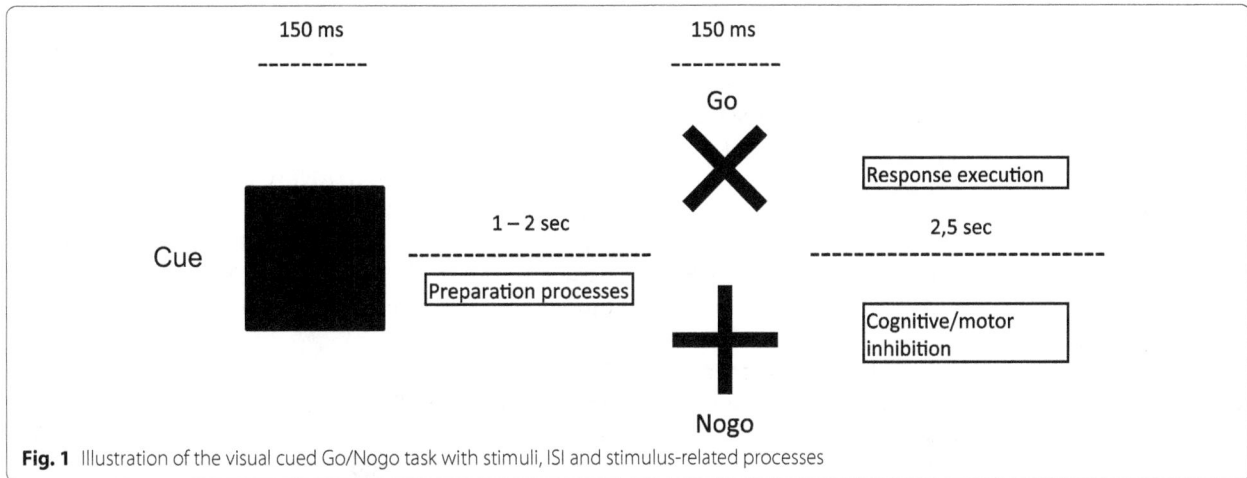

Fig. 1 Illustration of the visual cued Go/Nogo task with stimuli, ISI and stimulus-related processes

explained them that the square was supposed to help them prepare for the following stimulus presentation. Both speed and accuracy were encouraged.

For the sake of EEG recordings, the children sat in a sound attenuated room in a comfortable resting chair with headrest. Distance from the 17″ computer monitor was 120 cm.

Electrophysiological recording
Brain electrical activity was recorded with an ASA EEG/ERP system (ANT software, The Netherlands) from 14 channels (Fz, F3, F4, Cz, C3, C4, Pz, P3, P4, Oz, O3, O4 and M1–M2 for the left and right mastoids), embedded in a waveguard cap (10–20 system) and all referred to the mean of the two mastoids. Horizontal and vertical eye movements were monitored using two bipolar recordings: one between each outer eye canthus and one between a supraorbital electrode and an electrode positioned just below the lower eyelid on the left side. The ground was placed on the left wrist. All impedances were kept below 10 kΩ. After amplification (×20) and online filtering (0.1–100 Hz, as recommended in Duncan et al. [52]), the input signals were digitized with a sampling rate of 512 Hz and stored on the computer disk for off-line averaging.

After the experimental task, children were asked to keep their eyes open to record eye-blinking rate, during two blocks of 2 min, one with and one without white noise exposure (in counterbalanced order).

Data analysis
Neuropsychological assessment, IQ testing and CBCL
Independent samples t tests were used to assess group differences (ADHD vs. TDC) with regard to IQ, CBCL questionnaire as well as scores from the TAP and from the Counting Stroop.

In the TAP subtests, subject's median RT was chosen as a measure of response latencies because it is less sensitive than the mean to the enhanced intra-individual variability in response time usually observed in the ADHD population [12]. Another dependent variable, estimating the intra-individual variability, was the coefficient of variation (CV) of reaction times [64], a normalized measure of dispersion, defined as the ratio of the standard deviation (σ) to the mean (μ): $CV = \sigma/\mu$. The CV is useful because the standard deviation of data must be understood in the context of the mean of the data [65]. We also used hits, anticipations (in the phasic alert part of the Alertness part) and errors (in the Go/Nogo test) as measures of impulsivity [59].

Two variables were computed to investigate the classical interference effect in the Counting Stroop, i.e. the difference scores (e.g., [66]) between counting and interference conditions for total time ("time interference index") and for total number of non-corrected errors ("errors interference index").

Experimental task
Dependent variables were omissions (no responses to "Go" trials), false alarms ("FA cue", pushing when the cue is shown and "FA Nogo", pushing when "+" is shown), RTs and the RT variability.

Group assignation
Subjects were assigned to two kinds of groups. First, they were assigned according to their diagnosis status: "ADHD" or "TDC". Second, they were assigned according to their benefit from noise or not during the task. Therefore, we computed a NBI that calculated the difference of omissions, for each subject, in noise vs. no-noise conditions (i.e. the percentage of hits in the noise condition minus the percentage of hits in the no-noise condition).

Children with a higher NBI index (i.e. more hits/less omissions in the noise condition) were grouped as "noise beneficiaries" (n = 12) and the others (same or less hits/more omissions in the noise condition) were assigned to the "non-beneficiaries" group (n = 18). Mean and standard deviation (SD) for the NBI scores in each group are: ADHD (mean = 9.11, SD = 22.24); TDC (mean = −2.80, SD = 7.20), noise beneficiaries (mean = 15.20; SD = 19.71); noise non-beneficiaries (mean = −6.20; SD = 3.71).

A median split, another possible way to create two groups regarding noise benefit, might have assigned participants who made more omissions in the noise condition to the "noise beneficiaries" group. Therefore, the former method, although not perfect, was considered more appropriate. As gender influences symptom expression and the cognitive profile [58], we performed a *Chi* square test of independence to assess whether the gender ratio was different between the groups ("noise-beneficiaries" and "non-beneficiaries"). It showed that the gender ratio was not statistically different between the groups [*Chi* square (1) = .55, p = .46]. Age did not statistically differ between these groups [t(28) = −1.72; p = .10].

For all dependent variables, two mixed ANOVA's were performed with between Group factors: (1) ADHD vs. TDC and (2) "noise beneficiaries" vs. "non-beneficiaries". Within-subjects factors were block (first vs. second block) and condition (noise vs. no-noise).

Chi square test of independence was applied to examine the potential relation between ADHD and benefiting from noise. Aside from the Chi square test, an independent samples *t* test was used to assess the difference in the mean of the NBI score between ADHD and TDC groups. Pearson correlations were used to examine relationships between the NBI and neuropsychological scores.

Neurophysiological measures
Continuous EEG was segmented in 1200 ms epochs including a 200 ms pre-stimulus onset baseline. Averaged waveforms were computed for each subject and then across groups for each of the following trials: "Go" ("×"), only when the subject had responded, "Nogo" ("+"), only when the child did not respond and "cue" (square).

Blinks were corrected with the SOBI algorithm [67] to avoid rejecting too many epochs during averaging. By doing so, we kept at least 90 % of the epochs for each participant after averaging (with a rejection criterion at ±100 μV, as recommended by Duncan et al., [52]). Data were baseline corrected before statistical analysis. Mean amplitudes were individually identified by group, for each type of P300 (Cue, Go, Nogo) and at Cz and Pz. They were computed in a 300 ms temporal window centered on the most positive point visually inspected (on

the grand average) for each of the three kinds of trials (Cue P300, Go P300 and Nogo P300), for each group, for each condition (noise and no-noise) and for each electrode (Cz and Pz).

For each "Type of P300" (Cue P300, Go P300 and Nogo P300), two mixed ANOVA's were performed for mean amplitude with Groups: (1) ADHD vs. TDC and (2) "noise beneficiaries" vs. "noise non-beneficiaries" as between-subjects factors. "Site" (Cz, Pz) and condition (noise vs. no noise) were within-subject factors.

Eye-blink rates
Spontaneous eye-blink rates (after the task) were analyzed with Matlab 2012. A free Matlab script, "peakdet" ([68] cited in [69]), allowed us to count eye-blinks for each subject from their EEG recording.

We chose to register spontaneous eye-blinks after the main experiment (and not during) because our goal was to make an indirect inference between dopaminergic functioning and white noise. While eye-blinks during a task seem to reflect the transition of activation between different neural networks [70], spontaneous eye-blink rates reflect a more "natural-state" of dopaminergic functioning. The latter, therefore, was chosen because it was more related to our original hypotheses. Moreover, children were explicitly asked not to blink too much during the task. This could have biased our observations, contrary to the resting state condition (without such instruction).

A repeated measures ANOVA was performed for eye-blink rates with Groups: (ADHD vs. TDC) as between subject factor and condition (noise vs. no noise) as within-subjects factor.

All statistical analyses were performed using "Statistica 8.0". When necessary, post hoc Tukey tests were applied.

Results
IQ testing, CBCL questionnaire and neuropsychological assessment
As illustrated in Table 1, TDC (IQ = 111.2 ± 6.8) performed higher than children with ADHD (IQ = 102.9 ± 9.9) on estimated IQ measures [t(28) = −2.72; p = .01]. CBCL T-scores were significantly different between groups for the ADHD subscale only [t(28) = 4.51; p < .01].

In the Alertness TAP subtest, analyses disclosed larger mean median RTs in ADHD than in the TDC group in tonic [t(28) = 2.18; p = .04] and phasic alertness condition [t(28) = 2.24; p = .03]. Coefficient of variation was also higher in ADHD for tonic [t(28) = 2.42; p = .02] and phasic alertness [t(28) = 3.31; p < .001]. ADHD children had less correct responses [t(28) = −2.93; p = .01] and made more anticipations [t(28) = 2.89; p = .01] than the TDC group.

In the Go/Nogo TAP subtest, coefficient of variation [$t(28) = 2.21$; $p = .03$] and the number of errors [$t(28) = 2.48$; $p = .02$] were larger in the ADHD than in the TDC group.

In the Counting Stroop task, analyses disclosed significantly larger time interference [$t(28) = 4.46$; $p < .001$] and errors difference indices [$t(28) = 2.04$; $p = .05$] in ADHD than in TDC.

All results of the TAP tests and the Counting Stroop are shown in Table 2.

Cued Go/Nogo experimental task results

Relevant behavioral and electrophysiological data are presented according to the comparison between ADHD and TDC groups in Section 1 and according to the comparison between "noise-beneficiaries" and "non-beneficiaries" groups in Section 2. Block factor was included in each behavioral analysis but will not be presented, as the results were not relevant in this context.

Section 1: ADHD vs. TDC

Behavioral measures

Omissions

Children with ADHD made more omission errors than TDC [$F(1,28) = 5.69$, $p = .02$]. There was no main effect of Condition [$F(1,28) = 1.21$, $p = .28$], but a significant Group*Condition interaction (see Fig. 2) [$F(1,28) = 4.32$, $p = .04$] indicated that children with ADHD made more omissions than TDC in the no-noise condition only ($p = .02$). There was no other interaction (all Fs < 2.23).

RTs and RT variability

Children with ADHD were slower [$F(1,28) = 9.98$, $p = .004$] an more variable [$F(1,28) = 9.98$, $p = .04$] than TDC. All other factors did not reach significance and did not interact with each other (all Fs < 1).

FA cue

Children with ADHD committed more FA cues than TDC [$F(1,28) = 4.14$, $p = .051$]. No other factor reached significance and there was no interaction (all Fs < 2.96).

Table 2 Means, standard deviations and group comparison for TAP (tonic and phasic alert, Go/Nogo) and Counting Stroop tests

Measures	Group				t test	
	TDC N = 17		ADHD N = 13		t values	p
	Mean	SD	Mean	SD		
Alertness (tonic)[a]						
Median	305.35	71.12	421.00	203.96	2.18	.04*
CV	0.22	0.08	0.32	0.14	2.42	.02*
Hits	40.00	0.00	39.62	0.96	−1.66	.11
Anticipations	0.00	0.00	0.00	0.00	–	–
Alertness (phasic)[b]						
Median	281.94	55.20	353.38	115.81	2.24	.03*
CV	0.17	0.05	0.31	0.17	3.31	.00*
Hits	39.29	1.82	35.08	5.59	−2.93	.01*
Omissions	0.00	0.00	0.54	1.45	1.54	.13
Anticipations	5.00	4.55	12.08	8.69	2.89	.01*
Go/Nogo						
Median	521.88	79.15	584.83	92.01	1.97	.06
CV	0.24	0.06	0.29	0.05	2.21	.03*
Errors	2.59	2.12	5.23	3.68	2.48	.02*
Omission	0.71	1.21	3.15	5.16	1.90	.07
Stroop[c]						
Time interf. index	39.59	16.41	72.46	23.95	4.46	<.001*
Errors interf. index	0.35	0.70	2.08	3.40	2.04	.05*

[a] Scores of tonic alert in alertness task

[b] Scores of phasic alert in alertness task

[c] Scores representing the difference of performance between counting and interference conditions: *Time interf. index.* difference of total times; *Errors interf. index* difference of non-corrected errors

* p value indicating significant difference between groups; overall α = .0

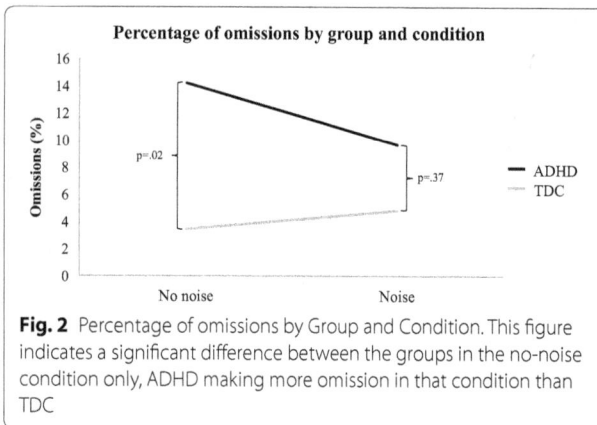

Fig. 2 Percentage of omissions by Group and Condition. This figure indicates a significant difference between the groups in the no-noise condition only, ADHD making more omission in that condition than TDC

FA nogo

No factor reached significance and there was no interaction (all Fs < 2.04).

Electrophysiological measures

Cue P300

Cue P300 amplitudes were similar regardless of the Group, Condition or Site and there was no interaction (all Fs < 2.88).

Go P300

Go P300 amplitudes were similar regardless of the Group, Condition or Site and there was no interaction (all Fs < 1).

Nogo P300

There was a Group*Site interaction [F(1,28) = 32.48, p < .001] and a three-way interaction Group*Condition* Site [F(1,28) = 5.04, p = .03], indicating that ADHD had a significant higher Nogo P300 than TDC but only at Pz in the noise condition (p = .05). No other factor reached significance and there was no interaction (all Fs < 3.75).

Section 2: Noise beneficiaries vs. noise non-beneficiaries

In this section, children who benefited from noise (noise-beneficiaries) were compared to those who did not (non-beneficiaries), independently of their diagnostic status. Given that we split our groups according to the fact that children benefited from noise on omissions errors, analyzing behavioral effects on these omissions would be redundant and was not included. Here we present analyses on electrophysiological because no relevant behavioral analysis reached significance. The clinical status * noise benefit * block * condition four-way mixed ANOVA would have allowed quantifying the interaction effect of clinical status and noise benefit on our dependent variables. However, we did not follow this approach because the two types of group assignment yielded an imbalanced design with cells with low sample sizes (see Table 4).

Electrophysiological measures

Go P300

There was a three-way interaction Group*Condition* Site [F(1,28) = 9.62, p = .005] indicating, as illustrated in Fig. 3, that the amplitude of the Go P300 increased marginally for noise beneficiaries at Cz in the noise relative to the no-noise condition (p = .06). All other factors did not reach significance and did not interact with each other (all Fs < 1.38).

There was no relevant result for Group, Condition or Site factors as regards Cue and Nogo P300.

The Noise Benefit Index (NBI) and its relationship to ADHD and cognitive functions

All significant correlations between NBI and neuropsychological tests (TAP and Counting Stroop) are presented in Table 3. Both markers of inattention (CV and hits from Phasic Alert test) and of motor and cognitive inhibition (respectively, anticipation from the Phasic Alert and the errors interference index from Stroop test) exhibited correlations with the NBI.

These correlations indicate a relationship between benefitting from noise and lower attention and inhibition (motor and cognitive) in the neuropsychological tests.

The Chi square test highlighted a significant relationship between the Group factor (ADHD or TDC) and benefitting from noise [Chi square (1) = 4.43 p = .035; see Table 4]. Children with ADHD had a significantly higher NBI score than TDC [t(28) = 2.08; p = .04].

Eye-blink rates

Children with ADHD made significantly more eye-blinks than TDC [F(1,28) = 5.94, p = .02]. There was no other significant effect or interaction (all Fs < 1.09).

Discussion

In this study, we first aimed to evaluate the potential cognitive benefit of white noise exposure during a visual cued Go/Nogo task in children with ADHD and TDC. The second objective was to examine, through the use of a new index (NBI), whether potential correlations could be observed between noise benefit in the visual cued Go/Nogo task and individual neuropsychological profiles. The third objective was to investigate whether this NBI had a neurophysiological correlate, i.e. whether differences in the P300 component can be observed between "noise-beneficiaries" and "non-beneficiaries". The fourth objective was to discuss, through the use of spontaneous eye-blink rates, the Moderate Brain Arousal model according to which white noise modulates dopaminergic functioning [38].

Regarding participant characteristics, ADHD and TDC differed in the CBCL only in the ADHD problems subscale, indicating a limited influence of comorbidities on

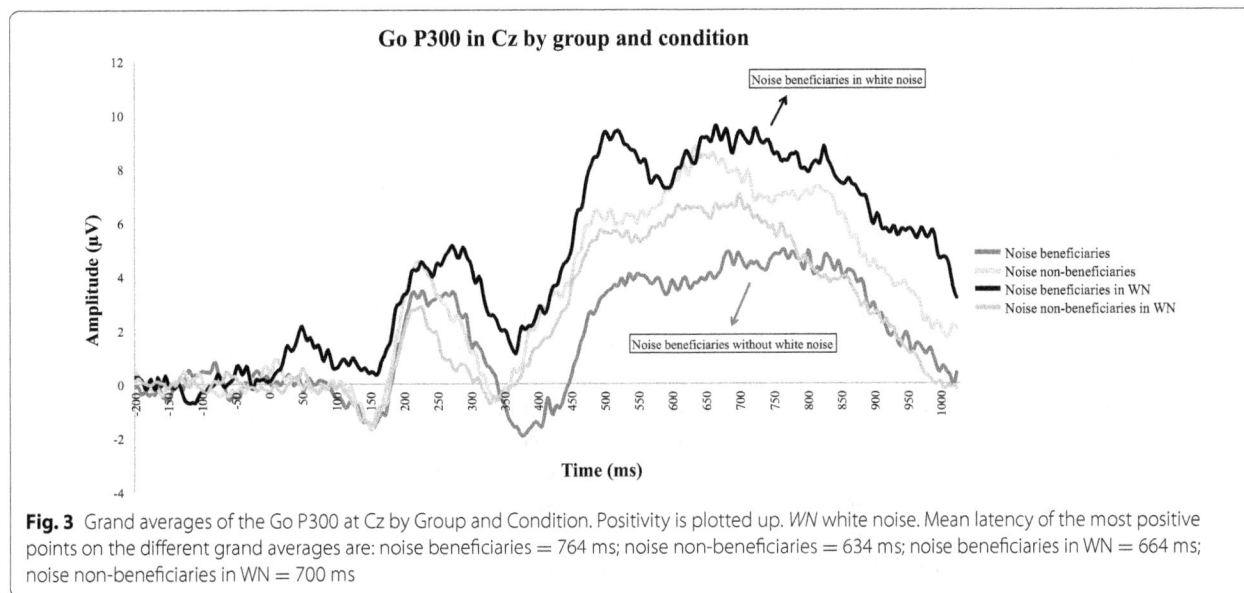

Fig. 3 Grand averages of the Go P300 at Cz by Group and Condition. Positivity is plotted up. *WN* white noise. Mean latency of the most positive points on the different grand averages are: noise beneficiaries = 764 ms; noise non-beneficiaries = 634 ms; noise beneficiaries in WN = 664 ms; noise non-beneficiaries in WN = 700 ms

Table 3 Significant correlation between NBI and neuropsychological tests

NBI[a] correlations	r	p	p corr[b]
Alertness (tonic)[c]			
CV	.62	<.01*	<.01*
Alertness (phasic)[d]			
Hits	−.50	<.01*	.02*
Anticipations	.45	.01*	.04*
Stroop[e]			
Errors interf. index	.69	<.01*	<.01*

[a] *NBI* Noise Benefit Index

[b] p value corrected for multiple comparison (for each cognitive function, p values were corrected according to the number of dependent variables)

[c] Scores of tonic alert (alertness task)

[d] Scores of phasic alert (alertness task)

[e] *Errors interf. index* difference of non-corrected errors between scores in counting and interference conditions

* p value indicating significant difference between groups; α = .05

Table 4 Repartition of each subject according to their categorization (ADHD or TDC) and to their benefit from noise during the visual cued Go/Nogo

Groups	Non-beneficiaries[a]	Noise-beneficiaries[b]
TDC	13	4
ADHD	5	8

[a] *Non-beneficiaries* all subjects who did not benefit from noise

[b] *Noise-beneficiaries* subjects who benefitted from noise

results. Results from the attentional and executive assessment showed significant differences between children with ADHD and TDC. Children with ADHD were slower and had higher RT variability on all neuropsychological tasks (phasic and tonic alert, Go/Nogo and our experimental task), confirming previous observations [71–73]. They made more omissions (phasic alert and Go/Nogo) and showed more impulsivity, as indexed by anticipations, Go/Nogo and interference in the Stroop.

Similar results were obtained in the experimental task. Children with ADHD made more omissions, more impulsive errors (i.e. FA cue) and had slower and more variable RTs than TDC. However, exposure to white noise during the experimental task showed a positive impact on cognitive performance in children with ADHD. To the best of our knowledge, this is the first demonstration of a beneficial effect of white noise in the Go/Nogo paradigm in a study comparing children with and without ADHD. Positive effects of white noise have already been documented on memory [22] and on Go/Nogo performance [26], but this last study was conducted with children teacher-rated inattentive. Taken together, results from the present study are in accordance with the optimal stimulation theory and the MBA model, both suggesting that the addition of extra-task stimulation is likely to improve cognitive functioning in ADHD. Moreover, these results help to clarify what kind of improvement might be expected (at 77 dB). Indeed, improvement was limited to omissions only (as in [26]). RTs and RT variability, as well as the number of false alarms (i.e., FA cue) remained significantly higher in children with ADHD compared to TDC, independent of the condition. Consequently, the beneficial effect of white noise on cognition is not generalizable to all attentional and executive functions but seems, in this task, to modulate vigilance more specifically. No Block effect was observed, which might have shown a larger beneficial effect of white noise exposure during the second half of the task, namely a real benefit in the wake of fatigue. A longer task might disclose such an effect, and this should be considered in future studies.

Electrophysiological data showed a significant Group*Condition*Site interaction with a higher Nogo P300 amplitude in ADHD than in TDC at Pz in the noise condition. This result might indicate enhanced inhibitory processes in children with ADHD in the noise condition. However, behavioral results did not show a similar effect, as we did not observe a difference between groups according to noise exposure. Possibly, this Nogo P300 underlines a positive neurophysiological effect of white noise that is not observed at the performance level (see e.g. [74]). More sensitive inhibition tasks (such as the stop-signal task [75, 76]) could be used in future studies. Electrophysiological data did not show other relevant difference between children with ADHD and TDC, regardless of the condition (noise or no-noise) and the type of P300—Cue P300, Go P300 and Nogo P300—that are associated with behavioral processes (preparatory processes, attentional and inhibitory processes respectively [51]. This suggests that despite the same amount of attentional resources allocated to these different cognitive processes in both groups [48], children with ADHD had worse behavioral performance. This observation highlights the heterogeneity of findings according to ERP research in ADHD [50]. With regard to the literature [48] and our behavioral results, we anticipated both a reduced Cue and Go P300 mean amplitudes in children with ADHD compared to TDC. Other studies have also found absence of effect on P300 amplitude despite a significant decline in performance in ADHD group [44, 77]. We suggest that this absence of neurophysiological difference can be explained by our non-comorbid group of children with ADHD. Indeed, Yoon et al. [78] showed that ADHD-comorbid (with ODD or CD) but not ADHD-pure children displayed significant P300 amplitude reduction compared to TDC.

When groups were assigned according to their noise benefit (noise-beneficiaries and non-beneficiaries), we demonstrated a significant relationship between group classification (ADHD or TDC) and benefiting (or not) from noise. In addition, we found significant correlations between benefitting from noise and markers of vigilance (RT variability, omissions) and motor/cognitive inhibition (anticipation errors and interference errors) in Stroop and TAP tasks (all correlations = p ≤ .01). These markers have been identified as core cognitive symptoms in ADHD [9].

Furthermore, noise-beneficiaries had a marginally larger Go P300 mean amplitude in the noise condition compared to the no-noise condition. This was not found in participants who didn't benefit from noise. Interestingly, white noise modulates only, at an electrophysiological level, the Go P300 mean amplitude (for noise-beneficiaries), which is associated with attentional processes (like vigilance); and white noise modulates only vigilance at a behavioral level (and not impulsive errors, RTs or RT variability) in children with ADHD. We propose two possible complementary explanations: (1) White noise, perceived as a potential distractor, could make noise beneficiaries (prone to distraction regarding their correlations with markers of vigilance) gathering up more attentional resources not to be distracted. (2) The perceptual load hypothesis [79] proposes that increasing perceptual load (adding "task irrelevant-distractors") reduces, or even eliminates, any distractor interference effect. Lavie [79] suggests that small increases in perceptual load may be beneficial for populations that are prone to distraction (e.g. children with ADHD). In our study, white noise, increasing general perceptual load, indeed reduces the inattention/improves vigilance (expressed in numbers of omissions) of children who are more easily distracted.

Finally, noise benefit on cognitive functioning supports the MBA model. However, it is unclear whether this noise improves performance through dopamine system modulation, as suggested by Sikstrom, Soderlund [38]. We addressed this issue by analyzing the spontaneous eye-blink rate, an indirect marker of dopamine functioning in the striatum [42, 43, 80, 81]. Spontaneous eye-blink rate measures showed that children with ADHD made more eye-blinks than TDC, which supports the relation between ADHD and dopaminergic system and could, therefore, be considered as a potential measure for future studies. However, noise did not significantly modulate eye-blink rate, which does not support the MBA model assumption. Yet, recent papers presented direct evidence that the central dopaminergic activity is involved in the modulation of P300 parameters [82, 83]. Given our finding of a modulation of the Go P300 by noise (for noise beneficiaries), the MBA model hypothesis is not to be ruled out but rather reviewed.

Limitations of the study

Some limitations of our study have to be mentioned including, first, the small number of participants. Second (probably related to the first), the three-way interaction showing a larger Go P300 for the noise beneficiaries in the noise condition was only a trend. Third, in ERP studies on cognition, it is recommended to use two-year groupings over the age of 8 years because of significant ERP changes over a short time period [84]. Due to the difficulty of recruiting (with respect to the exclusion criteria and the characteristics of the experiment) and the small number of subject, the groups would be too small to consider this recommendation. Future studies with larger samples are needed to further investigate these original and new findings. Fourth, our NBI was calculated according to the number of omissions to create groups, while other factors, such as RT-variability, are also considered as pathways that contribute to distinguishing children with and without ADHD [85]. From our point of view, choosing another component (such as RT-variability) remains interesting but omission was the only one, in this present study, that seemed to be modulated by noise exposure. Therefore, it was considered to be more relevant.

Conclusion and future direction

The finding of a white noise benefit in children with ADHD during a Go/Nogo task validates the optimal stimulation theory. However, the benefits of white noise are not to be generalized to all analyzed functions within this task and seem more specifically associated with vigilance improvement. The NBI allowed us to characterize a neuropsychological profile, related to that of ADHD, positively sensitive to noise at both behavioral and electrophysiological levels. We also provide neurophysiological correlates of noise benefit. The eye-blink rate investigation distinguishes ADHD between TDC groups, but was not sensitive to white noise, questioning the influence on dopaminergic functioning suggested by the MBA model. With regard to the literature, the type of extra-task stimulation has a different impact on cognitive functioning according to task requirements and interpersonal differences [38, 86]. Future research should manipulate these different parameters to better understand which stimulation improves/modulates the different executive or attentional function. The present study should be conducted in adults with and without ADHD to see if development is a crucial factor to take into account. It would be of interest to measure eye-blink rates during the task in a future study, and avoiding asking children explicitly to not blink during the test. Finally, while this study highlighted the potential benefit of adding stimulation in the environment, it is time to consider children's on-task behavior in a more ecologic environment (e.g., a virtual classroom) to fully understand what situational factors help moderating difficulties for children with ADHD [87, 88].

Authors' contributions

SB created the design of the study and the experimental paradigm, managed the acquisition of the data—gathering and testing (EEG and behavioral parts) the patients -, analyzed and interpreted the data, and wrote the first draft. HS has been involved in drafting and revising the manuscript, in the design regarding the neuropsychological testing and interpreting the behavioral data. GS acted as a collaborator, thinking about the design, the interpretation of the data and revising the manuscript. BD has been mainly involved in revising the manuscript and contributed on the interpretation of EEG data. PD helped in the construction of the paradigm in the EEG lab, during the

acquisitions and the analyses of the data. CC and ND both contributed equally for this study (both considered as last authors). They supervised each step of the work, criticizing and improving the design, the patients' selection, the drafts (revising), the statistical (and EEG) analyses and the interpretations of the results. All authors read and approved the final manuscript.

Author details
[1] Center for Research in Cognition and Neurosciences (CRCN), Université Libre de Bruxelles (ULB), Campus du Solbosch CP 191, Avenue F.D. Roosevelt 50, CP 151, 1050 Brussels, Belgium. [2] Research Unit in Cognitive Neurosciences (UNESCOG), Université Libre de Bruxelles (ULB), 1050 Brussels, Belgium. [3] Department of Neurology, Queen Fabiola Children's University Hospital (HUDERF), Université Libre de Bruxelles (ULB), Avenue Jean-Joseph Crocq, 15, 1020 Brussels, Belgium. [4] Laboratory of Cognitive and Sensory Neurophysiology, CHU Brugmann, Université Libre de Bruxelles (ULB), Place Van Gehuchten, 4, 1020 Brussels, Belgium. [5] Neuropsychology and Functional Neuroimaging Research Group (UR2NF), Université Libre de Bruxelles (ULB), 1050 Brussels, Belgium. [6] Department of Clinical and Cognitive Neuropsychology, Erasme Hospital, Université Libre de Bruxelles (ULB), Route de Lennik, 808, 1070 Brussels, Belgium. [7] Faculty of Teacher Education and Sports, Sogn og Fjordane, University College, Sogndal, Norway. [8] Inkendaal Rehabilitation Hospital, Vlezenbeek, Belgium.

Acknowledgements
We warmly thank the children and their parents who kindly took part in this research, as well as the schools and the teachers who agreed to collaborate in this study. The authors also thank Jeromy Hrabovecky for proofreading and language editing in this article. This study was supported by a grant from the Belgian Kids' Fund.

Competing interests
The authors declare that the research was conducted in the absence of any commercial, financial (and non-financial) relationships that could be construed as a potential competing interests.

References
1. APA. Diagnostic and statistical manual of mental disorders, 5th edition (DSM-V). Washington, DC: American Psychiatric Association; 2013.
2. Polanczyk G, Rohde LA. Epidemiology of attention-deficit/hyperactivity disorder across the lifespan. Curr Opin Psychiatry. 2007;20(4):386–92.
3. Polanczyk GV, Willcutt EG, Salum GA, Kieling C, Rohde LA. ADHD prevalence estimates across three decades: an updated systematic review and meta-regression analysis. Int J Epidemiol. 2014;43(2):434–42. doi:10.1093/ije/dyt261.
4. Willcutt EG. The prevalence of DSM-IV attention-deficit/hyperactivity disorder: a meta-analytic review. Neurotherapeutics. 2012;9(3):490–9. doi:10.1007/s13311-012-0135-8.
5. Danckaerts M, Sonuga-Barke EJ, Banaschewski T, Buitelaar J, Dopfner M, Hollis C, et al. The quality of life of children with attention deficit/hyperactivity disorder: a systematic review. Eur Child Adolesc Psychiatry. 2010;19(2):83–105. doi:10.1007/s00787-009-0046-3.
6. Jensen PS, Arnold LE, Swanson JM, Vitiello B, Abikoff HB, Greenhill LL, et al. 3-year follow-up of the NIMH MTA study. J Am Acad Child Adolesc Psychiatry. 2007;46(8):989–1002. doi:10.1097/CHI.0b013e3180686d48.
7. Kofler MJ, Rapport MD, Bolden J, Sarver DE, Raiker JS, Alderson RM. Working memory deficits and social problems in children with ADHD. J Abnorm Child Psychol. 2011;39(6):805–17. doi:10.1007/s10802-011-9492-8.
8. Barkley RA, Murphy KR. Impairment in occupational functioning and adult ADHD: the predictive utility of executive function (EF) ratings versus EF tests. Arch Clin Neuropsychol. 2010;25(3):157–73. doi:10.1093/arclin/acq014.
9. Rapport MD, Orban SA, Kofler MJ, Friedman LM. Do programs designed to train working memory, other executive functions, and attention benefit children with ADHD? A meta-analytic review of cognitive, academic,

and behavioral outcomes. Clin Psychol Rev. 2013;33(8):1237–52. doi:10.1016/j.cpr.2013.08.005.

10. Nigg JT. Is ADHD a disinhibitory disorder? Psychol Bull. 2001;127(5):571–98.

11. Willcutt EG, Doyle AE, Nigg JT, Faraone SV, Pennington BF. Validity of the executive function theory of attention-deficit/hyperactivity disorder: a meta-analytic review. Biol Psychiatry. 2005;57(11):1336–46. doi:10.1016/j.biopsych.2005.02.006.

12. Castellanos FX, Sonuga-Barke EJ, Scheres A, Di Martino A, Hyde C, Walters JR. Varieties of attention-deficit/hyperactivity disorder-related intra-individual variability. Biol Psychiatry. 2005;57(11):1416–23. doi:10.1016/j.biopsych.2004.12.005.

13. Faraone SV, Buitelaar J. Comparing the efficacy of stimulants for ADHD in children and adolescents using meta-analysis. Eur Child Adolesc Psychiatry. 2010;19(4):353–64. doi:10.1007/s00787-009-0054-3.

14. McInnes A, Bedard AC, Hogg-Johnson S, Tannock R. Preliminary evidence of beneficial effects of methylphenidate on listening comprehension in children with attention-deficit/hyperactivity disorder. J Child Adolesc Psychopharmacol. 2007;17(1):35–49. doi:10.1089/cap.2006.0051.

15. Banaschewski T, Coghill D, Santosh P, Zuddas A, Asherson P, Buitelaar J, et al. Long-acting medications for the hyperkinetic disorders. A systematic review and European treatment guideline. Eur Child Adolesc Psychiatry. 2006;15(8):476–95. doi:10.1007/s00787-006-0549-0.

16. Barkley RA, McMurray MB, Edelbrock CS, Robbins K. Side effects of methylphenidate in children with attention deficit hyperactivity disorder: a systemic, placebo-controlled evaluation. Pediatrics. 1990;86(2):184–92.

17. Catala-Lopez F, Hutton B, Nunez-Beltran A, Mayhew AD, Page MJ, Ridao M, et al. The pharmacological and non-pharmacological treatment of attention deficit hyperactivity disorder in children and adolescents: protocol for a systematic review and network meta-analysis of randomized controlled trials. Syst Rev. 2015;4:19. doi:10.1186/s13643-015-0005-7.

18. Subcommittee on Attention-Deficit/Hyperactivity D, Steering Committee on Quality I, Management, Wolraich M, Brown L, Brown RT, et al. ADHD: clinical practice guideline for the diagnosis, evaluation, and treatment of attention-deficit/hyperactivity disorder in children and adolescents. Pediatrics. 2011;128(5):1007–22. doi:10.1542/peds.2011-2654.

19. National Institute of Mental Health. Attention deficit hyperactivity disorder (NIH Pub. No. 08-3572). Washington. 2008. http://www.nimh.nih.gov/health/publications/attention-deficit-hyperactivity-disorder/complete-index.shtml.

20. Zentall S. Optimal stimulation as theoretical basis of hyperactivity. Am J Orthopsychiatry. 1975;45(4):549–63.

21. Antrop I, Stock P, Verte S, Wiersema JR, Baeyens D, Roeyers H. ADHD and delay aversion: the influence of non-temporal stimulation on choice for delayed rewards. J Child Psychol Psychiatry. 2006;47(11):1152–8. doi:10.1111/j.1469-7610.2006.01619.x.

22. Soderlund G, Sikstrom S, Smart A. Listen to the noise: noise is beneficial for cognitive performance in ADHD. J Child Psychol Psychiatry. 2007;48(8):840–7.

23. Cook A, Bradley-Johnson S, Johnson CM. Effects of white noise on off-task behavior and academic responding for children with ADHD. J Appl Behav Anal. 2013. doi:10.1002/jaba.79.

24. Sonuga-Barke EJ, Taylor E. The effect of delay on hyperactive and non-hyperactive children's response times: a research note. J Child Psychol Psychiatry. 1992;33(6):1091–6.

25. Antrop I, Roeyers H, Van Oost P, Buysse A. Stimulation seeking and hyperactivity in children with ADHD. Attention Deficit Hyperactivity Disorder. J Child Psychol Psychiatry. 2000;41(2):225–31.

26. Helps SK, Bamford S, Sonuga-Barke EJ, Soderlund GB. Different effects of adding white noise on cognitive performance of sub-, normal and super-attentive school children. PLoS One. 2014;9(11):e112768. doi:10.1371/journal.pone.0112768.

27. Sergeant J. The cognitive-energetic model: an empirical approach to attention-deficit hyperactivity disorder. Neurosci Biobehav Rev. 2000;24(1):7–12.

28. Moss F. Stochastic resonance and sensory information processing: a tutorial and review of application. Clin Neurophysiol. 2004;115(2):267–81. doi:10.1016/j.clinph.2003.09.014.

29. Sikström S, Söderlund GBW. Stimulus-dependent dopamine release in attention-deficit/hyperactivity disorder. Psychol Rev. 2007;114(4):1047–75.

30. Zentall SS, Zentall TR. Optimal stimulation: a model of disordered activity and performance in normal and deviant children. Psychol Bull. 1983;94(3):446–71.

31. Zentall SS, Shaw JH. Effects of classroom noise on performance and activity of second-grade hyperactive and control children. J Educ Psychol. 1980;72(6):830–40.

32. Zentall SS, Meyer MJ. Self-regulation of stimulation for ADD-H children during reading and vigilance task performance. J Abnorm Child Psychol. 1987;15(4):519–36.

33. Zentall SS, Falkenberg SD, Smith LB. Effects of color stimulation and information on the copying performance of attention-problem adolescents. J Abnorm Child Psychol. 1985;13(4):501–11.

34. Zentall S. Effects of color on performance and activity of hyperactive and nonhyperactive children. J Educ Psychol. 1986;78:159–65.

35. Abikoff H, Courtney ME, Szeibel PJ, Koplewicz HS. The effects of auditory stimulation on the arithmetic performance of children with ADHD and nondisabled children. J Learn Disabil. 1996;29(3):238–46.

36. Moss F, Ward LM, Sannita WG. Stochastic resonance and sensory information processing: a tutorial and review of application. Clin Neurophysiol. 2004;115(2):267–81. **(S1388245703003304 [pii])**.

37. Jepma M, Wagenmakers EJ, Band GP, Nieuwenhuis S. The effects of accessory stimuli on information processing: evidence from electrophysiology and a diffusion model analysis. J Cogn Neurosci. 2009;21(5):847–64. doi:10.1162/jocn.2009.21063.

38. Sikstrom S, Soderlund G. Stimulus-dependent dopamine release in attention-deficit/hyperactivity disorder. Psychol Rev. 2007;114(4):1047–75.

39. Solanto MV. Dopamine dysfunction in AD/HD: integrating clinical and basic neuroscience research. Behav Brain Res. 2002;130(1–2):65–71. **(S0166432801004314 [pii])**.

40. Soderlund GB, Sikstrom S, Loftesnes JM, Sonuga-Barke EJ. The effects of background white noise on memory performance in inattentive school children. Behav Brain Funct. 2010;6:55.

41. Palsson E, Soderlund G, Klamer D, Bergquist F. Noise benefit in prepulse inhibition of the acoustic startle reflex. Psychopharmacology. 2011;214(3):675–85. doi:10.1007/s00213-010-2074-6.

42. Blin O, Masson G, Azulay JP, Fondarai J, Serratrice G. Apomorphine-induced blinking and yawning in healthy volunteers. Br J Clin Pharmacol. 1990;30(5):769–73.

43. Colzato LS, van den Wildenberg WP, van Wouwe NC, Pannebakker MM, Hommel B. Dopamine and inhibitory action control: evidence from spontaneous eye blink rates. Exp Brain Res. 2009;196(3):467–74. doi:10.1007/s00221-009-1862-x.

44. Baijot S, Deconinck N, Slama H, Massat I, Colin C. Behavioral and neurophysiological study of attentional and inhibitory processes in ADHD-combined and control children. Acta Neurol Belg. 2013;. doi:10.1007/s13760-013-0219-1.

45. Banaschewski T, Roessner V, Dittmann RW, Santosh PJ, Rothenberger A. Non-stimulant medications in the treatment of ADHD. Eur Child Adolesc Psychiatry. 2004;13(Suppl 1):I102–16. doi:10.1007/s00787-004-1010-x.

46. van Leeuwen TH, Steinhausen HC, Overtoom CC, Pascual-Marqui RD, van't Klooster B, Rothenberger A, et al. The continuous performance test revisited with neuroelectric mapping: impaired orienting in children with attention deficits. Behav Brain Res. 1998;94(1):97–110. **(S0166-4328(97)00173-3 [pii])**.

47. Fallgatter AJ, Ehlis AC, Rosler M, Strik WK, Blocher D, Herrmann MJ. Diminished prefrontal brain function in adults with psychopathology in childhood related to attention deficit hyperactivity disorder. Psychiatry Res. 2005;138(2):157–69. doi:10.1016/j.pscychresns.2004.12.002.

48. Woltering S, Liu Z, Rokeach A, Tannock R. Neurophysiological differences in inhibitory control between adults with ADHD and their peers. Neuropsychologia. 2013;51(10):1888–95. doi:10.1016/j.neuropsychologia.2013.06.023.

49. Barry RJ, Johnstone SJ, Clarke AR. A review of electrophysiology in attention-deficit/hyperactivity disorder: II. Event-related potentials. Clin Neurophysiol. 2003;114(2):184–98. **(S1388245702003632 [pii])**.

50. Karayanidis F, Robaey P, Bourassa M, De Koning D, Geoffroy G, Pelletier G. ERP differences in visual attention processing between attention-deficit hyperactivity disorder and control boys in the absence of performance differences. Psychophysiology. 2000;37(3):319–33.

51. Banaschewski T, Brandeis D, Heinrich H, Albrecht B, Brunner E, Rothenberger A. Questioning inhibitory control as the specific deficit

of ADHD–evidence from brain electrical activity. J Neural Transm. 2004;111(7):841–64. doi:10.1007/s00702-003-0040-8.

52. Duncan CC, Barry RJ, Connolly JF, Fischer C, Michie PT, Naatanen R, et al. Event-related potentials in clinical research: guidelines for eliciting, recording, and quantifying mismatch negativity, P300, and N400. Clin Neurophysiol. 2009;120(11):1883–908. doi:10.1016/j.clinph.2009.07.045.

53. Pietrzak RH, Mollica CM, Maruff P, Snyder PJ. Cognitive effects of immediate-release methylphenidate in children with attention-deficit/hyperactivity disorder. Neurosci Biobehav Rev. 2006;30(8):1225–45.

54. APA APA. Diagnostic and statistical manual of mental disorders, 4th edition, Text Revision (DSM-IV-TR). Washington, DC: American Psychiatric Association; 2000.

55. Arffa S. The relationship of intelligence to executive function and non-executive function measures in a sample of average, above average, and gifted youth. Arch Clin Neuropsychol. 2007;22(8):969–78. doi:10.1016/j.acn.2007.08.001.

56. Barbey AK, Colom R, Solomon J, Krueger F, Forbes C, Grafman J. An integrative architecture for general intelligence and executive function revealed by lesion mapping. Brain. 2012;135(Pt 4):1154–64. doi:10.1093/brain/aws021.

57. Archenbach T, Edelbrock C. Manual for the child behaviour checklist and revised child behaviour profile. Burlington: University of Vermont Department of Psychiatry; 1991.

58. Hudziak JJ, Achenbach TM, Althoff RR, Pine DS. A dimensional approach to developmental psychopathology. Int J Methods Psychiatr Res. 2007;16(Suppl 1):S16–23. doi:10.1002/mpr.217.

59. Zimmermann P, Fimm, B. Tests d'évaluation de l'attention (TEA, version 1.6): Normes pour enfants et adolescents, Manuel supplémentaire. Herzogenrath: Psytest; 2004

60. Tucha L, Tucha O, Walitza S, Sontag TA, Laufkotter R, Linder M, et al. Vigilance and Sustained Attention in Children and Adults With ADHD. J Atten Disord. 2009;12(5):410–21.

61. Mary A, Slama H, Mousty P, Massat I, Capiau T, Drabs V, et al. Executive and attentional contributions to Theory of Mind deficit in attention deficit/hyperactivity disorder (ADHD). Child Neuropsychol. 2015;22(3):1–21. doi:10.1080/09297049.2015.1012491.

62. Tucha O, Prell S, Mecklinger L, Bormann-Kischkel C, Kubber S, Linder M, et al. Effects of methylphenidate on multiple components of attention in children with attention deficit hyperactivity disorder. Psychopharmacology. 2006;185(3):315–26.

63. Bush G, Frazier JA, Rauch SL, Seidman LJ, Whalen PJ, Jenike MA, et al. Anterior cingulate cortex dysfunction in attention-deficit/hyperactivity disorder revealed by fMRI and the Counting Stroop. Biol Psychiatry. 1999;45(12):1542–52.

64. Drechsler R, Brandeis D, Foldenyi M, Imhof K, Steinhausen HC. The course of neuropsychological functions in children with attention deficit hyperactivity disorder from late childhood to early adolescence. J Child Psychol Psychiatry. 2005;46(8):824–36. doi:10.1111/j.1469-7610.2004.00384.x.

65. Hendricks WA, Robey KW. The Sampling Distribution of the Coefficient of Variation. Ann Math Statist. 1936;7(3):129–32.

66. MacLeod CM. Half a century of research on the Stroop effect: an integrative review. Psychol Bull. 1991;109(2):163–203.

67. Belouchrani A, Abed-Meraim K, Cardoso J-F, Moulines E. A blind source separation technique using second-order statistics. IEEE Trans Signal Process. 1997;45(2):434–44.

68. Billauer E. Peakdet: peak detection using MATLAB. 2007. http://www.billauer.co.il/peakdet.html.

69. Kelley DJ, Oakes TR, Greischar LL, Chung MK, Ollinger JM, Alexander AL, et al. Automatic physiological waveform processing for FMRI noise correction and analysis. PLoS One. 2008;3(3):e1751. doi:10.1371/journal.pone.0001751.

70. Nakano T, Kato M, Morito Y, Itoi S, Kitazawa S. Blink-related momentary activation of the default mode network while viewing videos. Proc Natl Acad Sci USA. 2013;110(2):702–6. doi:10.1073/pnas.1214804110.

71. Castellanos FX, Sonuga-Barke EJS, Milham MP, Tannock R. Characterizing cognition in ADHD: beyond executive dysfunction. Trends Cogn Sci. 2006;10(3):117–23. doi:10.1016/j.tics.2006.01.011.

72. Sjowall D, Roth L, Lindqvist S, Thorell LB. Multiple deficits in ADHD: executive dysfunction, delay aversion, reaction time variability, and emotional deficits. J Child Psychol Psychiatry. 2013;54(6):619–27. doi:10.1111/jcpp.12006.

73. Mary A, Slama H, Mousty P, Massat I, Capiau T, Drabs V, et al. Executive and attentional contributions to theory of mind deficit in Attention Deficit Hyperactivity Disorder (ADHD). Child Neuropsychology. in revision.

74. Massat I, Slama H, Kavec M, Linotte S, Mary A, Baleriaux D, et al. Working memory-related functional brain patterns in never medicated children with ADHD. PLoS One. 2012;7(11):e49392. doi:10.1371/journal.pone.0049392.

75. Quay HC. Inhibition and attention deficit hyperactivity disorder. J Abnorm Child Psychol. 1997;25(1):7–13.

76. Rubia K, Russell T, Overmeyer S, Brammer MJ, Bullmore ET, Sharma T, et al. Mapping motor inhibition: conjunctive brain activations across different versions of go/no-go and stop tasks. Neuroimage. 2001;13(2):250–61. doi:10.1006/Nimg.2000.0685.

77. Novak GP, Solanto M, Abikoff H. Spatial orienting and focused attention in attention deficit hyperactivity disorder. Psychophysiology. 1995;32(6):546–59.

78. Yoon HH, Iacono WG, Malone SM, Bernat EM, McGue M. The effects of childhood disruptive disorder comorbidity on P3 event-related brain potentials in preadolescents with ADHD. Biol Psychol. 2008;79(3):329–36. doi:10.1016/j.biopsycho.2008.08.001.

79. Lavie N. Distracted and confused?: selective attention under load. Trends Cogn Sci. 2005;9(2):75–82. doi:10.1016/j.tics.2004.12.004.

80. Karson CN. Spontaneous eye-blink rates and dopaminergic systems. Brain. 1983;106(Pt 3):643–53.

81. Taylor JR, Elsworth JD, Lawrence MS, Sladek JR Jr, Roth RH, Redmond DE Jr. Spontaneous blink rates correlate with dopamine levels in the caudate nucleus of MPTP-treated monkeys. Exp Neurol. 1999;158(1):214–20. doi:10.1006/exnr.1999.7093.

82. Pogarell O, Padberg F, Karch S, Segmiller F, Juckel G, Mulert C, et al. Dopaminergic mechanisms of target detection—P300 event related potential and striatal dopamine. Psychiatry Res. 2011;194(3):212–8. doi:10.1016/j.pscychresns.2011.02.002.

83. Polich J. Updating P300: an integrative theory of P3a and P3b. Clin Neurophysiol. 2007;118(10):2128–48. doi:10.1016/j.clinph.2007.04.019.

84. Picton T, Bentin S, Berg P, Donchin E, Hillyard S, Johnson R, et al. Guidelines for using human event-related potentials to study cognition: recording standards and publication criteria. Psychophysiology. 2000;37(02):127–52.

85. de Zeeuw P, Weusten J, van Dijk S, van Belle J, Durston S. Deficits in cognitive control, timing and reward sensitivity appear to be dissociable in ADHD. PLoS One. 2012;7(12):e51416. doi:10.1371/journal.pone.0051416.

86. Benikos N, Johnstone SJ. Arousal-state modulation in children with AD/HD. Clin Neurophysiol. 2009;120(1):30–40. doi:10.1016/j.clinph.2008.09.026.

87. Kofler MJ, Rapport MD, Alderson RM. Quantifying ADHD classroom inattentiveness, its moderators, and variability: a meta-analytic review. J Child Psychol Psychiatry. 2008;49(1):59–69. doi:10.1111/j.1469-7610.2007.01809.x.

88. Imeraj L, Antrop I, Sonuga-Barke E, Deboutte D, Deschepper E, Bal S, et al. The impact of instructional context on classroom on-task behavior: a matched comparison of children with ADHD and non-ADHD classmates. J Sch Psychol. 2013;51(4):487–98. doi:10.1016/j.jsp.2013.05.004.

15

A functional magnetic resonance imaging investigation of visual hallucinations in the human striate cortex

Hina Abid[1], Fayyaz Ahmad[2*], Soo Y. Lee[3], Hyun W. Park[3], Dongmi Im[3], Iftikhar Ahmad[2] and Safee U. Chaudhary[4*]

Abstract

Purpose: Human beings frequently experience fear, phobia, migraine and hallucinations, however, the cerebral mechanisms underpinning these conditions remain poorly understood. Towards this goal, in this work, we aim to correlate the human ocular perceptions with visual hallucinations, and map them to their cerebral origins.

Methods: An fMRI study was performed to examine the visual cortical areas including the striate, parastriate and peristriate cortex in the occipital lobe of the human brain. 24 healthy subjects were enrolled and four visual patterns including hallucination circle (HCC), hallucination fan (HCF), retinotopy circle (RTC) and retinotopy cross (RTX) were used towards registering their impact in the aforementioned visual related areas. One-way analysis of variance was used to evaluate the significance of difference between induced activations. Multinomial regression and and K-means were used to cluster activation patterns in visual areas of the brain.

Results: Significant activations were observed in the visual cortex as a result of stimulus presentation. The responses induced by visual stimuli were resolved to Brodmann areas 17, 18 and 19. Activation data clustered into independent and mutually exclusive clusters with HCC registering higher activations as compared to HCF, RTC and RTX.

Conclusions: We conclude that small circular objects, in rotation, tend to leave greater hallucinating impressions in the visual region. The similarity between observed activation patterns and those reported in conditions such as epilepsy and visual hallucinations can help elucidate the cortical mechanisms underlying these conditions.

Trial Registration 1121_GWJUNG

Keywords: Functional magnetic resonance imaging (fMRI), Visual hallucinations, Visual cortex, Brodmann area, K-means clustering, Logistic regression

Background

Cerebrum forms the largest part of human brain. It comprises of an outer layer called the cerebral cortex which can be further divided into four lobes namely frontal, parietal, occipital and temporal lobe [1]. Cytoarchitectonically, the cerebral cortex has been classified into 52 cortical Brodmann areas (BA) of which the occipital lobe containing the visual cortex has BAs 17, 18 and 19 [2]. Visual tasks processing related area 'V1' is located in

BA 17 (striate cortex) while 'V2–V6' are located in BA 18 (parastriate cortex) and 19 (peristriate cortex). The ventral stream ('what pathway') initiates with V1, passes through V2 and V4, and leads into the inferior temporal cortex (IT cortex). The dorsal stream ('where pathway') starts at V1 and proceeds to V2, V6 and V5.

Upon absorption of light rays emitted by an object, the photoreceptors in the retina send a signal through the optic nerve via the optic chiasma into the intra laminar nucleus of the thalamus. The signal then enters V1 where the striate cortex processes the stimulus in the visual cortex of the brain in tandem with extrastriate cortex. As a result, increased blood-oxygen-level dependent (BOLD) activations can be measured in the corresponding areas

---

*Correspondence: dr.fayyaz@uog.edu.pk, safeeullah@lums.edu.pk
[2] University of Gujrat, Gujrat, Pakistan
[4] Lahore University of Managment Sciences, Lahore, Pakistan
Full list of author information is available at the end of the article

of the brain. The intensity of each activation depends on the physical form of the object presented to the subject [3, 4]. Causal networking among different brain localities has been determined by Ahmed et al. [5]. The neural activations are adjudged according to the object presented and their magnitude depends on the type of the stimulus [6, 7]. Functional magnetic resonance imaging (fMRI) enables us to capture such activations in the brain, during the working phase, for onwards analysis [8, 9]. Tootell et al. [10] have reported that middle temporal (MT) region of the brain responds selectively to moving (translating or rotating) and stationary visual stimuli. Howard et al. [11], have demonstrated the effectiveness of fMRI scanners in capturing visual hallucinations in the visual cortex of patients suffering from Charles Bonnet Syndrome (CBS). It is important to note here that sometimes non-existent objects are reportedly visualized by subjects which are primarily due to residual information present in the visual cortex from past experiences [12]. Research into such observations has shown activations in V1 region of the brain suggesting that the impact of hallucinatory patterns constitutes similar cortical characteristics as that of ordinary vision. Hallucinations have also been attributed to the specific anatomical structure of the brain as proposed in the neuroanatomical model [13].

Visual hallucinations are therefore those sensory perceptions that are felt in the absence of any physical stimulus. Visual hallucinations may instigate with auras preceding petit mal epilepsy [14], fortification patterns of migraine headaches [15], drug induced hallucinations [16]. The false images comprising a visual hallucination may have either formed or unformed appearances. A person suffering from hallucinations may report seeing huge shadows, flashes of light, haphazard or outlined patterns, and may even catch a glimpse of a departed loved one. The brain may also present an oversized projection of an article which in reality may just be a minute entity. Here, it must be noted that continual experience of visual hallucinations can translate into serious human ailments such as migraine pain and epilepsy [17].

Empirically, visual hallucinations can be investigated by exposing subjects to visual stimuli consisting of the hallucinogenic patterns which may activate visual cortex of the brain [18]. Bressloff et al. [19], presented four types of images including spirals, cobwebs, tunnels and lattices and identified them as the origin of hallucinations. Stripes, spirals, rings and collective burst type patterns excite the neurons in visual cortex when exposed to the human eye [20]. A mathematical theory of such geometric type patterns, giving rise to visual hallucination, was proposed by Ermentrout et al. [21]. Vincent et al. [22] used flickering checkerboard as stimuli and measured hallucinogenic activations in brain. However,

a mechanistic understanding of these induced hallucinations in the visual cortex remains elusive till date. Specifically, evaluation of hallucinogenic impacts (such as cortical magnification and retinotopy) of moving and stationary visual stimuli on BAs 17, 18 and 19 and statistical evaluation of incumbent BOLD signal data remains to be investigated.

In this study, we aim to determine if hallucinations can be induced by visual stimuli designed using cues provided by previous studies; evaluate significance and classify the hallucinogenic impacts of these visual stimuli on the visual cortical areas. Towards this goal, we induced visual hallucinations in healthy individuals by presenting them with four visual stimuli namely retinotopy cross (RTX), hallucination fan (HCF), retinotopy circle (RTC) and hallucination circle (HCC). HCF and HCC were in rotary motion about their axis while RTC and RTX were stationary. The activations registered in the visual cortex were measured using an fMRI scanner and contribution of each visual stimulus in activating the visual cortex was found to be significant corresponding to $p \leq 0.05$ (FWE-correction). Finally, the mixed activation data was clustered using K-means whereby it resolved into respective BAs (17, 18 and 19). Our results show that visual cortex exhibited significant activations upon presentation of each visual stimulus with highest activations observed for HCC proceeded by RTC, HCF and RTX in order. Application of least square difference (LSD) test on the activation data identified BA 17 to be the most significant contributor to induced visual hallucinations followed by BAs 18 and 19. Moreover, the mixed activation data obtained from presentation of four stimuli was separable into individual clusters with HCC and RTX significantly activating BAs 17–19 while RTC managing activations in BA 17 only.

Taken together, we conclude that small circular objects in rotation induce greater activations in the visual cortex of the brain. These activation patterns observed are similar to those reported in migraine pain and epilepsy. Hence, the proposed experimental and data analysis methodology can assist in enhancing the understanding of visual hallucinations in disease states by an accurate cortical mapping of the brain.

Methods
fMRI Experimental design and data acquisition
The fMRI scanning procedure was conducted at Korea Advanced Institute of Science and Technology (KAIST), South Korea. 24 healthy subjects (15 males, 9 females, mean age 21, SD 0.8), with normal color vision, were enrolled and scanned in the study. Each subject was exposed to a procedure comprising alternating rest and task conditions while being examined by an fMRI

scanner. The data obtained was preprocessed to identify and filter out datasets which contained head movement induced motion blur, background noise or low quality measurements. 4 subjects which produced the highest quality datasets were selected for onward methodological study and analysis.

Every experimental session lasted for 160 s and consisted of 8 blocks with each rest block leading a stimulus block. The duration of each rest and stimulus block was for 24 and 16 s, respectively. Within a single scanning session, 80 volume scans (32 with stimuli and 48 at rest) were obtained at intervals of 2 s. We applied cluster analysis on the resulting 80 data points corresponding to average activations in BA17, 18 and 19 voxels for the classification amongst HCC, HCF, RTC and RTX.

Four visual stimuli of different shapes and sizes were designed towards evaluating their potential hallucinogenic impact on the visual cortex. HCC comprised of concentric circles with varying diameters and colors (shades of grey). These circles were then set into synchronous rotation about the center point. RTC contained three static concentric circles with checkered boundaries and their center point indicated by a black spot. HCF pattern was a four-winged fan rotating about its center while the RTX was a stationary cross drawn using checkered lines (Fig. 1). Of the four sessions, each session was

confined to a single visual stimulus. The experimental sessions were designed such that RTX was presented first followed by HCF, RTC and HCC respectively. A scan was acquired every 2 s while the stimulus was being shown. This pattern was repeated for the remaining three sessions as well. During each scan, the subjects were directed to continually focus on the presented stimulus and encouraged to keep their minds relaxed during the rest phase. To ensure high quality data from scanning procedure, their heads were placed in a brace and adjusted before a scan was performed.

Image acquisition

The images were acquired using a 3 Tesla (FORTE, Oxford magnet, Varian Console, built up by ISOL) instrument, with a quadrature head coil to get an anatomic scan and a surface coil to obtain the functional scan. High-resolution anatomic images (structural resolution 1.25 mm isotropic voxels) were acquired using an MPRAGE sequence (echo time TE = 3.7 ms, TR = 8.1 ms, flip angle = 8°, FOV = 256 × 256 mm) and functional data were acquired using echo planar imaging (EPI, TE = 37 ms, phase encoding = top to bottom, flip angle = 70°, TR = 2000 ms, matrix = 128 × 128 mm, slices = 15, voxels = 3 mm × 3 mm, no gap) as shown Fig. 1.

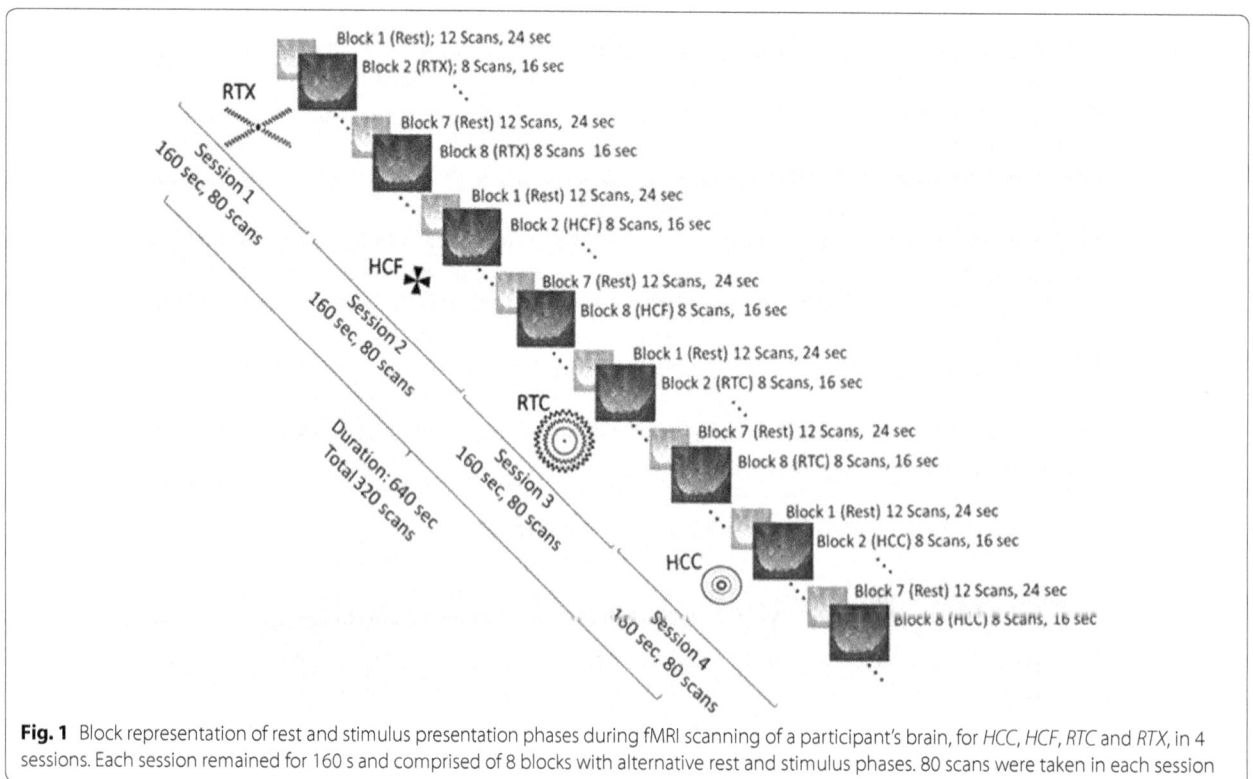

Fig. 1 Block representation of rest and stimulus presentation phases during fMRI scanning of a participant's brain, for *HCC*, *HCF*, *RTC* and *RTX*, in 4 sessions. Each session remained for 160 s and comprised of 8 blocks with alternative rest and stimulus phases. 80 scans were taken in each session

Image analysis

Data was analyzed using Statistical Parametric Mapping software (SPM8b; Wellcome Department of Cognitive Neurology, University College London, London, UK). Images realignment was performed to correct for the artifacts due to minor head vibrations and normalized to a standard Montreal Neurological Institute (MNI) template. Smoothing was done by 4-mm full width at half maximum smoothing to average the data with the neighboring data points. Images were analyzed using contrast vector C = [1 −1] corresponding to p < 0.05 [Family Wise Error (FWE) correction] (Fig. 3).

fMRI images configuration

Grey-scale fMRI images were used for onward investigations, with the darker regions having a higher pixel value while the lighter regions approaching to a zero on the pixel scale. A total of 80 scans were taken for each session so as to ascertain accuracy in the ensuing statistical analysis of these results. All volume scans were cut down into 15 slices. The dimension of a single volume was 128 × 128 × 15. The total number of voxels in a volume counted to 245,760. Each voxel in the study had a uniform size of 3 × 3 × 3 mm.

Statistical methods and techniques for fMRI data analysis

To test the variation and significance of data obtained after presentation of visual stimuli, analysis of variance (ANOVA) test [23] was employed. Upon ascertaining significance of impact on visual cortex, LSD [24] was applied to determine the individual contribution of each stimulus on the visual cortex. For classifying the mixed cortical activations into clusters, K-means clustering [25] was applied to the activation data. To compute the probabilistic relationship between each visual stimuli and BAs 17, 18 and 19, we used multinomial logistic regression (MLR) [26].

Results

Analysis of fMRI data obtained from presentation of four visual stimuli

Upon presentation of visual stimuli, BOLD signals were measured in the visual cortex. The axial slicing view of fMRI scans was observed and activations were registered only in the middle axial slices (MNI coordinates and cluster size in Table 1). The activation data obtained was continuous time-series fMRI data. These activations were evaluated using t test (p < 0.05 FEW-corrected), for each scan (task vs. rest state), and exhibited varying levels of activation in each case (Fig. 2). Highest activations were determined by comparing the averages of voxel activations induced by the four stimuli, in a participant's visual cortex, using general linear model (GLM) analysis. The distribution of voxel activations for a single participant, for each stimulus, is shown in Fig. 3. Highest activations were observed when HCC came into sight (average: 1190) followed by RTC (average: 1050), HCF (average: 796) and RTX (average: 475), in order as shown in box plot. The results also showed that HCF elicited the most variable response followed by RTC, HCC and RTX, in descending order. The participants reported magnified visualizations in cases of HCC and RTC stimuli. The four conditions can, therefore, be discriminated from each other based on the fMRI responses elicited from 3 visual areas. Importantly, the hallucinatory stimuli can excite more neurons than normal retinotopic stimuli.

Significance analysis of cortical activation data

To ascertain the significance of the stimulus-induced activations, ANOVA testing was employed. Our results (Table 2) show that all stimuli had exerted a significant impact on the visual cortex (p < 0.05). Furthermore, a pairwise comparison (using LSD test) was performed between the activation data of each stimulus towards computing the contribution of

Table 1 MNI coordinates of peak voxels within each cluster and T statistics from BA17 (Threshold = p < 0.05)

ROI	Stimulus	x	y	z	T value	Cluster size
R V1	HCC	11	−78	7	15.41	3941
L V1	HCC	−11	−81	8	15.62	1486
R V1	HCF	17	−83	11	17.47	4698
L V1	HCF	−7	−84	13	16.07	2254
R V1	RTC	14	−88	8	16.07	2251
L V1	RTC	−8	−75	15	17.47	4700
R V1	RTX	19	−74	12	15.62	893
L V1	RTX	−3	−76	6	22.50	1342

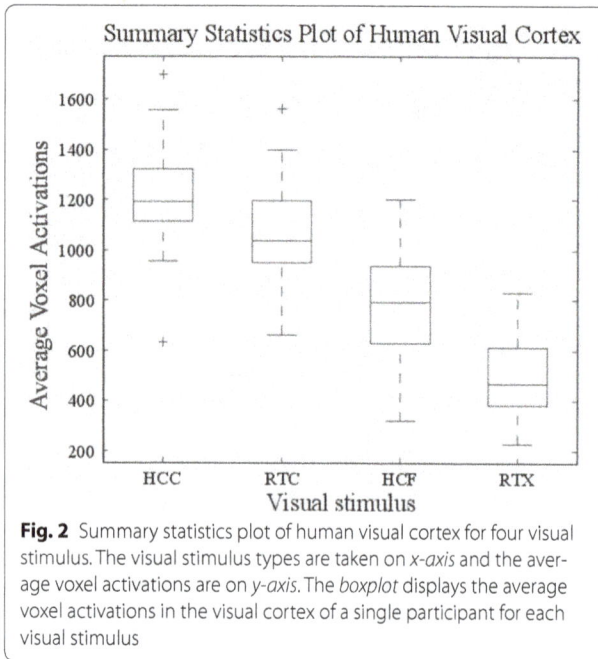

Fig. 2 Summary statistics plot of human visual cortex for four visual stimulus. The visual stimulus types are taken on *x-axis* and the average voxel activations are on *y-axis*. The *boxplot* displays the average voxel activations in the visual cortex of a single participant for each visual stimulus

largest, followed by RTC (HCC = 79.9757825, HCF = 39.9680400, RTX = 62.4324969), HCF (HCC = 40.0077425, RTC = 39.9680400, RTX = 22.4644569) and RTX (HCC = 17.5432856, RTC = 62.4324969, HCF = 22.4644569), in terms of magnitude (Table 3).

Classification of cortical activations by visual stimuli
To classify the cortical activation data generated by the presented visual stimuli, K-means clustering was employed. The data got separated into clusters 1 through 4 (Fig. 4). Activations generated by HCC and RTX clustered into clusters 1 and 4, respectively. However, there was a slight mixing between these clusters (Cluster 1; HCC = 76, RTX = 6, Cluster 4; HCC = 4, RTX = 74). Data corresponding to RTC and HCF stimuli clustered perfectly into clusters 2 and 3, respectively. The within sum of square (SSE) was used to measure the cluster cohesion and it was found to be the highest (12436.723) for cluster 2 (Table 4). Qualitative analysis of clustering results was performed by computing variations within and in between clusters (total sum of square), overall cluster cohesion (total within sum of squares) and cluster separation (between sum of square) (results shown in Table 5). Classification of the voxel activations data for

stimuli activating the visual cortex. HCC's pair-wise contribution (RTC = 79.9757825, HCF = 40.0077425, RTX = 17.5432856) was found to be the

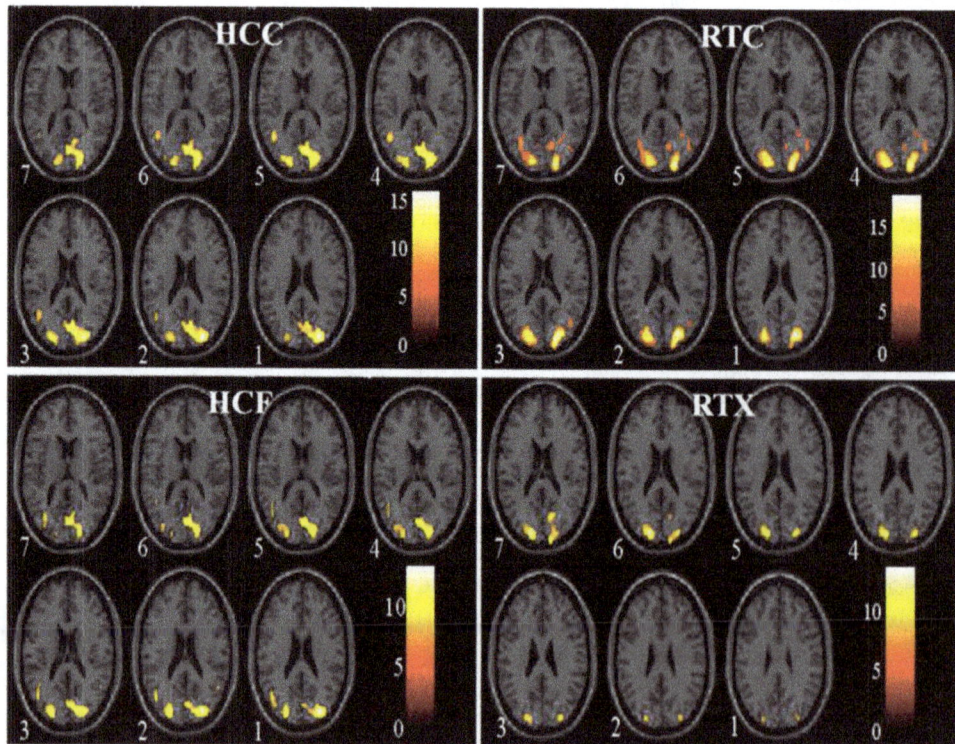

Fig. 3 Comparison of activated areas in the visual cortex of a subject. The figure shows a 2 × 2 display of statistical parameter maps (SPM) after presenting *HCC, RTC, HCF* and *RTX*. The significant activations are measured using t-scale at p < 0.05 (corrected)

Table 2 One way analysis of variance

Variation source	Sum of squares	df	Mean square	F	Sig.
Between groups	286,371.146	3	95,457.049	1056.665	0.000
Within groups	28,637.164	317	90.338		
Total	315,008.310	320			

The mean difference is significant at the 0.05 level

Table 3 LSD test for significance

(I) Factors	(J) Factor	Mean difer (I − J)	Std. error	Sig.
HCC	RTC	−79.9757825*	1.5028145	.000
	HCF	−40.0077425*	1.5028145	.000
	RTX	−17.5432856*	1.4981690	.000
RTC	HCC	79.9757825*	1.5028145	.000
	HCF	39.9680400*	1.5028145	.000
	RTX	62.4324969*	1.4981690	.000
HCF	HCC	40.0077425*	1.5028145	.000
	RTC	−39.9680400*	1.5028145	.000
	RTX	22.4644569*	1.4981690	.000
RTX	HCC	17.5432856*	1.4981690	.000
	RTC	62.4324969*	1.4981690	.000
	HCF	−22.4644569*	1.4981690	.000

* The mean difference is significant at the 0.05 level

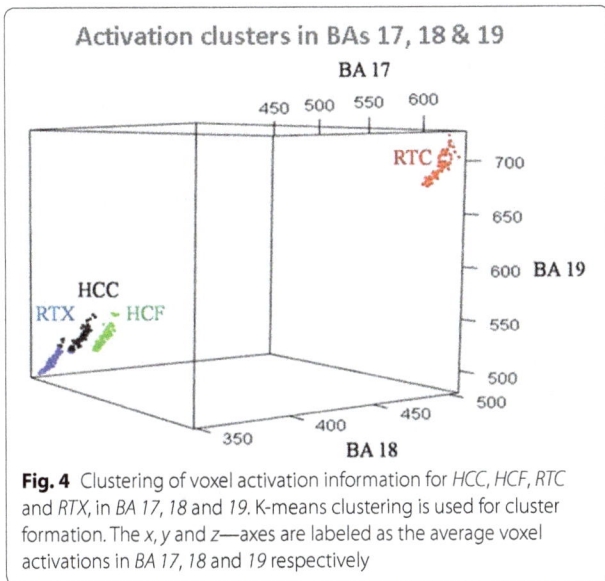

Fig. 4 Clustering of voxel activation information for *HCC, HCF, RTC* and *RTX*, in *BA 17, 18* and *19*. K-means clustering is used for cluster formation. The *x, y* and *z*—axes are labeled as the average voxel activations in *BA 17, 18* and *19* respectively

HCC, HCF, RTC and RTX into individual clusters determined the correlation in the three BA's. The impact of HCC on BAs (17, 18 and 19) was found out to be 460, 370 and 530, respectively. For RTC it was 640, 500 and 710; for HCF the impact was 490, 370 and 540 while for RTX

Table 4 Size of clusters, cluster means and within sum of squares

No. of cluster	Cluster size	Cluster means			Within sum of squares
		BA 17	BA 18	BA 19	
1	82	464.2945	370.8899	519.8890	7605.788
2	80	627.4581	496.4402	694.6261	12,436.723
3	80	488.8951	374.0905	524.2706	7108.980
4	78	457.0710	357.5852	495.6686	5530.045

Table 5 Sum of squares

Total SS	Within SS	Between SS
4,575,623	32,681.54	4,542,941

it was 460, 360 and, 500. The pair-wise activated voxels with respect to each BA (17, 18 and 19) have been plotted using a scatter matrix plot (Fig. 5; Table 6).

Probabilistic relationship of visual stimulus with BA 17, 18 and 19

To determine the probabilistic relationship between the each stimulus (HCC, RTC, HCF and RTC) and every Brodmann area (BA 17, 18 and 19), multinomial logistic regression (MLR) was employed. Inferior temporal gyrus (BA 20); a visual cortical area lying in the temporal lobe of the brain was used as a reference base category. Category 1 was reserved for BA 20 while BAs 17, 18 and 19 were encoded into categories 2, 3 and 4, respectively.

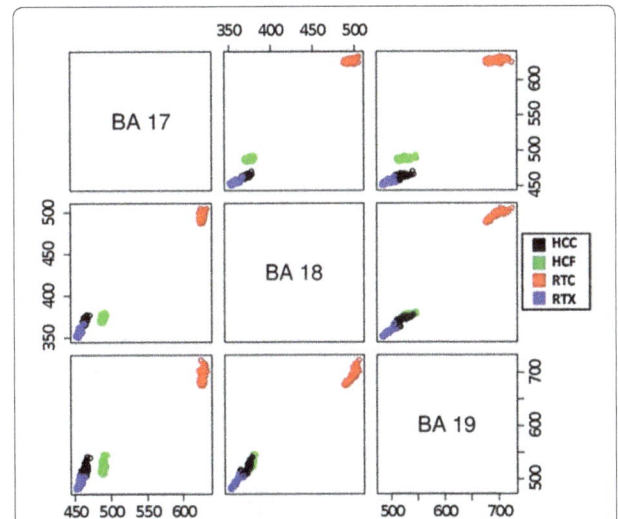

Fig. 5 Scatter matrix plot of activated information corresponding to visual cortical areas. The *plot* is a 3 × 3 display with *BA 17, 18* and *19* shown in *rows* (*columns*) 1, 2 and 3 respectively. The off diagonal cells represents the pairwise correlation of clustered points in BA's. The cells in lower triangle below the diagonal are the mirror images of the cells in the upper triangle above the diagonal of the *matrix plot*

Table 6 Allocation of points corresponding to each cluster

	Cluster 1	Cluster 2	Cluster 3	Cluster 4
HCC	76	0	0	4
HCF	0	80	0	0
RTC	0	0	80	0
RTX	6	0	0	74

MLR coefficient of HCC was found to be the highest for BA 17 (45.44663) and lowest for BA 19 (22.30781) suggesting that striate cortex was highly activated by HCC (Table 7). For RTC, HCF and RTX, their respective contribution in activating BA 17 was found to be 11.378715, 2.51319718 and 36.24384. For the activations in BA 19, RTC, HCF and RTX contributed 2.449028, 0.03642327 and 20.10646, respectively.

Discussion

This study aims to elucidate the cortical mechanisms underpinning visual hallucinations in the human brain thereby building an improved understanding of the condition. Towards this goal, experiments were designed around four visual stimuli (HCC, RTC, HCF and RTX), having different shapes and sizes with varying movements. These stimuli were presented to the participants and their fMRI scans were obtained. The resulting data was analyzed towards determining the impact of each visual stimulus on the visual cortex (i.e. BAs 17, 18 and 19). Significant activations were observed in the visual cortex upon presentation of each stimulus type, however, the magnitude of induced activations was observed to be different. For each participant, HCC induced the highest BOLD signal in the visual cortex followed by RTC, HCF and RTX during 80 scans. The results indicated that smaller objects having circular appearances in rotation create larger impacts in the visual cortex as compared to static non-circular objects. Furthermore, while visualizing HCC and RTC, the participants reported visual perceptions of enlarged visual stimuli which were in fact artificially induced hallucinations.

Table 7 Coefficients of multinomial logistic regression model

Y	Intercept	pHCC	pRTC	pHCF	pRTX
2[a]	−0.3372760	−45.44663	11.378715	−2.51319718	36.24384
	(0.4586571)[b]	(34.74687)	(9.509267)	(1.4800913)	(33.28803)
3	−0.5260880	33.22444	−4.316287	0.2773366	−29.71157
	(0.4831243)	(23.03927)	(8.545127)	(0.8823183)	(21.40103)
4	−0.2112646	22.30781	−2.449028	0.03642327	−20.10646
	(0.4322987)	(22.33585)	(8.040815)	(0.8376842)	(20.87877)

[a] Categories 2, 3 and 4 represents BA 17, 18 and 19 respectively

[b] Standard errors

Having induced hallucinating impacts in the visual cortex of the participants, we set out to analyze the continuous time-series fMRI data using specific statistical techniques. We investigated the patterns of activations by measuring impact of each visual stimulus on each Brodmann area. Clustering of the mixed task and rest state data helped us determine the activation correlation in the three BA's for hallucinating (HCC, RTC) and non-hallucinating (HCF, RTX) stimuli. The impact of HCC on BAs (17, 18 and 19) was found out to be 460, 370 and 530, respectively. For RTC it was 640, 500 and 710; for HCF the impact was 490, 370 and 540 while for RTX it was 460, 360 and, 500. These results, specifically for HCC and RTC, were interpreted to constitute a Brodmann area footprint as the requisite setting for experiencing visual hallucinations.

Similar studies conducted earlier have employed cobwebs, funnel, spirals and concentric circles towards inducing hallucinations [21]. In our experiments, we have designed and employed four unique visual stimuli comprising of circles (HCC, RTC) and crosses (RTX, HCF) and elicited their impact on visual cortex. The stimuli HCC and HCF were also set into motion while RTC and RTX were kept static. It might be of interest to evaluate the cortical impact of an expanded set of visual stimuli, with a broader range of optical properties. Stimuli design changes may include different shapes, sizes and, rates of rotation.

Furthermore, in case of diseases such as epilepsy and migraine, research has reported similar hallucinating impacts in the visual cortex of patients [27]. Patients are known to experience auras such as flickering, zig-zag lines, disks and balls of light [28]. These auras may be enlarged or diminished in size, stationary or moving and single or multiple. The magnified shapes that are seen by patients suffering from such pathologies are comparable to the hallucinating magnification reported by participants in our study [29]. Hence, the statistical evaluation methodology described in this work can specifically assist in eliciting the cortical mechanisms giving rise to enlargement of objects in epilepsy [27]. The study can be extended further by replacing the uncolored stimuli with colored ones, in varying shapes. This can help in benchmarking the hallucinating sensations induced in the subjects against those in the patients. Moreover, auditory, olfactory and tactile hallucination studies can also be carried out and their impacts can be measured in the respective BA's. Furthermore, our study can also be extended by employing more powerful data analysis tools such as structural equation modelling (SEM) and Bayesian techniques towards investigating the interplay between BAs during induced hallucinations.

Taken together, the proposed methodology can be employed in investigating the impact of a variety of stimuli on the visual cortex. Alongside, the findings from this study can assist in screening as well as prognosis of epileptic and migraine patients presenting specific hallucinating patterns in fMRI analysis.

Abbreviations

ANOVA: analysis of variance (statistical technique); BA: Brodmann area (brain cortical areas); EPI: echo planar imaging; fMRI: functional magnetic resonance imaging (technique to scan images); FOV: field of view; GLM: generalized linear model (a statistical technique); HCC: hallucination circle (visual stimulus); HCF: hallucination fan (visual stimulus); KAIST: Korea Advanced Institute of Science and Technology; LSD: least significant difference (statistical technique); MLR: multiple linear regression; MNI: Montreal Neurological Institute; MPRAGE: magnetization-prepared rapid gradient-echo; MSE: mean square error; MT: middle temporal (visual area); RTC: retinotopy circle (visual stimulus); RTX: retinotopy cross (visual stimulus); SPM: statistical parametric mapping; TE: echo time; TR: repetition time; V1: visual area 1; V2: visual area 2; V3: visual area 3; V4: visual area 4; V5: visual area 5; V6: visual area 6.

Authors' contributions

HA, FA and SYL conceived and designed the study. FA, DIM and SYL obtained the fMRI scans for the subjects. HA, IA, SUC and FA performed data analysis, visualization and interpretation of results. HA and SUC drafted and critically reviewed the manuscript. FA supervised the study. All authors read and approved the final manuscript.

Author details

[1] Quaid-e-Azam University, Islamabad, Pakistan. [2] University of Gujrat, Gujrat, Pakistan. [3] Korea Advanced Institute of Science and Technology, Daejeon, South Korea. [4] Lahore University of Managment Sciences, Lahore, Pakistan.

Acknowledgements

This work was supported by KAIST (Korea Advanced Institute of Science and Technology).

Competing interests

The authors declare that they have no competing interests.

Appendix: MATLAB program for extracting ROIs data

```
clear all;
    BrodmannAtlas         =         spm_read_vols(spm_
vol(`xxbrodmann.img'));
    BA 17 = ismember(BrodmannAtlas,17);
    V = spm_vol(`xxbrodmann.img');
    V.fname=`BA17.nii';
    V.private.dat.fname = V.fname;
    spm_write_vol(V,BA 17);
    BA 17;
    Temp_array = [];
    for i = 1:80
    filename = ([`.jnartx(new)' num2str(i)`.img']);
    nii = load_nii(filename);
    x = nii.img(:,:,:);
    t = x(BA 17);
    Temp_array = [Temp_array t];
    end
```

(The specified MATLAB program is to extract the data for Brodmann area 17).

Data for Brodmann areas 18 and 19 are extracted using similar code.

References

1. Finger S. Origins of neuroscience: a history of explorations into brain function. New York: Oxford University Press; 1994.
2. Garey LJ. Brodmann's localisation in the cerebral cortex—the principles of comparative localisation in the cerebral cortex based on cytoarchitectonics. New York: Springer Science; 2006.
3. Murray SO, et al. Shape perception reduces activity in human primary visual cortex. Proc Natl Acad Sci. 2002;99(23):15164–9.
4. Harter MR, White C. Effects of contour sharpness and check-size on visually evoked cortical potentials. Vis Res. 1968;8(6):701–11.
5. Ahmad F, et al. A shrinkage method for causal network detection of brain regions. Imag Sys Technol. 2013;23(2):140–6.
6. Watanabe T, et al. Task-dependent influences of attention on the activation of human primary visual cortex. Proc Natl Acad Sci USA. 1998;95(19):11489–92.
7. Ahmad F, et al. A novel method for detection of voxels for decision making: An fMRI study. Imag Sys Technol. 2016;26(2):163–7.
8. Engel S, Glover G, Wandell B. Retinotopic organization in human visual cortex and the spatial precision of functional MRI. Cereb Cortex. 1997;7(2):181–92.
9. Ahmad F, et al. A slice-wise latent structure regression method for the analysis of functional magnetic resonance imaging data. Concepts Magn Reson A. 2013;42(4):130–9.
10. Tootell RB, et al. Functional analysis of human MT and related visual cortical areas using magnetic resonance imaging. J Neurosci. 1995;15(4):3215–30.
11. Ffytche DH, et al. The anatomy of conscious vision: an fMRI study of visual hallucinations. Nat Neurosci. 1998;1(6):738–42.
12. Mundy-Castle AC. A case in which visual hallucinations related to past experience were evoked by photic stimulation. Electroencephalogr Clin Neurophysiol. 1951;3(3):353–6.
13. Allen P, et al. The hallucinating brain: a review of structural and functional neuroimaging studies of hallucinations. Neurosci Biobehav Rev. 2008;32(1):175–91.
14. Horowitz MJ, Adams JE, Rutkin BB. Evoked hallucinations in epilepsy. Psychiatr Specul. 1967;11:4.
15. Richards W. The fortification illusions of migraines. Sci Am. 1971;224(5):88–96.
16. Brawley P, Duffield J. The pharmacology of the hallucinogens. Pharmacol Rev. 1972;24(1):31–66.
17. Panayiotopoulos CP. Elementary visual hallucinations in migraine and epilepsy. J Neurol Neurosurg Psychiatr. 1994;57(11):1371–4.
18. Le Bihan D, et al. Activation of human primary visual cortex during visual recall: a magnetic resonance imaging study. Proc Natl Acad Sci USA. 1993;90(24):11802–5.
19. Bressloff PC, et al. What geometric visual hallucinations tell us about the visual cortex. Neural Comput. 2002;14(3):473–91.
20. Fohlmeister C, et al. Spontaneous excitations in the visual cortex: stripes, spirals, rings, and collective bursts. Neural Comput. 1995;7(5):905–14.
21. Ermentrout GB, Cowan JD. A mathematical theory of visual hallucination patterns. Biol Cybern. 1979;34(3):137–50.
22. Billock VA, Tsou BH. Neural interactions between flicker-induced self-organized visual hallucinations and physical stimuli. Proc Natl Acad Sci. 2007;104(20):8490–5.
23. Ostertagová E, Ostertag O. Methodology and application of oneway ANOVA. Am J Mech Eng. 2013;1(7):256–61.
24. Williams LJ, Abdi H. Fisher's least significant difference (LSD) test. Encycl Res Des. 2010;1:23–6.
25. Pang-Ning T, Steinbach M, Kumar V. Introduction to data mining. Boston: Addison-Wesley; (2005)
26. Agresti A. An introduction to categorical data analysis, vol. 135. New York: Wiley; 1996.

16

Oral administration of potassium bromate induces neurobehavioral changes, alters cerebral neurotransmitters level and impairs brain tissue of swiss mice

Jamaan Ajarem[1], Naif G. Altoom[1], Ahmed A. Allam[1,2], Saleh N. Maodaa[1], Mostafa A. Abdel- Maksoud[1*] and Billy KC. Chow[3]

Abstract

Background: Potassium bromate (KBrO$_3$) is widely used as a food additive and is a major water disinfection by-product. The present study reports the side effects of KBrO$_3$ administration on the brain functions and behaviour of albino mice.

Methods: Animals were divided into three groups: control, low dose KBrO$_3$ (100 mg/kg/day) and high dose KBrO$_3$ (200 mg/kg/day) groups.

Results: Administration of KBrO$_3$ led to a significant change in the body weight in the animals of the high dose group in the first, second and the last weeks while water consumption was not significantly changed. Neurobehavioral changes and a reduced Neurotransmitters levels were observed in both KBrO$_3$ groups of mice. Also, the brain level of reduced glutathione (GSH) in KBrO$_3$ receiving animals was decreased. Histological studies favoured these biochemical results showing extensive damage in the histological sections of brain of KBrO$_3$-treated animals.

Conclusions: These results show that KBrO$_3$ has serious damaging effects on the central nervous system and therefore, its use should be avoided.

Keywords: Organ toxicity, Dopamine, Serotonin, Acetylcholine, Reduced glutathione

Background

Potassium bromate (KBrO$_3$) is widely used as a flour improver that acts as a maturing agent [1]. During the last 90 years, it has been used as a food additive [2]. It acts principally in the late dough stage giving strength and elasticity to the dough during the baking process in addition to promoting the rise of bread. KBrO$_3$ is also used in cheese production, beer making and is commonly added to fish paste products [3]. Also, it is used in pharmaceutical and cosmetic industries and is a constituent of cold wave hair solutions [2]. Moreover, KBrO$_3$ can appear as a byproduct in an ozonization of water containing bromide. As a result of KBrO$_3$ biotransformation, free radicals' generation can cause oxidative damage to essential cellular macro molecules, leading to marked nephrotoxicity and cancer in experimental animals [4]. Indeed, many previous reports have documented that KBrO$_3$ can induce multiple organ toxicity in humans and experimental animals [5–7]. KBrO$_3$ is highly irritating and injurious to tissues especially those of the central nervous system (CNS) and kidneys [8]. Many cases of accidental poisoning in children resulting from ingestion of bromate solution and sugar contaminated with bromate were reported as the source of mild poisoning in New Zealand [9]. Consequently, KBrO$_3$ has been prohibited in several countries like United Kingdom, Nigeria and Canada [2]. Toxicological studies have convincingly shown that

*Correspondence: harrany@gmail.com
[1] Department of Zoology, College of Science, King Saud University, P.O. Box 2455, Riyadh 11451, Saudi Arabia
Full list of author information is available at the end of the article

$KBrO_3$ affects the neurobehavioral (motor equilibrium performance and spontaneous locomotor activity) status of guinea pigs [10]. $KBrO_3$ induced detrimental effects on auditory brainstem response of guinea pigs whereas it caused Otto-neurotoxicity mainly through the peripheral auditory nerve [11]. Behavioral changes are usually associated with a disturbance in neurotransmitters [12]. Acetylcholine, dopamine and serotonin are common neurotransmitters that can directly or indirectly influence neurons, thereby affecting behavior [13]. Behavioral changes are also associated with oxidative stress [14]. It is known that $KBrO_3$ induces oxidative stress in tissues [15–18] that could be the basis of bromate-induced behavioral changes. Moreover, $KBrO_3$ induces hemorrhage, neuronal degeneration and vacuolation of the brain tissue sections [19]. The present study attempts to assess the effect of oral administration of $KBrO_3$ on the behavioral changes, neurotransmitters, antioxidant status and brain histomorphology of white albino mice using two different doses of $KBrO_3$ to compare their effects.

Methods
Animals
Thirty (30) adult male albino mice (*Mice musculus*) with an average weight of 30.2 ± 4.24 g were obtained from animal house- College of pharmacy- King Saud University and maintained and monitored in a specific pathogen-free environment. All animal procedures were performed in accordance with the standards set out in the Guidelines for the Care and Use of Experimental Animals issued by the Committee for the Purpose of Control and Supervision of Experiments on Animals (CPCSEA). The study protocol was approved by the Animal Ethics Committee at King Saud University. All animals were allowed to acclimatize in plastic cages inside a well-ventilated room for one week prior to the experiment. The animals were maintained under standard laboratory conditions (temperature of 23 °C, relative humidity of 60–70 % and a 12-hour light/dark cycle), fed a diet of standard commercial pellets and given water ad libitum.

Potassium bromate preparation and dosing schedule
Potassium bromate salt, a product of British drug home limited, Poole England was supplied in its white crystalline form by ASILA chemicals (Saudi Arabia). It was then dissolved in water to prepare the 100 mg/kg dose and the 200 mg/kg dose. Animals were divided into 3 groups as follows: Group (I) control group (was given distilled water); Group (II) Low dose $KBrO_3$ group (was given 100 mg/kg); Group (III) High dose $KBrO_3$ group (was given 200 mg/kg). $KBro_3$ was orally administered daily through oral intubation at the two doses of 100 and 200 mg/kg/day for 42 days. The doses used in the current study were adjusted according to the LD50 calculations carried out by Kurokawa et al. [24].

Monitoring of water consumption and body weight changes
Daily water consumption was monitored for all animals in the three groups. The animals were weighed prior to the commencement of administration and in subsequent weeks during the experiment period. At the end of administration, the mice were sacrificed by cervical dislocation.

Behavioral studies
Ten animals from each group were used in the current study. For testing, the animals were brought in a room (25 °C) of dim red light reserved for that purpose. All tests were conducted blindly by the same experimenter [20]. Except for Morris maze experiment, all experiments were carried out during the 3rd and the 6th weeks.

T-maze conducting assay
All animal's groups were deprived from food all night before this examination. The elevated T-maze consists of three closed arms to be T like structure. The main arm ($100 \times 10 \times 20$ cm) and the two lateral arms ($40 \times 10 \times 20$ cm) at an elevation of 20 cm above the floor. At the end of the right lateral arm, the rodent food was placed. Hungry animals were placed in the terminal end of the main arm of the elevated T-maze facing the passage to the two lateral arms, and left to explore the maze for one min then the animal removed from the maze and kept in its cage for 2 hrs and replaced in the same position in the main arm and the behavior analyzed for 5 min. Both of the time spent exploring the arms to reach food, and the time spent in the food arm in seconds, were determined. The frequency and time of entering the food lateral arm was considered to be memory reflector.

Grip-strength meter assay
The Ugo Basile 47,200-Grip-Strength Meter (COMERIO-Varese, Italy) is suitable for mice and can automatically measures grip-strength (i.e. peak force and time resistance) of forelimbs in mice. The aim was to assess forelimbs muscle strength. Each animal was tested three times and the peak force of each mouse was recorded. The mean of three values of each mouse was recorded.

Rota-rod assay
The Ugo Basile Rota-rod instrument (COMERIO-Varese, Italy) has been used in this test. The mouse is placed on a horizontally oriented position and mechanically rotating at 15 rpm rod. The rod is suspended above a cage floor, which is high enough for avoidance of fall. Mice naturally

try to stay on the rotating rod, or Rota-rods, and avoid falling to the ground. The length of time that a given animal stays on this rotating rod is considered as a measure of their balance, coordination, and motor-activity.

Sample collection

For histological studies, brains were removed and cut into small pieces in sterile saline solution, fixed in 10 % neutral buffered formalin and embedded in paraffin. For biochemical investigations, samples were prepared by weighing 200 mg of longitudinal brain sections into a dry and clean Teflon digestion beaker, to which, 6 ml of HNO_3, 2 ml HCl and 2 ml HF were added. Samples were digested on the hot plate at 120–150 °C for 40 min. The resulting digest was filtered through whatman filtered paper no42. The filtered digest was transferred to a 50 ml plastic volumetric flask and completed to the mark using deionized water.

Histological studies

For the histological slides preparation, left loop of cerebellum, cerebral cortex and medulla oblongata of three sacrificed animals were fixed in 20 % formalin saline for 24 h. To remove the excess of the fixative, the tissues were washed and then dehydrated in ascending grades (70, 80, 90 and 95 %) of ethanol for 45 min each, then in two changes of absolute ethanol for 30 min each. This was followed by two changes of xylene for 30 min each. The tissues were then impregnated and embedded in paraplast plus. Sections (4–5 µm) were prepared with a microtome, de-waxed, hydrated and stained in Mayer's haemalum solution for 3 min. The sections were stained in Eosin for one min, washed in tap water and dehydrated in ethanol as described above.

Neurochemical studies

Dopamine and serotonin determination

The level of dopamine and serotonin was estimated in the brain using the modified method of Patrick et al. [21]. A 10 % homogenate of the brain has been re-centrifuged at 17,000 rpm at 4 °C for 5 min. The supernatants were filtered using 0.45 µm pore filters and analyzed by high performance liquid chromatography. The mobile phase consisted of 32 mM citric acid monohydrate, 12.5 mM disodium hydrogen orthophosphate, 7 % methanol, 1 mM octane sulfonic acid and 0.05 mM EDTA. The mobile phase was filtered through 0.22 µm filter and degassed under vacuum before use. Bondpak C18 column was used at a flow rate of 1.2 ml/min and the injection volume of the sample was 20 µl. The levels of dopamine and serotonin were calculated using a calibration curve and results were expressed as ng/mg tissue weight.

Determination of acetylcholine

The level of acetylcholine was estimated in the brain using a method that has been described previously [22]. In brief, dialysate samples were injected into the liquid chromatography/electrochemistry system assisted by a chromatography manager (Millennium; Waters, Milford, MA), and analyzed for acetylcholine. Acetylcholine was separated on a coiled cation exchanger acetylcholine column (analytical column) (Sepstik 530 × 1.0 mm I.D., packed with polymetric strong exchanger, 10 µm in diameter; BAS, West Lafayette, IN), followed by the post-immobilized enzyme reactor which consisted of choline oxidase/acetylcholine esterase. Acetylcholine was hydrolyzed by acetylcholine esterase to form acetate and choline in the post-immobilized enzyme reactor, and then choline was oxidized by choline oxidase to produce betaine and hydrogen peroxide (H_2O_2). H_2O_2 is detected via oxidation of horseradish peroxidase, which in turn entrapped in the redox polymer coated on the surface of the glassy carbon electrode (MF-9080; BAS), set at +100 mV (LC-4C; BAS) versus Ag/AgCl reference electrode. This reduction was analyzed with the detector (LC-4C; BAS) as a signal indicating acetylcholine on the chromatogram.

Reduced Glutathione (GSH) assay

Reduced glutathione content was determined according to the method of Beutler et al. [23] with some modification. Briefly, 0.20 ml of tissue supernatant was mixed with 1.5 ml of the precipitating solution which contains 1.67 % glacial metaphosphoric acid, 0.20 % Na-EDTA and 30 % NaCl. The mixture was allowed to stand for 5 min at room temperature and centrifuged at 1000 rpm for 5 min. One ml clear supernatant was mixed with 4 ml 0.30 M Na_2HPO_4 and 0.50 ml DTNB reagent (40 mg 5, 5′dithiobis-(2-nitrobenzoic acid dissolved in 1 % sodium citrate). The blank was prepared similarly whereas 0.20 ml water was used instead of the brain supernatant. The absorbance of the color was measure at 412 nm in a spectrophotometer.

Statistical analysis

Prior to further statistical analysis, the data were tested for normality using the Anderson–Darling test, as well as for homogeneity variances. The data was normally distributed and is expressed as the mean ± standard error of the mean (SEM). Significant differences among the groups were analysed by one- or two-way ANOVA followed by Tukey's post-test using SPSS software, version 17. Differences were considered statistically significant at $P < 0.05$.

Results

Effect of KBrO₃ on the body weight and water consumption of the treated mice

Figure 1a illustrates that during the first, the second and the last weeks of KBrO₃ treatment, the high dose of KBrO₃ (200 mg/kg) was accompanied with a decrease in body weight in comparison to both the control group and the low dose treated group. On the other hand, the low dose of KBrO₃ (100 mg/kg) effect on body weight decrease, was not significant. Water consumption was investigated to study its correlation with KBrO₃ dose. As illustrated in Fig. 1b, the means of water consumption were similar between all KBrO₃ exposure and control groups throughout the study.

KBrO₃ treatment can cause a disturbance in the behavior of the treated mice

When investigating the behavior of animals in the T-maze, bad memory and low smell ability of the KBrO₃

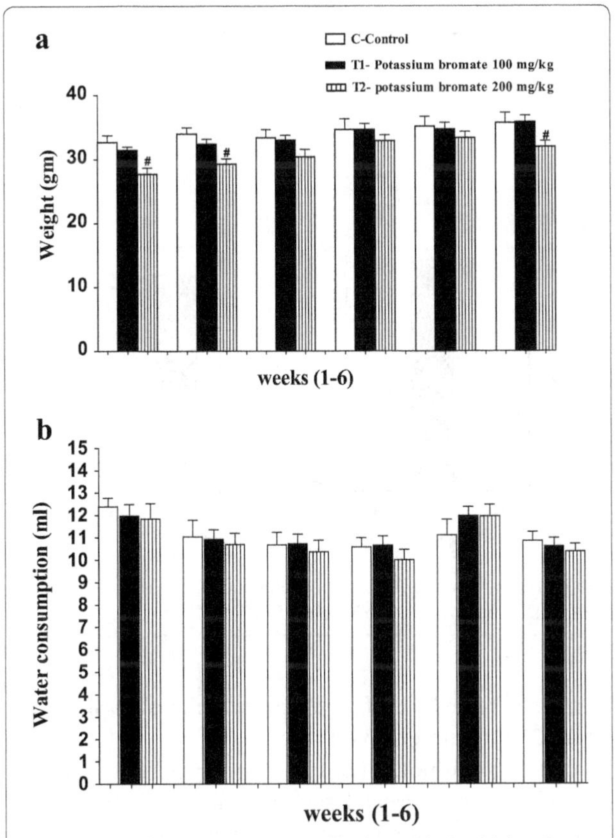

Fig. 1 Effect of KBrO₃ on the mean of body weight (gm) (**a**) and water consumption (ml) (**b**) in treated mice during six successive weeks using two different doses of KBrO₃. The data are the mean ± SEM for 10 mice per group for the control group (*open white bars*), low dose KBrO₃ treated group (*closed black bars*), and high dose KBrO₃ treated group (*hatched bars*). *P < 0.05 for low dose KBrO₃ treated group vs. control group; #P < 0.05 for high dose KBrO₃ treated group vs. control group; +P<0.05 for high dose KBrO₃ treated group vs. low dose KBrO₃ treated group

treated groups during both the 3rd week and the 6th week in comparison to the control group was recorded. This was represented in the reduction of the number of entrances to the main arm (Fig. 2a), the increase in the time consumed to reach to the food in the food arm (Fig. 2b), the decrease in both of the number of entrances to the food arm (Fig. 2c) and the number of entrances to the empty arm (Fig. 2d). Additionally, the Moris—maze examination confirmed the observed bad memory in T-maze. Learning ability was also limited in both of the KBrO₃ groups whereas they consumed much time to reach to the target (Fig. 3a) along four successive days. Still, the harmful effect of the high dose of KBrO₃ is much more significant than that of the low dose one.

The fore-limb muscles of the animals in the group of the KBrO₃ low dose recorded lower beaks in comparison to the control group in the grip strength examination scores. Moreover, the recorded beaks of the high dose KBrO₃ group appeared significantly lower than the control group during both the 3rd and the 6th weeks (Fig. 3b).

In rotator test, both of the KBrO₃ groups have exhibited a short time on the rod during both the 3rd and the 6th weeks in comparison to the animals of the control group. The staying times of the animals of the low dose KBrO₃ group on the rod were less than the time of the control group. For the high dose KBrO₃ group, the staying times of the animals on the rod were lower than that of the low dose group (Fig. 3c).

KBrO₃ treatment is associated with depletion of neurotransmitters in the brain of the treated mice

Dopamine is an important neurotransmitter that plays a number of important roles in the brain. Consequently, investigating the brain level of this molecule after KBrO₃ treatment is of special relevance. In comparison to the control group (49.089 ± 0.634), a significant (*P < 0.05*) depletion of dopamine concentration (39.338 ± 0.533) has been detected in the low dose KBrO₃ group. Also, a highly significant (#P < 0.05) reduction (26.672 ± 0.672) in the dopamine level in the high dose KBrO₃ group in comparison to the control group was recorded (Fig. 4a). Another important monoamine neurotransmitter is serotonin. Here, a significant (*P < 0.05*) reduction (2.331 ± 0.0664) in brain-serotonin concentration in the low dose KBrO₃ group in comparison to the control group (3.243 ± 0.0943) was detected. Additionally, a highly significant (#P < 0.05) decrease (1.756 ± 0.0525) in brain-serotonin concentration in the high dose KBrO₃ group in comparison to the control group was detected (Fig. 4b). Another organic molecule that acts as a neurotransmitter is acetylcholine. Indeed, acetylcholine

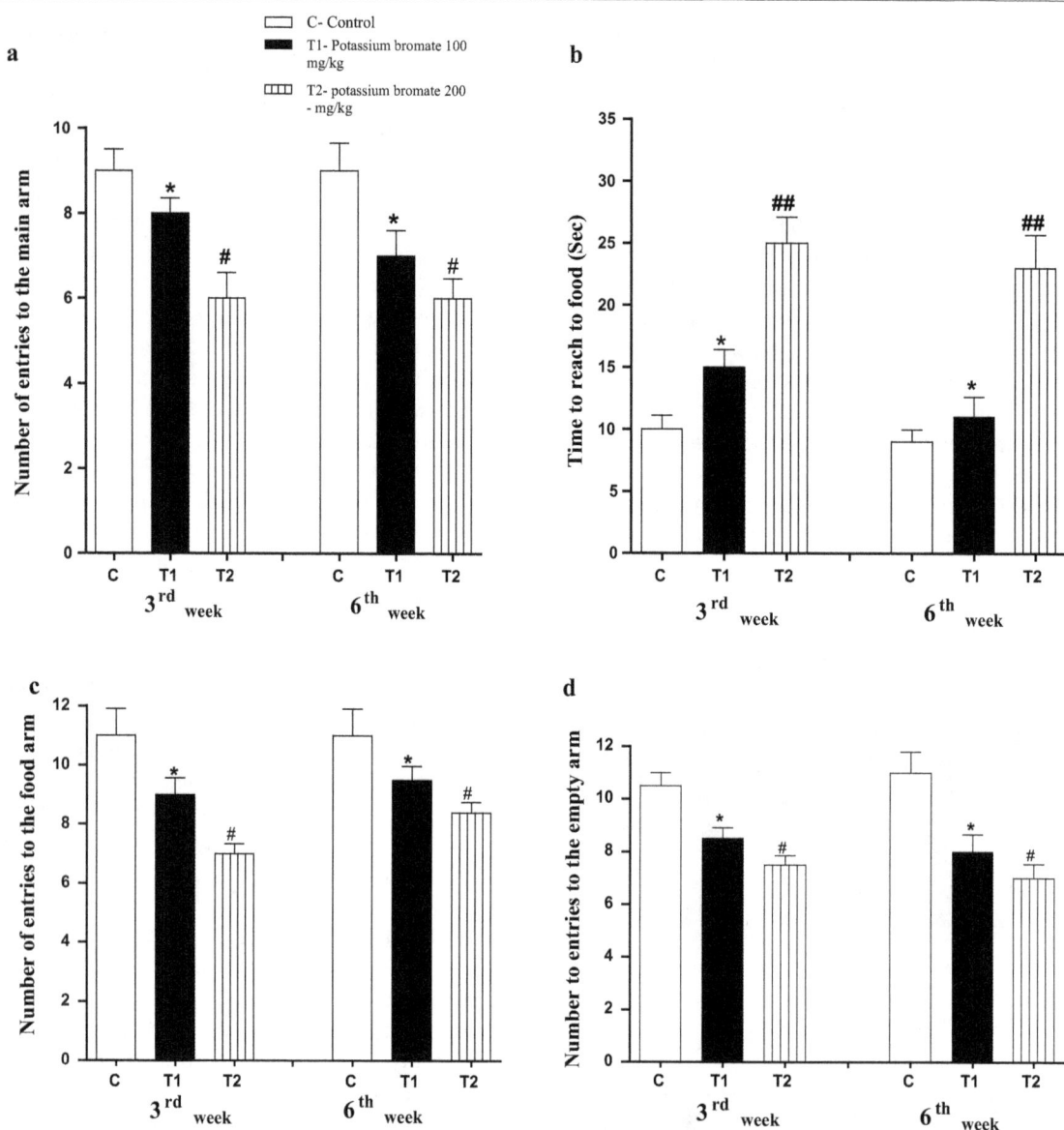

Fig. 2 Effect of KBrO₃ on the animal's behavior in T-maze. **a** The number of entrances of main arm. **b** The time consumed to reach to the food. **c** The number of entrances to the food arm. **d** The number of entrances to the empty arm. Data are expressed as mean ± SEM for 10 mice per group

concentrations showed similar results to that of both dopamine and serotonin. In comparison to the control group (65.678 ± 0.627), acetylcholine concentration in the brain of the low dose KBrO₃ group was significantly (*P < 0.05) reduced (47.936 ± 0.459). Again, the brain level of acetylcholine in the high dose KBrO₃ group was significantly (#P < 0.05) lower (37.16 ± 0.728) than that of both the control group and the low dose KBrO₃ group (Fig. 4c). This harmful effect of KBrO₃ was dominant during both the 3rd and the 6th weeks.

Decreased brain level of reduced glutathione (GSH) after KBrO₃ treatment in animals

Reduced glutathione (GSH) is an important antioxidant that plays a crucial role in nearly all living organisms. KBrO₃ treatment had a negative effect on the brain level of this important molecule. In the low dose KBrO₃ group, the brain level of GSH was significantly (*P < 0.05) reduced (250.31 ± 39.61) in comparison to the control group (420.63 ± 59.61). Also, a significant (#P < 0.05) reduction in the level of this crucial molecule was detected in the high dose KBrO₃ group (110.76 ± 15.87)

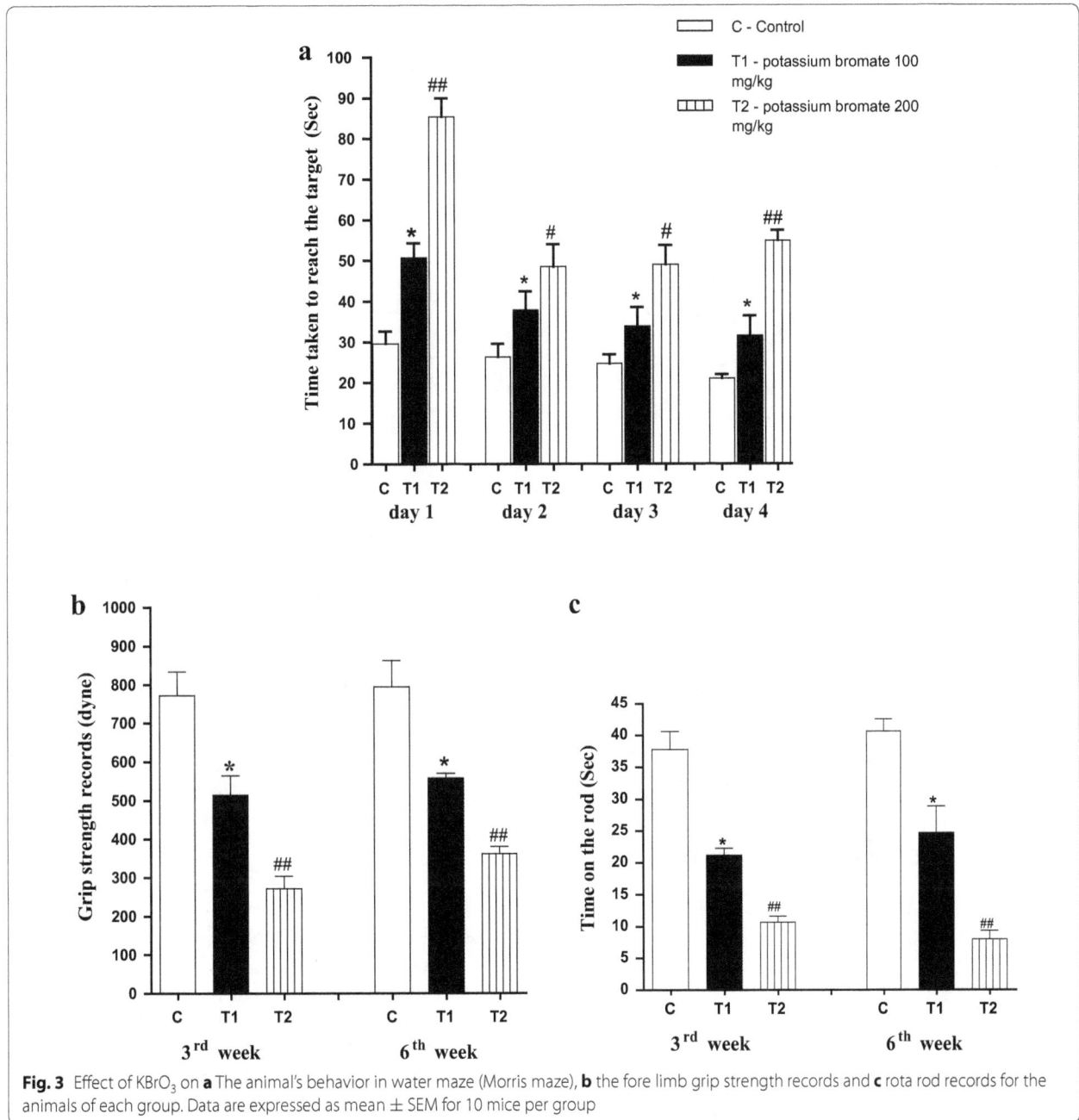

Fig. 3 Effect of KBrO$_3$ on **a** The animal's behavior in water maze (Morris maze), **b** the fore limb grip strength records and **c** rota rod records for the animals of each group. Data are expressed as mean ± SEM for 10 mice per group

in comparison to either the control group or the low dose KBrO$_3$ group (Fig. 5). Like neurotransmitters, the reducing effect of KBrO$_3$ on the glutathione level, was dominant during both the 3rd and the 6th weeks.

KBrO$_3$ treatment has induced brain histopathological changes in mice

In the control group, the normal pyramidal neurons exhibited their general characteristic shape with rounded, large and centrally located nuclei (Fig. 6). The normal

cells of the cerebral cortex had a spherical perikaryon whose nuclei were large. Also the neurons were arranged in a regular pattern (Fig. 6a, b). In both of KBrO$_3$ treated groups, pyknosis and chromatolysis have been observed in the pyramidal neurons (Fig. 6c, d, e, f).

In the cerebellum, the neuronal density in the molecular layer of control group was the highest compared to KBrO$_3$ treated groups. The normal Purkinje cells were arranged in a single row of large neurons with pear-shaped perikaryon and large nucleus. The lateral

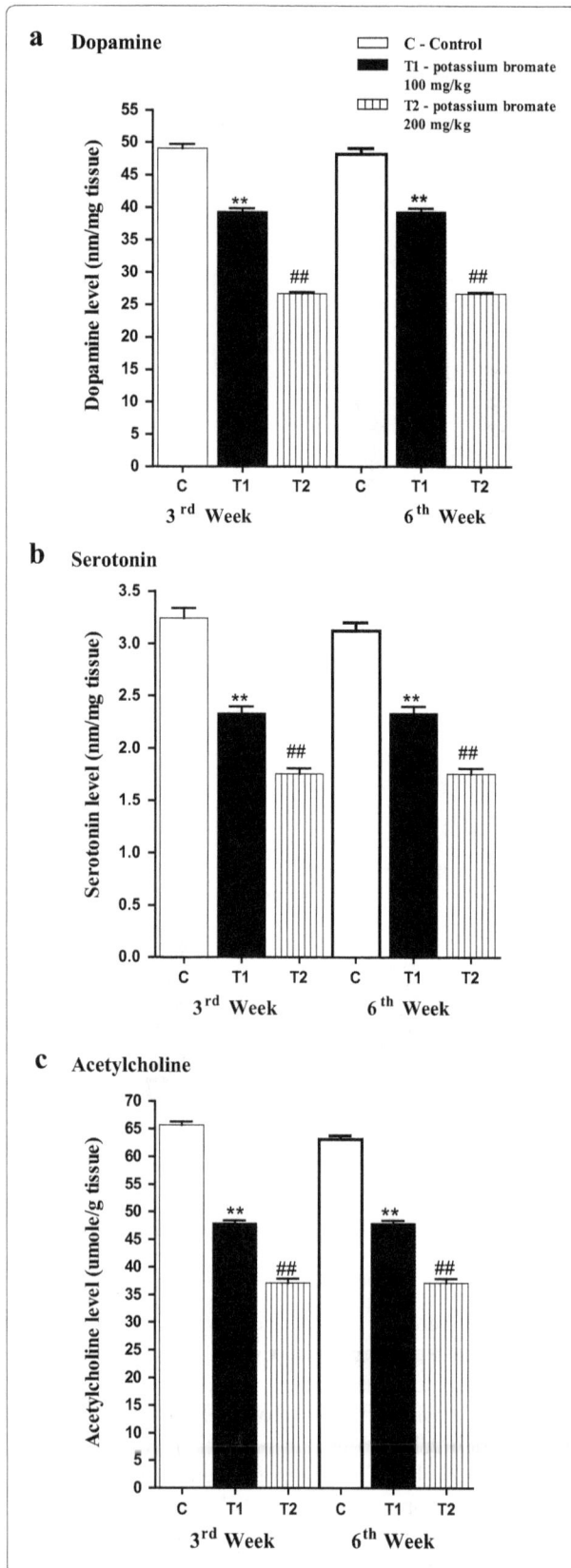

◀ **Fig. 4** Effect of KBrO$_3$ treatments on the level of neurotransmitters in the brain of treated mice. **a** Mean of Dopamine (nm/mg tissue) in brain tissue of treated mice during third and sixth weeks, **b** mean of Serotonin (nm/mg tissue) in brain tissue of treated mice during third and sixth weeks, **c** mean of Acetylcholine (umole/g tissue) in brain tissue of treated mice during third and sixth weeks. Data are expressed as mean ± SEM for 10 mice per group

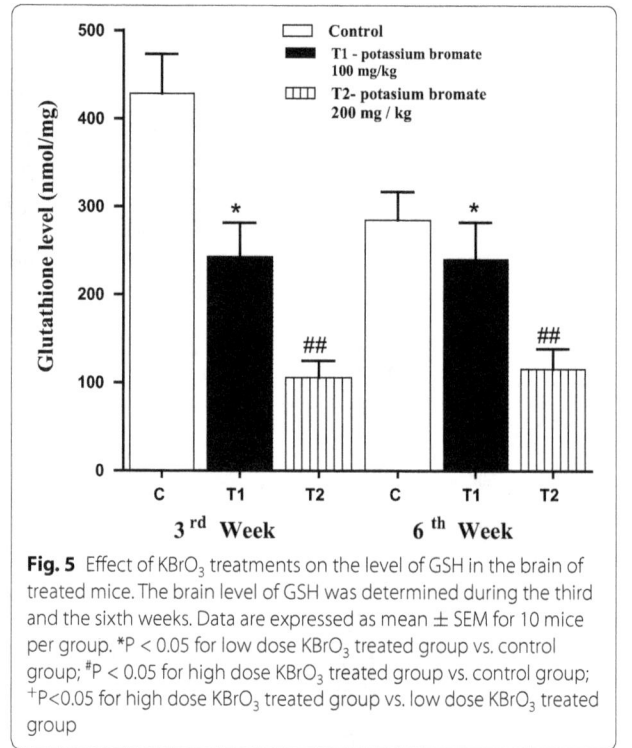

Fig. 5 Effect of KBrO$_3$ treatments on the level of GSH in the brain of treated mice. The brain level of GSH was determined during the third and the sixth weeks. Data are expressed as mean ± SEM for 10 mice per group. *P < 0.05 for low dose KBrO$_3$ treated group vs. control group; #P < 0.05 for high dose KBrO$_3$ treated group vs. control group; +P<0.05 for high dose KBrO$_3$ treated group vs. low dose KBrO$_3$ treated group

processes disappeared and the apical processes formed the permanent dendritic tree (Fig. 7a, b). On the other hand, in both of KBrO$_3$ treated groups, some degenerated Purkinje cells were detected and some were more spindle-shaped and small (Fig. 7c, d, e, f). In control group, the normal neurons in the medulla appeared large in size, polygonal, varied in shape and had round nuclei (Fig. 8a, b). In both of KBrO$_3$ treated groups, most of medulla neurons appeared small and pyknotic (Fig. 8c, d, e, f). Also, degenerated medullary neurons were observed (Fig. 8 d, f).

Discussion

Potassium bromate (KBrO$_3$) is widely used as improving additive for bread making [7] and marketed as a neutralizer in home permanent cold wave hair kits. Several cases of accidental poisoning in children resulting from the ingestion of KBrO$_3$ solution, were reported [9]. Due

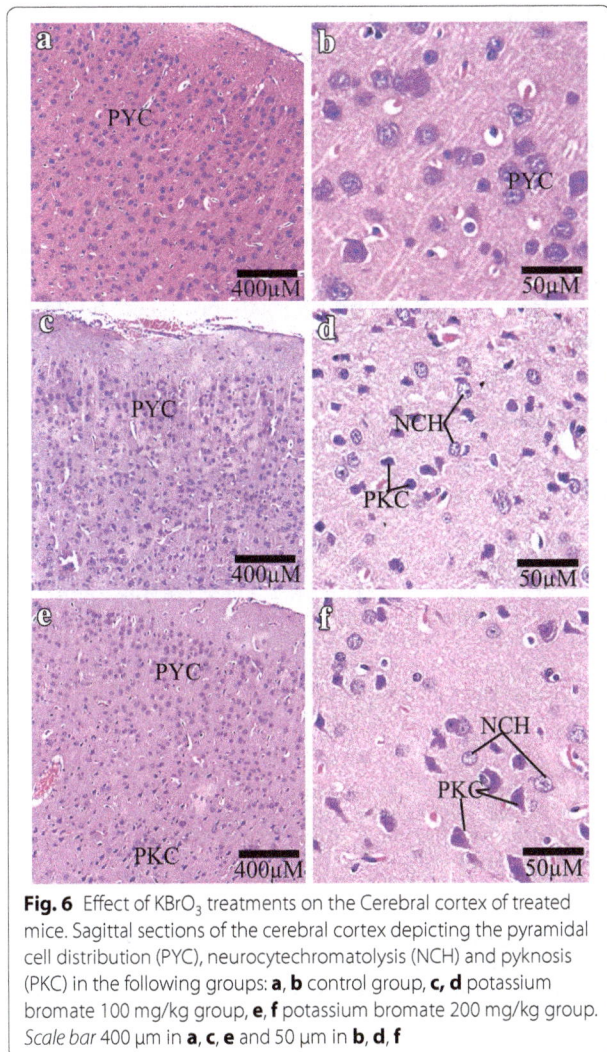

Fig. 6 Effect of KBrO$_3$ treatments on the Cerebral cortex of treated mice. Sagittal sections of the cerebral cortex depicting the pyramidal cell distribution (PYC), neurocytechromatolysis (NCH) and pyknosis (PKC) in the following groups: **a, b** control group, **c, d** potassium bromate 100 mg/kg group, **e, f** potassium bromate 200 mg/kg group. *Scale bar* 400 μm in **a, c, e** and 50 μm in **b, d, f**

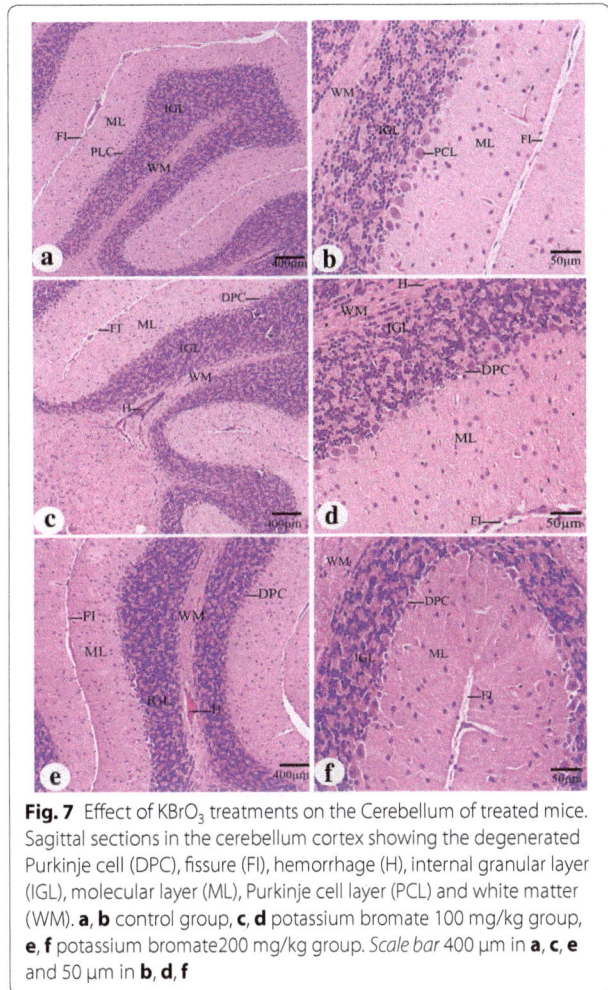

Fig. 7 Effect of KBrO$_3$ treatments on the Cerebellum of treated mice. Sagittal sections in the cerebellum cortex showing the degenerated Purkinje cell (DPC), fissure (FI), hemorrhage (H), internal granular layer (IGL), molecular layer (ML), Purkinje cell layer (PCL) and white matter (WM). **a, b** control group, **c, d** potassium bromate 100 mg/kg group, **e, f** potassium bromate 200 mg/kg group. *Scale bar* 400 μm in **a, c, e** and 50 μm in **b, d, f**

to its hazardous effects, it has been forbidden in various countries [2]. Toxicity studies in animals are commonly used to assess potential health risk in humans caused by intrinsic adverse effects of chemical compounds [24]. These adverse effects may manifest significant alterations in the levels of bio molecules, normal functioning and histomorphology of the organs [3]. The current study was designed to investigate some of the behavioral and biochemical changes induced by KBrO$_3$ intake in albino mice. We have observed that oral intubation of KBrO$_3$ at the dose of 200 mg/dl was accompanied with an obvious decrease in the body weight of the animals while the lower dose cannot do this effect. This is in agreement with the results obtained by Kurokawa et al. [25] who have reported a dose-dependent inhibition of body weight increase in both male and female F344 rats after oral administration of KBrO$_3$. Also, similar results were obtained with guinea pigs [11]. Water consumption was not affected by the oral administration of KBrO$_3$ with either the 100 or 200 mg/dl doses. These results agree with that of Dodd et al. [26] who have reported that only the 400 mg/L dose can result in a significant increase in water consumption and other lower doses cannot. Many environmental contaminants were reported to be associated with behavioral changes and this was elucidated in many studies before [27–31]. The abnormal pattern in open-field, social, learning and emotional behaviors were documented in Wister rats after receiving Sodium nitrite in the drinking water [32]. KBrO$_3$-mediated behavioral changes seen in the current study may be attributed partially to the harmful effect of KBrO$_3$ on the brain level of neurotransmitters. It was reported that abnormalities in the regulation of neurotransmitter release and/or abnormal levels of extracellular neurotransmitter concentrations are considered as core components of hypotheses on the neuronal foundations of behavioral

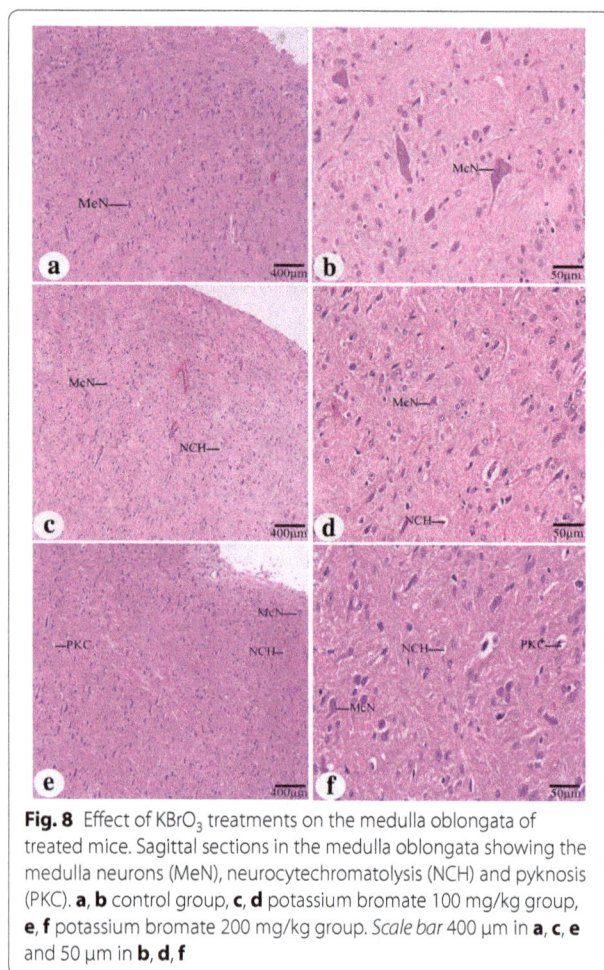

Fig. 8 Effect of KBrO$_3$ treatments on the medulla oblongata of treated mice. Sagittal sections in the medulla oblongata showing the medulla neurons (MeN), neurocytechromatolysis (NCH) and pyknosis (PKC). **a**, **b** control group, **c**, **d** potassium bromate 100 mg/kg group, **e**, **f** potassium bromate 200 mg/kg group. *Scale bar* 400 μm in **a**, **c**, **e** and 50 μm in **b**, **d**, **f**

antioxidant status and brain histomorphology of white albino rat and that using two different doses of KBrO$_3$ has different outcomes.

Conclusions

Potassium bromate has deleterious effects on the central nervous system of mice. It can disturb the neurotransmitters levels, antioxidant defence molecules and induce histopathological changes in cerebral tissue. Therefore, its use in human used- products should be stopped.

Abbreviations
EDTA: ethylene diamine tetra acetic Acid; ICP-MS: inductively coupled plasma mass spectrometer; GSH: reduced glutathione; KBrO$_3$: potassium bromate; CNS: central nervous system; H$_2$O$_2$: hydrogen peroxide.

Authors' contributions
JA and NA carried out the experimental work, participated in the design of the study. AA and SN provided expertise in the HPLC–MS analysis and participated in the design and coordination of the study. MA participated in the design of the study, revised the whole Ms and performed statistical revision. All authors read and approved the final manuscript.

Author details
[1] Department of Zoology, College of Science, King Saud University, P.O. Box 2455, Riyadh 11451, Saudi Arabia. [2] Department of Zoology, Faculty of Science, Beni-suef University, Beni-Suef, Egypt. [3] School of Biological Sciences, University of Hong Kong, Hong Kong, China.

Acknowledgements
We extend our appreciation to the Dean of Scientific Research, King Saud University, for funding the work through the research group project number RGP-VPP-240.

Competing interests
The authors declare no competing interests. This manuscript has not been published or submitted elsewhere. This work complies with the Ethical Policies of the Journal and has been conducted under internationally accepted ethical standards following relevant ethical review.

References
1. Vadlamani KR, Seib PA. Effect of zinc and aluminium ions in bread making. Cereal Chem. 1999;76:355–60.
2. Oloyede OB, Sunmonu TO. Potassium bromate content of selected bread samples in Ilorin, Central Nigeria and its effect on some enzymes of rat liver and kidney. Food Chem Toxicol. 2009;47:2067–70.
3. Ahmad MK, Mahmood R. Protective effect of taurine against potassium bromate-induced hemoglobin oxidation, oxidative stress, and impairment of antioxidant defense system in blood. Environ Toxicol. 2014. doi:10.1002/tox.22045.
4. Chipman JK, Davies JE, Parsons JL, Nair J, O'Neill G, Fawell JK. DNA oxidation by potassium bromate; a direct mechanism or linked to lipid peroxidation. Toxicology. 1998;126:93–102.
5. Farombi EO, Alabi MC, Akuru TO. Kolaviron modulates cellular redox status and impairment of membrane protein activities induced by potassium bromate KBr O3 in rats. Pharmacol Res. 2002;45:63–8.
6. Kujawska M, Ignatowicz E, Ewertowska M, Adamska T, Markowski J, Jodynis-Liebert J. Attenuation of KBr O$_3$-induced renal and hepatic toxicity by cloudy apple juice in rat. Phytother Res. 2013;27:1214–9.

and cognitive disorders and the symptoms of neuropsychiatric and neurodegenerative disorders [13]. GSH is the most abundant antioxidant molecule that is critical for protecting the brain from oxidative stress, acting as a free radical scavenger and inhibitor of lipid peroxidation. In the current study, the decrease in the brain level of the antioxidant molecule, GSH, could be considered as an important reason for the observed behavioral changes. Previous reports have documented a direct relationship between behavioral changes and oxidative stress [33, 34]. Oxidative stress can mediate neurodegeneration in hippocampus and behavioral changes of adult rats [35]. Concomitantly, KBrO$_3$ induced pathological changes on the histological level in the brain tissue of the treated rats which may be considered as another important causative factor for the negative behavioral changes. Previous studies have reported hemorrhage, neuronal degeneration and vacuolation of the brain tissue sections of rats after KBrO$_3$ treatment [19]. Taken together, our data illustrate that oral administration of KBrO$_3$ has a direct effect on the behavioral level, neurotransmitters content,

7. Ahmad MK, Khan AA, Ali SN, Mahmood R. Chemoprotective effect of taurine on potassium bromate-induced DNA damage, DNA-protein crosslinking and oxidative stress in rat intestine. PLoS One. 2015. doi:10.1371/journal.pone.0119137.

8. Robert IA, William BC. Carcinogenicity of potassium bromate in rabbit. Biol Edu. 1996;34:114–20.

9. Paul AH. Chemical food poisoning by potassium bromate. NZ Med J. 1966;65:33–40.

10. Young YH, Chuu JJ, Liu SH, Lin-Shiau SY. Toxic effects of potassium bromate and thioglycolate on vestibule ocular reflex systems of Guinea pigs and humans. Toxicol Appl Pharmacol. 2001;177:103–11.

11. Chuu JJ, Hsu CJ, Lin-Shiau SY. The detrimental effects of potassium bromate and thioglycolate on auditory brainstem response of Guinea pigs. Chin J Physiol. 2000;43:91–6.

12. Allain H, Schuck S. Neurotransmitters and behavioral disorders. Encephale. 1998;1:34–7.

13. Sarter M, Bruno JP, Parikh V. Abnormal neurotransmitter release underlying behavioral and cognitive disorders: toward concepts of dynamic and function-specific dysregulation. Neuropsychopharmacology. 2007;32:1452–61.

14. Kita T, Miyazaki I, Asanuma M, Takeshima M, Wagner GC. Dopamine-induced behavioral changes and oxidative stress in methamphetamine-induced neurotoxicity. Int Rev Neurobiol. 2009;88:43–64.

15. Sai K, Takagi A, Umemura T, Hasegawa R, Kurokawa Y. Relation of 8-hydroxydeoxyguanosine formation in rat kidney to lipid peroxidation, glutathione level and relative organ weight after a single administration of potassium bromate. J Cancer Res. 1991;82:165–9.

16. Watanabe T, Abe T, Satoh M. Two children with bromate intoxication dueto ingestion of the second preparation for permanent hair waving. Act Paediatr Jpn. 1992;34:601–5.

17. Parsons JL, Chipman JK. DNA oxidation by potassium bromate: a direct mechanism or linked to peroxidation. Toxicology. 1992;126:93–102.

18. Parsons JL, Chipman JK. The role of glutathione in DNA damage by potassium bromate in vitro. Mutagenesis. 2000;15:311–6.

19. Abuelgasim A, Omer R, Elmahdi B. Serrobiochemical Effects of Potassium Bromate on Wistar Albino Rats. Am J Food Technol. 2008;3:303–9.

20. Ajarem JS, Ahmad M. Behavioral and biochemical consequences of perinatal exposure of mice to instant coffee: a correlative evaluation. Pharmacol Biochem Behav. 1991;40:847–52.

21. Patrick OE, Hirohisa M, Masahira K, Koreaki M. Central nervous system bioaminergic responses to mechanic trauma. Surg Neurol. 1991;35:273–9.

22. Ichikawa J, Li Z, Dai J, Meltzer HY. Atypical antipsychotic drugs, quetiapine, iloperidone, and melperone, preferentially increase dopamine and acetylcholine release in rat medial prefrontal cortex: role of 5-HT1A receptor agonism. Brain Res. 2002;956:349–57.

23. Beutler E, Duron O, Kelly BM. Improved method for determination of blood glutathione. J Lab Clin Med. 1963;61:882–8.

24. Kurokawa Y, Maekawa A, Takahashi M, Hayashi Y. Toxicity and carcinogenicity of potassium bromate–a new renal carcinogen. Environ Health Perspect. 1990;87:309–35.

25. Kurokawa Y, Aoki S, Matsushima Y, Takamura N, Imazawa T, Hayashi Y. Dose-response studies on the carcinogenicity of potassium bromate in F344 rats after long-term oral administration. J Natl Cancer Inst. 1986;77:977–82.

26. Dodd DE, Layko DK, Cantwell KE, Willson GA, Thomas RS. Subchronic toxicity evaluation of potassium bromate in Fischer 344 rats. Environ Toxicol Pharmacol. 2013;36:1227–34.

27. Branchi I, Capone F, Alleva E, Costa LG. Poly brominated diphenyl ethers: neurobehavioral effects following developmental exposure. Neurotoxicology. 2003;24:449–62.

28. Eriksson P, Jakobsson E, Fredriksson A. Brominated flame retardants: a novel class of developmental neurotoxicants in our environment. Environ Health Perspect. 2001;109:903–8.

29. Eriksson P, Fischer C, Fredriksson A. Polybrominateddiphenyl ethers, a group of brominated flame retardants, can interact with polychlorinated biphenyls in enhancing developmental neurobehavioral defects. Toxicol Sci. 2006;94:302–9.

30. Viberg H, Fredriksson A, Eriksson P. Neonatal exposure to poly brominated diphenyl ether (PBDE 153) disrupts spontaneous behaviour, impairs learning and memory, and decreases hippocampal cholinergic receptors in adult mice. Toxicol Appl Pharmacol. 2003;192:95–106.

31. Viberg H, Johansson N, Fredriksson A, Eriksson J, Marsh G, Eriksson P. Neonatal exposure to higher brominated diphenyl ethers, hepta-, octa-, or nonabromodiphenyl ether, impairs spontaneous behavior and learning and memory functions of adult mice. Toxicol Sci. 2006;92:211–8.

32. Nyakas C, Buwalda B, Markel E, Korte SM, Luiten PG. Life-spanning behavioral and adrenal dysfunction induced by prenatal hypoxia in the rat is prevented by the calcium antagonist nimodipine. Eur J Neurosci. 1994;6:746–53.

33. Tasset I, Peña J, Jimena I, Feijóo M, Del Carmen Muñoz M, Montilla P, Túnez I. Effect of 17beta-estradiol on olfactory bulbectomy-induced oxidative stress and behavioral changes in rats. Neuropsychiatr Dis Treat. 2008;4:441–9.

34. da-Rosa DD, Valvassori SS, Steckert AV, Ornell F, Ferreira CL, Lopes-Borges J, Varela RB, Dal-Pizzol F, Andersen ML, Quevedo J. Effects of lithium and valproate on oxidative stress and behavioral changes induced by administration of m-AMPH. Psychiatry Res. 2012;15:521–6.

35. Selvakumar K, Bavithra S, Ganesh L, Krishnamoorthy G, Venkataraman P, Arunakaran J. Polychlorinated biphenyls induced oxidative stress mediated neurodegeneration in hippocampus and behavioral changes of adult rats: anxiolytic-like effects of quercetin. Toxicol Lett. 2013;222:45–54.

17

The neural correlates of mental arithmetic in adolescents: a longitudinal fNIRS study

Christina Artemenko[1,2*] iD, Mojtaba Soltanlou[2,3,4], Ann-Christine Ehlis[1,5], Hans-Christoph Nuerk[1,2,4†] and Thomas Dresler[1,5†]

Abstract

Background: Arithmetic processing in adults is known to rely on a frontal-parietal network. However, neurocognitive research focusing on the neural and behavioral correlates of arithmetic development has been scarce, even though the acquisition of arithmetic skills is accompanied by changes within the fronto-parietal network of the developing brain. Furthermore, experimental procedures are typically adjusted to constraints of functional magnetic resonance imaging, which may not reflect natural settings in which children and adolescents actually perform arithmetic. Therefore, we investigated the longitudinal neurocognitive development of processes involved in performing the four basic arithmetic operations in 19 adolescents. By using functional near-infrared spectroscopy, we were able to use an ecologically valid task, i.e., a written production paradigm.

Results: A common pattern of activation in the bilateral fronto-parietal network for arithmetic processing was found for all basic arithmetic operations. Moreover, evidence was obtained for decreasing activation during subtraction over the course of 1 year in middle and inferior frontal gyri, and increased activation during addition and multiplication in angular and middle temporal gyri. In the self-paced block design, parietal activation in multiplication and left angular and temporal activation in addition were observed to be higher for simple than for complex blocks, reflecting an inverse effect of arithmetic complexity.

Conclusions: In general, the findings suggest that the brain network for arithmetic processing is already established in 12–14 year-old adolescents, but still undergoes developmental changes.

Keywords: Functional near-infrared spectroscopy (fNIRS), Adolescents, Mental arithmetic, Arithmetic complexity, Longitudinal development, Natural setting

Background

Arithmetic processing consistently activates a fronto-parietal network in the adult brain, which includes parietal regions such as the superior parietal lobule (SPL) and inferior parietal lobule (IPL), and frontal regions such as the inferior frontal gyrus (IFG), middle frontal gyrus (MFG) and left superior frontal gyrus (for a meta-analysis see [1]; see also [2–4]). In children, arithmetic processing also generally recruits a similar fronto-parietal network ([5–7]; for a review see [8]); however, some differences have been reported between children and adults. Specifically, arithmetic processing seems to be less functionally specialized in children, which leads to less parietal activation especially in the intraparietal sulcus (IPS) for children compared to adolescents and for adolescents compared to adults [7, 9]. But since neurocognitive development does not necessarily progress linearly, it is not possible to generalize the neural and behavioral correlates of arithmetic processing from either adults or children to adolescents, an underrepresented age cohort in

*Correspondence: christina.artemenko@uni-tuebingen.de
†Hans-Christoph Nuerk and Thomas Dresler contributed equally and should be considered as shared senior authors
2 Department of Psychology, University of Tuebingen, Tuebingen, Germany
Full list of author information is available at the end of the article

neurocognitive research (for a review see [8]; for a meta-analysis see [10]). Therefore, the focus of the current study is to systematically investigate the neurocognitive correlates of arithmetic processing in adolescents by considering developmental activation changes as well as different complexity levels in all basic arithmetic operations.

Neurocognitive development of arithmetic processing in children and adolescents

During childhood, the neurocognitive underpinnings of arithmetic change with age and development: with increasing age, children show decreasing activation in bilateral SFG, MFG and the left IFG, indicating reduced reliance on working memory and attentional resources, and simultaneously increasing activation in the left supramarginal gyrus and IPS, which is a core area in number processing ([11]; see also [7, 9, 12, 13]; for meta-analyses see [14, 15]). This so-called *fronto-parietal shift* in brain activation can be considered to represent the increasing functional specialization of the parietal cortex for arithmetic processing accompanied by decreasing reliance on domain-general cognitive processes [16].

While there is broad evidence for the fronto-parietal shift during development, the specific activation changes seem to depend on age, arithmetic content and design. For instance, contradictory findings exist from cross-sectional to longitudinal studies on arithmetic development in 7–9 year-old children within 1 school year: Rosenberg-Lee et al. [17] found increased fronto-parietal activation in a cross-sectional study, while Qin et al. [18] found a general reduction of activation in the fronto-parietal network and increasing hippocampal activation in a longitudinal study.

In summary, there is evidence for the fronto-parietal activation shift during development in general. However, contradictory neural findings were reported for development during elementary school when arithmetic skills are taught, and furthermore children's arithmetic development is quite heterogeneous [15, 19], which limits the conclusions of cross-sectional designs. Finally, very little is known about arithmetic development in adolescents during secondary school when they already possess arithmetic knowledge. Therefore, we chose to investigate the neurocognitive underpinnings of arithmetic development during 1 year of secondary school in a longitudinal design.

Neurocognitive processing of arithmetic complexity in children

Besides interindividual differences in arithmetic skills during development, neurocognitive processing is also affected by arithmetic complexity which differs between problems (for an overview see [20, 21]). In mental arithmetic, complexity is increased when additional arithmetic procedures have to be applied (e.g., carry and borrow procedures) or when the numerical magnitude of the operands is relatively large (e.g., two-digit versus single-digit operands). Problems that require carrying in addition (unit sum is larger than 9) or borrowing in subtraction (subtrahend unit is larger than minuend unit) are more difficult for children than problems without these procedures (e.g., [22]). The carry and borrow effects are primarily associated with activation in frontal areas such as the left IFG, bilateral MFG and SFG, as well as with activation in parietal areas such as the left IPS in adults [23–27]. However, the neural correlates of the carry and borrow effects have so far not been investigated in children or adolescents.

Arithmetic complexity indexes not only the need for additional arithmetic procedures like carrying or borrowing, which recruit mainly domain-general processes in children [28], but also domain-specific attributes such as numerical magnitude. Indeed, arithmetic problems with relatively large operands are more difficult to solve than problems with relatively small operands as reflected by the problem size effect in children (e.g., [29]). On a neural level, the problem size effect in single-digit arithmetic in children was found to be associated with increased activation in the IPS, SPL, left MFG, and IFG in addition [17, 30, 31] and subtraction [30, 32], and in the left IPS and left DLPFC in multiplication [32]. Moreover, two-digit (as compared to single-digit) problems led to higher activation in IPS and angular gyrus (AG) in addition [5] and in the right MFG in multiplication [33]. Furthermore, with increasing problem size less activation in AG and superior temporal gyri was observed [5, 30].

To summarize, the literature suggests that carrying/borrowing and problem size both increase arithmetic complexity by enhancing domain-general and domain-specific processing demands, respectively. Although both types of arithmetic complexity are associated with distributed fronto-parietal activation, we expect the carry and borrow effects to be represented mostly in frontal and partially in parietal brain regions in children, while the opposite pattern is expected for the problem size effect. In this study, we will investigate both types of arithmetic complexity in different arithmetic operations, since brain activation patterns have been shown to be operation-specific, particularly in children and adolescents ([30, 32, 34]; but see [6]) and the effects of arithmetic complexity seem to depend on the operation (e.g., for multiplication see [35, 36]). The neural substrates of division have not been investigated in children and adolescents so far (except for a structural diffusion tensor imaging (DTI) study [37]). Therefore, arithmetic complexity will be addressed using all four basic arithmetic operations in the current study, i.e., the carry and borrow effects in addition and subtraction, and the problem size effect in multiplication and division.

An ecologically valid assessment of arithmetic processing in children

The typical arithmetic tasks used in neuroimaging studies differ from the tasks usually employed in schools, where children and adolescents typically have to *produce* written solutions for arithmetic problems, often in a time-restricted manner. Typical neuroimaging studies investigating the correlates of arithmetic in adults use verification or forced choice paradigms instead of written production paradigms (as an exception see e.g., [38] for an oral production paradigm) and fixed designs instead of self-paced designs (as an exception see e.g., [39] for a self-paced design). Importantly, these differences need to be considered, because they seem to evoke different cognitive processes as well.

First, verification and forced choice paradigms, which are particularly apt for movement-sensitive fMRI measurements, allow for shortcut strategies depending on the distractor, and include additional decision and recognition processes (cf. [25, 40–42]) not involved in the spontaneous calculation of arithmetic problems. Thus, these paradigms have little in common with the written production process usually employed in school. Second, in fixed designs, the average neural activation across trials is compared between conditions. If the reaction time differs between conditions, this can lead to systematic activation differences depending on task duration, while self-paced responses allow for a different number of trials within each block. Self-paced designs were further shown to be comparable to fixed designs in sensitivity and even superior in reproducibility and reliability [43].

In order to assess the neural activation patterns underlying calculation in a more natural setting, a written production paradigm within a self-paced block design was used in this study (cf. [33]). A written production paradigm as used in schools can be realized by using functional near-infrared spectroscopy (fNIRS) to assess task-related neural activation, since this method is relatively movement-insensitive, allows for natural body postures, and can be easily administered in students [44–46].

Objectives

The aim of this study is to understand arithmetic development and complexity in adolescents, by investigating arithmetic processing for all four basic operations with varying complexity in a natural setting, in a longitudinal design so that individual differences can be controlled. Specifically, we will address the following issues:

1. Do brain activity patterns change within frontal and parietal regions for all arithmetic operations over the course of 1 year? In line with the frontal-to-parietal shift hypothesis, a simultaneous decrease in frontal activation and increase in parietal activation is expected.
2. Do the neural correlates of the basic arithmetic operations in adolescents vary with arithmetic complexity? It is expected that the carry effect in addition and the borrow effect in subtraction mainly lead to larger frontal activation, while problem size effects in multiplication and division mainly lead to larger parietal activation associated with number magnitude processing.

These questions will be addressed by investigating all four basic arithmetic operations at differing complexity levels in 12–14 year-old adolescents in grades 6 and 7 in an fNIRS study. While basic arithmetic skills are mostly acquired in elementary school, it is unclear whether they still undergo further automatization in older children and adolescents. In order to assess arithmetic processing in a natural setting, a written production paradigm with self-paced responses will be used, and a standardized arithmetic test will serve for the evaluation of generalizability to arithmetic skills.

Methods
Participants

Twenty-six adolescents (20 male) were recruited through local schools and a university mailing list. Nineteen adolescents completed both measurements at the end of grades 6 and 7 (16 male; age in grade 6: $M \pm SD = 12.19 \pm 0.33$, range $= 11.75–12.75$ years; age in grade 7: $M \pm SD = 13.34 \pm 0.35$, range $= 12.75–13.92$ years). The time interval between the two measurements was 1 year (interval in months: $M \pm SD = 13.73 \pm 1.05$, range $= 12–15$ months). All adolescents attended a German secondary school, showed no history of neurological or mental disorders, and all except for three left-handed participants were right-handed. Non-verbal intelligence was assessed by the matrix reasoning subtest of HAWIK-IV and verbal intelligence by the similarities subtest of HAWIK-IV (Hamburg–Wechsler-Intelligenztest für Kinder-IV; [47]). The adolescents showed on average scores of 108.68 ± 10.91 for non-verbal intelligence and 110.00 ± 9.57 for verbal intelligence (IQ $\pm SD$). The standardized assessed arithmetic ability of the adolescents was 57.21 ± 8.70 (T score $\pm SD$), as assessed by the arithmetic subtest of DEMAT 5+ (Deutscher Mathematiktest für fünfte Klassen; [48]).

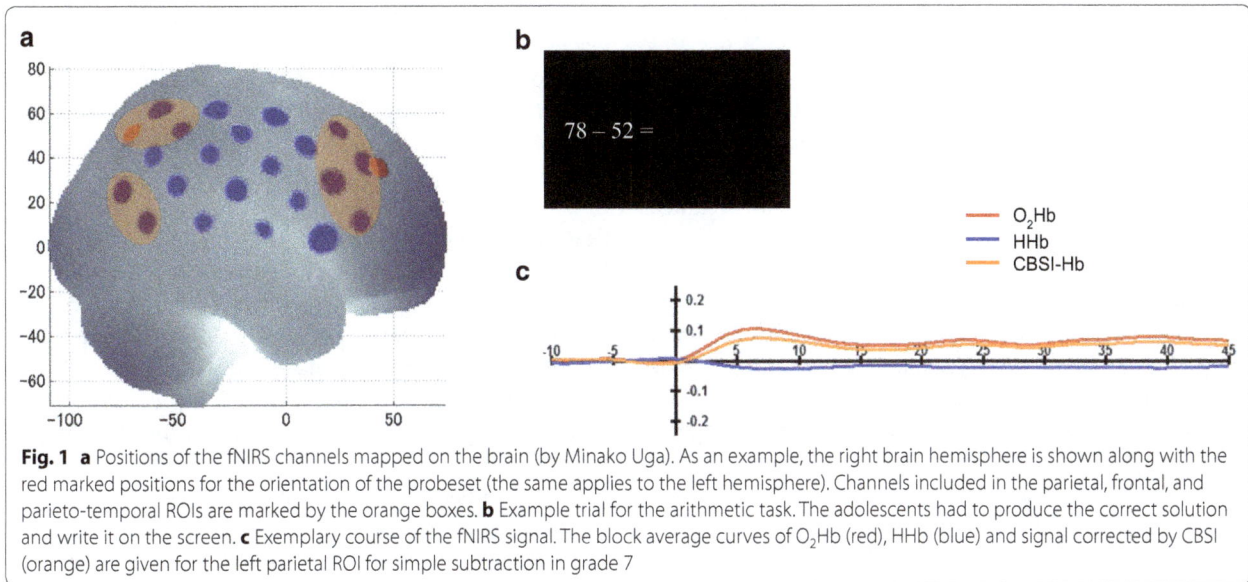

Fig. 1 **a** Positions of the fNIRS channels mapped on the brain (by Minako Uga). As an example, the right brain hemisphere is shown along with the red marked positions for the orientation of the probeset (the same applies to the left hemisphere). Channels included in the parietal, frontal, and parieto-temporal ROIs are marked by the orange boxes. **b** Example trial for the arithmetic task. The adolescents had to produce the correct solution and write it on the screen. **c** Exemplary course of the fNIRS signal. The block average curves of O_2Hb (red), HHb (blue) and signal corrected by CBSI (orange) are given for the left parietal ROI for simple subtraction in grade 7

Arithmetic tasks

All adolescents solved computerized addition, subtraction, multiplication, and division tasks which were presented in blocks with two complexity levels (simple, complex). The addition and subtraction tasks consisted of two two-digit operands with a two-digit solution. In simple blocks, the addition problems did not require the carry procedure and, accordingly, the subtraction problems did not require the borrow procedure. In complex blocks, the arithmetic problems requiring and not requiring the carry and borrow procedure were mixed, with no more than two no-carry or no-borrow problems in a row. The mixing of problems with and without carry or borrow procedure was meant to ensure that the adolescents had to decide whether or not to apply the carry or borrow procedure in each problem, and not just apply it during the whole block. The subtraction problems were constructed as the inverse of addition problems (e.g., $26 + 52 = 78 \rightarrow 78 - 52 = 26$). In the multiplication task, simple blocks included problems with two single-digit operands between 2 and 9 (solutions range between 12 and 72), while complex blocks included problems with one single-digit operand between 2 and 9 and one two-digit operand between 12 and 19 (solutions range between 32 and 162). The division problems were constructed as the inverse of multiplication problems (e.g., $8 \times 4 = 32 \rightarrow 32 : 4 = 8$).

The items were randomly chosen from a set of 50 items per operation and complexity level. In each stimulus set, the operands were matched in their numerical magnitude and parity. The units and decades of the operands were matched in their numerical magnitude and the position of the larger operand was counterbalanced in each

condition. Pure decades (e.g., 20), tie numbers (e.g., 44) and numbers sharing the same digit between operands or the solution (e.g., $34 + 38$) were excluded (for a similar procedure see [25]).

The arithmetic tasks were presented in a block design with a block length of 45 s, an inter-block-interval of 20 s, and four blocks per operation and complexity level, i.e., 32 blocks in total. Simple and complex blocks of all operations were pseudorandomized for each participant and presented in the same order at both measurement points. The arithmetic problems along with an equal sign were horizontally presented in white against black background on the left side of the computer screen (cf. Fig. 1b) using the software package Presentation (NeuroBehavioral Systems, Inc., Berkeley, USA). In a production paradigm, the adolescents were instructed to mentally solve the arithmetic problems and to write the solution on the touch screen using a contact pen (cf. [33]). The trace of the contact pen on the touch screen during the written responses was not visible to the adolescents and the screen remained black in order to emphasize mental arithmetic. Within a self-paced design, each trial followed after a fixed inter-trial-interval of 500 ms, after the button press or after the response time limit if no response was made. Therefore, the number of items within a block varied within and between participants. The time limits were chosen based on the study of Huber et al. [49], i.e., calculated by $M + 1$ SD regarding the sum of correctly and incorrectly solved trials within the time window: 5 and 6 s for simple and complex addition (a minimum of 9 simple and 8 complex trials per block), 6 and 9 s for simple and complex subtraction (a minimum of 8 simple and 5 complex trials per block), 7 and 25 s for simple and complex multiplication (a minimum of 7 simple and 2 complex trials per block), and 7 and 45 s for simple and complex division (a minimum of 7 simple and 1 complex trial per block), respectively. The testing phase was preceded by four practice trials for adolescents to become familiar with the arithmetic tasks. In total, the arithmetic tasks lasted 35 min and additionally included a break after two out of four runs.

Procedure

The measurements were conducted with adolescents at the end of grade 6 and 1 year later at the end of grade 7. In both experimental sessions, the adolescents solved computerized tasks for all four basic arithmetic operations during fNIRS recording in a dimly lit room. The adolescents were seated in front of the touch screen, which was placed in an angle of 37 degrees, and the fNIRS optodes were inserted into the cap on their head after pushing aside the hair at each position (for a picture of the general experimental setup, see Fig. 1c in the study of [33], p. 727). Additionally, arithmetic ability and intelligence were assessed in grade 6 before and after fNIRS measurement, respectively. The adolescents underwent further assessments in each session and performed two additional tasks during the fNIRS recording in grade 6 that are not part of this study.

fNIRS data acquisition

fNIRS was measured using the ETG-4000 Optical Topography System (Hitachi Medical Corporation, Tokyo, Japan). Continuous laser diodes with wavelengths of 695 ± 20 nm and 830 ± 20 nm were used as light sources. The sampling rate was 10 Hz. Two probesets with 22 channels and an inter-optode distance of 30 mm were integrated in an elastic cap in order to cover the left and right hemisphere. The probesets were placed into the cap by localizing the upper channels in the back at P3/P4 and orienting this channel row towards F3/F4 (according to the 10/20 system [50]; cf. Fig. 1a). Note that because of the constant optode distance, the brain areas underlying the channels varied depending on cap size (54, 56, 58 cm).

Analysis of behavioral data

As a behavioral measure in a self-paced design, the number of presented trials (i.e., the sum of presented trials during all experimental blocks of a certain condition) was calculated. Furthermore, the written solutions of the subjects were visualized with the help of a RON (ReadOut Numbers) program (Ploner, 2014) and manually analyzed for correctness. Response times (RT) were defined from stimulus onset to the final button press when the subject had finished producing the solution to the arithmetic problem. For RT analysis, only RTs of correct trials were

included and the median RT was calculated for each subject and condition. Accuracy (ACC) was calculated by the proportion of correctly solved trials. The behavioral data was statistically analyzed by a repeated-measures ANOVA with the within-subject factors grade (6, 7) and complexity (simple, complex) for each task.[1]

fNIRS data analysis

For each fNIRS channel, the optical data for the two wavelengths were transformed into relative concentration changes of oxygenated (O_2Hb) and deoxygenated haemoglobin (HHb). The analysis of the fNIRS data was conducted using custom MATLAB (The MathWorks, Inc., USA) scripts. For data preprocessing, a bandpass filter of 0.01–0.2 Hz was applied to the data [51]. In the next step, noisy fNIRS channels were interpolated by neighboring channels, and blocks containing uncorrectable artifacts were excluded from the analysis. Moreover, to deal with remaining motion artifacts, the signal was corrected by correlation-based signal improvement (CBSI) according to Cui et al. [52]. CBSI corrects the signal based on the assumption that simultaneous increases in O_2Hb and decreases in HHb are indicators of cortical activation [53] and is among the best methods for reducing motion artifacts [54], particularly in children and adolescents. Afterwards, the 45 s blocks were averaged across the four repetitions for each condition and baseline-corrected mean amplitudes of the hemodynamic responses were calculated channel-wise for each participant (baseline: 10 s).

Based on virtual registration [55–57] and according to the automated anatomic labeling (AAL) atlas [58], regions of interest (ROIs) were defined for left and right parietal areas (including SPL and IPL), frontal areas (including MFG and IFG), and parieto-temporal areas (including AG and middle temporal gyrus (MTG); cf. Fig. 1a for the position of the ROIs and Fig. 1c for an example signal within a ROI). Based on the individual activation peak within each ROI (cf. [59]), the contrasts for each grade and complexity level were calculated and the significance of activation was tested for each task using one-sample t-tests against zero (significance level of .05, False Discovery Rate (FDR) corrected for multiple statistical comparisons, cf. [60]). The main analysis focuses on the developmental fronto-parietal shift hypothesis and therefore was performed on the frontal

---

[1] The behavioral analysis is mainly based on the number of presented trials, since this reflects the most appropriate measure for self-paced written responses. The results for RT and ACC analyses should be regarded with caution, since the evaluation of the written responses was not objective due to technical problems with the touch monitor during the production paradigm. Because of these technical problems, the RT and ACC data of one subject is missing for grade 6.

Table 1 Behavioral results for the arithmetic tasks

Task	$N_{presented\ trials}$			RT			ACC		
	$F_{1,18}$	p	η_p^2	$F_{1,17}$	p	η_p^2	$F_{1,17}$	p	η_p^2
Addition									
Grade	2.93	.104	.140	1.49	.283	.081	3.98	.062	.190
Complexity	*166.33*	*<.001*	*.902*	*92.72*	*<.001*	*.845*	*15.63*	*.001*	*.479*
Grade × complexity	0.08	.783	.004	1.19	.291	.065	*7.75*	*.013*	*.313*
Subtraction									
Grade	1.61	.220	.082	1.43	.263	.073	*7.32*	*.015*	*.301*
Complexity	*299.87*	*<.001*	*.943*	*178.29*	*<.001*	*.913*	*7.20*	*.016*	*.297*
Grade × complexity	*6.61*	*.019*	*.269*	0.39	.539	.023	0.03	.877	.001
Multiplication									
Grade	0.00	.984	.000	0.73	.405	.041	3.24	.090	.160
Complexity	*191.66*	*<.001*	*.914*	*101.87*	*<.001*	*.857*	*55.25*	*<.001*	*.765*
Grade × complexity	1.27	.275	.066	0.24	.634	.014	0.16	.698	.009
Division									
Grade	0.03	.860	.002	0.69	.418	.039	1.15	.298	.063
Complexity	*150.03*	*<.001*	*.893*	*24.79*	*<.001*	*.593*	*67.90*	*<.001*	*.800*
Grade × complexity	0.47	.500	.026	0.58	.458	.033	0.66	.428	.037

Significant effects are shown in italics.

and parietal ROIs within a 2 grade (6, 7) × 2 complexity (simple, complex) × 2 ROI (frontal, parietal) × 2 hemisphere (left, right) repeated measures ANOVA for each task. Additionally, since some studies found temporal and AG activation to be associated with arithmetic during development (e.g., [32]), another analysis was performed on the parieto-temporal ROIs within a 2 grade (6, 7) × 2 complexity (simple, complex) × 2 hemisphere (left, right) repeated measures ANOVA for each task.

For significant effects of grade and arithmetic complexity, separate ANCOVAs were conducted by including the difference in the number of presented trials for the respective effect as a covariate. This procedure was conducted based on the self-paced design in accordance with Soltanlou et al. [33], but the results should be taken with caution, because the effect of the covariate was not independent from the investigated effects (see [61]). Furthermore, brain-behavior-correlations between the number of presented trials and cortical activation in each ROI were calculated for the effect of grade (grade 7 vs. grade 6) and the effect of arithmetic complexity (complex vs. simple) for each task. Results and discussion of the brain-behavior-correlations are reported in Additional file 1.

Results

Behavioral data

In general, better behavioral performance means that the adolescents solved more problems during the blocks (larger number of presented trials), were faster in solving

the problems (lower RT), and made fewer errors (larger ACC). Behavioral data was analyzed by a 2 grade (6, 7) × 2 complexity (simple, complex) ANOVA for each task (for statistical details see Table 1, see also Fig. 2).

In addition, there was a significant main effect of complexity for all measures, indicating a better performance on simple problems. Furthermore, a significant interaction of grade and complexity for ACC indicated that the adolescents were making fewer errors on simple problems from grade 6 to grade 7 (post hoc test: $p = .015$). No other effects were significant.

In subtraction, the main effect of grade was significant for ACC, indicating that the adolescents made fewer errors from grade 6 to grade 7. There was a significant main effect of complexity for all measures, indicating a better performance on simple problems. Furthermore, a significant interaction of grade and complexity for the number of presented trials indicated that the adolescents were only solving more simple problems from grade 6 to grade 7 (post hoc test: $p = .036$), which corresponds to the addition result for ACC.

In multiplication, there was a significant main effect of complexity for all measures, indicating a better performance for simple problems. No other effects were significant.

In division, there was a significant main effect of complexity for all measures, indicating a better performance for simple problems. No other effects were significant.

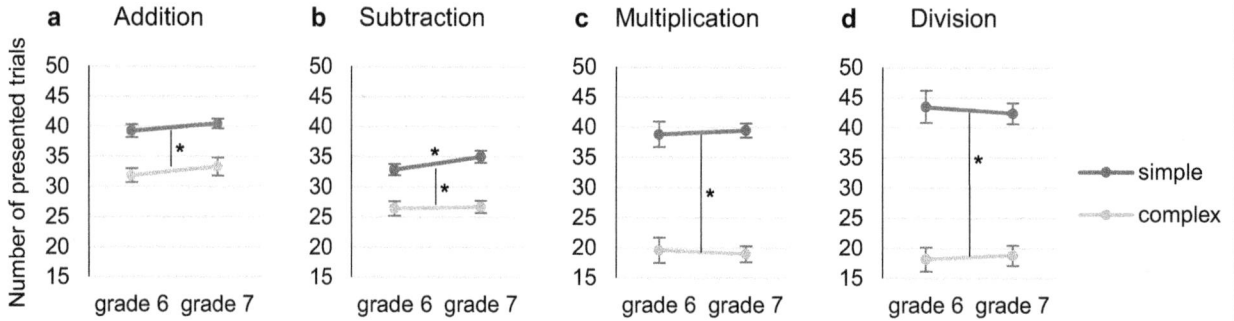

Fig. 2 Number of presented trials in the **a** addition, **b** subtraction, **c** multiplication, and **d** division tasks. Significant arithmetic complexity and grade effects are marked (*$p < .05$). Error bars indicate 1 SE of M

The standardized assessed arithmetic ability correlated positively with behavioral performance for all arithmetic tasks (average number of presented trials) in grade 6 ($r = .504$, $p = .028$) and showed a similar trend for grade 7 ($r = .443$, $p = .058$), indicating that arithmetic performance measured in the experimental task resembles the arithmetic skill of the adolescents.

fNIRS data

Cortical activation within the ROIs defined above was analyzed separately for complexity and grade level for each task (cf. Additional file 1: Figs. S1–S4). In all arithmetic tasks, significant activation was found in the bilateral parietal and bilateral frontal areas for simple and complex arithmetic in both grade levels ($ts(18) > 2.50$, FDR-corrected $ps < .05$). Additionally, significant deactivation was found in the left parieto-temporal area for complex addition in grade 6 ($t(18) = -2.32$, FDR-corrected $p < .05$; cf. Additional file 1: Fig. S1). There were no other areas with significant activation or deactivation (all FDR-corrected $ps > .05$).

Activation in MFG/IFG and SPL/IPL

First to examine our main question regarding the fronto-parietal shift in brain activation and arithmetic complexity effects in frontal (MFG/IFG) and parietal (SPL/IPL) brain regions, a 2 grade (6, 7) × 2 complexity (simple, complex) × 2 ROI (frontal, parietal) × 2 hemisphere (left, right) ANOVA was calculated for each task.

In addition, no significant effects were observed (all $ps > .1$).

In subtraction, there was a significant main effect of hemisphere ($F(1, 18) = 7.13$, $p = .016$, $\eta_p^2 = .284$) indicating that activation was larger in the left hemisphere than in the right hemisphere. Furthermore, the interaction of grade and ROI was significant ($F(1, 18) = 4.44$, $p = .050$, $\eta_p^2 = .198$) and a one-sided post hoc test based on our

directed hypothesis revealed that only frontal activation decreased from grade 6 to grade 7 ($p = .046$; cf. Fig. 3a). No other effects were significant (all $ps > .1$).

In multiplication, there was a significant main effect of hemisphere ($F(1, 18) = 7.23$, $p = .015$, $\eta_p^2 = .287$) indicating that activation was larger on the left hemisphere than on the right hemisphere. Furthermore, a significant main effect of complexity ($F(1, 18) = 5.20$, $p = .035$, $\eta_p^2 = .224$) and a significant interaction of complexity and ROI ($F(1, 18) = 5.74$, $p = .028$, $\eta_p^2 = .242$) were found, indicating that only parietal activation was increased for simple compared to complex problems (post hoc test: $p = .012$; cf. Fig. 3b). No other effects were significant (all $ps > .05$).

In division, there was a significant main effect of hemisphere ($F(1, 18) = 4.50$, $p = .048$, $\eta_p^2 = .200$) and a significant interaction of ROI and hemisphere ($F(1, 18) = 12.15$, $p = .003$, $\eta_p^2 = .403$) indicating that only parietal activation is larger on the left hemisphere than on the right hemisphere ($p = .005$). No other effects were significant (all $ps > .05$).

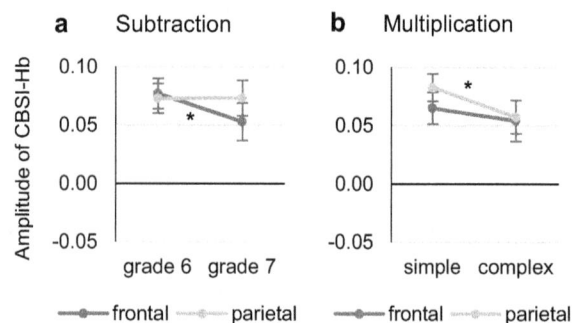

Fig. 3 Cortical activation in the frontal and parietal ROIs. **a** Significant reduction in frontal activation from grade 6 to grade 7 in the subtraction task (*$p < .05$). **b** Significantly increased parietal activation for simple compared to complex blocks in the multiplication task (*$p < .05$). Error bars indicate 1 SE of M

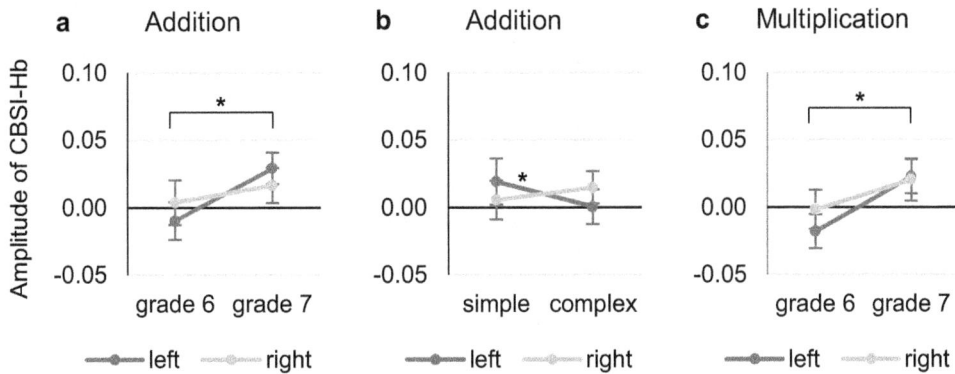

Fig. 4 Cortical activation in the parieto-temporal ROIs. **a** Significant change in parieto-temporal activation from grade 6 to grade 7 in the addition task (*p < .05). **b** Significantly increased left parieto-temporal activation for simple compared to complex blocks in the addition task (*p < .05). **c** Significant change in parieto-temporal activation from grade 6 to grade 7 in the multiplication task (*p < .05). Error bars indicate 1 SE of M

Activation in AG/MTG

Next to investigate developmental activation changes and arithmetic complexity effects for parieto-temporal brain regions (AG/MTG), an additional analysis was performed for parieto-temporal activation within a 2 complexity (simple, complex) × 2 grade (6, 7) × 2 hemisphere (left, right) ANOVA for each task. In the addition task, there was a significant main effect of grade ($F(1, 18) = 6.18$, $p = .023$, $\eta_p^2 = .256$) indicating that there was a change in the parieto-temporal region from deactivation in grade 6 to activation in grade 7 (cf. Fig. 4a). Furthermore, the addition task revealed a significant interaction effect of complexity and hemisphere ($F(1, 18) = 5.25$, $p = .034$, $\eta_p^2 = .226$) and a post hoc test revealed that only left parieto-temporal activation was higher for simple compared to complex problems ($p = .037$; cf. Fig. 4b). In the multiplication task, there was a significant main effect of grade ($F(1, 18) = 5.31$, $p = .033$, $\eta_p^2 = .228$) indicating that there was a change in the parieto-temporal region from deactivation in grade 6 to activation in grade 7 (cf. Fig. 4c). No other effects were significant (all $ps > .05$).

To summarize, grade effects were found for a reduction in frontal activation in subtraction and an increase in parieto-temporal activation in addition and multiplication, inverse arithmetic complexity effects were found for parietal activation in multiplication and left parieto-temporal activation in addition, and lateralization effects[2] were found for frontal activation in subtraction and multiplication and for parietal activation in subtraction, multiplication and division.

---

[2] Note that the lateralization effects got significant for all operations and the corresponding effect sizes were stronger when the left-handed participants were excluded from analyses (Addition: $F(1, 15) = 5.44$, $p = .034$, $\eta_p^2 = .266$; Subtraction: $F(1, 15) = 13.59$, $p = .002$, $\eta_p^2 = .475$; Multiplication: $F(1, 15) = 18.06$, $p = .001$, $\eta_p^2 = .546$; Division: $F(1, 15) = 10.87$, $p = .005$, $\eta_p^2 = .420$). This issue of handedness and cortical lateralization needs further investigation in future research.

Additional analysis of fNIRS data

Covariance analyses were conducted in order to account for the behavioral effects of grade and arithmetic complexity. Despite considering the behavioral effect, the effect of grade for parieto-temporal activation in the multiplication task was still significant ($F(1, 17) = 5.90$, $p = .027$, $\eta_p^2 = .258$) and in the addition task still marginal significant ($F(1, 17) = 3.26$, $p = .089$, $\eta_p^2 = .161$). On the other hand, the effect of grade for frontal activation in the subtraction task ($F(1, 17) = 2.27$, $p = .150$, $\eta_p^2 = .118$), the effect of arithmetic complexity for parietal activation in the multiplication task ($F(1, 17) = 1.07$, $p = .317$, $\eta_p^2 = .059$), and for left parieto-temporal activation in the addition task ($F(1, 17) = .46$, $p = .506$, $\eta_p^2 = .026$) did not reach significance when considering the behavioral effect.

Discussion

By investigating the neural underpinnings of calculation in adolescents, we observed activation within the bilateral fronto-parietal network for all basic arithmetic operations. Consistent with the general idea of a fronto-parietal shift with age and experience, the results provide further evidence for a reduction in activation of MFG/IFG from grades 6 to 7 for subtraction and a change in activation of AG/MTG for addition and multiplication. The activation of the left AG/MTG during addition was additionally modulated by arithmetic complexity. Potentially owing to the self-paced design, activation of SPL/IPL was found to be higher for simple than for complex multiplication, reflecting an inverse effect of arithmetic complexity.

In general, activation of the bilateral fronto-parietal network was found for all basic arithmetic operations. Overall, our findings are in line with previous studies showing that parietal regions (i.e., the SPL, IPL, and particularly the IPS) are associated with arithmetic in adults

[1, 62, 63]. Furthermore, it seems possible to generalize findings from exact addition in children and adolescents [5, 7, 45, 64] to arithmetic processing for all four basic operations. The present findings further corroborate previous studies [6, 65] which have observed overlapping frontal activation for all basic arithmetic operations in the MFG, IFG, and SFG. Taken together, the results show that adolescents rely on the bilateral fronto-parietal network of arithmetic processing to use the basic arithmetic operations in a natural setting. This activation pattern, however, is influenced by arithmetic development and complexity.

Developmental activation changes in arithmetic

During arithmetic development, brain activation for arithmetic processing is thought to rely less on frontal and more on parietal areas [11, 16]. From grade 6 to grade 7, the adolescents showed improved subtraction performance which was accompanied by reduced frontal activation in MFG/IFG. This result confirms decreasing frontal activation during development, as suggested by previous cross-sectional [11], longitudinal [18] and training data [12]. In line with these findings, children rely more on domain-general supportive frontal areas such as the IFG for working memory and cognitive control compared to adults [66]. Decreasing frontal activation was not observed for arithmetic operations other than subtraction, possibly because there was no general behavioral improvement in these operations from grade 6 to grade 7. In sum, the current data provide partial support for the developmental fronto-parietal shift during secondary school, since a reduction in frontal activation from grade 6 to grade 7 was found for subtraction, but not for other operations.

Contrary to predictions based on findings comparing children and adolescents to adults [9, 7, 11], no activation increase was observed within the SPL/IPL in any operation over the course of 1 year. Since explicit instruction and training for the basic arithmetic operations concludes earlier in elementary school education (in grade 4), adolescents are presumably proficient in arithmetic, and do not particularly practice or improve on these skills between grades 6 and 7. In light of the conflicting findings on changes in parietal activation during elementary school [17, 18, 32], the maturation of domain-specific processes might be related mostly to initial progress in learning arithmetic and less to general experience with numbers. Thus, the parietal activation increase during arithmetic development might occur earlier than in secondary school when arithmetic knowledge is already established.

In addition to the results for frontal and parietal brain regions, a change from AG/MTG deactivation in grade 6

to increased activation in grade 7 was observed for addition and multiplication. This resembles the finding from Rosenberg-Lee et al. [17] that right AG deactivation in grade 2 changed to above baseline activation in grade 3 for single-digit addition (see also [32]). Considering the role of the AG in the default mode network [67], deactivation in the AG most likely reflects increased task demands for arithmetic processing [68–70]. The same task may therefore become less demanding during development—similar to the way that task demands (and deactivation in the left AG) decline with increasing math competence in adults ([70–72]; for a review see [73]). Although behavioral improvement was only found for simple addition but not multiplication, the grade-related activation change in the AG/MTG might be related to the maturation of arithmetic fact retrieval processes [4]. Altogether, the current data show that arithmetic development during secondary school is to a certain extent accompanied by a reduction in frontal domain-general processing, but does not rely on increased parietal magnitude processing.

Regarding the findings for developmental changes in arithmetic, a note of caution is due since the probe placement varies with changes in head size during development. This is because the distance between the optodes is fixed and the probeset was oriented at parietal sites so that the position of frontal optodes in particular changes with head size. Head size increases by about 0.5 cm during 1 year in this age range (see [74]; see also Table 1 in [75] based on the data of [76]), corresponding to a deviation of 1 mm for the most frontal optodes. This deviation might have affected the frontal results for arithmetic development to some extent, but might be negligible, because fNIRS has a spatial resolution of 3 cm and brain weight does not substantially change between the age of 10 and 14 (see [77]). Thus, longitudinal research reflects a challenge for neuroimaging research.

Influence of complexity on arithmetic processing in adolescents

The neural correlates of arithmetic processing in adolescents vary with complexity. For instance, activation in the left AG/MTG was higher for simple compared to complex addition blocks, likely because the adolescents solved more simple than complex addition problems in a given length of time. This result corroborates previous findings on the problem size effect showing larger activation of the AG and superior temporal gyri for small problems [5, 30], which likely reflects the retrieval of exact arithmetic facts during single-digit addition problems (cf. [30, 78]). Interestingly, the left AG and MTG are known to belong to the network underlying verbally mediated arithmetic fact retrieval [4, 79]. In the current study, two-digit addition problems without carry procedure were used in the simple condition, so that the activation increase of the left AG/MTG for simple problems reflects separate arithmetic fact retrieval for the sum of the units and the sum of the decades (cf. [80]). Furthermore, the different activation levels of the left AG/MTG associated with arithmetic complexity indicate the increased task demand for complex compared to simple addition problems [67], because regions in the default mode network are generally less active when the task gets more complex [81].

Behaviorally, the carry/borrow effect in addition/subtraction and the problem size effect (comparing two-digit to single-digit problems) in multiplication/division increased task difficulty. However, surprisingly, increased arithmetic complexity was not found to be associated with increased frontal or parietal activation as previously observed (cf. [17, 30, 33, 72]). On the one hand, the self-paced block design might obscure these effects because activation may have increased not only due to difficulty in complex blocks but also due to the larger number of solved problems in simple blocks. It should be noted, however, that fixed-paced block designs or event-related designs are also problematic as arithmetic complexity is confounded with different durations for solving simple and complex problems, which can lead to more extensive activation for complex problems (cf. [82]) and to additional task-irrelevant activation (cf. [83]). On the other hand, the difference between simple and complex blocks in the present study might be too minor to be detected on the neural level, due to design specifications including a balanced problem size, the mix of carry/borrow and no-carry/borrow problems in complex blocks in addition and subtraction, as well as overlapping ranges of the problem size in multiplication and division (different from [33, 72]). Altogether, the specific design as well as properties of the stimulus material seem to have a crucial impact on the dependence of fronto-parietal activation on arithmetic complexity.

Number magnitude processing in a self-paced block design

Regarding arithmetic complexity, simple multiplication problems elicited larger parietal activation than complex multiplication problems. This inverse effect, in which decreased activation is associated with increased arithmetic complexity, might again be explained by the self-paced block design used here, since it was no longer significant when the number of presented problems was considered as a covariate. More problems were solved during simple than complex blocks, because the solutions for single-digit problems can be faster and relatively automatically retrieved from memory, while two-digit

problems mostly need to be solved by slower procedural strategies. Notably, the activation increase in SPL/IPL including the IPS, associated with automatized number magnitude processing [4, 84], was larger for simple blocks, i.e., when more problems were solved and thus elicited increased number magnitude processing. On the contrary, the question arises whether the higher parietal activation usually observed for more complex problems (e.g., [71]) is really due to the calculation procedures underlying their solution or rather due to the longer processing duration (cf. [83]). In sum, the function of the parietal cortex might additionally depend on the number of magnitudes to be processed, i.e., the number of arithmetic problems, besides the processing of number magnitude, i.e., problem size.

Conclusions and perspectives

In conclusion, the neural activation pattern within the fronto-parietal network of arithmetic processing was found to be similar across arithmetic operations, but still undergoes development in 12–4 year-old adolescents. Consistent with previous studies, a reduction in frontal activation was observed during development and arithmetic complexity was associated with reduced AG/MTG activation. In contrast to previous studies, however, arithmetic complexity elicited *less* parietal activation. We have argued that the current study differed from previous designs by using a self-paced written production paradigm, in which the complexity factor might be confounded with number of trials. Nevertheless, we wish to point out that the inverse arithmetic complexity effect observed in the current study is not just an artifact of the experimental design, but rather reflects the brain activation of adolescents in a natural setting.

More generally, we believe that this study shows that fNIRS seems suitable as an ecologically valid complementary method, especially for research in educational neuroscience [12], because arithmetic processes can be examined in a scholastic setting, where adolescents can solve arithmetic problems in the familiar style of written production (cf. [45, 46]; for a review see [85]).

Additional file

Additional file 1: Figure S1. Cortical activation in the addition task depending on arithmetic complexity and grade (*t* maps). Figure S2. Cortical activation in the subtraction task depending on arithmetic complexity and grade (*t* maps). Figure S3. Cortical activation in the multiplication task depending on arithmetic complexity and grade (*t* maps). Figure S4. Cortical activation in the division task depending on arithmetic complexity and grade (*t* maps). Figure S5. Brain-behavior-correlations for the effect of arithmetic complexity in the addition task.

Authors' contributions

All authors contributed to the study conception and design. Material preparation, data collection and analysis were performed by CA, MS and TD. The first draft of the manuscript was written by CA and all authors commented on previous versions of the manuscript. All authors read and approved the final manuscript.

Author details

[1] LEAD Graduate School & Research Network, University of Tuebingen, Tuebingen, Germany. [2] Department of Psychology, University of Tuebingen, Tuebingen, Germany. [3] Graduate Training Centre of Neuroscience/IMPRS for Cognitive and Systems Neuroscience, Tuebingen, Germany. [4] Leibniz-Institut für Wissensmedien, Tuebingen, Germany. [5] Department of Psychiatry and Psychotherapy, University of Tuebingen, Tuebingen, Germany.

Acknowledgements

We would like to thank Minako Uga and Ippeita Dan for their help in preparing the spatial registration and anatomical labeling of fNIRS channels. We also want to thank Samantha Speidel, Anne Büsemeyer and Joshua Schmid for assistance in the measurements, and Barbara Peysakhovich and Julianne Skinner for language proofreading of the paper.

Competing interests

The authors declare that they have no competing interests.

Funding

This research was funded by the LEAD Graduate School & Research Network [GSC1028], which is funded within the framework of the Excellence Initiative of the German federal and state governments supporting CA and TD. This research was further funded by a grant from the Science Campus Tuebingen, project 8.4 to HCN supporting MS. ACE was partly supported by the IZKF Tübingen (Junior Research Group, Grant 2115-0-0).

REFERENCES

1. Arsalidou M, Taylor MJ. Is $2 + 2 = 4$? Meta-analyses of brain areas needed for numbers and calculations. NeuroImage. 2011;54(3):2382–93. https://doi.org/10.1016/j.neuroimage.2010.10.009.
2. Dehaene S, Cohen L. Cerebral pathways for calculation: double dissociation between rote verbal and quantitative knowledge of arithmetic. Cortex. 1997;33(2):219–50. https://doi.org/10.1016/S0010-9452(08)70002-9.
3. Klein E, Moeller K, Glauche V, Weiller C, Willmes K. Processing pathways in mental arithmetic-evidence from probabilistic fiber tracking. PLoS ONE. 2013;8(1):e55455. https://doi.org/10.1371/journal.pone.0055455.
4. Klein E, Suchan J, Moeller K, Karnath HO, Knops A, Wood G, Willmes K. Considering structural connectivity in the triple code model of numerical cognition: differential connectivity for magnitude processing and arithmetic facts. Brain Struct Funct. 2016;221(2):979–95. https://doi.org/10.1007/s00429-014-0951-1.
5. Davis N, Cannistraci CJ, Rogers BP, Gatenby JC, Fuchs LS, Anderson AW, Gore JC. The neural correlates of calculation ability in children: an fMRI study. Magn Reson Imaging. 2009;27(9):1187–97. https://doi.org/10.1016/j.mri.2009.05.010.
6. Kawashima R, Taira M, Okita K, Inoue K, Tajima N, Yoshida H, Fukuda H. A functional MRI study of simple arithmetic—a comparison between children and adults. Cognit Brain Res. 2004;18(3):227–33. https://doi.org/10.1016/j.cogbrainres.2003.10.009.
7. Kucian K, von Aster M, Loenneker T, Dietrich T, Martin E. Development of neural networks for exact and approximate calculation: a FMRI study. Dev Neuropsychol. 2008;33(4):447–73. https://doi.org/10.1000/07565640021101474.
8. Peters L, De Smedt B. Arithmetic in the developing brain: A review of brain imaging studies. Dev Cognit Neurosci. 2017. https://doi.org/10.1016/j.dcn.2017.05.002.
9. Chang T-T, Metcalfe AWS, Padmanabhan A, Chen T, Menon V. Heterogeneous and nonlinear development of human posterior parietal cortex function. NeuroImage. 2016;126:184–95. https://doi.org/10.1016/j.neuroimage.2015.11.053.
10. Arsalidou M, Pawliw-Levac M, Sadeghi M, Pascual-Leone J. Brain areas needed for numbers and calculations in children: meta-analyses of fMRI studies. Dev Cognit Neurosci. 2017. https://doi.org/10.1016/j.dcn.2017.08.002.
11. Rivera SM, Reiss AL, Eckert MA, Menon V. Developmental changes in mental arithmetic: evidence for increased functional specialization in the left inferior parietal cortex. Cereb Cortex. 2005;15(11):1779–90. https://doi.org/10.1093/cercor/bhi055.
12. Soltanlou M, Artemenko C, Ehlis A-C, Huber S, Fallgatter AJ, Dresler T, Nuerk H-C. Reduction but no shift in brain activation after arithmetic learning in children: a simultaneous fNIRS-EEG study. Sci Rep. 2018. https://doi.org/10.1038/s41598-018-20007-x.
13. Soltanlou M, Sitnikova A, Nuerk H-C, Dresler T. Applications of functional near-infrared spectroscopy (fNIRS) in studying cognitive development: the case of mathematics and language. Front Psychol. 2018;9:277. https://doi.org/10.3389/fpsyg.2018.00277.
14. Houdé O, Rossi S, Lubin A, Joliot M. Mapping numerical processing, reading, and executive functions in the developing brain: an fMRI meta-analysis of 52 studies including 842 children. Dev Sci. 2010;13(6):876–85. https://doi.org/10.1111/j.1467-7687.2009.00938.x.
15. Kaufmann L, Wood G, Rubinsten O, Henik A. Meta-analyses of developmental fMRI studies investigating typical and atypical trajectories of number processing and calculation. Dev Neuropsychol. 2011;36(6):763–87. https://doi.org/10.1080/87565641.2010.549884.
16. Menon V. Developmental cognitive neuroscience of arithmetic: implications for learning and education. ZDM. 2010;42(6):515–25. https://doi.org/10.1007/s11858-010-0242-0.
17. Rosenberg-Lee M, Barth M, Menon V. What difference does a year of schooling make? Maturation of brain response and connectivity between 2nd and 3rd grades during arithmetic problem solving. NeuroImage. 2011;57(3):796–808. https://doi.org/10.1016/j.neuroimage.2011.05.013.
18. Qin S, Cho S, Chen T, Rosenberg-Lee M, Geary DC, Menon V. Hippocampal-neocortical functional reorganization underlies children's cognitive development. Nat Neurosci. 2014;17(9):1263–9. https://doi.org/10.1038/nn.3788.
19. Siegler RS. Emerging minds: the process of change in children's thinking. Oxford: Oxford University Press; 1996.
20. Nuerk H-C, Moeller K, Klein E, Willmes K, Fischer MH. Extending the mental number line. J Psychol. 2011;219(1):3–22. https://doi.org/10.1027/2151-2604/a000041.
21. Nuerk H-C, Moeller K, Willmes K. Multi-digit number processing. In: Cohen Kadosh R, Dowker A, editors. Oxford handbook of mathematical cognition. Oxford: Oxford University Press; 2015. p. 106–39.
22. Lemaire P, Callies S. Children's strategies in complex arithmetic. J Exp Child Psychol. 2009;103(1):49–65. https://doi.org/10.1016/j.jecp.2008.09.007.
23. Artemenko C, Soltanlou M, Dresler T, Ehlis A-C, Nuerk H-C. The neural correlates of arithmetic difficulty depend on mathematical ability: evidence from combined fNIRS and ERP. Brain Struct Funct. 2018. https://doi.org/10.1007/s00429-018-1618-0.
24. Klein E, Moeller K, Dressel K, Domahs F, Wood G, Willmes K, Nuerk H-C. To carry or not to carry–is this the question? Disentangling the carry effect in multi-digit addition. Acta Physiol. 2010;135(1):67–76. https://doi.org/10.1016/j.actpsy.2010.06.002.
25. Klein E, Nuerk H-C, Wood G, Knops A, Willmes K. The exact vs. approximate distinction in numerical cognition may not be exact, but only approximate: how different processes work together in multi-digit addition. Brain Cogn. 2009;69(2):369–81. https://doi.org/10.1016/j.bandc.2008.08.031.
26. Kong J, Wang C, Kwong K, Vangel M, Chua E, Gollub R. The neural substrate of arithmetic operations and procedure complexity. Cognit Brain Res. 2005;22(3):397–405. https://doi.org/10.1016/j.cogbrainres.2004.09.011.
27. Verner M, Herrmann MJ, Troche SJ, Roebers CM, Rammsayer TH. Cortical oxygen consumption in mental arithmetic as a function of task difficulty: a near-infrared spectroscopy approach. Front Hum Neurosci. 2013;7:1–9. https://doi.org/10.3389/fnhum.2013.00217.

28. Artemenko C, Pixner S, Moeller K, Nuerk H-C. Longitudinal development of subtraction performance in elementary school. Br J Dev Psychol. 2017. https://doi.org/10.1111/bjdp.12215.

29. De Brauwer J, Verguts T, Fias W. The representation of multiplication facts: developmental changes in the problem size, five, and tie effects. J Exp Child Psychol. 2006;94(1):43–56. https://doi.org/10.1016/j.jecp.2005.11.004.

30. De Smedt B, Holloway ID, Ansari D. Effects of problem size and arithmetic operation on brain activation during calculation in children with varying levels of arithmetical fluency. Neuroimage. 2011;57(3):771–81. https://doi.org/10.1016/j.neuroimage.2010.12.037.

31. Matejko AA, Ansari D. How do individual differences in children's domain specific and domain general abilities relate to brain activity within the intraparietal sulcus during arithmetic? An fMRI study. Hum Brain Mapp. 2017;3956:3941–56. https://doi.org/10.1002/hbm.23640.

32. Prado J, Mutreja R, Booth JR. Developmental dissociation in the neural responses to simple multiplication and subtraction problems. Dev Sci. 2014;17(4):537–52. https://doi.org/10.1111/desc.12140.

33. Soltanlou M, Artemenko C, Dresler T, Haeussinger FB, Fallgatter AJ, Ehlis A-C, Nuerk H-C. Increased arithmetic complexity is associated with domain-general but not domain-specific magnitude processing in children: a simultaneous fNIRS-EEG study. Cognit Affect Behav Neurosci. 2017. https://doi.org/10.3758/s13415-017-0508-x.

34. Chang T-T, Rosenberg-Lee M, Metcalfe AWS, Chen T, Menon V. Development of common neural representations for distinct numerical problems. Neuropsychologia. 2015;75:481–95. https://doi.org/10.1016/j.neuropsychologia.2015.07.005.

35. Domahs F, Delazer M, Nuerk H-C. What makes multiplication facts difficult: problem size or neighborhood consistency? Exp Psychol. 2006;53(4):275–82. https://doi.org/10.1027/1618-3169.53.4.275.

36. Domahs F, Domahs U, Schlesewsky M, Ratinckx E, Verguts T, Willmes K, Nuerk H-C. Neighborhood consistency in mental arithmetic: behavioral and ERP evidence. Behav Brain Funct BBF. 2007;3:66. https://doi.org/10.1186/1744-9081-3-66.

37. Van Beek L, Ghesquière P, Lagae L, De Smedt B. Left fronto-parietal white matter correlates with individual differences in children's ability to solve additions and multiplications: a tractography study. Neuroimage. 2014;90:117–27. https://doi.org/10.1016/j.neuroimage.2013.12.030.

38. Andres M, Pelgrims B, Michaux N, Olivier E, Pesenti M. Role of distinct parietal areas in arithmetic: an fMRI-guided TMS study. Neuroimage. 2011;54(4):3048–56. https://doi.org/10.1016/j.neuroimage.2010.11.009.

39. Gruber O, Indefrey P, Steinmetz H, Kleinschmidt A. Dissociating neural correlates of cognitive components in mental calculation. Cereb Cortex. 2001;11(4):350–9. https://doi.org/10.1093/cercor/11.4.350.

40. Hinault T, Lemaire P. What does EEG tell us about arithmetic strategies? A review. Int J Psychophysiol. 2016;106:115–26. https://doi.org/10.1016/j.ijpsycho.2016.05.006.

41. Moeller K, Klein E, Nuerk H-C. (No) small adults: children's processing of carry addition problems. Dev Neuropsychol. 2011;36(6):702–20. https://doi.org/10.1080/87565641.2010.549880.

42. Moeller K, Klein E, Nuerk H-C. Three processes underlying the carry effect in addition—evidence from eye tracking. Br J Psychol. 2011;102(3):623–45. https://doi.org/10.1111/j.2044-8295.2011.02034.x.

43. Krinzinger H, Koten JW, Hennemann J, Schueppen A, Sahr K, Arndt D, Willmes K. Sensitivity, reproducibility, and reliability of self-paced versus fixed stimulus presentation in an fMRI study on exact, non-symbolic arithmetic in typically developing children aged between 6 and 12 years. Dev Neuropsychol. 2011;36(6):721–40. https://doi.org/10.1080/87565641.2010.549882.

44. Bahnmueller J, Dresler T, Ehlis A-C, Cress U, Nuerk H-C. NIRS in motion-unraveling the neurocognitive underpinnings of embodied numerical cognition. Front Psychol. 2014;5:1–4. https://doi.org/10.3389/fpsyg.2014.00743.

45. Dresler T, Obersteiner A, Schecklmann M, Vogel ACM, Ehlis A-C, Richter MM, Fallgatter AJ. Arithmetic tasks in different formats and their influence on behavior and brain oxygenation as assessed with near-infrared spectroscopy (NIRS): a study involving primary and secondary school children. J Neural Transm. 2009;116(12):1689–700. https://doi.org/10.1007/s00702-009-0307-9.

46. Obersteiner A, Dresler T, Reiss K, Vogel ACM, Pekrun R, Fallgatter AJ. Bringing brain imaging to the school to assess arithmetic problem solving: chances and limitations in combining educational and neuroscientific research. ZDM. 2010;42(6):541–54. https://doi.org/10.1007/s11858-010-0256-7.

47. Petermann F, Petermann U, Wechsler D. Hamburg-Wechsler-Intelligenztest für Kinder-IV: HAWIK-IV. USA: Huber; 2007.

48. Götz L, Lingel K, Schneider W. DEMAT5+: Deutscher Mathematiktest für fünfte Klassen. Europe: Hogrefe; 2013.

49. Huber S, Moeller K, Nuerk H-C. Differentielle Entwicklung arithmetischer Fähigkeiten nach der Grundschule: Manche Schere öffnet und schließt sich wieder. Lernen Und Lernstörungen. 2012;1(2):119–34. https://doi.org/10.1024/2235-0977/a000014.

50. Jasper HH. The ten twenty electrode system of the international federation. Electroencephalogr Clin Neurophysiol. 1958;10:371–5.

51. Scholkmann F, Kleiser S, Metz AJ, Zimmermann R, Mata Pavia J, Wolf U, Wolf M. A review on continuous wave functional near-infrared spectroscopy and imaging instrumentation and methodology. Neuroimage. 2014;85:6–27. https://doi.org/10.1016/j.neuroimage.2013.05.004.

52. Cui X, Bray S, Reiss AL. Functional near infrared spectroscopy (NIRS) signal improvement based on negative correlation between oxygenated and deoxygenated hemoglobin dynamics. Neuroimage. 2010;49(4):3039–46. https://doi.org/10.1016/j.neuroimage.2009.11.050.

53. Obrig H, Villringer A. Beyond the visible—imaging the human brain with light. J Cereb Blood Flow Metab. 2003;23:1–18. https://doi.org/10.1097/01.WCB.0000043472.45775.29.

54. Brigadoi S, Ceccherini L, Cutini S, Scarpa F, Scatturin P, Selb J, Cooper RJ. Motion artifacts in functional near-infrared spectroscopy: a comparison of motion correction techniques applied to real cognitive data. Neuroimage. 2014;85:181–91. https://doi.org/10.1016/j.neuroimage.2013.04.082.

55. Rorden C, Brett M. Stereotaxic display of brain lesions. Behav Neurol. 2000;12(4):191–200. https://doi.org/10.1155/2000/421719.

56. Singh AK, Okamoto M, Dan H, Jurcak V, Dan I. Spatial registration of multichannel multi-subject fNIRS data to MNI space without MRI. Neuroimage. 2005;27(4):842–51. https://doi.org/10.1016/j.neuroimage.2005.05.019.

57. Tsuzuki D, Jurcak V, Singh AK, Okamoto M, Watanabe E, Dan I. Virtual spatial registration of stand-alone fNIRS data to MNI space. Neuroimage. 2007;34(4):1506–18. https://doi.org/10.1016/j.neuroimage.2006.10.043.

58. Tzourio-Mazoyer N, Landeau B, Papathanassiou D, Crivello F, Etard O, Delcroix N, Joliot M. Automated anatomical labeling of activations in SPM using a macroscopic anatomical parcellation of the MNI MRI single-subject brain. Neuroimage. 2002;15:273–89. https://doi.org/10.1006/nimg.2001.0978.

59. Arthurs OJ, Boniface SJ. What aspect of the fMRI BOLD signal best reflects the underlying electrophysiology in human somatosensory cortex? Clin Neurophysiol. 2003;114(7):1203–9. https://doi.org/10.1016/S1388-2457(03)00080-4.

60. Benjamini Y, Hochberg Y. Controlling the false discovery rate: a practical and powerful approach to multiple testing. J R Stat Soc B. 1995;57(1):289–300.

61. Miller GA, Chapman JP. Misunderstanding analysis of covariance. J Abnorm Psychol. 2001;110(1):40–8. https://doi.org/10.1037//0021-843X.110.1.40.

62. Baldo JV, Dronkers NF. Neural correlates of arithmetic and language comprehension: a common substrate? Neuropsychologia. 2007;45(2):229–35. https://doi.org/10.1016/j.neuropsychologia.2006.07.014.

63. Dehaene S, Molko N, Cohen L, Wilson AJ. Arithmetic and the brain. Curr Opin Neurobiol. 2004;14(2):218–24. https://doi.org/10.1016/j.conb.2004.03.008.

64. Meintjes EM, Jacobson SW, Molteno CD, Gatenby JC, Warton C, Cannistraci CJ, Jacobson JL. An fMRI study of magnitude comparison and exact addition in children. Magn Reson Imaging. 2010;28(3):351–62. https://doi.org/10.1016/j.mri.2009.11.010.

65. Fehr T, Code C, Herrmann M. Common brain regions underlying different arithmetic operations as revealed by conjunct fMRI-BOLD activation. Brain Res. 2007;1172:93–102. https://doi.org/10.1016/j.brainres.2007.07.043.

66. Cantlon JF, Libertus ME, Pinel P, Dehaene S, Brannon EM, Pelphrey KA. The neural development of an abstract concept of number. J Cognit Neurosci. 2009;21(11):2217–29. https://doi.org/10.1162/jocn.2008.21159.

67. Uddin LQ, Supekar K, Amin H, Rykhlevskaia E, Nguyen DA, Greicius MD, Menon V. Dissociable connectivity within human angular gyrus and intraparietal sulcus: evidence from functional and structural connectivity. Cereb Cortex. 2010;20(11):2636–46. https://doi.org/10.1093/cercor/bhq011.

68. Grabner RH, Ansari D, Koschutnig K, Reishofer G, Ebner F. The function of the left angular gyrus in mental arithmetic: evidence from the associative confusion effect. Hum Brain Mapp. 2013;34(5):1013–24. https://doi.org/10.1002/hbm.21489.

69. Rosenberg-Lee M, Chang TT, Young CB, Wu S, Menon V. Functional dissociations between four basic arithmetic operations in the human posterior parietal cortex: a cytoarchitectonic mapping study. Neuropsychologia. 2011;49(9):2592–608. https://doi.org/10.1016/j.neuropsychologia.2011.04.035.

70. Wu SS, Chang TT, Majid A, Caspers S, Eickhoff SB, Menon V. Functional heterogeneity of inferior parietal cortex during mathematical cognition assessed with cytoarchitectonic probability maps. Cereb Cortex. 2009;19(12):2930–45. https://doi.org/10.1093/cercor/bhp063.

71. Grabner RH, Ansari D, Reishofer G, Stern E, Ebner F, Neuper C. Individual differences in mathematical competence predict parietal brain activation during mental calculation. NeuroImage. 2007;38(2):346–56. https://doi.org/10.1016/j.neuroimage.2007.07.041.

72. Soltanlou M, Jung S, Roesch S, Ninaus M, Brandelik K, Heller J, Moeller K. Behavioral and neurocognitive evaluation of a web-platform for game-based learning of orthography and numeracy. In: Buder J, Hesse FW, editors. Informational environments: effects of use, effective designs. New York: Springer; 2017. https://doi.org/10.1007/978-3-319-64274-1.

73. Zamarian L, Ischebeck A, Delazer M. Neuroscience of learning arithmetic—evidence from brain imaging studies. Neurosci Biobehav Rev. 2009;33(6):909–25. https://doi.org/10.1016/j.neubiorev.2009.03.005.

74. Roche AF, Mukherjee D, Guo SM, Moore WM. Head circumference reference data: birth to 18 years. Pediatrics. 1987;79(5):706–12.

75. Weaver DD, Christian JC. Familial variation of head size and adjustment for parental head circumference. J Pediatr. 1980;96(6):990–4. https://doi.org/10.1016/S0022-3476(80)80623-8.

76. Nellhaus G. Head circumference from birth to eighteen years: practical composite international and interracial graphs. Pediatrics. 1968;41(1):106–14.

77. Dekaban AS, Sadowsky D. Changes in brain weight during the span of human life: relation of brain weight to body height and body weight. Ann Neurol. 1978;4:345.

78. Stanescu-Cosson R, Pinel P, van De Moortele PF, Le Bihan D, Cohen L, Dehaene S. Understanding dissociations in dyscalculia: a brain imaging study of the impact of number size on the cerebral networks for exact and approximate calculation. Brain A J Neurol. 2000;123:2240–55. https://doi.org/10.1093/brain/123.11.2240.

79. Polspoel B, Peters L, Vandermosten M, De Smedt B. Strategy over operation: neural activation in subtraction and multiplication during fact retrieval and procedural strategy use in children. Hum Brain Mapp. 2017. https://doi.org/10.1002/hbm.23691.

80. Klein E, Moeller K, Nuerk H-C, Willmes K. On the neuro-cognitive foundations of basic auditory number processing: an fMRI study. Behav Brain Funct. 2010;6:42. https://doi.org/10.1186/1744-9081-6-42.

81. Pletzer B, Kronbichler M, Nuerk H-C, Kerschbaum HH. Mathematics anxiety reduces default mode network deactivation in response to numerical tasks. Front Hum Neurosci. 2015;9:202. https://doi.org/10.3389/fnhum.2015.00202.

82. Delazer M, Domahs F, Bartha L, Brenneis C, Lochy A, Trieb T, Benke T. Learning complex arithmetic—an fMRI study. Cognit Brain Res. 2003;18:76–88. https://doi.org/10.1016/j.cogbrainres.2003.09.005.

83. Basho S, Palmer ED, Rubio MA, Wulfeck B, Müller RA. Effects of generation mode in fMRI adaptations of semantic fluency: paced production and overt speech. Neuropsychologia. 2007;45(8):1697–706. https://doi.org/10.1016/j.neuropsychologia.2007.01.007.

84. Klein E, Willmes K, Dressel K, Domahs F, Wood G, Nuerk H-C, Moeller K. Categorical and continuous-disentangling the neural correlates of the carry effect in multi-digit addition. Behav Brain Funct. 2010;6(1):70. https://doi.org/10.1186/1744-9081-6-70.

85. Grabner RH, Ansari D. Promises and potential pitfalls of a "cognitive neuroscience of mathematics learning". ZDM. 2010;42(6):655–60. https://doi.org/10.1007/s11858-010-0283-4.

18

Selective impairment of attentional set shifting in adults with ADHD

Aquiles Luna-Rodriguez[1]* ⓘ, Mike Wendt[2], Julia Kerner auch Koerner[3,5], Caterina Gawrilow[4,5] and Thomas Jacobsen[1]

Abstract

Background: Task switch protocols are frequently used in the assessment of cognitive control, both in clinical and non-clinical populations. These protocols frequently confound task switch and attentional set shift. The current study investigated the ability of adult ADHD patients to shift attentional set in the context of switching tasks.

Method: We tested 38 adults with ADHD and 39 control adults with an extensive diagnostic battery and a task switch protocol without proactive interference. The experiment combined orthogonally task-switch vs. repetition, and attentional set shift vs. no shift. Each experimental stimulus had global and local features (Hierarchical/"Navon" stimuli), associated with corresponding attentional sets.

Results: ADHD patients were slower than controls in task switch trials with a simultaneous shift of attention between global/local attentional sets. This also correlated significantly with diagnostic scales for ADHD symptoms. The patients had more variable reaction times, but when the attentional set was kept constant neither were they significantly slower nor showed higher task switch costs.

Conclusion: ADHD is associated with a deficit in flexible deployment of attention to varying sources of stimulus information.

Keywords: ADHD, Attentional set, Task switching, Cognitive control, Executive function

Background

Daily life difficulties experienced by individuals suffering under ADHD symptoms have frequently been linked to deficits in executive functions, a class of mental processes assumed to organize cognitive activity in the service of goal-directed behavior (e.g., [1–8]). Although the concept of executive functions is not well defined, a core aspect thereof relates to the ability to adjust mental sets according to changing task requirements and context conditions. A prevalent means of investigating such adjustment is the task switching (TS) paradigm (overview in [9, 10]). In standard task switching studies, participants execute two different tasks, usually involving the same set of stimuli, in varying sequences. Response performance is typically worse in task switch trials (i.e., trials preceded by a trial associated with the other task) than in task repetition trials (i.e., trials preceded by a trial associated with the same task). Although these *task switch costs* have been attributed to executive processes of task-set reconfiguration, they may also be accounted for in terms of stimulus- and task-specific proactive interference.

ADHD-related impairment in conditions associated with TS has been reported in several studies (e.g., [11–13]). In light of the fact that a deficit in TS performance may arise from a multitude of processes involved in task switching, the current study examined evidence for ADHD-related impairment concerning a particular component of task-set reconfiguration. In many TS experiments the tasks between which participants switch differ with regard to the relevant perceptual features of the stimulus. Participants may switch between color and shape identification tasks [14, 15], between reporting the

*Correspondence: luna@hsu-hh.de
[1] Experimental Psychology Unit, Helmut-Schmidt-University/
University of the Federal Armed Forces Hamburg, Holstenhofweg 85,
22043 Hamburg, Germany
Full list of author information is available at the end of the article

number of -identical- stimulus elements vs. their identity [11, 12, 16], or between classifying digits vs. letters [13, 17]. TS in these situations may involve a shift of the attentional set (AtS), that is, reconfiguring attentional weights assigned to relevant and irrelevant stimulus features. This contrasts with conditions in which two different tasks have to be applied to the same perceptual attributes of the stimulus. For instance, [18] asked children with and without ADHD to switch between classifying a digit stimulus as either odd/even or smaller/larger than 5, and failed to find a difference in TS costs. Crucially, in the former case TS performance may be supported by deploying attention to the perceptually distinct attributes of the stimulus that define the target information of the current task (see [19] for a demonstration of dissociable attentional sets in the domain of spatial stimulus selection). Enhancement of switch costs for individuals with ADHD might thus go back to a deficit in flexible adjustment of attention, that is, in efficient re-weighting of attentional weights assigned to changing perceptual attributes.

Findings obtained in a recent Eriksen Flanker Task study [20] involving a manipulation of the ratio of congruent and incongruent trials, are in line with the notion of a deficit in flexible adjustment of attention in patients with ADHD. Specifically, whereas the control group showed a higher congruency effect in blocks with 80% congruent stimuli than in blocks with 20% congruent, in the ADHD group, the congruency effect was low regardless of the congruent/incongruent ratio. This suggests that control participants adjusted their attention depending on distractor utility (cf. [21], overview in [22]), while the ADHD group appeared to maintain a strong attentional focus regardless of context conditions.

Because in selective attention tasks, such as Eriksen Flanker, the target stimulus contains all information needed for successful task performance, these tasks can be accomplished by maintaining a strongly focused state of attention regardless of contextual changes. Deficits in flexible attentional adjustment should be associated with more detrimental consequences, however, if task-relevant stimulus information must be extracted from frequently changing stimulus features. As noted above, this is the case in TS studies which involve tasks associated with different target stimulus features. In light of the fact that tasks combined in TS experiments are associated with a multitude of additional processing differences (i.e., cognitive operations of stimulus classification and response selection), however, it is conceivable that TS performance can be accomplished by relying on biasing processing independently of stimulus perception (e.g., [23]).

Standard TS protocols may thus not constitute an optimal means to assess attentional adjustment. To investigate a possible impairment in adjusting the set of stimulus

selection, we followed the approach of [21]. This study used hierarchical stimuli [24], either big letters made out of small letters or big numbers made out of small numbers (see "Apparatus and stimuli"). The tasks were digit and letter identification, and each could be performed with two AtS levels, either global or local (big and small, respectively). With this method, task switch costs could be compared in conditions with and without the need to shift the AtS. In addition, congruency effects, exerted by the irrelevant stimulus level, served as indication for the degree of processing the irrelevant level. Task switch costs and congruency effects were larger when switching between tasks was associated with shifting attention between stimulus levels (mixed levels condition) than when target levels were kept constant (constant levels condition), suggesting a specific cost of shifting the set of stimulus selection as well as a lower degree of shielding performance against interference from information presented on the irrelevant level after a level switch.

Assuming that ADHD is associated with a particular deficit in flexible adoption of (task-specific) sets of stimulus selection one would predict particular enhancement of switch costs and congruency effects in the mixed levels condition for patients with ADHD compared to controls. By contrast, switching between the same tasks should not be particularly impaired when target levels are kept constant.

Interpretation of task switch costs in terms of executive functioning is usually rendered difficult by stimulus-specific effects of interference between tasks. TS performance seems particularly impaired if a stimulus is processed that was previously presented in the context of the other task (e.g., [25]), possibly reflecting stimulus-based cuing of task-set conflict rather than impaired cognitive reconfiguration. Unlike standard TS protocols that involve frequent occurrences of all stimuli in the context of both tasks, the procedure used in the current study avoids such proactive interference by presenting qualitatively different stimuli in the two tasks (i.e., global digits made up of local digits vs. global letters made up of local letters [21]).

Methods
Participants
Demographic data of our sample is displayed in Table 1. Thirty-eight adults (M age = 36.14 years, SD = 12.17; 17 women) with a diagnosis of ADHD as their primary disorder, were recruited in a Hamburg neurological outpatient practice which is specialized in the diagnosis and treatment of ADHD in adults. During a regular appointment in the practice patients were informed about the possibility to participate in the experiment right away or make an appointment. Patients were included into

Table 1 Demographic description of the sample by group

	ADHD group (n = 38)	Control group (n = 39)	Group difference
Gender (n and % of women)	17 (44.7%)	19 (48.7%)	0.903[a]
M-age (SD)	36.14 (12.71)	33.61 (9.81)	0.330[b]
Country of birth Germany	35 (92.1%)	32 (82.1%)	0.331[a]
Highest educational level			0.947[a]
Primary school (Grundschule)	1 (2.6%)	0 (0.0%)	
Secondary school (Haupt- and Realschule)	10 (26.3%)	10 (25.6%)	
Secondary school and vocational training (Haupt-, Realschule mit Berufsabschluss, Gymnasium)	3 (7.9%)	4 (10.3%)	
University entrance degree (Fachhochschulreife, Abitur)	13 (34.2%)	13 (33.3%)	
University degree (Hochschulabschluss, Fachhochschulabschluss)	10 (26.4%)	11 (28.2%)	
Ph.D. (promotion)	1 (2.6%)	1 (2.6%)	
Other psychological diagnoses (%)	12 (31.6%)	2 (5.1%)	0.007[a]
Psychotherapy	24 (63.2%)	4 (10.3%)	< 0.001[a]

[a] χ^2, [b] p-value of t test

the sample if they had received a clinical diagnosis of ADHD. Fourteen patients received their diagnoses before the age of 18 years. Twelve patients reported to have comorbid diagnoses. Thirty-three patients were treated with extended-release methylphenidate, two with Serotonin–Noradrenalin-Reuptake-Inhibitors and four were not taking medication. Patients were instructed to take their medication as usual and during the experiment 26 patients were under the influence of their medication (i.e., had taken extended-release Methylphenidate within 12 h before the experiment or Serotonin–Noradrenalin-Reuptake-Inhibitors in the last-2 weeks). Twenty-four patients had received or were receiving psychotherapy.

The adults without ADHD of the control group were recruited using various strategies. We asked adults without any disorders that were accompanying patients into the practice to participate, we posted calls for participants on a website for job advertisements and addressed people waiting in local employment offices to recruit a diverse sample comparable to the sample with ADHD. Participants in the control group were excluded if they received clinically relevant (t-score above 65, t-scores have a mean of 50 and a standard deviation of 10) scores in two or three symptom scales of the CAARS inattention/memory problems, hyperactivity/restlessness and impulsivity/emotional lability. Two participants were excluded due to this criterion. The final control group included 39 control adults (M age = 33.61 years, SD = 9.81, 19 women). Two participants reported to have received psychological diagnoses in the past (depression and adjustment disorder) and four reported psychotherapy. We compared the group with ADHD with the group without ADHD with regards to gender, age, country of birth, degree of education and did not find any significant

group differences (see Table 1). As expected, patients reported more comorbid diagnoses and more psychological treatment.

The experiment and the diagnostic procedure were performed by trained student assistants in a quiet room of the neurological outpatient practice. The window blinds were closed to avoid distraction and ensure the same lighting conditions for all participants. After giving informed consent the participants were briefly interviewed about their demographics and ADHD diagnosis before they performed in the experiment. Subsequently, participants were asked to fill out the questionnaires (Conners' Adult ADHD Rating Scales [CAARS], Brief-Symptom-Inventory [BSI], Self-Control Scale [SCS-K-D]) as well as to take part in an IQ screening (Wechsler Adult Intelligence Scale fourth edition [WAIS-IV]) and in the tests of attention (test battery for attentional performance [TAP]). Finally, the last part of the session was the clinical interview (Wender-Reimherr-Interview [WRI]). After completion, participants received their reimbursement and were informed about the possibility to receive a written report about the results of the study in general. The session took approximately 2 h.

Diagnostic measures
The following table displays the results of the diagnostic measures. To avoid habituation or practice effects diagnostic measured used in this study differed from the diagnostic measures usually applied in the neurological outpatient practice.

Conners' Adult ADHD Rating Scales (CAARS)
The CAARS is a clinical questionnaire assessing attention problems in adults [26]. We used the German version

[27]. The scales inattention/memory problems, hyperactivity/restlessness, impulsivity/emotional lability and problems with self-concept assess the current symptoms. Furthermore, there are three scales assessing the DSM-IV symptoms of inattention and hyperactivity/impulsivity and an ADHD index. We used the long self-report version with 66 items. The scales show high internal consistency (Cronbachs Alpha > 0.85) and an average test–retest reliability of 0.88 [27]. Groups differed highly significant in all scales of the CAARS (Table 2).

Wender-Reimherr-Interview (WRI)
The WRI has been published in German as part of the Homburger ADHD-Scales for adults test battery (HASE) [28]. The WRI is based on the American WRI [29]. In a structured interview psychopathological items are rated by the interviewer on a scale from 0 (*not present*) to 2 (*medium or high*). The 28 items are part of seven subscales: inattention, hyperactivity, hot temper, mood instability, over reactivity, disorganization, impulsivity. The score is a sum of all items. Furthermore, there is a global

Table 2 Diagnostic data of the sample by group

	ADHD group (n = 38)	Control group (n = 39)	Group difference
CAARS			
Inattention/memory problems (t-value)	70,63 (16,26)	44.21 (8.09)	< 0.001
Hyperactivity/restlessness (t-value)	66.24 (14.38)	48.69 (8.80)	< 0.001
Impulsivity/emotional lability (t-value)	67.03 (17.31)	44.64 (6.50)	< 0.001
Problems with self-concept	10.24 (5.01)	4.10 (2.57)	< 0.001
DSM: inattention	15.05 (6.11)	3.87 (2.77)	< 0.001
DSM: hyperactivity/impulsivity	12.11 (6.13)	4.36 (3.33)	< 0.001
ADHD index	19.66(7.60)	6.74 (3.56)	< 0.001
WRI			
Inattention	7.53 (2.90)	1.41 (1.65)	< 0.001
Hyperactivity	3.11 (2.08)	0.69 (1.15)	< 0.001
Hot temper	3.87 (2.23)	1.00 (1.43)	< 0.001
Mood instability	5.05 (2.68)	1.56 (1.68)	< 0.001
Over reactivity	2.68 (2.11)	0.69 (1.26)	< 0.001
Disorganization	5.61 (3.36)	1.72 (1.69)	< 0.001
Impulsivity	5.26 (2.87)	2.79 (2.35)	< 0.001
WRI global score	11.55 (5.28)	3.13 (3.11)	< 0.001
TAP—working memory			
Correct hits	11.63 (3.95)	13.38 (1.89)	0.017
Errors of omission	3.95 (0.64)	1.89 (0.30)	0.017
BSI			
Somatization	0.63 (0.69)	0.23 (0.42)	0.004
Obsessive–compulsive	1.65 (0.97)	0.45 (0.48)	< 0.001
Interpersonal sensitivity	1.36 (1.14)	0.38 (0.45)	< 0.001
Depression	1.27 (1.06)	0.22 (0.29)	< 0.001
Anxiety	1.03 (0.81)	0.32 (0.37)	< 0.001
Hostility	1.18 (0.90)	0.25 (0.25)	< 0.001
Phobic anxiety	0.64 (0.95)	0.15 (0.19)	0.003
Paranoid ideation	1.18 (1.00)	0.31 (0.38)	< 0.001
Psychoticism	0.96 (0.94)	0.21 (0.29)	< 0.001
SCS-K-D	38.89 (3.33)	38.54 (2.82)	0.614
WAIS-IV matrices (raw score)	18.47 (4.95)	18.79 (3.81)	0.750
WAIS-IV vocabulary (raw score)	36.92 (11.97)	37.15 (10.83)	0.929
WAIS-IV estimated IQ	91.97 (15.33)	92.15 (11.29)	0.953

CAARS Conners' Adult ADHD Rating Scales, *WRI* Wender-Reimherr-Interview, *TAP* test battery for attentional performance, *BSI* brief-symptom-inventory, *SCS-K-D* Self-Control Scale, *WAIS-IV* Wechsler Adult Intelligence Scale fourth edition

rating for each scale judging symptom on a scale from 0 (*not present*) to 4 (*severe*). The WRI Global Score is a sum of the seven global ratings. Groups differed significantly in all scales and the global score of the WRI (Table 2). The interrater reliability for diagnoses of ADHD is kappa = 1.0; ICC = 0.92. The reliability for the total score is $\alpha = 0.82$ [28].

Test battery for attentional performance (TAP)

The subtest working memory from the TAP 2.3 [30] was administered. This working memory 2-back task, asked participants to press a button whenever the one-digit-number appeared on the screen was the same as the one before the last one. Patients had less correct hits and more errors of omission (Table 2). The split-half reliability for working memory was determined on the basis of odd–even splits with r being 0.847 for median reaction time, 0.885 for errors and 0.742 for omissions [30].

Brief-symptom-inventory (BSI)

The BSI [31] provides an overview of self-reported clinically relevant psychological symptoms in adolescents and adults. The BSI is the short version of the SCL-R-90 [32], which measures the same dimensions. Items for each dimension of the BSI were selected based on a factor analysis of the SCL-R-90, with the highest loading items on each dimension selected for the BSI [33, 34]. The BSI requires only 8–10 min to complete and consists of 53 items covering nine symptom dimensions: somatization, obsessive–compulsive, interpersonal sensitivity, depression, anxiety, hostility, phobic anxiety, paranoid ideation and psychoticism. The BSI has internal consistencies from $\alpha = 0.63$ to $\alpha = 0.85$ and retest-reliabilities from $r = 0.73$ to $r = 0.92$. Groups differed significantly in all scales of the BSI (Table 2).

Self-Control Scale (SCS-K-D)

The SCS-K the German adaption of the Brief Self-Control Scale (BSCS, [35]. The unidimensional questionnaire assesses self-control with 13 items which are rated on a 5-point, Likert scale with possible answers ranging from 1 (*not at all like me*) to 5 (*very much like me*). The internal consistency is $\alpha = 0.81$. Patients and controls did not differ in self-control (Table 2).

Wechsler Adult Intelligence Scale fourth edition (WAIS-IV)

We used two subtests from the German version of the WAIS-IV [36]: Matrix reasoning and vocabulary. These two subtests have been shown to form a good indicator for general cognitive abilities testing in an economic way ($r = 0.86$ with the full test battery, [37]). The internal consistency of this two-test short form is high $r = 0.94$ [37].

A full IQ can be estimated by using these two subtests. The estimated full IQ in our sample was surprisingly low (Table 2), given the educational level. This could be due to the fact that in a complete administration of the WAIS-IV, three other subtests are administered before the matrix reasoning and vocabulary subtest. Therefore, participants could be less experienced with the format of the test if only the two subtests are administered [37]. However and most importantly, groups did not differ in the estimated IQ or in the raw scores of the two subtests used (Table 2).

Reaction time experiment
Apparatus and stimuli

Stimuli were presented using a standard PC with a 23-inch LCD screen (1920 × 1080 pix., latency < 3 ms), viewed at a distance of approx. 55 cm. The experiment was implemented with MATLAB R2010a and Psychtoolbox 3.0. Responses were recorded with a 1-ms time resolution QWERTZ keyboard. The stimuli were composed of the characters 1, 2, 3, 4, A, B, C and D. Each of these characters could occur on the global and on the local level. The stimuli were adapted from the font Silkscreen, one of the smallest raster fonts. Each character consists of a 5 × 5 pixel matrix (no anti-aliasing) but the ones used here were all 4 × 5 pixels in size (except '1' hich was 3 × 5 pix.). The local characters consisted of 4 × 5 matrices of black squares with white fringes. The global level used the local level matrices as "pixels". The background was white. The local and global levels of each stimulus were both either digits or letters, never a mix of digit and letter. 25% of the stimuli were congruent across the global/local level (for example, a global letter 'B' made out of local letters 'B'). Between both levels, the stimuli had an appearance of "self-similarity" and the size difference was as small as possible (Fig. 1). The stimuli were presented in the form of 217 × 301 pixel bitmap pictures (local characters 0.71° × 0.88° visually, global characters 3.4° × 5.2°); the rest of the screen was a dark grey background. Each participant had two tasks, "digit" and "letter", presented in a random order with equal probability. The relevant level of the stimuli was mapped to the response keys 'F', 'V', 'N' and 'J' in the intuitive left-to-right fashion: 1, A: F; 2, B: V; 3, C: N, and 4, D: J. The response keys were pressed by the participant's middle and index fingers of both hands. Half of the experimental blocks had a constant AtS level for both tasks, either global or local. The other half has a mixed AtS levels, either global-number/local-letter or local-number/global-letter. Balancing which constant set, which mixed sets and whether participants start with constant or mixed sets, resulted in eight different versions of the experiment.

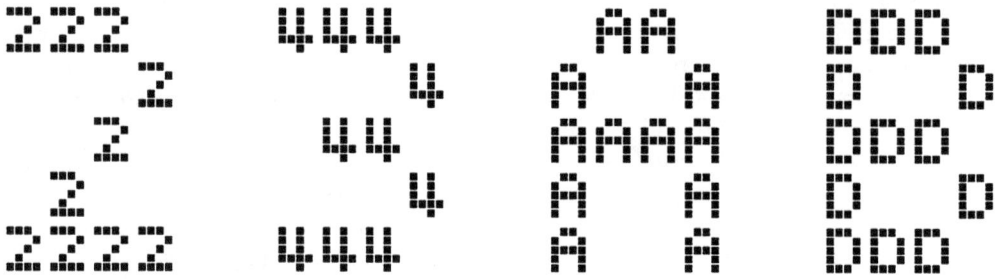

Fig. 1 Examples of the stimuli used in the experiment. Left to right, the first and third stimuli are congruent in the global/local target levels, the second and fourth are incongruent

Procedure

Each trial presented first a task cue ("Zahl" or "Buchst.", German for "number" and "letter" respectively) and then the hierarchical stimulus. Each trial consisted of a 500 ms blank screen, 200 ms cue, and a 200 ms presentation of the stimulus. The trial ended when a response key was pressed. The participants performed three 30-items long practice blocks, first the number task, then the letter task, and finally both tasks mixed. This was followed by four 80-trials experimental blocks. After this, the AtS was changed from constant to mixed levels (or vice versa). Participants were accordingly instructed, and performed another four experimental blocks (without previous practice). During the whole experiment, a 900 ms feedback was given for each false response, and after each experimental block the mean reaction time and error percentage was shown.

Results

The first three trials of each block, trials with an incorrect response and trials immediately following these were excluded from analysis. Response times were aggregated according to the within-subject factors constant vs. mixed level, task switch vs. repetition and congruent vs. incongruent stimulus. Unless otherwise noted, all the following statistics were based on repeated-measures analysis of variance (ANOVAs) with two-tailed significance values. ANOVAs were conducted on the mean reaction times of correct responses and on the average error proportions. In the reaction time analysis, the three main within-subjects factors were highly significant. Constant level was faster than mixed level, $F(1,75)=67,236$, $p<0.001$, $\eta_p^2=0.473$. Task repetition was faster than task switch, $F(1,75)=134,350$, $p<0.001$, $\eta_p^2=0.642$. Congruent stimuli were responded to faster than incongruent ones, $F(1,75)=30.127$, $p<0.001$, $\eta_p^2=0.287$. Averaged over the within-subject factors, patients with ADHD were slower than controls, $F(1,75)=4.516$, $p<0.037$, $\eta_p^2=0.057$.

The only within-subjects factor that interacted significantly with the between-subjects factor ADHD/control was TS repetition/switch, $F(1,75)=134.350$, $p<0.001$, $\eta_p^2=0.642$; more interestingly, a three way interaction between constant/mixed target levels, task repetition/switch and ADHD/control was also significant, $F(1,75)=4.600$, $p<0.035$, $\eta_p^2=0.058$. Inspection of Fig. 2 shows that both groups of participants were associated with larger TS costs in the mixed target levels condition than in the constant target levels condition but this difference was more pronounced for the patient group (Table 3).

This interpretation was confirmed by conducting separate ANOVAs for the constant and the mixed levels conditions. The interaction between repetition/switch and ADHD/control was highly significant in the mixed levels case, $F(1,75)=11.846$, $p<0.001$, $\eta_p^2=0.136$, but not significant in the constant level case, $F(1,75)=0.595$, $p<0.443$, $\eta_p^2=0.008$. Due to the experiment's design, it is conceivable that the presence of TS costs (without AtS shift) was an artifact. Half of the participants started with mixed

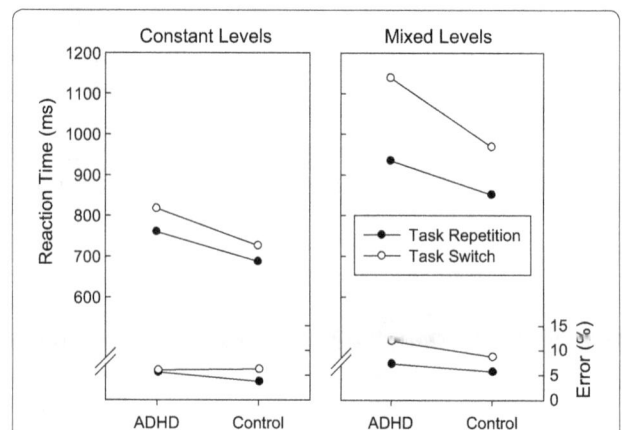

Fig. 2 Mean reaction times and mean error percentages as a function of group (patients with ADHD, controls), target levels (constant, mixed), and task sequence (repetition, switch)

Table 3 Repeated measures ANOVA of mean reaction times

	F	p	$\eta^2 p$
ADHD/control	4.516	0.037	0.057
Constant/mixed	67.236	<0.001	0.473
Constant/mixed * ADHD/control	0.645	0.424	0.009
Repetition/switch	134.350	<0.001	0.642
Repetition/switch * ADHD/control	8.232	0.005	0.099
Congruency	30.127	<0.001	0.287
Congruency * ADHD/control	0.058	0.810	0.001
Constant/mixed * repetition/switch	51.464	<0.001	0.407
Constant/mixed * repetition/switch * ADHD/control	4.600	0.035	0.058
Constant/mixed * congruency	12.647	0.001	0.144
Constant/mixed * congruency * ADHD/control	0.046	0.831	0.001
Repetition/switch * congruency	5.171	0.026	0.064
Repetition/switch * congruency * ADHD/control	0.090	0.764	0.001
Constant/mixed * repetition/switch * congruency	2.227	0.140	0.029
Constant/mixed * repetition/switch * congruency * ADHD/control	0.001	0.972	<0.001

levels, it is possible that in the following half of the experiment—unrequired—attention to the irrelevant AtS persisted. We examined therefore the constant level half of the experiment only in the participants that started with that condition (17 ADHD and 21 control participants). There was a trend towards TS costs for both groups, but no significant differences between ADHD patients and controls ($F(1,36) = 1.463$, $p < 0.234$, $\eta_p^2 = 0.039$).

We also examined the aggregated average error rate for each participant and factor combination (see Fig. 2). Again, all within-subjects main factors were highly significant and consistent with the reaction times [$F(1,75) = 16.164$, $p < 0.001$, $\eta_p^2 = 0.177$; $F(1,75) = 44.573$, $p < 0.001$, $\eta_p^2 = 0.373$; and $F(1,75) = 58.379$, $p < 0.001$, $\eta_p^2 = 0.438$, for constant/mixed target levels, task repetition/switch, and congruent/incongruent, respectively]. The interaction between ADHD/control and task repetition/switch was not significant, $F(1,75) = 0.764$, $p < 0.385$, $\eta_p^2 = 0.010$. The three-way interaction between ADHD/control, task repetition/switch, and constant/mixed target levels was not significant, $F(1,75) = 2.262$, $p < 0.137$, $\eta_p^2 = 0.029$. More importantly however, these last two interactions were numerically consistent with the reaction times, i.e., longer reaction times correspond to higher error rates. Separate ANOVAs for the constant levels condition and the mixed levels condition revealed that the interaction between repetition/switch and ADHD/control was significant in the constant levels $F(1,75) = 4.325$, $p < 0.041$, $\eta_p^2 = 0.055$, but not in the mixed levels, $F(1,75) = 0.401$, $p < 0.528$, $\eta_p^2 = 0.005$. As can be seen in Fig. 2, switch costs in the ADHD group were almost completely absent when the target level was kept constant.

A typical result found in the literature on executive control is that patients with ADHD show more reaction time variability. Although many studies report results in the form of standard deviations, this may be misleading because slower responses have higher numerical values, and tend to result in higher standard deviations. We opted instead to compute standard deviations for each participant and factor combination, and divided these values by the corresponding averages to obtain coefficients of variability, thus controlling the effect of speed differences; we then analyzed these coefficients with ANOVA using the same factors as in the reaction time analyses. Comparing ADHD patients with controls, the first show a significantly higher variability in response times, $F(1,75) = 10.727$, $p < 0.001$, $\eta_p^2 = 0.125$. The only other significant effect was that the mixed target levels condition had more variable response times than the fixed one, $F(1,75) = 24.152$, $p < 0.001$, $\eta_p^2 = 0.244$. No significant interaction with ADHD/control was found.

A final important question in this study is whether TS and AtS shift are related in general to ADHD deficits. We calculated a crude measure of performance in these executive functions simply by subtracting for each participant the average reaction time in task repetitions from the average in task switches (i.e., TS costs), and calculated this measure separately for the constant and mixed target levels halves of the experiment. Since these values are not corrected for age, sex or any other variable, we correlated these measurements with the raw values (no T-correction) of the scales attention, hyperactivity and impulsivity of the CAARS and WRI-HASE diagnostic tests. The results are displayed in Table 4.

Table 4 Pearson correlations between task switch-costs under constant/mixed target levels and diagnostic scales

	TS-cost constant		TS-cost mixed	
	r	Significance	r	Significance
CAARS inattention	0.282	0.0904	0.367	0.0113[a]
CAARS hyperactivity	0.329	0.0280[a]	0.253	0.1578
CAARS impulsivity	0.342	0.0211[a]	0.366	0.0113[a]
WRI inattention	0.222	0.2596	0.405	0.0031[b]
WRI hyperactivity	0.148	0.2701	0.172	0.2701
WRI impulsivity	0.220	0.2596	0.207	0.2596

Significance values are Holm–Bonferroni corrected for 12 comparisons, alpha 0.05

TS task switching, *AtS* attentional set, *CAARS* Conners' Adult ADHD Rating Scales, *WRI* Wender-Reimherr-Interview

[a] Correlation is significant at the 0.05 level (two-tailed)

[b] Correlation is significant at the 0.01 level (two-tailed)

TS cost in the constant target level condition correlated significantly with the CAARS Hyperactivity and Impulsivity scales, mixed level TS correlated significantly with the CAARS inattention and impulsivity scales, but only the TS cost in the mixed condition had a significant correlation with the WRI-HASE attention scale. The diagnostic scales correlated among themselves in a much stronger way (not shown in the table, inattention $r = 0.772$, $p < 0.01$, hyperactivity $r = 0.759$, $p < 0.01$, impulsivity $r = 0.566$, $p < 0.01$.

Discussion

Comparing the performance of persons with and without ADHD, patients were slower in task switch trials only when attention shifted to different stimulus features. When the attentional set was kept constant, task switch costs were present but not larger for patients than controls.

ADHD symptoms have long been assumed to be associated with a deficit in executive functioning, particularly with the flexible deployment of attention to varying sources of stimulus information. Findings of enhanced task switch costs may not be indicative of a deficit in AtS, however, because in standard task switching protocols, switches between tasks are often confounded with switches between perceptual features of the stimuli. Our experiment disentangled AtS from other components of task-set switch. The digit task had as targets 1, 2, 3 and 4, while the letter task used the letters A, B, C and D. Using stimuli with global and local features, half of the trial blocks had a constant target level (both tasks either local or global) while the other half required shifting the AtS on each task switch. The stimuli never combined digits and letters. In light of the heterogeneity of findings

obtained in task switching studies involving patients with ADHD [11–13, 15, 18, 38, 39], lack of "pure" TS costs differences between patients with ADHD and controls has to be considered with caution. It must be emphasized that TS in the current study differed from usual TS protocols by the fact that the stimuli were strictly task-unique. Such conditions might not be associated with substantial demands of executive task-set reconfiguration. Also, this method avoided the occurrence of stimulus-related proactive interference, presumably a major source of task switch costs [25]. By consequence, task switch costs tended to be very small and may not be informative about the ability to shift task-sets or inhibit interference from the irrelevant task-set (cf. [21]).

Identifying deficits in executive functioning constitutes a major challenge in clinical (neuro)psychology. It has been criticized, in this connection, that commonly used procedures are characterized by lack of theoretical justification and more specific assessment of separable components of executive functions are desirable [40, 41] This seems to apply, particularly, to task switching performance as a diagnostic means, which has been found to be impaired in ADHD in some previous studies [8, 11, 15] but has been associated with comparably low effect sizes in meta-analyses [1, 42] Alongside with the search for discriminative subtypes in ADHD [43], isolating more specific components of task-set shift, as attempted in the current study with regard to shifting the attentional set, seems a valuable method to improve this situation, and allows a more detailed description of which cognitive processes may be affected.

The present study is consistent with the literature on ADHD showing more variable response times in TS experiments [44]. Also, we replicated previous findings on a student sample [21], demonstrating increased costs of switching tasks and increased congruency effects between global and local stimulus levels when task switching was associated with a shift of the attentional set.

However, patients did not display a larger difference in the size of the congruency effect in the mixed levels vs. the constant level condition than the control group. This result is reminiscent of previous findings of dissociations between overt responding to the global or local stimulus level and interference exerted by the other level (e.g., [45, 46]). Although we cannot rule out power problems, there is thus so far no indication of an impairment in shielding the processing of target stimulus information against distracting stimulus features. This pattern of findings is consistent with the observation in [20] that patients with ADHD showed no deficit regarding selective processing of target stimulus information but were reluctant to attenuate processing selectivity when the distractor stimuli were useful.

A strength of the current study is the representativeness of the sample and the well-matched control group. We had about an equal number of male and female patients [47, 48]. The educational level was very heterogeneous in both groups and the patients did not differ from controls with regards to IQ [49]. However, they did show high comorbid symptoms although they were being treated [50].

Concerning the relevance of our results for general ADHD symptoms, TS costs both in the constant and mixed target levels cases, correlated with the symptom scales of two ADHD diagnostic scales. Besides the unclear importance of TS without AtS shift, we deem our results robust enough to claim that attentional set shift is impaired in ADHD patients.

Abbreviations

ADHD: attention deficit hyperactivity disorder; ANOVA: analysis of variance; AtS: attentional set; BSCS: Brief Self-Control Scale; BSI: brief symptom inventory; CAARS: Conners' Adult ADHD Rating Scales; DSM-IV: diagnostic and statistical manual of mental disorders, revision IV; HASE: Homburger ADHS-Skalen für Erwachsene (German version of WRI); SCS-K-D: Self-Control Scale; TAP: test battery for attentional performance; TS: task switch/task switching; WAIS-IV: Wechsler Adult Intelligence Scale, edition IV; WRI: Wender-Reimherr-Interview.

Authors' contributions

All authors contributed to the conception of the research. ALR, MW, JKK and TJ organized and planed data collection. ALR and JKK were involved in data collection. MW and TJ supervised data collection. ALR and JKK analyzed the data with contributions from MW and TJ. ALR wrote the manuscript. MW, JKK, and TJ contributed parts of it. MW and TJ revised the manuscript. All authors read and approved the final manuscript.

Author details

[1] Experimental Psychology Unit, Helmut-Schmidt-University/University of the Federal Armed Forces Hamburg, Holstenhofweg 85, 22043 Hamburg, Germany. [2] Faculty of Human Sciences, Medical School Hamburg, Hamburg, Germany. [3] Educational Psychology, Helmut-Schmidt-University/University of the Federal Armed Forces Hamburg, Hamburg, Germany. [4] School Psychology, Eberhard Karls Universität Tübingen, Tübingen, Germany. [5] Center for Individual Development and Adaptive Education of Children at Risk (IDeA), Frankfurt, Germany.

Acknowledgements

We specially thank Dr. Heinrich Goossens-Merkt and his team, who recruited the patients and provided rooms in the neurological outpatient practice. We also thank Dr. Detlef Steuer for his advice in statistics. Finally, we thank our assistants Ruth Wewers, Stina Klein, Henning Schmidt, Moritz Held and Julian Protzer, for their help in literature research, participant recruiting, data collection, typing, checking data and checking again.

Competing interests

The authors declare that they have no competing interests.

Funding

This research was funded by a grant within the Priority Program SPP 1772 of the German Research Foundation (Deutsche Forschungsgemeinschaft) to Thomas Jacobsen (JA 1009/13-1).

References

1. Willcutt EG, Doyle AE, Nigg JT, Faraone SV, Pennington BF. Validity of the executive function theory of attention-deficit/hyperactivity disorder: a meta-analytic review. Biol Psychiatry. 2005;57:1336–46.
2. Barkley RA. Behavioral inhibition, sustained attention, and executive functions: constructing a unifying theory of ADHD. Psychol Bull. 1997;121(1):65–94.
3. Bayliss D, Roodenrys S. Executive processing and attention deficit hyperactivity disorder: an application of the supervisory attentional system. Dev Neuropsychol. 2000;17(2):161–80.
4. Houghton S, Douglas G, West J, Whiting K, Wall M, Langsford S, Powell L, Carroll A. Differential patterns of executive function in children with attention-deficit hyperactivity disorder according to gender and subtype. J Child Neurol. 1999;14:801–5.
5. Klorman R, Hazel-Fernandez LA, Shaywitz SE, Fletcher JM, Marchione KE, Holahan JM, Stuebing KK, Shaywitz BA. Executive functioning deficits in attention-deficit/hyperactivity disorder are independent of oppositional defiant or reading disorder. J Am Acad Child Adolesc Psychiatry. 1999;38(9):1148–55.
6. Pennington BF, Ozonoff S. Executive functions and development psychopathology. J Child Psychol Psychiatry. 1996;37:51–87.
7. Schachar RJ, Tannock R, Logan G. Inhibitory control, impulsiveness, and attention deficit hyperactivity disorder. Clin Psychol Rev. 1993;13(8):721–39.
8. Rauch WA, Gold A, Schmitt K. To what extent are task-switching deficits in children with attention-deficit/hyperactivity disorder independent of impaired inhibition. ADHD Atten Defic Hyperact Disord. 2012;4:179–87. https://doi.org/10.1007/s12402-012-0083-5.
9. Kiesel A, Steinhauser M, Wendt M, Falkenstein M, Jost K, Philipp AM, Koch I. Control and interference in task switching—a review. Psychol Bull. 2010;136(5):849.
10. Vandierendonck A, Liefooghe B, Verbruggen F. Task switching: interplay of reconfiguration and interference control. Psychol Bull. 2010;136(4):601–26.
11. Cepeda NJ, Cepeda ML, Kramer AF. Task switching and attention deficit hyperactivity disorder. J Abnorm Child Psychol. 2000;28:213–26.
12. Kramer AF, Cepeda NJ, Cepeda ML. Methylphenidate effects on task-switching performance in attention-deficit/hyperactivity disorder. J Am Acad Child Adolesc Psychiatry. 2001;40:1277–84.
13. White HA, Shah P. Training attention-switching ability in adults with ADHD. J Atten Disord. 2006;10:44–53.
14. Goschke T. Intentional reconfiguration and involuntary persistence in task set switching. In: Monsell S, Driver J, editors. Control of cognitive processes: attention and performance XVIII. Cambridge: MIT Press; 2000. p. 331–55.
15. King JA, Colla M, Brass M, Heuser I, von Cramon DY. Inefficient cognitive control in adult ADHD: evidence from trial-by-trial Stroop test and cued task switching performance. Behav Brain Funct. 2007;3:42.
16. Allport A, Styles EA, Hsieh S. Shifting intentional set: exploring the dynamic control of tasks. In: Umiltà C, Moscovitch M, editors. Conscious and nonconscious information processing: attention and performance XV. Cambridge: MIT Press; 1994. p. 421–52.
17. Rogers R, Monsell S. Costs of a predictable switch between simple cognitive tasks. J Exp Psychol Gen. 1995;124:207–31.
18. Hung CL, Huang CJ, Tsai YJ, Chang YK, Hung TM. Neuroelectric and behavioral effects of acute exercise on task switching in children with attention-deficit/hyperactivity disorder. Front Psychol. 2016;7:1589.
19. Wendt M, Kähler ST, Luna-Rodriguez A, Jacobsen T. Adoption of task-specific sets of visual attention. Front Psychol. 2017. https://doi.org/10.3389/fpsyg.2017.00687.
20. Merkt J, Singmann H, Bodenburg S, Goossens-Merkt H, Kappes A, Wendt M, Gawrilow C. Flanker performance in female college students with ADHD—a diffusion model analysis. ADHD Atten Defic Hyperact Disord. 2013. https://doi.org/10.1007/s12402-013-0110-1.
21. Wendt M, Luna-Rodriguez A, Jacobsen T. Shifting the set of stimulus selection when switching between tasks. Psychol Res. 2018;82(1):134–45. https://doi.org/10.1007/s00426-017-0890-6.
22. Bugg JM, Crump MJC. In support of a distinction between voluntary and

stimulus-driven control: a review of the literature on proportion congruent effects. Front Psychol. 2012;3:367. https://doi.org/10.3389/fpsyg.2012.00367.

23. Meiran N, Kessler Y, Adi-Japha E. Control by action representation and input selection (CARIS): a theoretical framework for task switching. Psychol Res. 2008;72:473–500.

24. Navon D. Forest before trees: the precedence of global features in visual perception. Cogn Psychol. 1977;9(3):353–83.

25. Waszak F, Hommel B, Allport DA. Task-switching and long-term priming: role of episodic stimulus-task bindings in task-shift costs. Cogn Psychol. 2003;46:361–413.

26. Conners K, Erhardt D, Sparrow E. Conners' adult adhd rating scales (CAARS). Toronto: Multi-Health Systems; 1999.

27. Christiansen H, Hirsch O, Abdel-Hamid M, Kis B. Conners Skalen zu Aufmerksamkeit und Verhalten für Erwachsene. [Conners' Adult ADHD Rating Scales]. Bern, Switzerland: Verlag Hans Huber, Hogrefe. 2014.

28. Rösler M, Retz-Junginger P, Retz W, Stieglitz R-D. Homburger ADHS-Skalen für Erwachsene (HASE) [Homburger ADHD-scales for adults test battery]. Göttingen: Hogrefe. 2007.

29. Wender PH. Attention-deficit hyperactivity disorder in adults. Oxford: University Press; 1995.

30. Zimmermann P, Fimm B. Testbatterie zur Aufmerksamkeitsprüfung (TAP) [test battery for attentional performance] (version 2.3). Würselen, Germany: Psytest. 2006.

31. Franke GH. Brief Symptom inventory von L. R. Derogatis (Kurzform der SCL-90-R—German version). Göttingen, Germany: Beltz Test GmbH. 2000.

32. Derogatis LR. Manual for the symptom checklist 90 revised (SCL-90-R). Derogatis: Baltimore; 1986.

33. Derogatis LR. Brief symptom inventory (BSI), administration, scoring, and procedures manual. 3rd ed. Minneapolis: Pearson Assessments; 1993.

34. Derogatis LR, Cleary PA. Confirmation of the dimensional structure of the SCL-90: a study in construct validation. J Clin Psychol. 1977;33:981–9. https://doi.org/10.1002/1097-4679(197710)33:4%3c981:AID-JCLP2270330412%3e3.0.CO;2-0.

35. Tangney JP, Baumeister RF, Boone AL. High self-control predicts good adjustment, less pathology, better grades, and interpersonal success. J Pers. 2004;72(2):271–324.

36. Petermann F, Petermann U. Wechsler adult intelligence scale (WAIS-IV, German version). Frankfurt/Main: Pearson Assessment and Information; 2012.

37. Daseking M, Petermann F, Waldmann HC. Schätzung der allgemeinen Intelligenz mit einer Kurzform der WAIS-IV bei neurologischen Fragestellungen [estimation of general intelligence in neurological settings by a short form of the WAIS-IV]. Aktuelle Neurologie. 2014;41:349–55. https://doi.org/10.1055/s-0034-1382050.

38. Mor B, Yitzhaki-Amsalem S, Prior A. The joint effect of bilingualism and ADHD on executive functions. J Atten Disord. 2015;19:527–41.

39. Oades RD, Christiansen H. Cognitive switching processes in young people with attention deficit/hyperactivity disorder. Arch Clin Neuropsychol. 2008;23:21–32.

40. Chan RCK, Shum D, Toulopoulou T, Chen EYH. Assessment of executive functions: review of instruments and identification of critical issues. Arch Clin Neuropsychol. 2008;23:201–16.

41. Miyake A, Freidman NP, Emerson MJ, Witzki AH, Howerter A, Wager TD. The unity and diversity of executive functions and their contributions to the complex "frontal lobe" tasks: a latent variable analysis. Cogn Psychol. 2000;41:49–100.

42. Pauli-Pott U, Becker K. Neuropsychological basic deficits in preschoolers at risk for ADHD: a meta-analysis. Clin Psychol Rev. 2011;31(4):626–37. https://doi.org/10.1016/j.cpr.2011.02.005.

43. Roberts BA, Martel MM, Nigg JT. Are there executive dysfunction subtypes within ADHD? J Atten Disord. 2017;21:284–93.

44. Kofler MJ, Rapport MD, Sarver DE, Raiker JS, Orban SA, Friedman LM, Kolomeyer EG. Reaction time variability in ADHD: a meta-analytic review of 319 studies. Clin Psychol Rev. 2013;33:795–811.

45. Lamb MR, Yund EW. The role of spatial frequency in the processing of hierarchically organized stimuli. Percept Psychophys. 1993;54:773–84. https://doi.org/10.3758/BF03211802.

46. Lamb MR, Roberstson LC, Knight RT. Attention and interference in the processing of global and local information: effects of unilateral temporo-parietal lesions. Neuropsychologia. 1989;27:471–83. https://doi.org/10.1016/0028-3932(89)90052-3.

47. de Zwaan M, Gruss B, Müller A, Graap H, Martin A, Glaesmer H, Hilbert A, Philipsen A. The estimated prevalence and correlates of adult ADHD in a German community sample. Eur Arch Psychiatry Clin Neurosci. 2012;262:79–86.

48. Simon V, Czobor P, Bálint S, Mészáros A, Bitter I. Prevalence and correlates of adult attention-deficit hyperactivity disorder: meta-analysis. Br J Psychiatry. 2009;194:204–11.

49. Bridgett DJ, Walker ME. Intellectual functioning in adults with ADHD: a meta-analytic examination of full scale IQ differences between adults with and without ADHD. Psychol Assess. 2006;18:1–14. https://doi.org/10.1037/1040-3590.18.1.1.

50. Sobanski E, Brüggemann D, Alm B, Kern S, Deschner M, Schubert T, Philipsen A, Rietschel M. Psychiatric comorbidity and functional impairment in a clinically referred sample of adults with attention-deficit/hyperactivity disorder (ADHD). Eur Arch Psychiatry Clin Neurosci. 2007;2007(254):371–7. https://doi.org/10.1007/s00406-007-0712-8.

19

Left centro-parieto-temporal response to tool–gesture incongruity: an ERP study

Yi-Tzu Chang[1,2], Hsiang-Yu Chen[2,3], Yuan-Chieh Huang[4], Wan-Yu Shih[5], Hsiao-Lung Chan[6], Ping-Yi Wu[7], Ling-Fu Meng[2,8*], Chen-Chi Chen[9] and Ching-I Wang[2]

Abstract

Background: Action semantics have been investigated in relation to context violation but remain less examined in relation to the meaning of gestures. In the present study, we examined tool–gesture incongruity by event-related potentials (ERPs) and hypothesized that the component N400, a neural index which has been widely used in both linguistic and action semantic congruence, is significant for conditions of incongruence.

Methods: Twenty participants performed a tool–gesture judgment task, in which they were asked to judge whether the tool–gesture pairs were correct or incorrect, for the purpose of conveying functional expression of the tools. Online electroencephalograms and behavioral performances (the accuracy rate and reaction time) were recorded.

Results: The ERP analysis showed a left centro-parieto-temporal N300 effect (220–360 ms) for the correct condition. However, the expected N400 (400–550 ms) could not be differentiated between correct/incorrect conditions. After 700 ms, a prominent late negative complex for the correct condition was also found in the left centro-parieto-temporal area.

Conclusions: The neurophysiological findings indicated that the left centro-parieto-temporal area is the predominant region contributing to neural processing for tool–gesture incongruity in right-handers. The temporal dynamics of tool–gesture incongruity are: (1) firstly enhanced for recognizable tool–gesture using patterns, (2) and require a secondary reanalysis for further examination of the highly complicated visual structures of gestures and tools. The evidence from the tool–gesture incongruity indicated altered brain activities attributable to the N400 in relation to lexical and action semantics. The online interaction between gesture and tool processing provided minimal context violation or anticipation effect, which may explain the missing N400.

Keywords: Action semantics, Tool–gesture incongruity, N300, N400, Late negative complex

Background

A goal-directed action semantic involves comprehension of the object and its corresponding actions with respect to the context. In previous studies of action semantics, participants were mostly asked to determine the compatibility of the actions in a given situation [1–12]. Presentations of conditions violating action-semantics have often involved orientation or functional mismatch to properly execute the functions of the tools [1, 2], illogical tool substitution (e.g. cutting bread or playing cello with a saw instead of a bread knife or a bow [3–7]), or inappropriate body movements in a given context (e.g., a woman who's looking at her watch, and carrying a suitcase while walking on a treadmill [4]). Concurrent event-related brain potentials (ERPs) have been analyzed to reveal the neural bases of the cognitive processes of action semantics [1–12]. Although context appears to be an indispensable factor processed with action as a meaningful unit, the gesture itself, which is a fundamental component of a valid action, has largely been ignored in the research field of action semantics. Thus, the present study aims to uncover the neural cognitive processes of tool–gesture incongruity.

*Correspondence: lfmeng@mail.cgu.edu.tw
[2] Department of Occupational Therapy & Graduate Institute of Behavioral Science, Chang Gung University, Taoyuan, Taiwan
Full list of author information is available at the end of the article

ERPs for action semantics

Since gesture semantics is part of action semantics, a brief review of previous studies on action semantics is provided here. Among previous studies examining action semantics [1–12], the N400 is the most reported neural index revealing the congruency effect of action semantics. On the other hand, some researchers have also reported similar N300/N400 peaking earlier at 300 ms after stimulus onset, which has been assumed to reflect picture-related or action-specific semantic processing [5, 7, 8]. In terms of the N400 component, it was observed at first over the centro-parietal scalp areas in response to word stimuli derived from reading sentences in linguistic paradigms with semantically anomalous endings [13]. Later, similar N400 with more frontal distribution than the linguistic N400 have been reported as the action N400 from non-linguistic materials [1–4, 7, 8]. The N400 is therefore regarded as a neural index which can be elicited across stimuli if they are potentially meaningless and incomprehensible.

More consideration of the enhanced N400

Several underlying factors can influence the magnitude of the N400 in our consideration. The first is the extent of context violation. During sentence reading tasks, it has been reported that the magnitude of the N400 would be influenced by the cloze probability of a word [13, 14]. For instance, words that complete sentences in a nonsensical fashion (low cloze-probability; e.g., The bill was due at the end of the hour) elicit much larger N400 waves than those semantically appropriate words do (high cloze-probability; e.g., The bill was due at the end of the month) in a text [14]. Comprehension of linguistic and non-linguistic semantics is processed based on broad similarities, thus the neural activity patterns resulting from semantically anomalous information in a linguistic domain may show up along with non-linguistic domains such as action semantics. Second, the structural complexity of the background or peripheral context may also be a determining factor. The more abundant the structure is, the more the visual cues and/or that artifacts are provided, thereby influencing the effect of congruity. Third, whether the stimuli are presented in dynamic-, serial-, or static-, influences the topographical distribution and the magnitude of N300/N400 component [3, 7, 8, 10, 11]. For instance, Wu and Coulson [10] reported reduced N400 amplitude for serial cartoon segments, compared to static image paradigms. Taken together, the N400 appears to be a high-context-dependent component. In this regard, the present study intends to minimize the peripheral factors such as illogical context violation or redundant background information, thereby manifesting the congruency effect of tool–gesture semantics.

Gesture semantics in previous ERP researches

Here we further review those studies using gestures as the main stimuli. Gestures, which are central to communication, have been found to trigger the N300 and N400 during the process of discriminating the semantics of hand postures [15]. Shibata et al. [16] used EPRs to evaluate the appropriateness of cooperative actions using pass-and-receive paradigms. Pictorial stimuli were presented in a series: first, a preshaped passing hand (e.g., an object placed at the hollow of the palm), then a receiving hand (e.g., palm down as the appropriate receiving action, palm up as inappropriate one), followed by a blank interval. It was found that an inappropriate receiving action elicited a more widely distributed cortical response than did an appropriate action, and the maximum N400 was located in the parietal region. The parietal N400, which is different from the fronto-central N400 reported for the context-violation paradigm, was thought to be semantics processing related to the prediction of interpersonal actions between two people.

Bach et al. [1] further investigated the appropriateness of tool-use actions by classifying mismatch conditions into "functional mismatch," which involves instruments paired with normally inappropriate target objects (e.g., screwdriver to keyhole) and "orientation mismatch," which relates to inconsistent spatial properties between the motor action and the target (e.g., orthogonal orientation between insertion and slot). The results of the varied latency of N400 indicated that action and object semantics derive from different sub-processes related to functional and orientation domains, respectively. In line with Bach et al. [1], Balconi and Caldiroli [2] reported a topographical difference in object-related action comprehension, where the significant N400 was observed in the fronto-central area for incorrect object use and predominantly in the temporo-parietal area for unusual object use.

More currently, Proverbio et al. [17, 18] proposed a left hemispheric asymmetry in the activation of premotor and somatosensory areas involved in object perception, which was associated with tool manipulability. They further used the ERPs to examine the neural responses to the visual presentation pictures depicting unimanual (e.g., a hammer) and bimanual (e.g., a handlebar) tools [19]. In the time window of 230–260 ms, the N2 amplitude was elicited at the left parietal cortex, followed by N400 (350–450 ms) at the right parietal cortex. Regardless of the time series, both components were found to be activated in the left premotor cortex. Specifically, only unimanual tools were related to the activation of the left postcentral gyrus in the second time window. This pattern of results suggests a role of the left hemisphere in the neural representation of grasping in right handed people, especially for the N2 component.

Though electrophysiological responses to appropriateness between action and tool have been assessed, the paradigms were quite divergent, hence, less consistent inferences could be concluded. Further, no straightforward evidence up to present has been proposed for understanding the compatibility of tools and manipulation of hand gestures. The present study would be the first to report brain activities involved in tool–gesture congruency, using the tool–gesture paradigm without the confounding factor of context violation and the effect of anticipation.

Late waveforms beyond N400

In addition to the N400 component, a late positive complex (LPC) after N400 has been observed in some recent studies [1, 5, 10, 12], while late negativity has been found in others [7, 8, 16]. Regardless of its polarities, researchers have assumed this late effect as a reevaluation of the available knowledge of goal-related requirements related to real-world actions [5] or decision-making-related processes [10]. The continued late effect suggests that N400 is not the final stage of the semantic process [14, 20]. Using EPRs enables us to investigate tool–gesture semantics in good time domain analysis, and whether later effect of tool–gesture compatibility occurs after 400 ms can therefore be determined.

In sum, the primary goal of this study is to investigate tool–gesture incongruity using an intra-gesture experimental design with the ERP technique. Based on previous literature, we preliminarily hypothesize that incorrect tool–gesture pairs elicit greater negative N400 amplitude than correct tool–gesture pairs do. Furthermore, a late waveform is expected because the task is relatively difficult and requires a greater degree of visual and cognitive deconstruction than those in previous studies. By means of the ERP recordings, the present study should reveal tool–gesture semantics processing with respect to tool manipulation.

Methods

Participants

Twenty healthy university students (nine male) aged 18–24 years (mean = 20.25 years, SD = 1.55), all of whom are right-handed, were recruited in this study (laterality quotient = 83.00 ± 18.66 for handedness based on the Edinburgh Handedness Inventory) [21]. Inclusion criteria for all participants included normal or corrected-to-normal vision. Participants who had suffered from neurologic diseases, hospitalized, under medication, consumed alcohol or tobacco within 6 weeks prior to the experiment were excluded.

The present study recruited healthy adults participating according to their free will via the Internet and was carried out with a non-invasive method. All participants were provided with verbal and written instructions of all the details of the experiment. After understanding and providing consent to participate in this study, personal information was then provided and the questionnaires used in this study were filled in thereafter. All participants could withdraw at any time. The participants did not expect to obtain any benefit from being in this research study. Each participant received a reasonable fee as compensation for their inconvenience and commute expenses.

Stimuli

Six commonly used tools, including a pair of chopsticks, a pair of scissors, a pen, a hammer, a toothbrush, and a spoon, were used as the stimuli (Fig. 1). Each frame combined a hand gesture and one of the tools together as a unit. In correct conditions, the tool was manipulated by a gesture that enabled its functional use, whereas in incorrect conditions, the tool was manipulated by an unusual or incomprehensible hand gesture that lacked a goal-directed function. To be more precise, participants were shown images of tools being manipulated with (1). correct gestures: a pen, toothbrush, chopstick, and spoon held in a tripod grasp, a hammer held in a power grasp, and a pair of scissors held with the thumb in the front hole as mover, the index and middle finger in the back hole as stabilizer (Fig. 1 upper section), or (2). incorrect gestures: a pen, toothbrush, chopstick, and spoon held in a tight fist or hook grasp, a hammer and a pair of scissors held in a disoriented manner that disabled the tool's normal functions (Fig. 1 shows the lower section). Each frame was repeated 20 times. A total of 240 trials composed of tools with correct gestures (120 trials) and incorrect gestures (120 trials) were presented to the participants.

We also invited another 24 college students to judge whether each frame was a correct or incorrect pair. Accuracy was 95% for the correct condition and 89% for the incorrect condition (for more detail please see Appendix). Based on previous studies, we choose static images to minimize the effect of anticipation which may result from sequential presentation. All stimuli were photographed with a 3-megapixel digital camera and edited with Microsoft Window's built-in Paint software. The stimuli were 15 cm × 15 cm high-resolution photos presented in random order at the center of a 17-inch, 1024 × 768 pixel desktop computer screen. The stimuli were modified referring to the images proposed by Wu et al. (Fig. 1) [22]. Moreover, besides the gesture and the tool themselves, any other visual hints from the

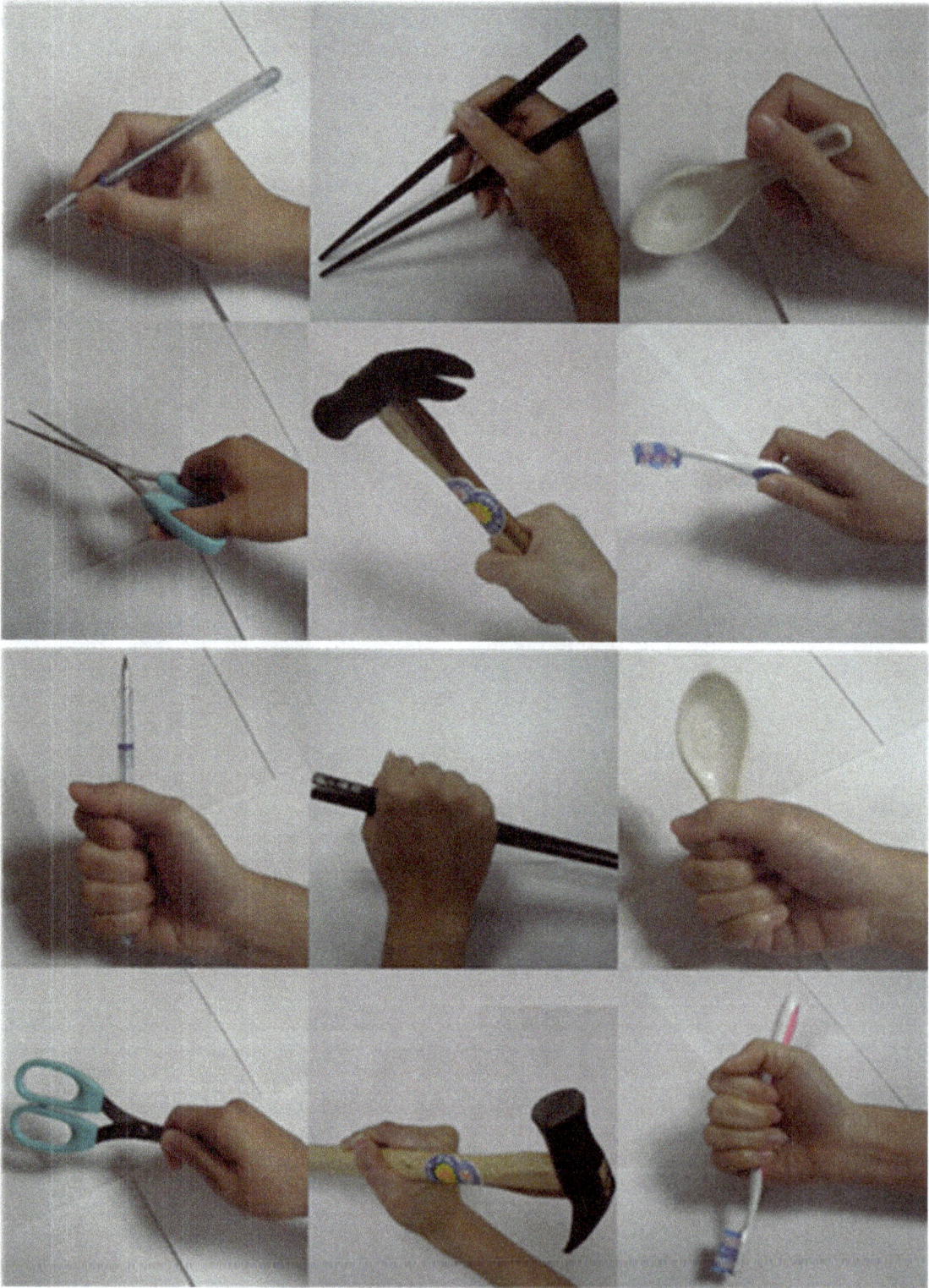

Fig. 1 Examples of congruent (upper part) and incongruent (lower part) tool–gesture pairs used in this study

background were removed. With the high commonality of pictorial structure between each stimulus, the core neural activities indicating tool–gestures semantics should be revealed. This experimental design enabled us to test whether gestures can affect comprehension in the absence of other sources of semantic input and assess how gestures undergo action semantic processing.

Procedure

Participants were seated in a dimly lit room approximately 1 m from the computer monitor used for stimuli presentation, and they were fitted with a 32-electrode cap. Each participant was asked to complete 2 blocks of tool–gesture judgment tasks using the contrary respond mode. Each frame was presented for 300 ms. A time window of 1700 ms was allowed for valid responses after stimulus onset. The inter-trial interval (ITI) was 2000 ms. Six additional trials were used in a practice block.

During the first block, participants were asked to judge the tool–gesture pair by pressing button '1' with the index finger for "correct" and button '2' with the middle finger for "incorrect" using their right hand. To counterbalance behavioral response, contrary response mode was used in the second block (by asking participants to press button '2' with their middle fingers for "correct" and '1' with the index finger for "incorrect" using their right hand). Approximately 3–4 min were needed to accomplish the experiment for each block. Short pauses were allowed between blocks to avoid visual fatigue or other factors that could contaminate the EEG recording. During the experiment, a black background was maintained to avoid background variability. The procedure was modified referring to the previous study by Wu et al. [22].

EEG acquisition and analysis

The EEG was recorded by BrainVision Recorder (version 1.10; Brain Products, Germany) from 32 electrodes distributed based on the 10–20 system (including electrodes from F3/F4, F7/F8, FC1/FC2, FC5/FC6, C3/C4, T7/T8, TP9/TP10, CP1/CP2, CP5/CP6, P3/P4, P7/P8, O1/O2, FPZ, FZ, FCZ, CZ, PZ, and OZ). Eye artifacts were monitored with four EOG electrodes: two located at the outer canthi of the right and left eyes, and two above and below the center of the right eye. The impedances were kept below 10 kΩ. During recording, all electrodes were referenced to the FCz electrode. The EEG was continuously sampled at 1000 Hz with a band pass filter of 0.01–70 Hz and stored for off-line analysis. Resolution of the amplifier was 0.1 μV.

The offline analysis was then conducted using the BrainVision Analyzer software (version 1.05; Brain Products, Germany). Epochs were started at 200 ms and continued to 1000 ms, following stimulus-locked rules.

Incorrect behavioral responses and reactions beyond 1700 ms after stimulus onset were eliminated manually. At least 100 trials were maintained for each condition. Averages were aligned to a 200 ms pre-stimulus baseline. The band pass filter was 0.1–30 Hz (12 dB/octave). Offline data were re-referenced to the average of the TP9 and TP10 electrodes. Segments contaminated by artifacts as amplitudes exceeding ± 100 μV at 4 EOG electrodes, and ± 60 μV at the resting electrodes were detected and excluded for the following analysis. Prior to averaging, ocular artifacts were also corrected by independent component analysis (ICA). Bipolar vertical EOG (VEOG) and horizontal EOG (HEOG) channels were calculated as the difference between VEOU/VEOD and HEOL/HEOR electrodes, respectively. Thirty channels including VEOG and HEOG, and excluding VEOU, VEOD, HEOL and HEOR, were entered into the ICA analysis, resulting in 30 independent components. The components resembling blinks and eye movements were blocked through the inspection of topographic maps and the time course with the EOG channels. Segments were averaged separately for each congruent or incongruent condition.

After group averaging from data of all 20 participants, mean amplitudes for 3 visually prominent components were calculated by self-programmed MATLAB (Mathworks, USA), including N300 (220–360 ms), N400 (400–550 ms) and the late negative complex (LNC, 720–800 ms). The focus of the analyses was the mean amplitudes of these three components in different regions. Twenty-one electrodes were classified into 7 regions for further analysis, including the left-fronto-central area (F7, F3, FC5), left-centro-parieto-temporal area (T7, C3, CP5), left-parieto-occipital area (P3, P7, O1), midline (Fz, Cz, Pz), right-fronto-central area (F8, F4, FC6), right-centro-parieto-temporal area (T8, C4, CP6), and right-parieto-occipital area (P4, P8, O2).

Statistical analysis

For behavioral data and electrophysiological data, differences were assessed using paired sample t tests to correctness (correct/incorrect) as the factor. We further report the effect size of Cohen's d value to reveal the strength of the relationship between conditions [23]. Statistical differences achieved significance when $p < 0.05$ (two-tailed). p values were adjusted for multiple testing with the Hochberg method for electrophysiological data.

Results

Behavioral results

In general, participants responded accurately when deciding the correctness of the tool–gesture stimuli. The participants demonstrated a higher accuracy rate (AR) and faster reaction time (RT) for the correct condition. The mean AR and RT were 96.08 ± 2.90% and 678.33 ± 104.31 ms for correct tool–gesture pairs, and 93.42 ± 4.50% and 701.60 ± 92.42 ms for incorrect tool–gesture pairs, respectively. The differences in both AR and RT between correct and incorrect conditions reached a significant level [t(19) = 2.791, p = 0.012, ES(d) = 0.70 for AR; t(19) = − 3.251, p = 0.004, ES(d) = 0.24 for RT].

Event-related potentials results

Figure 2 shows the averaged ERP waveforms for correct and incorrect tool–gesture stimuli. In the time period of 220-360 ms after stimulus appearance, correct pictures (mean = − 1.54 µV, SD = 2.06) elicited more negative N300 than incorrect pictures (mean = − 1.03 µV, SD = 2.02) did in the left centro-parieto-temporal area [t(19) = − 2.687, Hochberg adjusted p = 0.015, ES(d) = 0.60]. The result indicates the left centro-parieto-temporal N300 was elicited when participants saw comprehensible tool–gesture pairs. None of the other areas showed significant N300 components (all Hochberg adjusted p > 0.05). Contrary to our expectations, none of the areas demonstrated significant congruency

effects for N400 (all Hochberg adjusted p > 0.05). From 720 to 800 ms epochs, correct pictures (mean = 1.10 µV, SD = 2.92) evoked a greater late negativity complex than incorrect pictures (mean = 1.87 µV, SD = 2.47) did in the left centro-parieto-temporal area [t(19) = − 1.979, p = 0.024, ES(d) = 0.55)].

Discussion

This study investigates action semantic processing for tool–gesture incongruity using an intra-gesture experimental design with the ERP technique. Unlike previous studies exploring the action semantics [1–12], the present study deliberately designed and controlled the stimuli to minimize the effect of context violation and anticipation, for the purpose of revealing the core neural activities indicating tool–gesture semantics. According to the present findings, participants were less accurate and approximately 20 ms slower in discerning incorrect tool–gesture pairs. Two main findings were derived from our ERP data: correct tool–gesture pairs elicited (1). more negative N300, and (2). more negative late negativity complex (LNC) than incorrect pairs did in the left

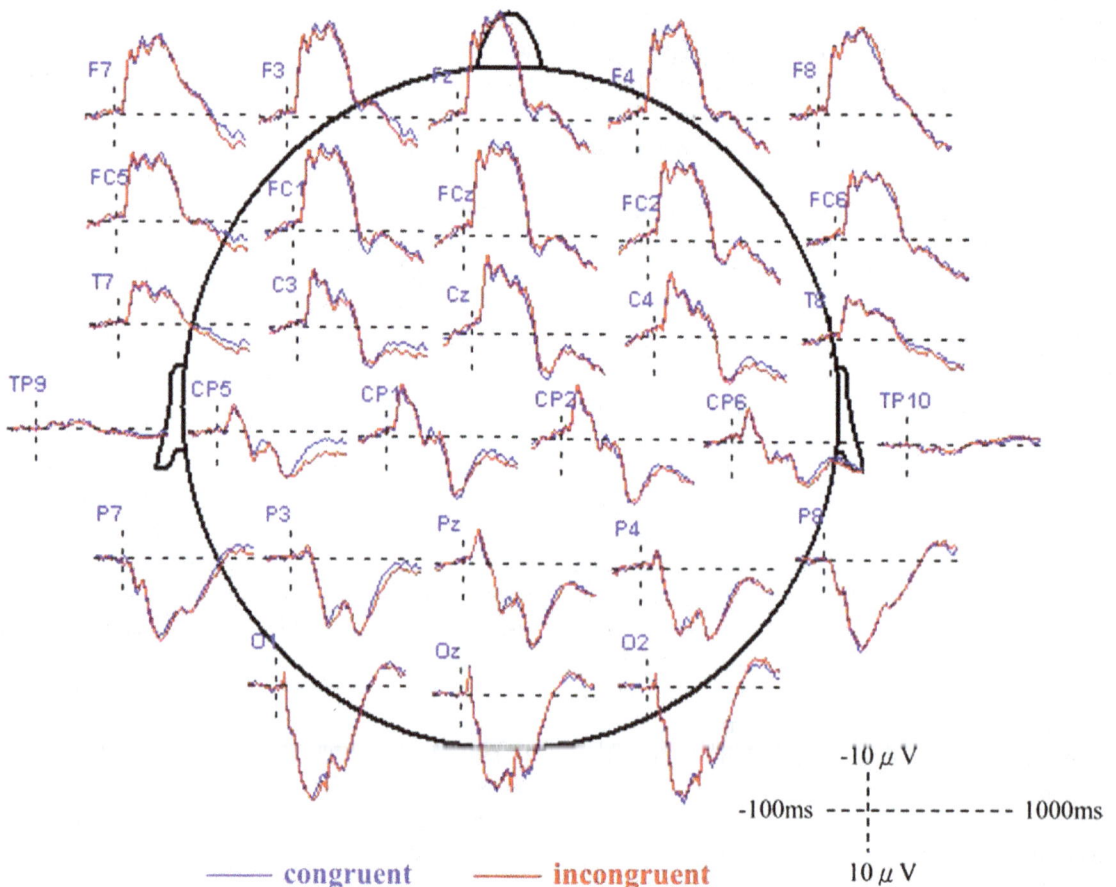

Fig. 2 Grand averaged ERPs for correct (blue) and incorrect (red) tool–gesture stimuli

centro-parieto-temporal area. However, we did not find the typical N400 component for the semantic processing of linguistic material [13, 24–26] or action-related material [1–4, 11, 16, 20]. Our results imply that the neural mechanism for comprehending tool–gesture semantics is different from those for understanding action semantics with respect to context.

Raised N300: object recognition of semantic memories

In this study, we found more negative N300 elicited by correct tool–gesture pairs in the left centro-parieto-temporal area; this may represent the neural processes for perceptual object recognition [5, 7, 8, 13, 27, 28] and structural description matching [29, 30]. The present finding was in line with Proverbio et al. [17, 18], who reported left hemispheric asymmetry in the activation of premotor areas involved in object perception in right handers, which was associated with tool manipulability, specifically for gestures. In addition, the anterior temporal cortex has been suggested as a primary semantic source of top-down influences involved in object recognition [31]. In brief, the result from the present study indicates that object recognition, which is mainly addressed by the left centro-parieto-temporal area, is the first stage of neural processing of tool–gesture incongruity in right handers.

Among previous studies investigating action semantics using neurolinguistic paradigms, the enhanced recognition potential (RP, or N250) between 250 and 350 ms with an occipitally distribution has been reported for visually recognized and semantically comprehended actions within the context reference [3, 4]. Consistent with the above findings, the present study found that when the tools were accompanied by a gesture that conveyed the functional meaning (the *correct* condition in this study), the visually recognizable characters lead to an increase in N300 amplitude. Whereas in *incorrect* conditions, the tools were manipulated with an unusual or incomprehensible hand gesture, which lowered the possibility for recognizing the congruence between tool and gesture in visual processing, hence resulting in decreased N300.

In this study, the effects resulting from contextual violations and incongruent contexts were minimized. Thus, the participants therefore had to pay more attention to the structural matching between the tools and the gestures to make the right judgment. Buxbaum et al.'s study [32] inferred that the hand shaping for object use additionally requires access to stored knowledge about the skilled manipulation specific to a given object. Note this inference is in accordance with the reported finding of the observed enhanced N300 when semantic expectations matched the baseline. Some authors therefore have suggested the N300 as an index in the rapid matching of

visual input to stored semantic knowledge [13, 27, 33]. This idea was also supported by an object and action identification study, wherein an increased N3 complex was observed for successful category decisions with intact known objects rather than scrambled ones [34]. Therefore, an increased N300 effect for correct tool–gestures is consistent with the findings for object identification tasks, which suggests that N300 is involved in perceptual object categorization of visual stimuli based on semantic memories.

Reasons for the lack of N400

Since N400 has been considered as a strong neural index across linguistic and action semantic researches [1–14], we were looking forward to verifying the role of N400 as a representative component initially. In light of action semantics, Reid and Striano [11] interpreted the N400 response as the rapid indexing of neural system activities, discerning semantic information in actions, and anticipating information within goal-directed actions [14]. Based on our experimental design, however, insignificant N400 waves between conditions were reported. According to the present findings, we inferred that understanding the way gestures undergo action semantic processing with tools is different from understanding action semantics with context violation. We suggest it is the substantially structural similarities, the subtle distinctions between the correct and incorrect tool–gesture pairs, which may have bothered the participants' ability to rapidly match the semantic information conceptually, as suggested by Reid and Striano [11], hence resulting in the insignificance of N400 between conditions.

Another possible explanation for the diminished N400 may be related to stimulus repetition and familiarity. Because of the small set of only six (tools), participants could become familiar with how to categorize them easily (as incorrect) after a few repetitions. It is possible that the repetition and familiarity effects had the power of reducing the incongruence effect.

Enhanced LNC for the secondary reanalysis of tool–gesture incongruity

The present findings indicate that a quick matching of N300 or N400 appears to be insufficient for understanding tool–gesture incongruity. Rather, a LNC should be responsible for the secondary reanalysis of the functional semantics and consistency between gesture and tool. Late deflections in context deviation paradigms in previous studies were interpreted as a reanalysis or reevaluation process, which have mainly been reported with broad neural activities across the frontal to parietal lobes [5–7, 12, 24]. The time-serial result was in line with the notion that brain dynamics for tool–gesture semantic processing is similar to that of lexical semantics in the later stage; however, the dominant area for the secondary reanalysis of tool–gesture incongruity has mainly been addressed by the left centro-parieto-temporal area [3, 7, 8, 11].

Late negative complex (LNC) has been investigated in memory studies and found to reflect processes that are engaged in the tasks of color source retrieval [35], when task-relevant memory features require more evaluation [36], and in action monitoring and contextual retrieval [37]. In this study, functional construction of tool–gesture stimuli is considered to be formed by previous knowledge rather than anticipation. Hence, the online interaction between gesture and tool may be inclined toward the memory retrieval process rather than prediction. The increased late effect indexes the efforts when participants reintegrate the information of the tool and the manipulated hand gesture as a whole. This retrieval process helps to build meaning by mental spatial manipulation based on users' prior experience and object knowledge.

The LNC contributes particular meaning, apart from that reported in previous studies, to the tool–gesture stimuli. We propose that discriminating between the incorrect and the correct tool–gesture pair in such a high similarity condition is relatively mind-consuming for visual perception, thus a visually-dependent secondary reanalysis of the functional semantics and consistency between gesture and tool is necessitated. In addition to the perquisite knowledge of tool-identification and ideo-motor praxis, it is the resemblance of the pictorial stimuli that prompted a more skilled visual analysis to reevaluate the compatibility and the visual-spatial construction of the tool–gesture pair as a unit. More visual and cognitive loading therefore facilitated the left centro-parieto-temporal neural activities during gesture-semantic judgment.

Limitations

Several limitations and underlying factors may have influenced the outcomes and the inferences of the present study. First, the stimulus set was small (only six tools with twelve stimuli were used). The more times each visual stimulus was repeated, the high familiarity of the incorrect pairs might have decreased such difficulty in categorization/recognition. Second, in an object-related action comprehension study, Balconi and Caldiroli [2] found N400-like event-related potentials with different topographical distributions for "unusual" or "incorrect" object use. However, this study provided the dichotomous decision of "correct" or "incorrect" rather than subdividing these visual stimuli into more detailed categories, as in Balconi and Caldiroli's research. A more

detailed categorization may help future studies of brain topography related to action semantics.

Third, because a gesture is a component comprised of complex dual orientation and function meanings, it is difficult to discriminate function mismatches from orientation mismatches such as those studied in Bach et al. [1]. Fourth, could presentation of hand gesture itself (e.g., a picture showing only tripod grasp or power grasp without tools) elicit differential brain activities for visual analysis? The findings from an additional control experiment (unpublished data) demonstrated that within each time window of interest, neural activities for only a hand gesture without tool presentation were insignificant between correct and incorrect conditions. The result from the control experiment helped us to rule out the confounding possibility of the gesture itself. Fifth, longer reaction times and lower accuracy rates indicate the difficulty of judging incorrect tool–gesture pairs. The difficulty of the task itself may have strengthened the anticipated results. Rigorous experimental designs are needed for future studies. Lastly, the present findings demonstrating the left-hemispheric dominance of tool–gesture incongruity may be generalized to right-handers only. Using the transcranial magnetic stimulation (TMS)-induced motor evoked potentials (MEPs) technique, Sartori et al. [38] reported that regardless of the laterality of the hand being observed, the motor resonance is noted in the observer's dominant effector for both left- and right-handers. Due to the concern about effector-independent motor representations, the current finding of left-hemispheric dominance of tool–gesture incongruity might be reversed in left-handers. Recruiting left-handers would help further clarify such issue.

Conclusion

This study focused on tool–gesture action semantics congruency. Our study showed conclusively that the left centro-parieto-temporal area was the dominant brain region contributing to the neural processing of tool–gesture action semantics in right handers. The temporal brain dynamics indicate that the N300 was evoked and indexed as the neural processing of object recognition based on semantic memory in the first stage. Later, a late negative complex (LNC) was evoked and indexed as the visually-dependent memory retrieval process for the secondary reevaluation of tool–gesture compatibility. Unlike previous studies reporting consistent N400 across the investigation of linguistic or action semantics [1–14], the tool–gesture paradigm from the present study reports no N400 response. The reason for the lack of N400 may be related to the absence of context violation, the effect of anticipation, and the high similarities of the visual-spatial constructions of the stimuli used in this study. The specific relationship between the activated cortical area and types of linguistic and/or action semantic violations merit further discussion.

Authors' contributions
LF conceived and planned the research as well as funding application. LF, HY, and PY contributed to the study design. HY and CC contributed to experiment conduction and data collection. YC, HY, WY, HL, and CI contributed to the signal processing. YT, YC, and CI contributed to the data analysis and statistical analysis. YT and LF contributed to the data interpretation and the manuscript drafting. Administrative affairs were helped by YC, CC, YT, and CI. All authors read and approved the final manuscript.

Author details
[1] Department of Educational Psychology and Counseling, National Taiwan Normal University, Taipei, Taiwan. [2] Department of Occupational Therapy & Graduate Institute of Behavioral Science, Chang Gung University, Taoyuan, Taiwan. [3] Faculty of Psychology, Technische Universität Dresden, Dresden, Germany. [4] Department of Clinical Psychology, Fu Jen Catholic University, New Taipei, Taiwan. [5] Institute of Neuroscience, National Yang-Ming University, Taipei, Taiwan. [6] Department of Electrical Engineering, Chang Gung University, Taoyuan, Taiwan. [7] Division of Occupational Therapy, Department of Physical Medicine and Rehabilitation, Center for Neural Regeneration, Taipei Veterans General Hospital, Taipei, Taiwan. [8] Division of Occupational Therapy, Department of Rehabilitation, Chiayi Chang Gung Memorial Hospital, Chiayi, Taiwan. [9] Health Center, Taipei Fuhsing Private School, Taipei, Taiwan.

Acknowledgements
The authors sincerely thank the participants in this study.

Competing interests
The authors declare that the research was conducted in the absence of any commercial or financial relationships that could be construed as a potential competing interests.

Funding
Preparation of this article was supported by National Science Council in Taiwan (NSC 101-2511-S-182-006-MY3) and the Broad Medical Research Program in Chang Gung University, Taiwan (BMRP424).

Appendix
See Table 1.

Table 1 Accuracy of the judgment of tool–gesture pairs (N = 24)

Categorization	Accuracy	
	Correct	Incorrect
Correct		
Chopsticks	20/24	4/24
Scissors	24/24	0/24
Hammer	23/24	1/24
Spoon	22/24	2/24
Pen	24/24	0/24
Toothbrush	24/24	0/24
Incorrect		
Chopsticks	1/24	23/24
Scissors	12/24	12/24
Hammer	1/24	23/24
Spoon	2/24	22/24
Pen	0/24	24/24
Toothbrush	0/24	24/24

References
1. Bach P, Gunter TC, Knoblich G, Prinz W, Friederici AD. N400-like negativities in action perception reflect the activation of two components of an action representation. Soc Neurosci. 2009;4:212–32. https://doi.org/10.1080/17470910802362546.
2. Balconi M, Caldiroli C. Semantic violation effect on object-related action comprehension. N400-like event-related potentials for unusual and incorrect use. Neuroscience. 2011;197:191–9. https://doi.org/10.1016/j.neuroscience.2011.09.026.
3. Proverbio AM, Riva F. RP and N400 ERP components reflect semantic violations in visual processing of human actions. Neurosci Lett. 2009;459:142–6. https://doi.org/10.1016/j.neulet.2009.05.012.
4. Proverbio AM, Riva F, Zani A. When neurons do not mirror the agent's intentions: sex differences in neural coding of goal-directed actions. Neuropsychologia. 2010;48:1454–63. https://doi.org/10.1016/j.neuropsychologia.2010.01.015.
5. Sitnikova T, Holcomb PJ, Kiyonaga KA, Kuperberg GR. Two neurocognitive mechanisms of semantic integration during the comprehension of visual real-world events. J Cogn Neurosci. 2008;20:2037–57. https://doi.org/10.1162/jocn.2008.20143.
6. Ganis G, Kutas M. An electrophysiological study of scene effects on object identification. Cogn Brain Res. 2007;16:123–44.
7. Mudrik L, Lamy D, Deouell LY. ERP evidence for context congruity effects during simultaneous object-scene processing. Neuropsychologia. 2010;48:507–17. https://doi.org/10.1016/j.neuropsychologia.2009.10.011.
8. West WC, Holcomb PJ. Event-related potentials during discourse-level semantic integration of complex pictures. Cogn Brain Res. 2002;13:363–75. https://doi.org/10.1016/S0926-6410(01)00129-X.
9. Kelly SD, Kravitz C, Hopkins M. Neural correlates of bimodal speech and gesture comprehension. Brain Lang. 2004;89:253–60. https://doi.org/10.1016/S0093-934X(03)00335-3.
10. Wu YC, Coulson S. Meaningful gestures: electrophysiological indices of iconic gesture comprehension. Psychophysiology. 2005;42:654–67. https://doi.org/10.1111/j.1469-8986.2005.00356.x.
11. Reid VM, Striano T. N400 involvement in the processing of action sequences. Neurosci Lett. 2008;433:93–7. https://doi.org/10.1016/j.neulet.2007.12.066.
12. Sitnikova T, Kuperberg G, Holcomb PJ. Semantic integration in videos of real-world events: an electrophysiological investigation. Psychophysiology. 2003;40:160–4. https://doi.org/10.1111/1469-8986.00016.
13. Kutas M, Hillyard SA. Reading senseless sentences: brain potentials reflect semantic incongruity. Science. 1980;207:203–5. https://doi.org/10.1126/science.7350657.
14. Kutas M, Federmeier KD. Thirty years and counting: finding meaning in the N400 component of the event-related brain potential (ERP). Annu Rev Psychol. 2011;62:621–47. https://doi.org/10.1146/annurev.psych.093008.131123.

15. Gunter TC, Bach P. Communicating hands: ERPs elicited by meaningful symbolic hand postures. Neurosci Lett. 2004;372:52–6. https://doi.org/10.1016/j.neulet.2004.09.011.

16. Shibata H, Gyoba J, Suzuki Y. Event-related potentials during the evaluation of the appropriateness of cooperative actions. Neurosci Lett. 2009;452:189–93. https://doi.org/10.1016/j.neulet.2009.01.042.

17. Proverbio AM, Adorni R, D'Aniello GE. 250 ms to code for action affordance during observation of manipulable objects. Neuropsychologia. 2011;49:2711–7. https://doi.org/10.1016/j.neuropsychologia.2011.05.019.

18. Proverbio AM. Tool perception suppresses 10–12 Hz μ rhythm of EEG over the somatosensory area. Biol Psychol. 2012;91:1–7. https://doi.org/10.1016/j.biopsycho.2012.04.003.

19. Proverbio AM, Azzari R, Adorni R. Is there a left hemispheric asymmetry for tool affordance processing? Neuropsychologia. 2013;51:2690–701. https://doi.org/10.1016/j.neuropsychologia.2013.09.023.

20. Amoruso L, Gelormini C, Aboitiz F, Alvarez González M, Manes F, Cardona J, Ibanez A. N400 ERPs for actions: building meaning in context. Front Hum Neurosci. 2013. https://doi.org/10.3389/fnhum.2013.00057.

21. Oldfield R. The assessment and analysis of handedness: the Edinburgh inventory. Neuropsychologia. 1971;9:97–113. https://doi.org/10.1016/j.neulet.2012.11.043.

22. Wu PY, Meng LF, Cheng FY, Chiu PY. Gesture-object incongruence and N400. In: 2004 1st International Congress of Neuroscience, Taipei, Taiwan. (Proceedings & Poster session).

23. Cohen J. Statistical power analysis for the behavioral sciences. 2nd ed. Hillsdale: Lawrence Earlbaum Associates; 1988.

24. Arzouan Y, Goldstein A, Faust M. Brainwaves are stethoscopes: ERP correlates of novel metaphor comprehension. Brain Res. 2007;1160:69–81. https://doi.org/10.1016/j.brainres.2007.05.034.

25. Rutter B, Kröger S, Hill H, Windmann S, Hermann C, Abraham A. Can clouds dance? part 2: an ERP investigation of passive conceptual expansion. Brain Cogn. 2012;80:301–10. https://doi.org/10.1016/j.bandc.2012.08.003.

26. Kutas M, Hillyard SA. Brain potentials during reading reflect word expectancy and semantic association. Nature. 1984;307:161–3. https://doi.org/10.1038/307161a0.

27. Schendan HE, Kutas M. Neurophysiological evidence for the time course of activation of global shape, part, and local contour representations during visual object categorization and memory. J Cogn Neurosci. 2007;19:734–49. https://doi.org/10.1162/jocn.2007.19.5.734.

28. Federmeier KD, Kutas M. Meaning and modality: influences of context, semantic memory organization and perceptual predictability on picture processing. J Exp Psychol Learn. 2001;27:202–24. https://doi.org/10.1037//0278-7393.27.1.202.

29. Doniger GM, Foxe JJ, Murray MM, Higgins BA, Snodgrass JG, Schroeder CE, et al. Activation timecourse of ventral visual stream object-recognition areas: high density electrical mapping of perceptual closure processes. J Cogn Neurosci. 2000;12:615–21. https://doi.org/10.1162/089892900562372.

30. Schendan HE, Kutas M. Neurophysiological evidence for two processing times for visual object identification. Neuropsychologia. 2002;40:931–45. https://doi.org/10.1016/S0028-3932(01)00176-2.

31. Chiou R, Lambon Ralph MA. The anterior temporal cortex is a primary semantic source of top-down influences on object recognition. Cortex. 2016;79:75–86. https://doi.org/10.1016/j.cortex.2016.03.007.

32. Buxbaum LJ, Kyle KM, Tang K, Detre JA. Neural substrates of knowledge of hand postures for object grasping and functional object use: evidence from fMRI. Brain Res. 2006;1117:175–85. https://doi.org/10.1016/j.brainres.2006.08.010.

33. Maguire MJ, Magnon G, Ogiela DA, Egbert R, Sides L. The N300 ERP component reveals developmental changes in object and action identification. Dev Cogn Neurosci. 2013;5:1–9. https://doi.org/10.1016/j.dcn.2012.11.008.

34. Schendan HE, Lucia LC. Object-sensitive activity reflects earlier perceptual and later cognitive processing of visual objects between 95 and 500 ms. Brain Res. 2010;1329:124–41. https://doi.org/10.1016/j.brainres.2010.01.062.

35. Nie A, Guo C, Liang J, Shen M. The effect of late posterior negativity in retrieving the color of Chinese characters. Neurosci Lett. 2013;534:223–7. https://doi.org/10.1016/j.neulet.2012.11.043.

36. Johansson M, Mecklinger A. The late posterior negativity in ERP studies of episodic memory:action monitoring and retrieval of attribute conjunctions. Biol Psychol. 2003;64:91–117. https://doi.org/10.1016/S0301-0511(03)00104-2.

37. Herron JE. Decomposition of the ERP late posterior negativity: effects of retrieval and response fluency. Psychophysiology. 2007;44:233–44. https://doi.org/10.1111/j.1469-8986.2006.00489.x.

38. Sartori L, Begliomini C, Castiello U. Motor resonance in left- and right-handers: evidence for effector-independent motor representations. Front Hum Neurosci. 2013. https://doi.org/10.3389/fnhum.2013.00033.

20

Magnitude processing of symbolic and non-symbolic proportions: an fMRI study

Julia Mock[1*†], Stefan Huber[1†], Johannes Bloechle[1,2], Julia F. Dietrich[1], Julia Bahnmueller[1,3], Johannes Rennig[1,2], Elise Klein[1] and Korbinian Moeller[1,3]

Abstract

Background: Recent research indicates that processing proportion magnitude is associated with activation in the intraparietal sulcus. Thus, brain areas associated with the processing of numbers (i.e., absolute magnitude) were activated during processing symbolic fractions as well as non-symbolic proportions. Here, we investigated systematically the cognitive processing of symbolic (e.g., fractions and decimals) and non-symbolic proportions (e.g., dot patterns and pie charts) in a two-stage procedure. First, we investigated relative magnitude-related activations of proportion processing. Second, we evaluated whether symbolic and non-symbolic proportions share common neural substrates.

Methods: We conducted an fMRI study using magnitude comparison tasks with symbolic and non-symbolic proportions, respectively. As an indicator for magnitude-related processing of proportions, the distance effect was evaluated.

Results: A conjunction analysis indicated joint activation of specific occipito-parietal areas including right intraparietal sulcus (IPS) during proportion magnitude processing. More specifically, results indicate that the IPS, which is commonly associated with absolute magnitude processing, is involved in processing relative magnitude information as well, irrespective of symbolic or non-symbolic presentation format. However, we also found distinct activation patterns for the magnitude processing of the different presentation formats.

Conclusion: Our findings suggest that processing for the separate presentation formats is not only associated with magnitude manipulations in the IPS, but also increasing demands on executive functions and strategy use associated with frontal brain regions as well as visual attention and encoding in occipital regions. Thus, the magnitude processing of proportions may not exclusively reflect processing of number magnitude information but also rather domain-general processes.

Keywords: Proportions, Fractions, Decimals, Magnitude processing, fMRI

Background

Fractions, ratios, and proportions are among the most ubiquitous forms of numerical information encountered in everyday life. Yet, they are also one of the most difficult concepts to learn and even adults frequently fail to process them correctly [1, 2]. Therefore, understanding the processing and acquisition of fractions and proportions poses one of the most challenging problems in numerical cognition research as well as mathematics education [3].

In teaching and learning fractions, symbolic and non-symbolic presentation formats are often presented side by side to successfully foster conceptual understanding of proportional relations [4–6]. The present study aims at exploring why these pedagogic approaches might be successful from a neurocognitive perspective. To this end, we aimed at broadening the understanding of mechanisms underlying proportion processing by investigating the neural correlates of processing symbolic fractions and non-symbolic proportions in the human brain. In particular, a shared neural correlate for the magnitude processing of fractions and proportions, independent of

*Correspondence: j.mock@iwm-tuebingen.de
†Julia Mock and Stefan Huber contributed equally to this work and should be considered shared first authors
[1] Leibniz-Institut für Wissensmedien, Schleichstraße 6, 72076 Tuebingen, Germany
Full list of author information is available at the end of the article

their presentation format, might explain the efficacy of these pedagogic approaches.

Before the details of the current study will be outlined, we will give a brief summary of recent advances in numerical cognition research by describing (i) neural networks involved in number processing in general, (ii) processes of symbolic and non-symbolic quantities and their underlying neural correlates in particular, and (iii) argue how our investigation of a common neural substrate for both symbolic and non-symbolic proportion processing can be informative for a better understanding of relative magnitude processing.

Neural networks involved in number processing

Previous studies on number processing showed that the intraparietal sulcus (IPS) is crucially involved in the processing of absolute quantity and number magnitude [7–10]. To evaluate the processing of magnitude information conveyed by natural numbers and fractions, the numerical distance effect in magnitude comparison tasks has been employed repeatedly. The numerical distance effect reflects the finding of shorter and more accurate responses with larger numerical distance between two to-be-compared numbers (e.g., 1_9 vs. 4_5; [11]). Importantly, the presence of the numerical distance effect is considered to indicate number magnitude processing in the task at hand [11, 12].

Behavioral results on the distance effect were substantiated by findings showing that activation within the IPS was negatively correlated with numerical distance in number magnitude comparison tasks for natural numbers (e.g., [13], but see [14]). This indicates that the IPS seems to play a crucial role in the representation and processing of number magnitude information [13–17].

However, although neuroimaging research on number processing primarily focused on parietal cortex and especially on the IPS, a rather complex system of functional brain networks was observed to contribute to numerical cognition in general [18, 19]. Besides the IPS, numerical distance was also shown to negatively correlate with activation in bilateral prefrontal and precentral cortex, indicating fronto-parietal networks of number magnitude processing [9, 20]. However, recent research suggests an even broader network to be involved in numerical cognition.

For instance, there is evidence that early perceptual numerical features are decoded in the ventral visual stream, including V1 and the inferior temporal cortex (ITC), before visual-spatial features of numerical quantity are processed in the IPS and the superior parietal lobule (SPL; [18, 21]). Moreover, it was suggested that a widespread fronto-parietal network, comprising IPS, supramarginal gyrus, supplementary motor areas, and

dorsolateral prefrontal cortex (DLPFC), is involved in planning, executing, and monitoring arithmetic procedures as well as maintaining intermediate results [18, 22–24]. Additionally, DLPFC as well as anterior cingulate cortex (ACC) were also associated with processes of cognitive control to optimize performance by monitoring and adapting task execution as well as inhibiting undesired responses [18, 25–27]. Furthermore, the angular gyrus (AG) was also argued to be involved in verbal retrieval of math facts ([10, 28, 29], but see [15, 30]). Finally, the anterior insula and ventrolateral prefrontal cortex were suggested to be involved in processes of guiding and maintaining goal-directed attention [18, 19].

Thus, although parietal regions, and in particular the IPS, play a central role in numerical cognition, there is growing evidence that cognitive processes such as working memory, cognitive control, and executive functions associated with frontal, temporal, and insular cortex are also vital to access numerical information, employ representations of numerical knowledge, and manipulate quantities during calculations.

Neural processing of symbolic numbers and non-symbolic quantities

While the IPS is thought to comprise a notation-independent representation of the magnitude information conveyed by numerals [20, 31], words [9, 32], or non-symbolic arrays as quantities [33, 34], Sokolowski and colleagues [35] observed several additional areas jointly activated in processing symbolic as well as non-symbolic quantities. As a result of a meta-analysis, the authors reported joint activation of bilateral inferior parietal lobule (IPL) and precuneus as well as left superior parietal lobule (SPL) and right superior frontal gyrus (SFG) during the processing of both symbolic and non-symbolic numbers. Furthermore, Holloway and colleagues [36] reported a right-sided dominance of joint processing of symbolic and non-symbolic magnitude in right IPL and SPL. Several other studies also indicated that this region is involved in processing symbolic [9, 20, 31, 37] and non-symbolic numerical magnitude [8, 33, 38]. Furthermore, Holloway and colleagues [36] found joint activations for symbolic and non-symbolic magnitude in the inferior frontal gyrus (IFG) extending to middle frontal gyrus, right anterior insula, ACC, and SFG. Thereby, these findings imply that these brain regions comprise format-independent processing of symbolic and non-symbolic magnitudes.

However, recent research also indicated that symbolic and non-symbolic magnitudes are processed by both overlapping but also distinct neural systems [8, 35, 36]. The processing of non-symbolic magnitude was observed to involve visual cortex areas due to greater visual demands such as the individuation and summation of non-symbolic items [36]. The meta-analysis of Sokolowski and colleagues [35] revealed a right-lateralized fronto-parietal network including right SPL, IPL, precuneus, SFG, and insula as well as middle occipital gyrus involved in non-symbolic number processing compared to symbolic numbers.

In contrast, stronger activation for processing symbolic compared to non-symbolic numbers was found in right supramarginal gyrus, IPL, and left AG. Holloway and colleagues [36] also reported involvement of left AG as well as superior temporal gyrus during symbolic compared to non-symbolic number processing. These regions have repeatedly been reported to be important during exact calculation [28, 34] and arithmetic fact retrieval [29, 39].

Thus, previous research suggests that the human brain seems to represent numerical magnitude both format-dependent as well as format-independent, and thus, abstract [35].

Neural correlates of processing symbolic fractions and non-symbolic proportions
Recent studies indicated that the same brain regions associated with processing absolute magnitude are also involved in processing fractions and proportions, and thus, relative magnitude in general [40–43]. Importantly, the magnitude of a fraction (e.g., ¼) might be represented by the numerical magnitude of the fraction as a whole (e.g., .25) or involve separate representations of the magnitudes of numerator and denominator. Ischebeck and colleagues [41] found that activation within the right IPS, right medial frontal gyrus, and middle occipital gyrus was only modulated by the overall numerical distance between fractions and was not influenced by numerator or denominator distances. Therefore, these authors concluded that fraction magnitude is represented holistically at the neural level.

Moreover, Jacob and Nieder [42] provided evidence that the processing of fraction magnitude within the IPS seems to be independent of presentation format. Using a functional MRI adaptation (fMRA) paradigm, participants were habituated to a given fraction number (e.g., $^1/_6$) and were then presented with either a deviant fraction number (e.g., ½) or fraction word (e.g., 'one-half'). During adaptation, the blood oxygen level-dependent (BOLD) signal decreased. When presented with deviants, signal in bilateral IPS, bilateral prefrontal cortex, and a small cluster in the right cingulate cortex recovered as a function of numerical distance between deviant and adapted fraction magnitude. This effect was independent of presentation format. This suggests that the same populations of neurons seem to code the same fraction magnitude, irrespective of presentation format.

Jacob and Nieder [43] also observed that the BOLD signal in bilateral IPS and lateral prefrontal cortex decreased during the adaptation phase in an fMRA experiment using non-symbolic proportions (e.g., proportions of line lengths or numerosities). Again, BOLD signal recovered when presented with a deviant stimulus as a function of the distance between the deviant and the adapted proportion with strongest effects in bilateral anterior IPS. Further clusters of activations were found in bilateral prefrontal and precentral regions with seemingly right-lateralized dominance.

Taken together, previous work indicates that a network comprising bilateral IPS, prefrontal cortex, middle occipital gyrus, and cingulate cortex, which was reported to be activated for processing absolute numerical magnitude, is also activated when relative magnitude needs to be processed, irrespective of presentation format (for a brief overview see [13]).

The present study
So far, a common neural substrate for processing proportion magnitude was observed only for (i) symbolic fractions and fraction words [42], (ii) proportional line lengths and non-symbolic numerosities [43], and (iii) different pairs of symbolic fractions ([41], e.g., same denominator: 2/7 vs. 5/7; same nominator: 3/5 vs. 3/8; mixed pairs: 2/3 vs. 1/5). Thus, it has not yet been investigated systematically whether both symbolic and non-symbolic proportions have a common neural substrate for relative magnitude processing reflected by shared activation for processing relative magnitude independent of presentation format. However, this is an important question: in teaching and learning settings, symbolic and non-symbolic presentation formats of fractions and proportions are often used side by side to introduce and foster the understanding of proportional relations. To allow for a better and easier-to-grasp conceptual understanding of proportionality aspects, symbolic fractions in particular are often presented and illustrated using non-symbolic pie charts and proportional dot patterns [4, 5, 44–47]. Additionally, understanding of fraction magnitude is usually supported by references to its respective equivalent in decimal notations [48]. Furthermore, non-symbolic proportions can be displayed either discretely involving countable units such as patterns of, for instance, blue and yellow dots or continuously without segmentation as in pie charts to support the conceptual understanding of fractions. Therefore, the current study aimed at investigating whether magnitude processing of symbolic and non-symbolic proportions has a common neural substrate. We conducted an fMRI study using magnitude

comparison tasks with symbolic (e.g., fractions and decimals) and non-symbolic proportions (e.g., dot patterns and pie charts), respectively.

As an indicator of magnitude-related processing, we specifically considered the numerical distance effect in our analyses. In a two-stage procedure, we first evaluated distance-related activations in proportion processing in different formats before addressing the issue of a common neural substrate underlying both symbolic and non-symbolic proportion processing.

Because of the similarity of decimals to integers, we expected activation in areas typically associated with the processing of symbolic numbers for the processing of decimals. These areas involve bilateral IPS, left AG, and supramarginal gyrus [21, 35, 36]. Additional to activations in bilateral IPS, we expected stronger frontal activations in SMA, DLPFC, and ACC for the processing of fraction magnitude due to higher cognitive and working memory demands reflecting additional computations necessary for accessing fraction magnitude [18, 25, 26, 41]. For proportions reflected by dot patterns, comparable cognitive and working memory demands were expected, and thus, activations in frontal areas such as DLPFC and ACC in addition to IPS [43]. Furthermore, we hypothesized that dot patterns should elicit stronger activations in visual-occipital areas because of higher visual demands as well as right IPS due to their non-symbolic nature [8, 33, 36, 38]. For pie charts, we expected activations in a fronto-parietal network including SMA, DLPFC and IPS as well as in occipital brain regions due to necessary visual processing and evaluations of part-whole relations as well as the resulting working memory demands.

As all previous studies on processing fractions or non-symbolic proportions showed an involvement of bilateral intraparietal cortex with a right-lateralized preference as well as activations in PFC, we also expected to find joint magnitude-related fronto-parietal activation in bilateral IPS and PFC for all four presentation formats.

Methods
Participants
Twenty-four right-handed volunteers (13 female, mean age = 23.2 years; $SD = 2.99$ years) participated in the study. All participants were university students. After being informed about the experimental procedure, they gave their written consent in accordance with the protocol of the local Ethics Committee of the Medical Faculty of the University of Tuebingen. All participants reported normal or corrected to normal vision and no previous history of neurological or psychiatric disorders. They received monetary compensation for their participation.

Design and procedure
We employed a block design with alternating comparison task blocks in four conditions (i.e., fraction, decimal, pie chart, dot pattern comparison tasks). Blocks were presented in pseudo-random order. In total, we ran 24 blocks (six blocks per condition) consisting of one practice trial and four critical trials each. Thus, the experiment consisted of six practice and 24 experimental trials per condition (24 practice and 96 experimental trials in total). Each task block was built as follows: at the beginning of each block, a cue indicating the upcoming proportion type for the next five trials was presented for 500 ms. Subsequently, a black screen was presented for 4000 ms. The cue was the fraction 1/4 shown in the different presentation formats in the center of the screen against grey background. Afterwards, critical trials were presented starting with a black fixation cross against grey background for 500 ms, followed by the presentation of a proportion stimulus for up to 5000 ms. Participants had to respond within this time limit by pressing one of two MRI compatible response buttons with either their left (indicating left proportion larger) or right thumb (indicating right proportion larger). When participants responded faster than the given 5000 ms, a mask was presented in the remaining time (visual noise consisting of blue, yellow, and grey pixels). Then the next trial was presented. The procedure of the beginning of a block is shown in Fig. 1. There was no jitter between successive stimuli. At the end of each block, a black screen was shown for 6000 ms.

Stimuli
We applied four different presentation formats of proportions: fractions, decimals, pie charts, and dot patterns (see Fig. 2). For each of these four presentation formats, we constructed 30 items. Proportions were presented in pairs with the magnitude of the first proportion ranging from .13 to .86 and of the second proportion ranging from .22 to .89. Absolute distances between proportions ranged from .02 to .69.

We first generated the symbolic fraction items and converted them into the other presentation formats. Numerators of the fractions ranged from 1 to 8 and denominators from 2 to 9. Fractions were constructed such that in half of the items the comparison of numerators and denominators was either congruent or incongruent with the comparison of overall fraction magnitude. In this context, congruency means that separate comparisons of numerator and denominator magnitudes yielded the same answer as the comparison of the overall magnitudes of fraction pairs (e.g., 1/5 < 2/9 with 1 < 2 and 5 < 9). In incongruent pairs,

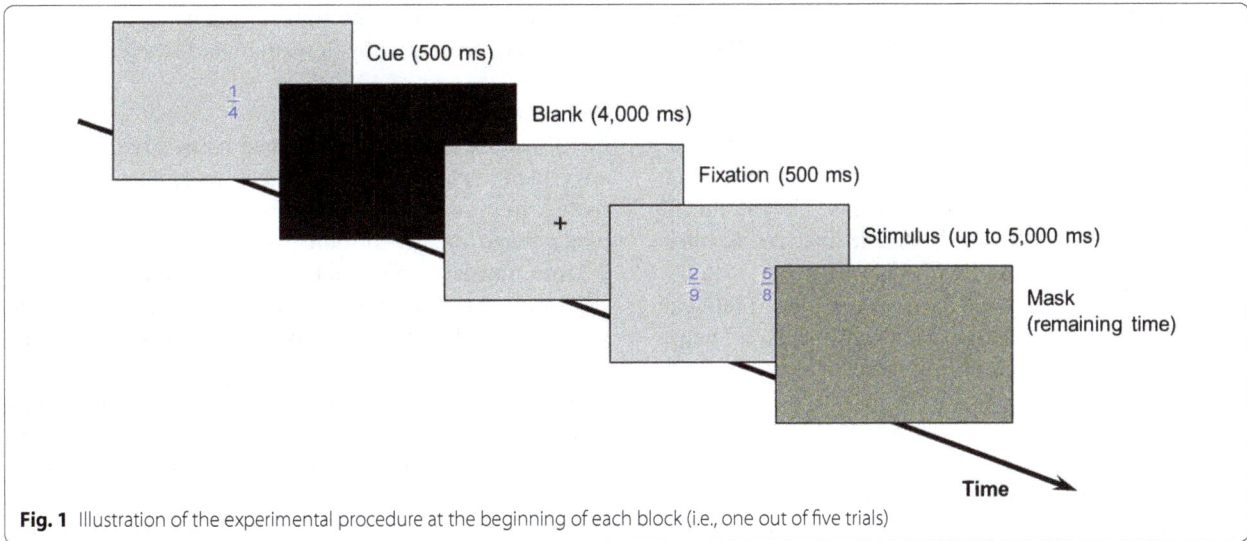

Fig. 1 Illustration of the experimental procedure at the beginning of each block (i.e., one out of five trials)

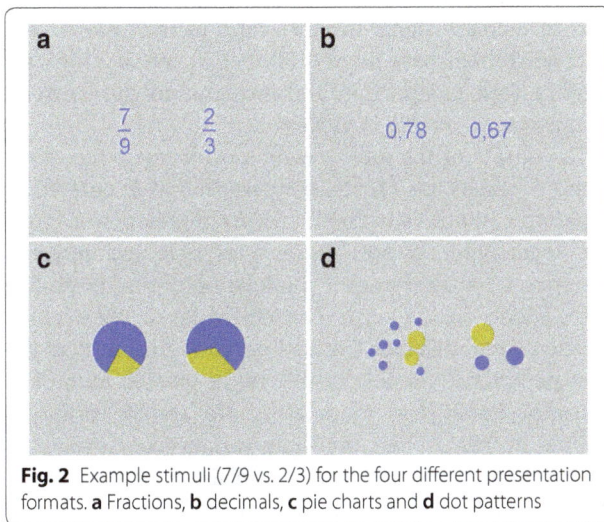

Fig. 2 Example stimuli (7/9 vs. 2/3) for the four different presentation formats. **a** Fractions, **b** decimals, **c** pie charts and **d** dot patterns

separate comparisons of numerator and denominator magnitudes yielded opposing answers as compared to the overall magnitude of the fractions (e.g., $5/9 < 2/3$, but $5 > 2$ and $9 > 3$). Hence, participants could not solve the task correctly, when relying on the magnitude of numerators or denominators only. In the next step, we constructed decimals by dividing numerators by denominators and rounding up the result to two digits after the decimal mark. Fractions as well as decimals were presented in blue (RGB-values: 53, 85, 204; font type: Arial; font size: 80) on a grey background (RGB-values: 204, 204, 204). One proportion was located on the left half (x/y-coordinates: 356/384 px), whereas the other one was located on the right half

(x/y-coordinates: 668/384 px) of the screen (screen resolution: $1024 \times$ px).

Pie charts were drawn by dividing circles into two pie segments according to the magnitude of the respective fraction items. For instance, 5/9 was drawn by coloring 5/9 of the pie in blue (same blue as for fractions) and 4/9 in yellow (RGB-values: 203, 187, 0). The same grey as for fractions and decimals was used as a background color. Moreover, the location of the yellow part varied pseudo-randomly. We varied the size of the circles such that in half of the items the larger proportion was also larger according to the visual area of the blue pie segment, whereas in the other half of the items it was smaller. Thereby, we ensured that participants could not select the larger proportion by relying only on the visual area of pie segments. The diameter of pies ranged from 95 to 289 px.

Dot patterns were drawn on an invisible rectangular area of size 491×363 px in the center of the left and the right side of the screen. Location of dots was varied randomly in these invisible rectangular areas. Diameter of dots varied randomly from 21 to 98 px. Dot patterns were colored according to the fractions they denoted using the same colors as for pie charts. For instance, the dot pattern of 5/9 was drawn by coloring five dots in blue and four dots in yellow (and thus, 5 out of 9 dots were colored in blue). Moreover, we equated the sum of the yellow and blue areas of the dots across the two dot patterns which had to be compared to ensure that participants could not rely on visual area when comparing the dot patterns.

fMRI data acquisition

MRI data were acquired using a 3T Siemens Magnetom TrioTim MRI system (Siemens AG,

Erlangen, Germany). A high resolution T1-weighted anatomical scan (TR $= 2300$ s, matrix $= 256 \times 256$, 176 slices, voxel size $= 1.0 \times 1.0 \times 1.0$ mm^3; FOV $= 256$ mm^2, TE $= 2.92$ ms; flip angle $= 8°$) was collected at the end of the experimental session. All functional measurements covered the whole brain using standard echo-planar-imaging (EPI) sequences (TR $= 2400$ ms; TE $= 30$ ms; flip angle $= 80°$; FOV $= 220$ mm^2, 88×88 matrix; 42 slices, voxel size $= 2.5 \times 2.5 \times 3.0$ mm^3, gap $= 10\%$).

FMRI data was acquired in a single run. Total scanning time was approximately 20 min. We included pauses between blocks in which a black screen was presented for 6000 ms.

Behavioral data analysis

We analyzed both reaction times and accuracy. A first inspection of the distribution of reaction times showed that they were strongly skewed to the right. To approach normal distribution while conserving statistical power, we used the inverse transformation and transformed reaction times into speed with measurement unit 1/sec [49].

We analyzed speed by running a linear mixed effects model (LME) and accuracy by running a generalized linear mixed model (GLME) with logit as link function and assuming a binomial error distribution. We ran (G)LME instead of analysis of variances (ANOVA) to be able to include random effects for both, participants and items to take into account that besides drawing only a sample of participants, we also included only a sample of all possible items [50]. Moreover, running ANOVA on accuracy (or error data) can result in spurious effects [51]. In the LME, we included fixed effects of condition (fractions, decimals, pie charts, and dot patterns) and distance between proportions as well as their interaction, random intercepts for participants as well as items (crossed random effects), and a random slope for condition (i.e., a maximal model; [52]). In the GLME, we included the same fixed effects and random intercepts for participants and items. Moreover, we effect-coded the predictor condition and centered the continuous predictor distance.

We considered only correctly solved trials in the analysis of speed. Additionally, we removed trials with absolute z-scaled residuals of the full model larger than ± 3. In total, we considered 82.6% of all trials for the analysis of speed.

Statistical analyses were run using R [53] and the R package lme4 for running (G)LME [54]. p values for fixed effects of LME were calculated running F tests using the Kenward–Roger approximation for degrees of freedom [55]. For GLME, we ran likelihood ratio tests (LRT). These methods are available via the R package afex [56]. Post-hoc tests were run using the R package multcomp

[57] and corrected for multiple testing using the false discovery rate procedure by Benjamini and Hochberg [58].

fMRI data analysis

fMRI data analysis was performed using SPM12 (http://www.fil.ion.ucl.ac.uk/spm). Images were slice-time corrected, motion corrected, and realigned to each participant's mean image. Motion parameters did not exceed 2.5 mm translation in total (i.e., they did not exceed voxel size) and a head rotation of 1.5 degree in pitch, roll, and yaw in total. Therefore, none of the participants had to be excluded from the analyses because of head movements. The mean image was co-registered with the whole-brain volume. Imaging data was then normalized into standard stereotaxic MNI space (Montreal Neurological Institute, McGill University, Montreal, Canada). Images were resampled every 2.5 mm using 4th degree spline interpolation to obtain isovoxel and then smoothed with a 8 mm full-width half-maximum (FWHM) Gaussian kernel to accommodate inter-subject variation in brain anatomy and to increase signal-to-noise ratio in the images. The data were high-pass filtered (128 s) to remove low-frequency noise components and corrected for autocorrelation assuming an AR(1) process.

The onsets of the four presentation formats (i.e., fractions, decimals, pie charts, dot patterns) were entered as separate conditions in the GLM. As regressors of interest, logarithmic overall distance as first and reaction times as second parametric modulation of the conditions were added on the single-participant level. We decided to use overall distance (instead of reaction times) as the first parametric modulator due to its specific numerical features. Parametric modulators are serially orthogonalised in SPM. Therefore, only variance not explained by the first modulator can be explained by the second modulator. Consequently, logarithmic distance entered the model first, because its inherent numerical quality was of particular interest. Generally, no supra-threshold activation was found for the parametric modulation of RT unless stated otherwise. Movement parameters estimated at the realignment stage of preprocessing were included as covariates of no interest. Brain activation was convolved over all experimental trials with the canonical haemodynamic response function (HRF) as implemented in SPM12 and its time and dispersion derivatives.

We performed a three-stage analysis. First, we evaluated activation associated with the distance effect in all four presentation formats, respectively, to examine specific magnitude-related brain activation in proportion processing. Second, in an exploratory analysis, we examined format-specific activations of both symbolic and non-symbolic relative magnitudes. Third, analogous to previous studies on proportion processing [42, 43], a conjunction analysis was calculated as implemented in SPM12 (conjunction null, see [59]) to identify brain activation common in all four presentation formats during magnitude processing.

The SPM Anatomy Toolbox [60], available for all published cytoarchitectonic maps (http://www.fz-juelich.de/ime/spm_anatomy_toolbox), was used for anatomical localization of effects where applicable. In areas not yet implemented, the anatomical automatic labelling tool (AAL) in SPM12 (http://www.cyceron.fr/web/aalanatomical_automatic_labeling.html) was used.

If not stated otherwise, thresholds for statistical inference were set at FWE-corrected $p < .05$ at the voxel level, corrected for multiple comparisons at the cluster level to FWE-corrected $p < .05$ with a cluster size of $k = 10$ voxels.

An uncorrected statistical threshold of $p < .001$ was chosen for the conjunction analysis because four conditions of interest needed to significantly modulate the fMRI signal in a given region in the conjunction analysis. The effective p value for a conjunction analysis is the square of the p values for each component. Therefore, a more liberal threshold for such a conservative statistical procedure is justified [36].

Results
Behavioral results
Mean speed of participants in the four conditions for fractions, decimals, pie charts, and dot patterns, respectively, was: $M_{fractions} = .57$ ($SD = .15$) items/sec, $M_{decimals} = 1.14$ ($SD = .17$) items/sec, $M_{pies} = .91$ ($SD = .17$) items/sec, and $M_{dots} = .60$ ($SD = .20$) items/sec. Moreover, mean accuracy in the four conditions for fractions, decimals, pie charts, and dot patterns, respectively, were: $M_{fractions} = 81.1\%$ ($SD = 10.9\%$), $M_{decimals} = 99.2\%$ ($SD = 1.5\%$), $M_{pies} = 91.5\%$ ($SD = 4.8\%$), and $M_{dots} = 72.5\%$ ($SD = 12.6\%$).

In the next step, we ran a LME with condition, distance between proportions as well as their interaction as fixed effects and speed as dependent variable testing for statistical significance of these differences. All three F tests were highly significant [condition: $F(3, 27.97) = 112.77$, $p < .001$, distance: $F(1, 49.81) = 133.76$, $p < .001$, and condition × distance: $F(3, 30.48) = 20.06$, $p < .001$]. This indicated that participants' speed differed between conditions. Pairwise post hoc comparisons revealed that except for the difference between fractions and dot patterns ($p = .567$) speed in all conditions differed significantly from each other (all $p < .001$). Additionally, the significant distance indicated that across all conditions speed increased with the overall numerical distance, slope $= .55$ items/sec ($SE = .05$). However, the significant interaction indicated that distance effects varied between conditions. Mean distance effects (SE in parenthesis) in

the separate conditions were for fractions: .52 (.07) items/sec, $z = 7.42$, $p < .001$, for decimals: .20 (.05) items/sec, $z = 3.85$, $p < .001$, for pies: .77 (.07) items/sec, $z = 10.39$, $p < .001$, and for dots: .69 (.09) items/sec, $z = 7.40$, $p < .001$, respectively. This indicated that we observed significant distance effects in all four presentation formats. Post-hoc analyses indicated that the distance effect for decimals differed significantly from distance effects of all other presentation formats ($p < .001$). Moreover, distance effects of fractions and pie charts differed significantly from each other ($p = .013$). Other pairwise comparisons were not significant ($p > .139$). Figure 3a gives an overview of the distance effects for speed data.

We also evaluated performance differences in accuracy between conditions by running a GLME with the same factors. Again, all three LRT for fixed effects were significant [condition: $\chi^2(3) = 210.64$, $p < .001$, distance: $\chi^2(1) = 100.75$, $p < .001$, and condition × distance: $\chi^2(3) = 10.28$, $p = .016$]. Estimated log odds (SE in parenthesis) of the four conditions were for fractions: 1.96 (.19), in % = 87.6%, for decimals: 6.63 (1.26), in % = 99.9%, for pie charts: 3.641 (.34), in % = 97.4%, and for dots: 1.30 (.17), in % = 78.6%, respectively. Pairwise post hoc comparisons revealed that log odds of all conditions differed from each other significantly (all $p < .021$). Moreover, the significant distance effect indicated that participants' accuracy increased with the overall numerical distance between two proportions, slope in log odds $= 13.69$, $SE = 2.87$. However, again the significant interaction between condition and distance indicated that distance effects differed between conditions. Mean distance effects in log odds (SE in parenthesis) in the separate conditions were for fractions: 9.37 (1.60), $z = 5.86$, $p < .001$, for decimals: 20.57 (10.52), $z = 1.96$, $p = .051$, for pie charts: 16.75 (3.02), $z = 5.55$, $p < .001$, and for dots: 8.05 (1.25), $z = 6.46$, $p < .001$, respectively. Pairwise post hoc comparisons revealed that only distance effects for dot patterns and pie charts differed significantly ($p = .033$), whereas all other comparisons were not significant (all $p > .067$). Distance effects for different conditions are shown in Fig. 3b.

Imaging results
Evaluating magnitude processing in different presentation formats
Fractions Numerical distance in fraction processing was associated with significantly increasing activation in right IPS, bilateral SMA and bilateral frontal gyrus for decreasing distance (see Table 1 and Fig. 4).

Dot patterns Numerical distance in processing dot patterns was associated with activation in bilateral IPS, left ACC, right SFG as well as visual cortex such as left

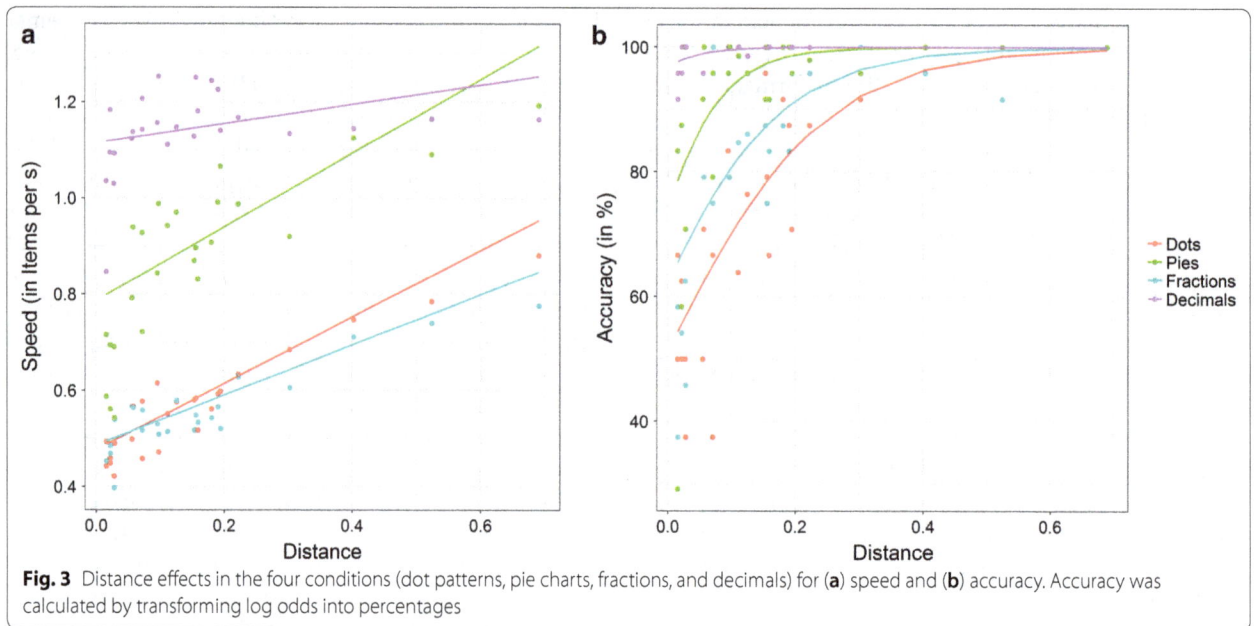

Fig. 3 Distance effects in the four conditions (dot patterns, pie charts, fractions, and decimals) for (**a**) speed and (**b**) accuracy. Accuracy was calculated by transforming log odds into percentages

middle and right inferior occipital gyrus with decreasing distance (see Table 1 and Fig. 4).

Pie charts Numerical distance in the processing of pie charts revealed activation in bilateral IPS, large bilateral occipital regions extending to parietal and temporal areas and bilateral IFG with decreasing distance. Further activation was observed in bilateral insula, bilateral precentral gyrus and bilateral MCC (Table 1 and Fig. 4).

Decimals Numerical distance in decimal processing was associated with activation in bilateral IPS, left occipito-temporal regions, left fusiform gyrus and frontal areas with a left-lateralized dominance with decreasing distance. Further clusters of activated voxels were observed in left insula and bilateral precentral gyrus (see Table 1 and Fig. 4).

Specific correlates of symbolic and non-symbolic proportional magnitudes

Additionally, an exploratory analysis of specific activations associated with processing symbolic and non-symbolic proportional magnitudes was conducted. Because the activation for theses contrasts did not survive FWE correction on a whole brain level, activations were thresholded at a whole-brain p value of $< .001$ uncorrected and only reported when they remained significant for multiple comparisons at the cluster-level at $p < .05$ FWE-corrected. This analysis revealed the following results.

Symbolic vs. non-symbolic magnitudes Distance in processing of symbolic (i.e., fractions and decimals) versus non-symbolic magnitudes (i.e., pie charts and dot patterns) indicated higher activation in bilateral middle frontal gyrus, left SFG, right SMA and left AG (see Table 2 and Fig. 5) with decreasing numerical distance.

Non-symbolic vs. symbolic magnitudes Numerical distance in non-symbolic versus symbolic magnitudes was associated with higher activations in a widespread temporal network extending to parietal and occipital cortex, left middle occipital gyrus, right MCC, insula and SFG (see Table 2 and Fig. 5).

Conjunction analysis of the distance effect

As previous studies evaluated shared neural correlates of magnitude processing for fractions and fraction words, we conducted a conjunction analysis ([41, 42]; conjunction null, see [59]) to evaluate the hypothesis of a common neural correlate of magnitude processing for symbolic and non-symbolic proportions. The conjunction analysis revealed significant joint activation in right SPL (hIP3) as well as bilateral occipital regions (see Table 3 and Fig. 6).

Discussion

The present study aimed at investigating whether the processing of symbolic and non-symbolic proportions draws on a common underlying neural substrate. Recent neuroimaging evidence indicated that symbolic fractions [41, 42] and non-symbolic proportions [43]

Table 1 Distance effect in proportion magnitude comparison for different presentation formats

Contrast	Brain region	MNI (x, y, z)			k	t
Fractions	RH inferior parietal lobule (hIP2)	43	− 42	53	31	5.43
	RH inferior parietal lobule (hIP3)[a]	46	− 45	55		
	RH supplementary motor area	8	23	45	101	7.59
	LH supplementary motor area[a]	− 7	18	48		
	LH middle frontal gyrus	− 47	28	33	176	6.58
	LH inferior frontal gyrus[a]	− 40	21	33		
	LH middle frontal gyrus	− 27	8	50	29	5.92
	RH precentral gyrus	36	3	30	23	5.73
	LH superior medial gyrus	− 7	33	40	11	5.66
	RH inferior frontal gyrus	46	31	25	90	6.98
	RH superior frontal gyrus	21	21	55	34	5.90
Dot patterns	RH superior parietal lobule (hIP3)	33	− 52	60	94	6.05
	LH superior parietal lobule	− 30	− 57	63	73	6.37
	RH superior frontal gyrus	26	3	63	41	6.54
	LH anterior cingulate gyrus	− 15	26	28	13	5.97
	RH calcarine gyrus	12	− 70	18	13	5.27
	LH caudate	− 20	6	18	12	5.69
	LH calcarine gyrus	− 17	− 75	10	1953	7.75
	LH middle occipital gyrus[a]	− 42	− 80	0		
	LH cuneus[a]	− 2	− 75	18		
	RH inferior occipital gyrus[a]	43	− 75	− 8		
Pie charts	RH middle occipital gyrus	28	− 75	33	2094	9.69
	RH superior occipital gyrus[a]	26	− 75	38		
	RH inferior occipital gyrus[a]	43	− 75	− 5		
	RH inferior temporal gyrus[a]	46	− 80	− 3		
	RH inferior parietal lobule (hIP2)[a]	41	− 40	48		
	RH superior parietal lobule (hIP3)[a]	28	− 60	60		
	LH superior parietal lobule	− 22	− 65	63	247	6.62
	LH inferior parietal lobule (hIP3)[a]	− 35	− 50	53		
	RH middle cingulate cortex	8	16	45	836	11.46
	LH middle cingulate cortex[a]	− 5	18	45		
	RH precentral gyrus	46	6	28	532	9.32
	RH inferior frontal gyrus[a]	48	28	25		
	RH insula	36	21	3	397	8.93
	RH inferior frontal gyrus[a]	33	26	− 5		
	LH insula	− 32	18	3	204	9.36
	LH inferior frontal gyrus	− 60	11	25	72	6.41
	LH precentral gyrus	− 45	1	40	37	5.43
	LH inferior occipital gyrus	− 42	− 75	− 10	1086	11.79
	LH middle occipital gyrus[a]	− 42	− 85	8		
	LH superior occipital gyrus[a]	− 25	− 80	25		
	LH calcarine gyrus	− 15	− 72	10	706	8.68
	RH calcarine gyrus[a]	16	− 67	13		

Table 1 (continued)

Contrast	Brain region	MNI (x, y, z)			k	t
Decimals	RH inferior parietal lobule (hIP2)	48	−40	45	95	5.96
	RH postcentral gyrus[a]	43	−32	60		
	LH inferior parietal lobule (hIP3)	−37	−52	58	21	5.41
	LH superior parietal lobule[a]	−30	−57	63		
	LH inferior parietal lobule	−27	−45	48	12	5.45
	LH supramarginal gyrus	−60	−45	30	24	5.59
	LH lingual gyrus	−15	−55	−10	468	7.38
	LH fusiform gyurs[a]	−37	−37	−23		
	RH inferior temporal gyrus	51	−62	−10	50	5.83
	RH fusiform gyrus[a]	41	−57	−13		
	LH inferior occipital gyrus	−45	−75	−13	344	7.60
	LH middle occipital gyrus[a]	−50	−75	−3		
	LH middle temporal gyrus[a]	−52	−70	13		
	LH Superior temporal gyrus	−42	−35	3	60	7.05
	LH middle temporal gyrus	−55	−55	15	45	5.72
	LH superior temporal gyrus[a]	−57	−45	15		
	RH temporal pole	51	16	−23	15	5.89
	LH middle temporal gyrus	−57	−37	8	14	5.50
	LH precentral gyrus	−40	−2	40	59	5.81
	LH inferior frontal gyrus	−45	28	−3	47	5.56
	LH inferior frontal gyrus	−42	13	15	29	6.66
	RH superior frontal gyrus	21	−15	75	25	6.21
	RH precentral gyrus	43	−17	58	16	5.32
	LH Middle frontal gyrus	−45	26	40	16	5.81
	LH middle frontal gyrus	−35	21	30	12	5.71
	LH posterior insula	−30	−20	13	28	5.72
	LH insula	−35	21	3	10	5.17
	LH cuneus	−2	−77	18	742	7.51
	LH calcarine gyrus[a]	−15	−72	13		
	LH superior occipital gyrus[a]	−12	−80	23		
	RH lingual gyrus	18	−47	−3	43	6.60
	LH putamen	−30	−12	−8	18	5.71
	LH paracentral lobule	−10	−32	75	13	5.11

Activations were thresholded at a whole-brain FWE-corrected p value of < .05 with a cluster size of k = 10 voxels and reported only when they remained significant following FWE-correction for multiple comparisons at the cluster-level at $p < .05$ FWE. Cerebellar activations are not reported due to incomplete coverage of the cerebellum depending on individual head size

k cluster size; LH left hemisphere; MNI Montreal Neurological Institute; RH right hemisphere; t t value

[a] Minor maximum

are processed within a fronto-parietal network including the IPS. Synced with evidence on whole number processing (e.g., [10, 13] for overviews) this suggests that both absolute and relative magnitude information seem to be processed within this brain area. Nevertheless, a systematic evaluation of brain areas jointly activated when processing symbolic *and* non-symbolic proportion magnitude was missing so far. Therefore, we systematically evaluated the neural correlates of processing symbolic fractions and decimals as well as

non-symbolic dot patterns and pie charts in the same experiment. Most importantly, we observed evidence for a common neural substrate in right IPS as well as bilateral visual cortex for processing relative magnitude irrespective of presentation format. In the following, we will first discuss this joint activation found for symbolic and non-symbolic proportions before addressing distance-related activation observed for symbolic and non-symbolic formats and in each presentation format separately.

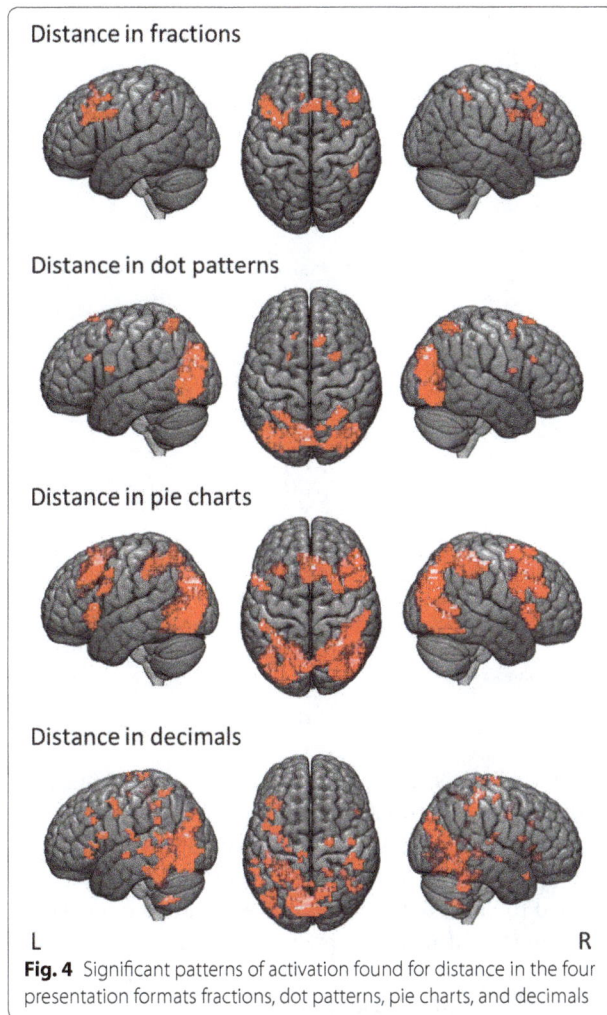

Fig. 4 Significant patterns of activation found for distance in the four presentation formats fractions, dot patterns, pie charts, and decimals

A common neural substrate for processing relative magnitude

We observed a common neural substrate for processing symbolic and non-symbolic proportions in an occipito-parietal network comprising the right IPS. Within this network, IPS activation seems to reflect processing of abstract relative magnitude (e.g. [9, 16, 34, 37]), whereas activation in occipital areas might rather reflect higher order visual processing as well as decoding of the visual form [15, 18, 21], which helps to process semantic features of quantity.

Recent research revealed a right-hemispheric preference for the processing of absolute number magnitude [9, 31, 32]. As such, the right IPS seems to specifically underlie the semantic representation of numerical distances [61]. This right-hemispheric preference for the processing of magnitude was reported for both symbolic and non-symbolic quantities (e.g., [8]). Importantly, our data showed joint activation for magnitude processing of symbolic and non-symbolic proportions

in an occipito-parietal network including the right IPS. Thus, besides absolute magnitude also relative magnitude information seems to be processed in right IPS, irrespective of presentation format. Importantly, this seems to reflect a neural correlate of an abstract concept for relative magnitude. This is in line with propositions of the triple code model of numerical cognition that numerical magnitude and mental arithmetic are represented and processed within the IPS [10, 13, 62, 63]. Importantly, recent evidence suggested that the respective parietal cortex areas might subserve an abstract, notation-independent representation for both absolute and relative magnitude ([9, 41–43, 64], but see [65] for a more detailed discussion of this point). The results of our conjunction analysis support this assumption. Moreover, our data also extended previous research on proportion processing because so far only the processing of either symbolic fractions [41], fractions and fraction words [42] or non-symbolic proportions [43] was investigated on the neural level. In the present study, we systematically investigated common neural activation for the processing of both symbolic and non-symbolic formats. Our results are also in line with recent research suggesting that humans (and animals) are not necessarily born with a "sense of number"—the ability to perceive, manipulate and understand discrete numerosities [66–68]—but rather a generalized and abstract "sense of magnitude" for the processing of both, numerosities and continuous magnitudes (e.g., size, area, and density; for a review, see [69]). As the present study found a shared neural correlate for both discrete (e.g., fractions and dot patterns) as well as continuous relative magnitudes (e.g., decimals and pie charts) in symbolic and non-symbolic presentation formats, the results further support the idea of such a generalized magnitude system.

Additionally, we found activation in bilateral visual cortex (bilateral superior, bilateral inferior, right middle occipital gyrus). These brain regions are involved in higher order visual processing and decoding of the visual form [15, 18, 21]. Furthermore, the ventral visual stream is anchored in the lateral occipital cortex (LOC; [19]). This stream plays an important role in number representation and magnitude manipulation as it interacts with the IPS for the semantic representation and procedural manipulation of quantity [19]. Importantly, the ventral visual stream areas in the occipital gyrus are not only co-activated with the IPS during numerical and arithmetic processing, but their activation also increases with task complexity [19, 70, 71]. Hence, our data point to higher order visual processing during relative magnitude processing in the ventral visual stream which may reflect the complexity of accessing relative magnitude information.

Table 2 Activations for distance in symbolic vs. non-symbolic as well as non-symbolic vs. symbolic presentation formats

Contrast	Brain region	MNI (x, y, z)			k	t
Symbolic vs. non-symb.	LH superior frontal gyrus	− 20	21	43	286	6.45
	LH middle frontal gyrus[a]	− 50	23	33		
	LH angular gyrus	− 37	− 60	28	273	4.59
	LH middle occipital gyrus[a]	− 42	− 72	33		
	RH supplementary motor area	21	13	33	229	6.77
	RH middle frontal gyrus[a]	26	8	28		
Non-symb. vs. symbolic	RH inferior temporal gyrus	48	− 72	− 5	1046	6.05
	RH middle occipital gyrus[a]	33	− 75	15		
	RH superior parietal lobule[a]	21	− 72	43		
	LH middle occipital gyrus	− 40	− 75	3	587	5.47
	RH middle cingulate cortex	8	13	43	390	5.76
	RH insula	43	23	0	221	4.54
	RH putamen[a]	28	3	10		
	RH caudate nucleus[a]	16	13	8		
	RH superior frontal gyrus	23	6	63	132	5.31

Activations were thresholded at a whole-brain p value of <.001 uncorrected with a cluster size of k = 10 voxels and reported only when they remained significant following FWE-correction for multiple comparisons at the cluster-level at p < .05 FWE-corrected. Cerebellar activations are not reported due to incomplete coverage of the cerebellum depending on individual head size

k cluster size; LH left hemisphere; MNI Montreal Neurological Institute; RH right hemisphere; t t value

[a] Minor maximum

This task complexity might also be reflected by the distance effect, an effect that is often associated with task difficulty as difficulty increases when the distance between two to-be-compared numbers decreases [11]. The distance effect for symbolic and non-symbolic proportions was observed in the behavioral data. We found differences in distance effects for error rates and reaction times between the different presentation formats. While error rates and reaction times were highest for fractions

and dot patterns, comparing pie charts—and even more so decimals—led to faster and more accurate responses. Increasing response times and error rates might reflect influences of task difficulty. Therefore, behavioral data seemed to indicate that accessing magnitude information of proportional relations might not be the only mechanisms involved. This is also reflected in the neural data.

The IPS was previously associated with tasks requiring specific attention due to higher levels of difficulty [72–74]. In studies on number processing the distance effect is a prominent paradigm (e.g., [9, 41]). However, this effect is strongly modulated by difficulty: as the distance between two numerals decreases, error rates as well as response times, and hence, difficulty increases. Thus, the observed activation in IPS during numerical tasks might also be driven by task difficulty. Yet, previous studies found activations in the IPS for either passive listening to number words [75] or passive viewing of symbolic numbers versus letters and colors [37]. Therefore, we are confident that particularly activation in right intraparietal regions, as observed in the present conjunction analysis, reflects processing of (relative) magnitude information over and beyond influences of task difficulty.

Specific activations for symbolic and non-symbolic presentation formats

The contrast between symbolic (i.e., fractions and decimals) and non-symbolic presentation formats (i.e., dot patterns and pie charts) indicated activation in a

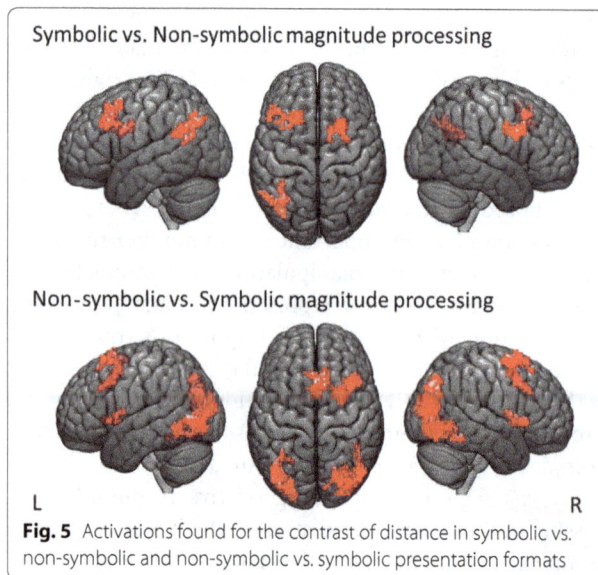

Fig. 5 Activations found for the contrast of distance in symbolic vs. non-symbolic and non-symbolic vs. symbolic presentation formats

Table 3 Joint activations across the four conditions (i.e., fractions, decimals, dot patterns, pie charts) for distance as revealed by the conjunction analysis

Contrast	Brain region	MNI (x, y, z)			k	t
Conjunction	RH superior parietal lobule (hIP3)	31	− 60	60	46	4.50
	LH calcarine gyrus	− 17	− 75	13	276	5.55
	RH calcarine gyrus[a]	16	− 67	18		
	LH cuneus[a]	− 2	− 75	20		
	RH superior occipital gyrus[a]	23	− 75	28		
	LH inferior occipital gyrus	− 40	− 72	− 8	76	4.76
	LH superior occipital gyrus	− 25	− 70	30	73	4.60
	RH middle occipital gyrus	46	− 82	0	22	3.88
	RH inferior occipital gyrus[a]	43	− 80	− 3		

Activations were thresholded at a whole-brain p value of < .001 uncorrected with a cluster size of k = 10 voxels. Cerebellar activations are not reported due to incomplete coverage of the cerebellum depending on individual head size

k cluster size; LH left hemisphere; MNI Montreal Neurological Institute; RH right hemisphere; t t value

[a] Minor maximum

fronto-parietal network comprising left AG, left superior and middle frontal gyrus, and right SMA. In line with previous research, activation found for symbolic vs. nonsymbolic proportions showed a left-lateralized preference [34].

The left AG has been previously associated with verbally-mediated processes such as the retrieval of arithmetic facts and symbolic numerical processing [10, 28, 29, 36]. Holloway and colleagues [36] argued that the left AG mediates the mapping between a visual form and its semantic referent, that is, between numerical symbols and their magnitudes. However, recent research indicated that the AG plays a more domain-general attentional role that may not be specific to math fact retrieval [30, 76]. In particular, Bloechle and colleagues [30] proposed that the left AG adjusts and adapts relative attentional demands in the neural networks associated with fact retrieval and magnitude manipulation. For accessing magnitude information of decimals a symbol-to-referent mapping in the left AG seems plausible. However, accessing the magnitude of a fraction might require additional computational steps. This might involve increased attentional effort or more demanding symbol-to-referent mapping during the

decoding of several numerals of the fraction itself. Thus, the role of the left AG in our data might reflect both scenarios—higher attentional demands or symbol-to-referent mapping.

Furthermore, activation of the left SFG and right SMA may be assumed to reflect goal creation, procedural steps as well as the generation of strategies for solving multistep problems during the processing of symbolic proportions [13].

In contrast, processing non-symbolic proportions indicated specific activation within the ventral visual stream (bilateral middle occipital gyrus, right inferior temporal gyrus, and right superior parietal lobule), right insula, left MCC, and right SFG. The large cluster of bilateral occipital activation might reflect higher visual demands of the non-symbolic presentation formats. Furthermore, activation of the ventral visual stream might point to the involvement of visuo-spatial functions and covert shifts of attention during processing non-symbolic proportions [19]. In particular, the superior parietal lobe was repeatedly reported for non-symbolic number processing [8, 33, 36, 38] and suggested to host a visual-spatial representation of quantity [21].

Moreover, higher activation of areas associated with cognitive control comprising, amongst others, MCC and SFG might indicate that accessing magnitude information of non-symbolic proportions required stronger involvement of cognitive control processes and performance monitoring than of symbolic proportions [77]. Furthermore, we suggest that the involvement of the SFG might reflect the application of strategies for solving multi-step problems [13]. Together with higher activation of areas subserving cognitive control, the right insula was suggested to be involved in initiating motivated behavior

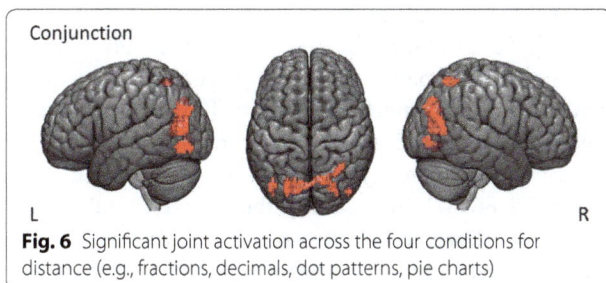

Conjunction

L   R

Fig. 6 Significant joint activation across the four conditions for distance (e.g., fractions, decimals, dot patterns, pie charts)

[78], execution of responses [79], and error processing ([80]; see also [13]).

Distance-related activation = magnitude-related representation?

We also evaluated magnitude-related activation in proportion processing by specifically focusing on the neural correlates of distance in the respective presentation formats. Our findings indicated that processing relative magnitude of symbolic and non-symbolic proportions might not exclusively reflect domain-specific magnitude-related processing. Rather, our results suggest that the idea of a unique reflection of (relative) magnitude processing by distance may be too simplistic. In fact, magnitude processing of proportions might not only reflect specific processing of magnitude information, but may also reflect influences of other less domain-specific cognitive processes involved in distance-related processing. In particular, it seems that different presentation formats contain different cognitive components to different degrees. In the following, we will discuss these differing components as indicated by observed activation of associated brain areas in the current study.

Activation in (intra)parietal cortex

Bilateral IPS was repeatedly reported active for processing absolute magnitude [9, 10, 16, 37]. In line with this idea, we found that magnitude processing of *decimals* was associated with activation in the bilateral IPS, most probably reflecting the processing of number magnitude information [8, 61, 64]. In fact, magnitude processing of decimals is very similar to processing absolute magnitude because skipping the leading 0 and just comparing the digits following the decimal point leads to a correct result [64]. Thus, no computation of part-whole relations, and thus, relative magnitude is necessary to access magnitude information of decimals compared to the other presentation formats used in this study. Consequently, the involvement of intraparietal regions typically involved in processing absolute magnitude comes as no surprise.

In line with previous research, our data also revealed activation in right IPS for the magnitude processing of *fractions* [41]. Because the right IPS was repeatedly reported to be activated during absolute number magnitude processing in number comparison tasks [8, 31, 32, 61], our data on the processing of relative magnitude extend these previous findings. In particular, our results indicate that in addition to absolute numerical magnitude, relative magnitude of symbolic proportions is also processed in the IPS. This is significant because additional computational steps may be necessary to access magnitude information of proportions. These findings, thus, further support previous results suggesting that the

right IPS is systematically involved in the processing of number magnitude, regardless of number format [8] or notation [9].

For the magnitude processing of *dot patterns* we found activation in the bilateral SPL extending to the IPS in the right hemisphere, which has been repeatedly reported for non-symbolic number processing [8, 33, 36, 38]. While activation of the right IPS might indicate additional computations of part-whole relations necessary for accessing relative magnitude information, activation of bilateral SPL rather reflects the involvement of visuospatial functions such as saccades and covert shifts of attention [19]. This finding seems plausible for this presentation format because eye-movements and attention shifts are particularly necessary to capture discrete quantities and the part-whole relation reflected by proportional dot patterns.

Moreover, we found activation in bilateral IPS and SPL for the magnitude processing in *pie charts*. It has been shown that bilateral IPS is activated during estimation strategies and approximation processes for symbolic and non-symbolic presentation formats [34, 81, 82]. To a certain degree, activation in bilateral superior and inferior parietal lobes might also indicate the involvement of mental rotation strategies [83, 84]. Thus, parietal activation might reflect an additional distance effect caused by the angular degrees between the to-be-compared blue parts of the pie charts. However, as we found joint activation for all presentation formats in right IPS (with the other three formats not requiring mental rotation), parietal activation in magnitude processing of pie charts should reflect not only mental rotation strategies, but at least partially the processing of relative magnitude information as well. This might indicate the involvement of estimation, approximation and mental rotation strategies during accessing relative magnitude information for this specific presentation format.

Activation in frontal cortex areas

Furthermore, we observed activation in bilateral inferior and middle frontal gyrus as well as SMA for the magnitude processing of *fractions*. Activation in frontal areas is commonly associated with rather domain-general supplementary executive processes such as strategy choice and procedural planning in numerical cognition [29, 62, 85]. Furthermore, increasing demands on working memory, performance monitoring, goal-directed problem solving, and interference control loads were associated with neural activation in a network comprising these frontal brain regions including IFG, ACC, MCC, and insula [18, 86, 87]. Importantly, the insular-cingulate salience network which initiates control signals during arithmetic problem solving is anchored in the anterior insula and ACC [19, 88]. In line with this rationale, participants may have applied different strategies which involve executive processes for accessing relative magnitude information of fractions. Observed activation in frontal areas might reflect increasing demands on such executive processes during magnitude computation of fractions, and thus, might reflect the active magnitude computation of the given part-whole relation. These computations can be very demanding, and thus, lead to high loads on executive functions. Hence, activation of frontal areas might reflect aspects of difficulty in actually computing relative fraction magnitude and, consequently, additional computational strategies necessary for doing so.

Importantly, it was shown that context-dependent shifts in strategy might also cause differences in activation of frontal brain regions [89]. Thus, frontal areas might be activated differently according to which strategy is applied for accessing relative magnitude information for the respective proportion and how high the demand on executive functions actually is. This is also reflected by the results of our conjunction analysis as we did not find joint frontal activation for all presentation formats. However, each presentation format elicited separate activation in specific frontal brain regions. Yet, these brain regions apparently did not overlap. Hence, different strategies seemed to be applied for accessing magnitude information of the respective presentation formats which, in turn, may have led to distinct activations in frontal areas.

Magnitude processing of *decimals* elicited activation in IFG, MFG and insula exclusively in the left hemisphere. IFG is typically involved in processing simple numerical tasks with low working memory or procedural requirements, while MFG and insula rather tend to support working memory systems and goal-directed attention maintenance [13, 18, 23].

For *pie charts*, computations of part-whole relations and visual strategies might play a crucial role for accessing relative magnitude information. Again, applying these visual estimation strategies and computations might have led to increased working memory demands as reflected by activation of bilateral IFG [90, 91]. Thus, activation in bilateral IFG, bilateral MCC as well as bilateral insula observed for magnitude processing of *pie charts* may indicate the involvement of the salience network as well as working memory and goal-directed attention processes also in this presentation format [19, 88].

We observed activation in left ACC and the right SFG for the magnitude processing of *dot patterns*. These activations indicated specific demands on working memory and cognitive control when accessing magnitude information of proportional dot patterns [13, 41]. In particular, the involvement of the SFG may further reflect the generation of strategies for solving multi-step problems

[13]. Hence, to access magnitude information of proportional dot patterns, participants seem to apply multi-step strategies for summation and quantification of non-symbolic part-whole relations, which in turn lead to increased working memory and cognitive control demands.

Activation of occipital brain areas

Previous studies showed that high attentional loads in visual processing, encoding, and reanalysis, as well as visual manipulations evoke activations in occipital areas [16, 92, 93]. We found activation in these brain regions for magnitude processing of both *pie charts* as well as *dot patterns*. Thus, accessing magnitude information of pie charts seems to recruit a wide range of executive processes and visual strategies, which are associated with a wide range of brain activations in fronto-parietal and occipital regions.

Magnitude processing of *dot patterns* was associated with activation of occipital brain regions involved in processing visual information. This activation in bilateral occipital gyri, thus, might reflect the specific processing demands on visual information to access magnitude information in this presentation format. Activation in visual cortex might be even stronger when participants drive their attention to a specific object, i.e. proportional dot patterns or pie charts [94]. Thus, to derive relative magnitude information of dot patterns and pie charts participants seemed to strongly rely on visual strategies. In particular, accessing magnitude information for nonsymbolic proportions might be associated with increasing visual processing demands, and thus, with increasing activation in visual areas.

Furthermore, we also found activation in the left occipital gyrus extending to fusiform gyrus, occipitotemporal areas as well as middle and superior temporal gyrus associated with magnitude processing of *decimals*. Interestingly, the ventral visual stream areas consisting, amongst others, of lateral occipital cortex, fusiform gyrus and inferior temporal cortex were co-activated with the IPS during arithmetic processing [19]. In this context, activation in occipitotemporal regions including the fusiform gyrus might indicate the involvement of the visual number form area during magnitude processing [62]. Although speculative, an explanation for this finding might be that participants had to visually encode more digits in trials with smaller distance. The smaller the distance, the further to the right in the digit string the decisive digit is to be found (e.g., .24_.75 vs. .53_.56). Thus, more digits had to be encoded visually to access the respective magnitude information. Visually encoding digits might in turn have led to increased activation in the visual number form area and the occipital gyrus. Additionally, activation in left superior temporal regions, which are typically involved in reading processes [95, 96], may reflect the connection between numerical symbols and their quantitative referents [36]. Interestingly, however, we failed to find activation in the visual number form area associated with the magnitude processing of fractions. This might indicate that the difficulty of this specific presentation format and cognitive demands during the additional computational steps for accessing magnitude information of fractions might be predominant over visual encoding processes. Furthermore, although previous studies suggested that fractions are represented holistically in the human brain [41], our results suggest that access to the magnitude information of a fraction seems to involve additional computational steps as reflected by activation of frontal working memory and cognitive control areas rather than a simple symbol-to-referent mapping. This might also explain why we did not observe any activation in the visual number form area for magnitude processing of fractions.

Practical implications of our study

From a more practical perspective, the neurocognitive results presented here might indicate that a shared use of symbolic and non-symbolic presentation formats could be supportive for teaching and learning fractions because they activate a joint neural correlate reflecting abstract relative magnitude processing. Moreover, it is known that learning with multiple representations can enhance students' understanding of new concepts [97]. However, teaching fractions currently focuses strongly on memorization of procedures and not on conceptual understanding [98, 99]. Yet, in order to choose the appropriate procedure to solve fraction problems, these procedures should be underpinned by good conceptual knowledge about fractions [100]. An intervention study of Gabriel and colleagues [6] showed that the use of non-symbolic presentation formats to represent and manipulate fractions improved students' conceptual understanding of fractions and their magnitudes. Additionally, an intelligent tutoring system as described by Rau and colleagues [4] enhanced the conceptual understanding of fraction magnitude by specifically associating symbolic fractions with non-symbolic presentation formats. After working with this tutoring system as part of their regular mathematics instructions, 4th- and 5th-grade students improved significantly in their conceptual understanding of fractions (for an overview, see [99]).

Although speculative, these positive effects when jointly using symbolic and non-symbolic presentation formats for teaching conceptual understanding of fractions, might be partly based on a shared neural correlate for relative magnitude processing. However, the benefit of

jointly using symbolic and non-symbolic formats might be additionally driven by complementary mechanisms in relative magnitude processing of different presentation formats: in addition to the shared neural correlate, all presentation formats showed distinct and specific activation patterns in the current study, which points to different additional (sub)processes that are linked to each presentation format. Because these (sub)processes differ for all presentation formats, non-symbolic presentation formats might complement symbolic formats and vice versa for conceptual understanding. Thereby, children who do not excel at understanding a particular presentation format might be able to compensate for these difficulties by means of other formats. The processing pathways for the presentation formats seem to differ partially depending on the format but to finally converge to abstract magnitude processing in the right IPS.

Thus, the present findings seem to support previous findings of intervention studies on the conceptual understanding of fractions and proportions from a neurocognitive perspective and vice versa.

Conclusion

Regions around the IPS are commonly associated with the processing of absolute magnitude (e.g., [8, 9]). However, recent research indicated that also relative magnitude information is associated with activation in parietal brain regions [41–43, 64]. Thus, brain areas involved in processing absolute magnitude of numbers were also activated during processing relative magnitude of symbolic fractions as well as non-symbolic proportions. Here, we investigated systematically whether the processing of symbolic and non-symbolic proportions draws on shared underlying neural correlates. Results of the present study indicated joint activation of specific occipito-parietal areas, including right IPS for both symbolic and non-symbolic proportions. In particular, the right IPS is associated with number magnitude processing [8, 9, 32, 61], while the occipital activation during magnitude processing rather reflects the higher order visual processing, which contributes to building semantic representations of quantity [15, 18, 21]. Thus, our findings indicate a shared neural substrate for a format-independent, abstract concept of relative magnitude.

Yet, our results may also be influenced by task difficulty. Nevertheless, activations in the IPS cannot be attributed to task difficulty exclusively, but also reflected specific processing of relative magnitude information. Furthermore, influences of task difficulty might rather be reflected by observed activation in frontal areas due to increasing demands on executive functions. Interestingly, we did not observe joint frontal activation for all presentation formats although all presentation formats elicited significant activation in frontal brain regions. This might indicate that participants applied different strategies depending on the respective presentation format. For instance, while demands on cognitive control and working memory may be lower for magnitude processing of decimals, magnitude processing of fractions might rather be associated with additional computational steps, and thus, with higher demands on working memory and cognitive control. Furthermore, participants might use estimation strategies for magnitude processing of pie charts whereas summation and quantification strategies might support magnitude processing of dot patterns.

Nevertheless, the present data provide evidence for a shared neural correlate for processing relative magnitude, irrespective of symbolic or non-symbolic presentation format.

Authors' contributions
KM and EK conceived the study. KM, EK, and SH participated in its design. JB, JB, and JR performed data collection. JM, SH, and JFD performed processing and statistical analyses. JM and SH drafted the manuscript; all other authors revised it critically. All authors contributed to the interpretation of the data. All authors read and approved the final manuscript.

Author details
[1] Leibniz-Institut für Wissensmedien, Schleichstraße 6, 72076 Tuebingen, Germany. [2] Division of Neuropsychology, Hertie-Institute for Clinical Brain Research, Otfried-Müller-Straße 27, 72076 Tuebingen, Germany. [3] Eberhardt-Karls University Tuebingen, 72074 Tuebingen, Germany.

Acknowledgements
Not applicable.

Competing interests
The authors declare that they have no competing interests.

Funding
JM was supported by the German Research Foundation (DFG; CR-110/8-1). SH, JB, JB, and JR were supported by the Leibniz-Competition Fund providing funding to EK. JFD was supported by the German Research Foundation (DFG; MO 2525/2-1). EK was supported by a Margarete von Wrangell fellowship from the Ministry of Science, Research and the Arts Baden-Württemberg as well as the European Social Fund (ESF). KM is principal investigator at the LEAD Graduate School [GSC1028], a project of the Excellence Initiative of the German federal and state governments.

References
1. Gigerenzer G. Calculated risk: how to know when numbers deceive you. New York: Simon & Schuster; 2002.
2. Siegler RS, Fazio LK, Bailey DH, Zhou X. Fractions: the new frontier for theories of numerical development. Trends Cogn Sci. 2013;17:13–9.
3. NMAP. Foundations for success: the final report of the National Mathematics Advisory Panel. Washington, DC: US Department of Education; 2008.
4. Rau MA, Aleven V, Rummel N, Rohrbach S. Sense making alone doesn't do it: fluency matters too! ITS support for robust learning with multiple representations. In: Cerri S, Clancey W, Papadourakis G, Panourgia K, editors. Intell. Tutoring Syst. 7315th ed. Berlin/Heidelberg: Springer; 2012. p. 174–84.
5. Rau MA, Aleven V, Rummel N. Successful learning with multiple graphical representations and self-explanation prompts. J Educ Psychol. 2015;107:30–46.
6. Gabriel F, Coche F, Szucs D, Carette V, Rey B, Content A. Developing children's understanding of fractions: an intervention study. Mind Brain Educ. 2012;6:137–46.
7. Nieder A. Counting on neurons: the neurobiology of numerical competence. Nat Rev Neurosci. 2005;6:177–90.
8. Piazza M, Pinel P, Le Bihan D, Dehaene S. A magnitude code common to numerosities and number symbols in human intraparietal cortex. Neuron. 2007;53:293–305.
9. Pinel P, Dehaene S, Rivière D, Le Bihan D. Modulation of parietal activation by semantic distance in a number comparison task. Neuroimage. 2001;14:1013–26.
10. Dehaene S, Piazza M, Pinel P, Cohen L. Three parietal circuits for number processing. Cogn Neuropsychol. 2003;20:487–506.
11. Moyer RS, Landauer TK. Time required for judgements of numerical inequality. Nature. 1967;215:1519–20.
12. Meert G, Grégoire J, Noël M-P. Rational numbers: componential versus holistic representation of fractions in a magnitude comparison task. Q J Exp Psychol. 2009;62:1598–616.
13. Arsalidou M, Taylor MJ. Is 2+2=4? Meta-analyses of brain areas needed for numbers and calculations. Neuroimage. 2011;54:2382–93.
14. Bugden S, Price GR, McLean DA, Ansari D. The role of the left intraparietal sulcus in the relationship between symbolic number processing and children's arithmetic competence. Dev. Cogn. Neurosci. 2012;2:448–57.
15. Jolles D, Supekar K, Richardson J, Tenison C, Ashkenazi S, Rosenberg-Lee M, et al. Reconfiguration of parietal circuits with cognitive tutoring in elementary school children. Cortex. 2016;83:231–45.
16. Pinel P, Piazza M, Le Bihan D, Dehaene S. Distributed and overlapping cerebral representations of number, size, and luminance during comparative judgments. Neuron. 2004;41:983–93.
17. Menon V, Rivera SM, White CD, Glover GH, Reiss AL. Dissociating prefrontal and parietal cortex activation during arithmetic processing. Neuroimage. 2000;12:357–65.
18. Fias W, Menon V, Szucs D. Multiple components of developmental dyscalculia. Trends Neurosci. Educ. 2013;2:43–7.
19. Menon V. Arithmetic in the child and adult brain. In: Dowker A, editor. Cohen Kadosh R. Oxford Handb. Numer. Cogn. Oxford: Oxford University Press; 2015. p. 502–30.
20. Ansari D, Garcia N, Lucas E, Hamon K, Dhital B. Neural correlates of symbolic number processing in children and adults. Neuroreport. 2005;16:1769–73.
21. Ansari D. Effects of development and enculturation on number representation in the brain. Nat. Rev. Neurosci. 2008;9:278–91.
22. van Dijck J-P, Gevers W, Fias W. Numvbers are associated with different types of spatial information depending on the task. Cognition. 2009;113:248–53.
23. Majerus S, D'Argembeau A, Martinez Perez T, Belayachi S, Van der Linden M, Collette F, et al. The commonality of neural networks for verbal and visual short-term memory. J. Cogn. Neurosci. 2010;22:2570–93.
24. Hitch GJ. Role of short-term working memory in mental arithmetic. Cogn. Psychol. 1978;10:302–23.
25. Cohen Kadosh R, Henik A, Rubinstein O, Mohr H, Dori H, Van de Ven V, et al. Are numbers special? The comparison systems of the human brain investigated by fMRI. Neuropsychologia. 2005;43:1238–48.
26. Kaufmann L, Koppelstaetter F, Delazer M, Siedentopf C, Rhomberg P, Golaszewski S, et al. Neural correlates of distance and congruity effects in a numerical Stroop task, an event-related fMRI study. Neuroimage. 2005;25:888–98.
27. Ansari D, Grabner RH, Koschutnig K, Reishofer G, Ebner F. Individual differences in mathematical competence modulate brain responses to arithmetic errors: an fMRI study. Learn. Individ. Differ. 2011;21:636–43.
28. Dehaene S, Spelke ES, Pinel P, Stanescu R, Tsivkin S. Sources of mathematical thinking: behavioral and brain-imaging evidence. Science. 1999;284:970–4.

29. Grabner RH, Ansari D, Koschutnig K, Reishofer G, Ebner F, Neuper C. To retrieve or to calculate? Left angular gyrus mediates the retrieval of arithmetic facts during problem solving. Neuropsychologia. 2009;47:604–8.

30. Bloechle J, Huber S, Bahnmueller J, Rennig J, Willmes K, Cavdaroglu S, et al. Fact learning in complex arithmetic - the role of the angular gyrus revisited. Hum. Brain Mapp. 2016;37:3061–79.

31. Chochon F, Cohen L, van de Moortele PF, Dehaene S. Differential contributions of the left and right inferior parietal lobules to number processing. J. Cogn. Neurosci. 1999;11:617–30.

32. Dehaene S. The organization of brain activations in number comparison: event-related potentials and the additive-factors method. J. Cogn. Neurosci. 1996;8:47–68.

33. Piazza M, Izard V, Pinel P, Le Bihan D, Dehaene S. Tuning curves for approximate numerosity in the human intraparietal sulcus. Neuron. 2004;44:547–55.

34. Venkatraman V, Ansari D, Chee MWL. Neural correlates of symbolic and non-symbolic arithmetic. Neuropsychologia. 2005;43:744–53.

35. Sokolowski HM, Fias W, Mousa A, Ansari D. Common and distinct brain regions in both parietal and frontal cortex support symbolic and non-symbolic number processing in humans: A functional neuroimaging metaanalysis. Neuroimage. 2017;146:376–94.

36. Holloway ID, Price GR, Ansari D. Common and segregated neural pathways for the processing of symbolic and nonsymbolic numerical magnitude: an fMRI study. Neuroimage. 2010;49:1006–17.

37. Eger E, Sterzer P, Russ MO, Giraud AL, Kleinschmidt A. A supramodal number representation in human intraparietal cortex. Neuron. 2003;37:719–25.

38. Ansari D, Dhital B, Siong SC. Parametric effects of numerical distance on the intraparietal sulcus during passive viewing of rapid numerosity changes. Brain Res. 2006;1067:181–8.

39. Delazer M, Ischebeck A, Domahs F, Zamarian L, Koppelstaetter F, Siedentopf C, et al. Learning by strategies and learning by drill - evidence from an fMRI study. Neuroimage. 2005;25:838–49.

40. Ischebeck A, Koschutnig K, Reishofer G, Butterworth B, Neuper C, Ebner F. Processing fractions and proportions: An fMRI study. Int. J. Psychophysiol. 2010;77:227.

41. Ischebeck A, Schocke M, Delazer M. The processing and representation of fractions within the brain. An fMRI investigation. Neuroimage. 2009;47:403–13.

42. Jacob SN, Nieder A. Notation-independent representation of fractions in the human parietal cortex. J. Neurosci. 2009;29:4652–7.

43. Jacob SN, Nieder A. Tuning to non-symbolic proportions in the human frontoparietal cortex. Eur. J. Neurosci. 2009;30:1432–42.

44. Siegler RS, Fuchs L, Jordan NC, Gersten R, Ochsendorf R. The center for improving learning of fractions: a progress report. In: Chinn S, editor. Routledge Int. Handb. Dyscalculia Math. Learn. Difficulties. New York: Routledge; 2015. p. 292–303.

45. Rau MA, Aleven V, Rummel N. Interleaved practice in multi-dimensional learning tasks: which dimension should we interleave? Learn Instr. 2013;23:98–114.

46. Rau MA, Aleven V, Rummel N. Intelligent tutoring systems with multiple representations and self-explanation prompts support learning of fractions. In: Dimitrova V, Mizoguchi R, Du Boulay B, editors. 14th Int. Conf. Artif. Intell. Educ. Amsterdam: IOS Press; 2009. p. 441–8.

47. Matthews PG, Chesney DL. Fractions as percepts? Exploring cross-format distance effects for fractional magnitudes. Cogn Psychol. 2015;78:28–56.

48. Common Core State Standards Initiative. Common Core State Standards for Mathematics 2010. http://www.corestandards.org/. Accessed cited 6 Mar 2018.

49. Ratcliff R. Methods for dealing with reaction time outliers. Psychol Bull. 1993;114:510–32.

50. Baayen RH, Davidson DJ, Bates DM. Mixed-effects modeling with crossed random effects for subjects and items. J Mem Lang. 2008;59:390–412.

51. Jaeger TF. Categorical data analysis: away from ANOVAs (transformation or not) and towards logit mixed models. J Mem Lang. 2008;59:434–46.

52. Barr DJ, Levy R, Scheepers C, Tily HJ. Random effects structure for confirmatory hypothesis testing: keep it maximal. J Mem Lang. 2013;68:255–78.

53. R Core Team. R: A language and environment for statistical computing. Vienna: R Foundation for Statistical Computing; 2015.

54. Bates D, Maechler M, Bolker B, Walker S. Fitting linear mixed-effects models using lme4. J Stat Softw.67:1–48.

55. Judd CM, Westfall J, Kenny DA. Treating stimuli as a random factor in social psychology: a new and comprehensive solution to a pervasive but largely ignored problem. J Pers Soc Psychol. 2012;103:54–69.

56. Singmann H, Bolker B, Westfall J. afex: analysis of factorial experiments. R package version 0.2015. p. 13–145.

57. Hothorn T, Bretz F, Westfall P. Simultaneous inference in general parametric models. Biom J. 2008;50:346–63.

58. Benjamini Y, Hochberg Y. Controlling the false discovery rate: a practical and powerful approach to multiple testing. J R Stat Soc Ser B. 1995;57:289–300.

59. Nichols T, Brett M, Andersson J, Wager T, Poline JB. Valid conjunction inference with the minimum statistic. Neuroimage. 2005;25:653–60.

60. Eickhoff SB, Stephan KE, Mohlberg H, Grefkes C, Fink GR, Amunts K, et al. A new SPM toolbox for combining probabilistic cytoarchitectonic maps and functional imaging data. Neuroimage. 2005;25:1325–35.

61. Mussolin C, Noel MP, Pesenti M, Grandin C, De Volder A. Neural correlates of the numerical distance effect in children. Front Psychol. 2013;4:1–9.

62. Dehaene S, Cohen L. Towards an anatomical and functional model of number processing. Math Cogn. 1:83–120.

63. Dehaene S, Cohen L. Cerebral pathways for calculation: double dissociation between rote verbal and quantitative knowledge of arithmetic. Cortex. 1997;33:219–50.

64. DeWolf M, Chiang JN, Bassok M, Holyoak KJ, Monti MM. Neural representations of magnitude for natural and rational numbers. Neuroimage. 2016;141:304–12.

65. Cohen Kadosh R, Walsh V. Numerical representation in the parietal lobes: Abstract or not abstract? Behav. Brain Sci. 2009;32:313–28.

66. Dehaene S. The number sense: How the mind creates mathematics. Oxford: Oxford University Press; 1997.

67. Cantlon JF, Platt ML, Brannon EM. Beyond the number domain. Trends Cogn. Sci. 2009;13:83–91.

68. Feigenson L, Dehaene S, Spelke E. Core systems of number. Trends Cogn. Sci. 2004;8:307–14.

69. Leibovich T, Katzin N, Harel M, Henik A. From, "sense of number" to "sense of magnitude": The role of conitnuous magnitudes in numerical cognition. Behav. Brain Sci. 2017;40:e164.

70. Keller K, Menon V. Gender differences in the functional and structural neuroanatomy of mathematical cognition. Neuroimage. 2009;47:342–52.

71. Rosenberg-Lee M, Tsang JM, Menon V. Smybolic, numeric, and magnitude representations in the parietal cortex. Behav. Brain Sci. 2009;32:350–1.

72. Shuman M, Kanwisher N. Numerical magnitude in the human parietal lobe: tests of representational generality and domain specificity. Neuron. 2004;44:557–69.

73. Culham JC, Brandt SA, Cavanagh P, Kanwisher N, Dale AM, Tootell RB. Cortical fMRI activation produced by attentive tracking of moving targets. J. Neurophysiol. 1998;80:2657–70.

74. Culham JC, Kanwisher N. Neuroimaging of cognitive functions in human parietal cortex. Curr. Opin. Neurobiol. 2001;11:157–63.

75. Klein E, Moeller K, Nuerk H-C, Willmes K. On the neuro-cognitive foundations of basic auditory number processing: an fMRI study. Behav. brain Funct. 2010;6:42.

76. Rosenberg-Lee M, Chang TT, Young CB, Wu S, Menon V. Functional dissociations between four basic arithmetic operations in the human posterior parietal cortec: A cytoarchitectonic mapping study. Neuropsychologia. 2011;49:2592–608.

77. MacDonald AW, Cohen JD, Stenger VA, Carter CS. Dissociating the role of the dorsolateral prefrontal and anterior cingulate cortex in cognitive control. Science. 2000;288:1835–8.

78. Uddin LQ, Menon V. The anterior insula in autism: under-connected and under-examined. Neurosci. Biobehav. Rev. 2009;33:1198–203.

79. Huettel AS, Guzeldere G, McCarthy G. Dissociating the neural mechanisms of visual attention in charge of detection using functional MRI. J. Cogn. Neurosci. 2001;13:1006–18.

80. Hester R, Fassbender C, Garavan H. Individual differences in error processing: A review and reanalysis of three event-related fMRI studies using GO/NOGO task. Cereb. Cortex. 2004;14:986–94.

81. Castelli F, Glaser DE, Butterworth B. Discrete and analogue quantity processing in the parietal lobe: a functional MRI study. Proc. Natl. Acad. Sci. U. S. A. 2006;103:4693–8.

82. Piazza M, Mechelli A, Price CJ, Butterworth B. Exact and approximate judgements of visual and auditory numerosity: An fMRI study. Brain Res. 2006;1106:177–88.

83. Alivisatos B, Petrides M. Functional activation of the human brain during mental rotation. Neuropsychologia. 1997;35:111–8.

84. Jordan K, Heinze H-J, Lutz K, Kanowski M, Jäncke L. Cortical Activations during the Mental Rotation of Different Visual Objects. Neuroimage. 2001;13:143–52.

85. Klein E, Suchan J, Moeller K, Karnath HO, Knops A, Wood G, et al. Considering structural connectivity in the triple code model of numerical cognition: differential connectivity for magnitude processing and arithmetic facts. Brain Struct. Funct. 2016;221:979–95.

86. Peterson BS, Kane MJ, Alexander GM, Lacadie C, Skudlarski P, Leung H-C, et al. An event-related functional MRI study comparing interference effects in the Simon and Stroop tasks. Cogn. Brain Res. 13:427–40.

87. Lui X, Banich MT, Jacobson BL, Tanabe JL. Common and distinct neural substrates of attentional control in an integrated Simon and spatial Stroop task as assessed by event-related fMRI. Neuroimage. 2004;22:1097–106.

88. Supekar K, Menon V. Developmental maturation of dynamic causal control signals in higher-order cognition: a neurocognitive network model. PLoS Comput. Biol. 2012;8:1002374.

89. Wagner AD, Desmond JE, Glover GH, Gabrieli JDE. Prefrontal cortex and recognition memory: functional-MRI evidence for context-dependent retrieval processes. Brain. 1998;121:1985–2002.

90. Bunge SA, Kahn I, Wallis JD, Miller EK, Wagner AD. Neural circuits subserving the retrieval and maintenance of abstract rules. J. Neurophysiol. 2003;90:3419–28.

91. Taillan J, Ardiale E, Anton JL, Nazarian B, Félician O, Lemaire P. Processes in arithmetic strategy selection: a fMRI study. Front. Psychol. 2015;6:1–12.

92. Somers DC, Dale AM, Seiffert AE, Tootell RBH. Functional MRI reveals spatially specific attentional modulation in human primary visual cortex. Proc. Natl. Acad. Sci. U. S. A. 2006;96:1663–8.

93. Wood G, Nuerk HC, Willmes K. Neural representations of two-digit numbers: A parametric fMRI study. Neuroimage. 2006;29:358–67.

94. Müller NG, Kleinschmidt A. Dynamic interaction of object-and space-based attention in retinotopic visual areas. J. Neurosci. 2003;23:9812–6.

95. Raij T, Uutela K, Hari R. Audiovisual integration of letters in the human brain. Neuron. 2000;28:617–25.

96. Van Atteveldt N, Formisano E, Goebel R, Blomert L. Integration of letters and speech sounds in the human brain. Neuron. 2004;43:271–82.

97. Ainsworth S. DeFT: A conceptual framework for considering learning with multiple representations. Learn. Instr. 2006;16:183–98.

98. Lortie-Forgues H, Tian J, Siegler RS. Why is learning fraction and decimal arithmetic so difficult? Dev. Rev. 2015;38:201–21.

99. Obersteiner A, Dresler T, Bieck SM, Moeller K. Understanding Fractions: Integrating Results from Mathematics Education, Cognitive Psychology, and Neuroscience. In: Norton A, Alibali MW, editors. Constr. Number - Merging Perspect. from Psychol. Math. Educ. Heidelberg: Springer; 2018.

100. Swan M. Dealing with misconceptions in mathematics. In: Gates P, editor. Issues Math. Teach. London: Routledge/Falmer; 2001. p. 147–65.

21

Reversal of reserpine-induced depression and cognitive disorder in zebrafish by sertraline and Traditional Chinese Medicine (TCM)

Shuhui Zhang[1†], Xiaodong Liu[1†], Mingzhu Sun[3†], Qiuping Zhang[2†], Teng Li[3], Xiang Li[1], Jia Xu[2], Xin Zhao[3*], Dongyan Chen[2*] and Xizeng Feng[1*]

Abstract

Background: With increased social pressure, individuals face a high risk of depression. Subsequently, depression affects cognitive behaviour and negatively impacts daily life. Fortunately, the Traditional Chinese Medicine Jia Wei Xiao Yao (JWXY) capsule is effective in reducing depression and improving cognitive behaviour.

Methods: The constituents of JWXY capsule were identified by ultra-performance liquid chromatography and quadrupole time-of-flight mass spectrometry analyses. We analysed behaviours of depression-like zebrafish in the novel tank with an automatic 3D video-tracking system and conducted the colour preference test, as well detected physiological changes after sertraline and JWXY capsule treatments.

Results: Both sertraline and JWXY capsule rescued the decreased locomotive behaviour and depression phenotype of zebrafish caused by reserpine. JWXY capsule especially improved the inhibited exploratory behaviour caused by reserpine. In addition, with the onset of depressive behaviour, zebrafish exhibited alterations in cognitive behaviour as indicated by colour preference changes. However, compared with sertraline, JWXY capsule was more efficaciously in rescuing this change in the colour preference pattern. Moreover, an increased level of cortisol, increased expression of tyrosine hydroxylase (TH) and decreased monoamine neurotransmitters, including serotonin (5-HT) and noradrenaline, were involved in the depressive behaviours. In addition, sertraline and JWXY capsule rescued the depressive phenotype and cognitive behaviour of zebrafish by altering the levels of endogenous cortisol and monoamine neurotransmitters.

Conclusions: JWXY capsule was more effectively than sertraline in rescuing reserpine-induced depression and cognitive disorder in zebrafish. Potentially, our study can provide new insights into the clinical treatment of depression and the mechanism of action of JWXY capsule.

Keywords: Depression behaviour, TCM, Colour preference, Monoamines, Zebrafish

*Correspondence: zhaoxin@nankai.edu.cn; chendy@nankai.edu.cn; xzfeng@nankai.edu.cn
†Shuhui Zhang, Xiaodong Liu, Mingzhu Sun and Qiuping Zhang contributed equally to this work
[1] State Key Laboratory of Medicinal Chemical Biology, The Key Laboratory of Bioactive Materials, Ministry of Education, College of Life Science, Nankai University, Tianjin 300071, China
[2] Tianjin Key Laboratory of Tumor Microenvironment and Neurovascular Regulation, Department of Histology and Embryology, School of Medicine, Nankai University, Tianjin 300071, China
[3] The Institute of Robotics and Automatic Information Systems, Nankai University, Tianjin 300071, China

Background

Major depressive disorder (MDD), one of the most common brain disorders, usually has a high rate of comorbidity with other psychiatric disorders [1]. Depressive disorder, characterised by decreased activity, a significant and lasting low mood, and slowed thinking and cognitive function [2, 3], markedly reduces quality of life. Psychiatric disorders such as psychosis, depression, and other mood disorders may have multigenic and multifactorial aetiologies [4]. Fortunately, improvements in the diagnosis and treatment of depression are increasing. Monoamines play a key role in the regulation of brain functions in animals and humans [5]. Monoamine neurotransmitters, including serotonin (5-HT), dopamine (DA) and noradrenaline (NA), are implicated in the regulation of a large number of processes, such as motor control, social behaviour, cognition, sleep, appetite, and anxiety in vertebrates [6–9]. In zebrafish, 5-HT and DA are the two most studied monoamines [10, 11]. Serotonin (5-hydroxytryptamine, 5-HT) serves as both a neurotransmitter and hormone; in higher vertebrates, 5-HT acts throughout the body, including the central nervous system (CNS), peripheral nervous system, cardiovascular system, and endocrine system; it also participates in sensory perception and many behaviours [12]. Serotonin is involved in many behavioural functions, including the organization of defence, and its putative pathological correlate, anxiety and stress disorders [13]. Anxiety-like behaviour positively correlates with 5-HT content in the novel tank test [14]. Stress levels can be measured by the whole-body cortisol concentration [15]. Some compounds cause Parkinson's disease-like behaviour due to decreased dopamine levels and locomotor activity [16, 17]. Thus, the study of monoamine neurotransmitters in the brain is indispensable for the treatment of depression.

For depression, the most widely used therapy is antidepressants, including monoamine oxidase inhibitors (MAOIs), tricyclic antidepressants (TCAs), serotonin and norepinephrine reuptake inhibitors (SNRIs) and selective serotonin reuptake inhibitors (SSRIs) [18]. For example, sertraline is one a SSRI. Although these antidepressant drugs are effectively relieve depression, they have several concerning side effects, such as headache, agitation or sedation, vomiting, and fatigue [19, 20]. Therefore, identifying a better antidepressant is necessary; this need has led researchers to focus on natural medicine, including Traditional Chinese Medicine (TCM). TCM has a long history of prevention and treatment of depression dating as far back as 2000 years ago. When treating depression, TCM starts at the whole-body level, considering not only the psychological problems that result from a patient's nervous system disorder but also the changes in the Zang-Fu organs, qi and blood [18]. TCM, such as Jia Wei

Xiao Yao (JWXY) capsule, can provide a reliable clinical curative effect comparable to that of Western medicine. In addition, TCM is much more affordable and has fewer side effects. However, a lack of rigorous clinical research has counteracted the unique advantage of TCM and seriously impeded its worldwide popularization and application. JWXY capsule can soothe the liver and reduce heat, strengthen the spleen and nourish the blood. Based on experiences with TCM, JWXY capsule exerts various actions, including soothing the liver and improving the circulation of qi to relieve depression. In China, JWXY capsule has been commonly recognized as a safe and effective prescription in the treatment of depressive disorder [18, 21–23]. However, the effects and mechanism of action of JWXY capsule remain poorly understood.

In the literature, several assays have been reported to measure behavioural learning changes in adult zebrafish such as the rotating escape test, bite test, novel tank test, place preference test, T-maze, plus maze and Y-maze assays [24, 25]. Most of tools used to assess learning and memory in animal models involve visual stimuli, including colour preferences. Zebrafish can discriminate colours and display spontaneous approach or avoidance behaviours. Some studies support colour-based learning and memory paradigms or experiments involving aversion, anxiety or fear in zebrafish [26, 27]. Zebrafish show a preference for blue and green and avoided yellow and red [28]. The zebrafish visual system includes retinas with cones sensitive to red, green, blue, and ultraviolet; moreover zebrafish are diurnal animals, which makes them an ideal model for developing research on cognitive responses to visual signals [29, 30].

In cognitive research, the zebrafish has become increasingly popular and has advantages in behavioural brain research due to its elaborate brain structure, simplicity and neurochemistry, which offers translational relevance to humans [31–33]. In addition, the zebrafish is an ideal and promising model organism for pharmacology [4, 18, 34–36], disease [35, 37], embryology and development studies [38, 39] because it shares many genes, protein products and molecular pathways with mammals [40]. There are also studies on the relationship between emotion regulation and colour preference in zebrafish [41]. Zebrafish may become a translationally relevant study species for the analysis of the mechanisms of learning and memory changes associated with psychopharmacological treatment of anxiety/depression [42].

Compared with 2D approaches, a 3D approach improves data integrity by using two videos and may help reduce the number of experimental subjects. We used two cameras covering the dorsal and lateral view to record fish behaviour in a novel tank. A 3D approach integrates the position information from the top and front views, which is essential to measure depression-like behaviour in zebrafish [43]. 2D approaches have also played a pivotal role in elucidating the neurobehavioural underpinnings of fish behaviour [43]. Hence, we utilized a camera from the top view to record the preference of zebrafish for different colours after pharmacological manipulations.

Reserpine causes depression by depleting monoamines and is widely used to induce depression-like phenotypes by pharmacological manipulation in zebrafish [5]. Therefore, in this study, we performed comparative analysis of the curative effect of sertraline and JWXY capsule treatment for reserpine-induced depression-like behaviour in zebrafish by examining behaviour and the concentrations of three monoamine neurotransmitters and the hormone cortisol. Sertraline and JWXY capsule rescued depressive behaviour and colour preference, accompanied by changes in monoamines and cortisol. The purpose of our study was to evaluate the effects of sertraline and JWXY capsule on behaviour, cognitive ability and biochemical parameters in zebrafish with depression induced by reserpine.

Methods
Zebrafish
Zebrafish (AB strain) were maintained in a fish-farming system at the State Key Laboratory of Medicinal Chemical Biology, Nankai University. The room was maintained at a constant temperature of 28.5 °C on a constant light cycle (14 h light/10 h dark), and the water (KCl 0.05 g/L, NaHCO$_3$ 0.025 g/L, NaCl 3.5 g/L, and CaCl$_2$ 0.1 g/L) was circulated continuously. The zebrafish were fed freshly hatched brine shrimp twice daily. All of the experimental protocols and procedures involving zebrafish were approved by the Committee for Animal Experimentation of the College of Life Science at Nankai University (no. 2008) and were performed in accordance with the NIH Guide for the Care and Use of Laboratory Animals (no. 8023, revised in 1996).

Behavioural test apparatuses and behavioural parameters
Behavioural apparatuses were designed according to previous studies [44, 45]. A novel tank, composed of transparent Plexiglass, was a 5 L rectangular box (23 cm length * 15 cm width * 15 cm depth) used to assess the depressive behaviour of zebrafish. We divided the tank into two equal horizontal portions virtually by marking a midline on the outside walls. The region above this midline indicated the "top" of the novel tank, while the area below indicated the "bottom" of the novel tank. The novel tank was placed over a light source, a light-emitting diode (LED) array, with an acrylic diffuser located above the tank. The light source was composed of white light (500

lux) arrays and a transparent platform. Two charge-coupled device (CCD) cameras (MV-VS078FM, Microvision, 10 frames/s) were placed to obtain the top (dorsal) view and side (lateral) view of the moving zebrafish (Fig. 1b). The offset cross maze and T-maze (Fig. 1c) were designed based on previous research and composed of transparent Plexiglass. Every arm of the offset cross maze is 20 cm * 8.8 cm. The sides of the four arms are covered with four different colours (blue, green, red and yellow) made from polypropylene. The centre Section (8.8 cm * 8.8 cm) of the cross maze is a starting place for the fish indicated by None. The two opposite arms of the maze are 20 cm * 8.8 cm each and are covered with two different colours (blue and yellow) of polypropylene on the sides. The last arm is 20 cm * 8.8 cm and uncoloured. The last arm and centre Section (8.8 cm * 8.8 cm) of the T-maze is a starting place for the fish indicated by No. The maze is 10 cm deep and filled with 6.5 cm system water. A CCD camera (MV-VS078FM, Microvision, 10 frames/s) was fixed above the maze to obtain the top view of the moving zebrafish (Fig. 1c). A daylight lamp (500 lux) or natural light served as the light source. All apparatuses rested on a level, stable surface and were placed in a relatively sound-proof room to minimize the effect of noise when behavioural tests were conducted. A big black cloak forming a space covered all the experimental apparatuses to eliminate environmental interference.

Briefly, the behavioural parameters were defined according to the literature and previous research [44, 45]. The definitions of behavioural parameters that described depression in the novel tank are shown in Table 1. The definitions of behavioural parameters that described colour preferences in the maze are provided in Table 2.

Chemical and experimental design
Reserpine (purity ≥ 98.0%) was purchased from Shanghai Macklin Biomedical Co., Ltd. The reserpine concentration of 40 µg/mL in this study was chosen based on previous research concerning the effective doses of reserpine for the depressive behaviour of zebrafish [5, 45]. Sertraline hydrochloride (purity > 98.0%) was purchased from TCI Co., Ltd. (Shanghai, China). Preliminary experiments proved that the effective concentration of sertraline hydrochloride was 0.1 µg/mL. The experimental doses of reserpine (40 µg/mL) or sertraline hydrochloride (0.1 µg/mL) were obtained by weighing and adding dry powder to system water. JWXY capsule (Z10960066) was purchased from Sichuan Baoxing Pharmaceutical Co., LTD (Sichuang, China). The composition of JWXY capsule is as follows: *Bupleuri Radix, Angelicae Sinensis Radix, Paeoniae Radix Alba, Atractylodis Macrocephalae Rhizoma* (stir-baking with bran), *Poria, Glycyrrhizae Radix Et Rhizoma, Menthae Haplocalycis Herba,*

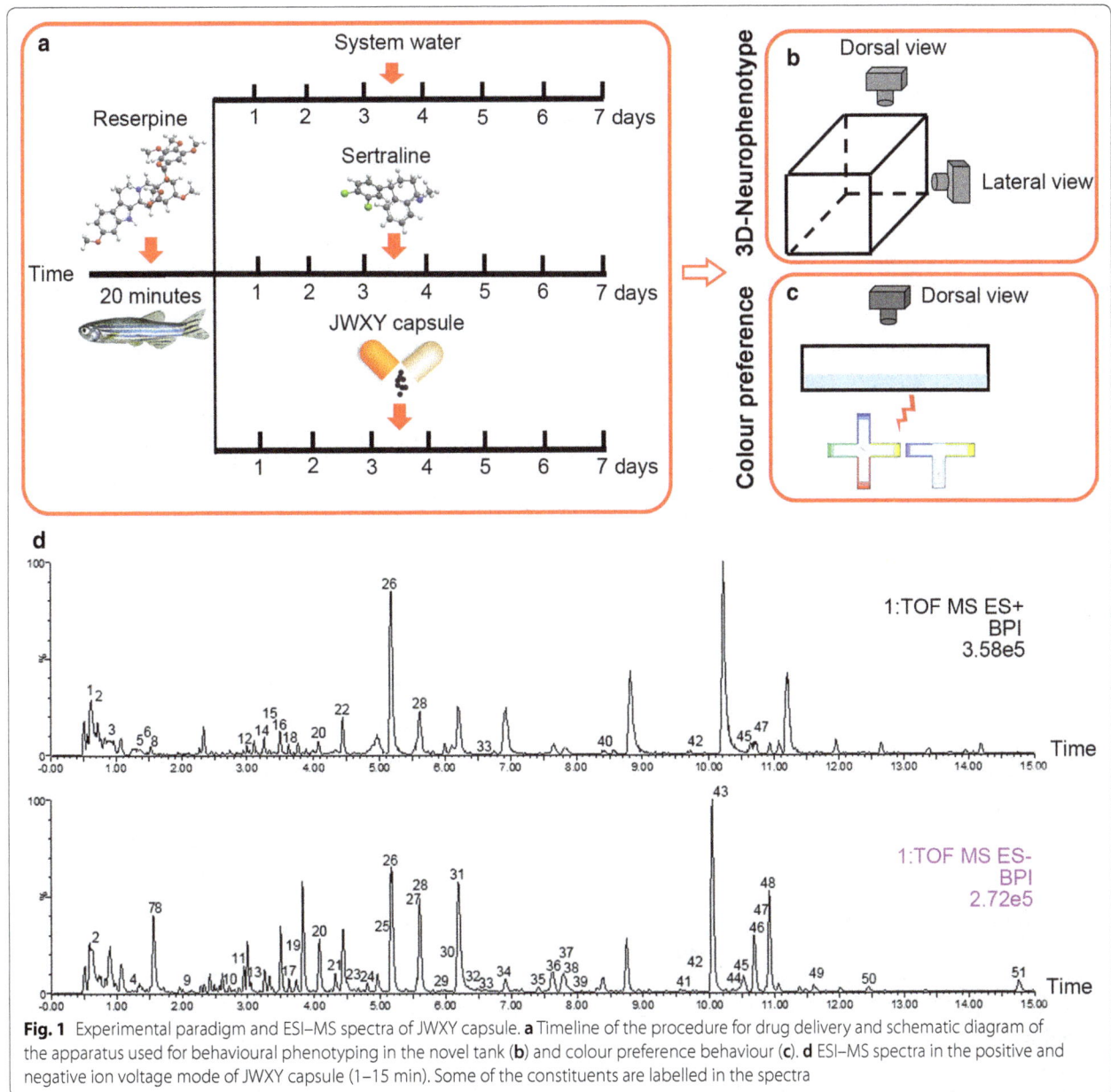

Fig. 1 Experimental paradigm and ESI–MS spectra of JWXY capsule. **a** Timeline of the procedure for drug delivery and schematic diagram of the apparatus used for behavioural phenotyping in the novel tank (**b**) and colour preference behaviour (**c**). **d** ESI–MS spectra in the positive and negative ion voltage mode of JWXY capsule (1–15 min). Some of the constituents are labelled in the spectra

Moutan Cortex, and *Gardeniae Fructus* (processed with ginger juice). Based on preliminary experiments, the effective concentration of JWXY capsule was 100 µg/mL. We opened the capsule and grinded the dry powdered contents. Then, the powdered medicine was weighed and dissolved in system water to obtain a solution with a concentration of 100 µg/mL. Experimental solutions were sonicated for 30 min to dissolve the medication.

A total of 48 experimentally naïve, adult zebrafish (9 months old, male:female = 1:1) were used in our study. All zebrafish were housed in groups of 2 zebrafish per 4 L tank (filled with system water maintained at

28 °C) on a 14:10 h light cycle. The 48 zebrafish were first tested by 3D neurophenotyping in the novel tank and colour preference behaviour in the maze (defined as control). Then, all 48 zebrafish were exposed 40 µg/mL reserpine for 20 min and tested by behavioural apparatuses (defined as acute). Next, acute zebrafish were separated into three groups according to the experimental design. The three groups were exposed to system water (indicated as the model), 0.1 µg/mL sertraline hydrochloride (indicated as sertraline) and 100 µg/mL JWXY capsule (indicated as JWXY) for 7 days and then subjected to behavioural testing (Fig. 1a). Solutions were

Table 1 The definitions of behavioural parameters in the novel tank

Behavioural parameters	Definition
Total distance travelled (m)	The total distance in the novel tank
Average velocity (cm/s)	The direction and magnitude of zebrafish speed in the novel tank
Turn angle (°)	The total turning angle of zebrafish in the novel tank
Angular velocity (°/s)	The direction and magnitude of zebrafish angular speed in the novel tank
Meandering (°/s)	The degree of turning vs. travel distance
Average entry duration in the top (s)	The amount of time spent at the top of the novel tank during each crossing
Distance travelled in the top (m)	The total distance moved in the defined top part in the novel tank
Time spent in the top (s)	The total time spent in the top part of the novel tank
Latency to enter the top (s)	The amount of time to first cross from the bottom part to the top of the novel tank
Number of entries to the top	The number of crosses from the bottom part to the top of the novel tank
Time spent ratio of top: bottom	The ratio of the time spent on top over bottom
Distance travelled ratio of top: bottom	The ratio of the total distance moved in the top part vs. the bottom
Entries ratio of top: bottom	The number of crosses from the bottom part to the top of the novel tank
Freezing bouts (frequency)	The total number of instances of immobility (> 1 s) during the 5 min test in the novel tank
Freezing duration (s)	The duration of all freezing bouts in the novel tank

Table 2 The definitions of behavioural parameters in the maze

Behavioural parameters	Definition
Time (%)	The ratio of the time zebrafish spent in each arm (colour) to the total time spent in the maze
Distance (%)	The ratio of the distance zebrafish travelled in each arm (colour) to the total distance travelled in the maze

refreshed every day after feeding with fresh brine shrimp.

Behavioural testing

All zebrafish used in our study were acclimated to the laboratory environment. Before the behavioural test at every endpoint, zebrafish were given 1 h to acclimate to the tank environment. Behavioural testing was performed between 9:00 am and 16:00 pm, i.e., the middle of the light phase of the light cycle, with tanks filled with system water at a temperature ranging from 26 to 28 °C. Zebrafish behaviours were recorded for 5 min by CCD cameras and evaluated by analysing the behavioural endpoints in Tables 1 and 2.

Enzyme-linked immunosorbent assay (ELISA)

Cortisol was extracted from zebrafish whole-body homogenates. Adult zebrafish in different treatment groups were weighed and stored at − 80 °C. The whole zebrafish was dissected into small pieces on ice and homogenised in 500 μL ELISA Buffer, followed by sonication on ice for 30 s. Diethyl ether was added to samples, which were shaken for 10 min and centrifuged at 2000 rpm for 15 min at 4 °C. After storing the samples at − 80 °C for 15 min, the supernatant was transferred

into new tubes. After the diethyl ether evaporated, the extracts were dissolved in 500 μL ELISA Buffer and analysed by using the Cortisol ELISA Kit (Cayman, 500360).

The NA, 5-HT and DA concentrations of adult zebrafish brains were analysed by a NA ELISA Kit (CUSABIO, Wuhan, China), 5-HT ELISA Kit (CUSABIO, Wuhan, China), and DA ELISA Kit (CUSABIO, Wuhan, China), respectively. Zebrafish brain tissue was rinsed with $1 \times PBS$, homogenised in 1 mL $1 \times PBS$ and stored overnight at − 20 °C. After two freeze–thaw cycles, homogenates were centrifuged at $5000g$ for 5 min at 4 °C. The supernatant was transferred into new tubes and assayed immediately according to the manufacturer's instruction.

Western blot

Total protein was extracted from adult zebrafish brain tissue with radioimmunoprecipitation assay (RIPA) (CWBIO, Beijing, China) buffer containing phenylmethylsulfonyl fluoride (PMSF) (Sigma-Aldrich). Protein concentrations were quantified using a BCA Protein Assay Kit (CWBIO). Proteins were separated in 10% sodium dodecyl sulphate-polyacrylamide gel electrophoresis (SDS-PAGE) and transferred to a polyvinylidene fluoride (PVDF) membrane that was blocked with Tris-buffered saline (TBS) containing 5% skim milk for 1 h at room temperature. Membranes were incubated with mouse anti-TH (1:1000; Millipore) and mouse anti- glyceraldehyde 3-phosphate dehydrogenase (GAPDH) (1:5000; Proteintech) overnight primary antibodies at 4 °C. After being washed with TBS containing 0.05% Tween-20 (TBST), the membrane was incubated with anti-mouse HRP-conjugated secondary antibody (1:3000; CWBIO). The membrane was then washed with TBS containing 0.05% Tween-20, and Super Signal West Pico chemiluminescent substrate (Thermo Scientific) was used for detection.

UPLC and Q-TOF-MS analyses
We opened the JWXY capsule and ground the dry powdered contents. The powdered medicine was dissolved in system water to obtain a solution. Next, we used the mixed solution for ultra-performance liquid chromatography (UPLC) and quadrupole time-of-flight mass spectrometry (Q-TOF-MS) analyses.

A Waters Acquity UPLC System (Waters, MA, USA) equipped with a photodiode array detector was used. The system was controlled by Masslynx V4.1 software (Waters Co.). An Acquity BEHC18 column (2.1 × 100 mm, 1.7 μm; Waters Co.) was used for separations. Using Rongchang capsule as an example, a gradient elution of 0.1% formic acid in water (A) and 0.1% formic acid in acetonitrile (B) was performed as follows: 2% B was obtained from 0 to 1 min, 2–10% B from 1 to 3 min, 10–15% B from 3 to 7 min, 15–30% B from 7 to 15 min, 30–50% B from 15 to 20 min, 50–80% B from 20 to 23 min, and 80–100% B from 23 to 24 min; In adition, 100% B was maintained from 24 to 25 min; 100–2% B was obtained from 25 to 27 min; and 2% B was maintained from 27 to 30 min. Other samples were slightly adjusted based on their ingredients and chemical polarity. The flow rate was 0.40 mL/min, and the column temperature was maintained at 35 °C. Accurate mass measurements and MS/MS were performed on a Waters Q-TOF Premier with an electrospray ionisation (ESI) system (Xevo G2-Q Tof, Waters MS Technologies, Manchester, UK). The electrospray ionisation mass spectrometry (ESI–MS) spectra were acquired in both the negative and positive ion voltage modes. The capillary voltages were set to 2.0 kV for the negative mode and 3.0 kV for the positive mode. The sample cone voltage was set to 40 V. High-purity nitrogen was used as the nebulisation and auxiliary gas. The nebulisation gas was set at a flow rate of 800 L/h at 450 °C, the cone gas was set at a flow rate of 50 L/h, and the source temperature was 120 °C. The Q-TOF Premieracquisition rate was 0.1 s, with a 0.2-s scan delay. The instrument was operated with the first resolving quadrupole in a wide pass mode (50–2000 Da) and with the collision cell operating at two alternative energies (i.e., 20 and 50 eV). Leucine enkephalin (200 pg/mL) was used as the lock mass ([M−H]$^-$ 554.2615, [M+H]$^+$556.2771).

Data analyses
Data represents the mean ± SEM (standard error of the mean). One-way ANOVA was performed to assess differences between groups, followed by post hoc Tukey HSD tests for data with a normal distribution. A nonparametric Kruskal–Wallis test followed by Dunn's multiple comparisons tests ($*p < 0.05$) was used for data that violated the assumption of normality. We used GraphPad Prism 7.0 to obtain statistical charts and graphs.

Results
Establishment of the experimental procedure and analyses of JWXY capsule constituents
All herbs in JWXY capsule are presented in Additional file 1: Table S1. We utilized a solution of capsule contents to conduct a novel tank assay and colour preference behavioural experiment. UPLC and Q-TOF-MS analyses were conducted for JWXY capsule analysis. Protonated [M+H]$^+$ or deprotonated [M−H]$^-$ ions were obtained with as much characteristic fragment information as possible to deduce the molecular and elemental compositions of every constituent. The inferred chemical structure was compared with published data and reported natural product information. The ESI–MS spectra were acquired in both the positive and negative ion voltage modes for each capsule. Here, we show the results of JWXY capsule in the positive and negative ion voltage mode (Fig. 1d). A total of 57 compounds were identified in JWXY capsule. Detailed identification results are presented in Additional file 1: Table S2, Figures S1–S8.

Both sertraline and JWXY capsule rescued the decreased locomotive behaviour of zebrafish caused by reserpine
The locomotive behaviour of zebrafish was measured by the total distance travelled, average velocity, turn angle and angular velocity. Compared with the control, acute treatment (20 min) with reserpine resulted in suppression of the total distance travelled and average velocity. Then, after treatment with system water for 7 days, the total distance travelled and average velocity were more significantly reduced (model). The turn angle and angular velocity showed the same trend. However, total distance travelled was rescued after treatment with sertraline and JWXY capsule for 7 days (Fig. 2b). Moreover, the average velocity revealed that sertraline and JWXY capsule significantly rescued the reduced activity caused by reserpine (Fig. 2c). Likewise, the turn angle and angular velocity demonstrated that sertraline and JWXY capsule rescued the effects of reserpine on zebrafish behaviour (Fig. 2d,

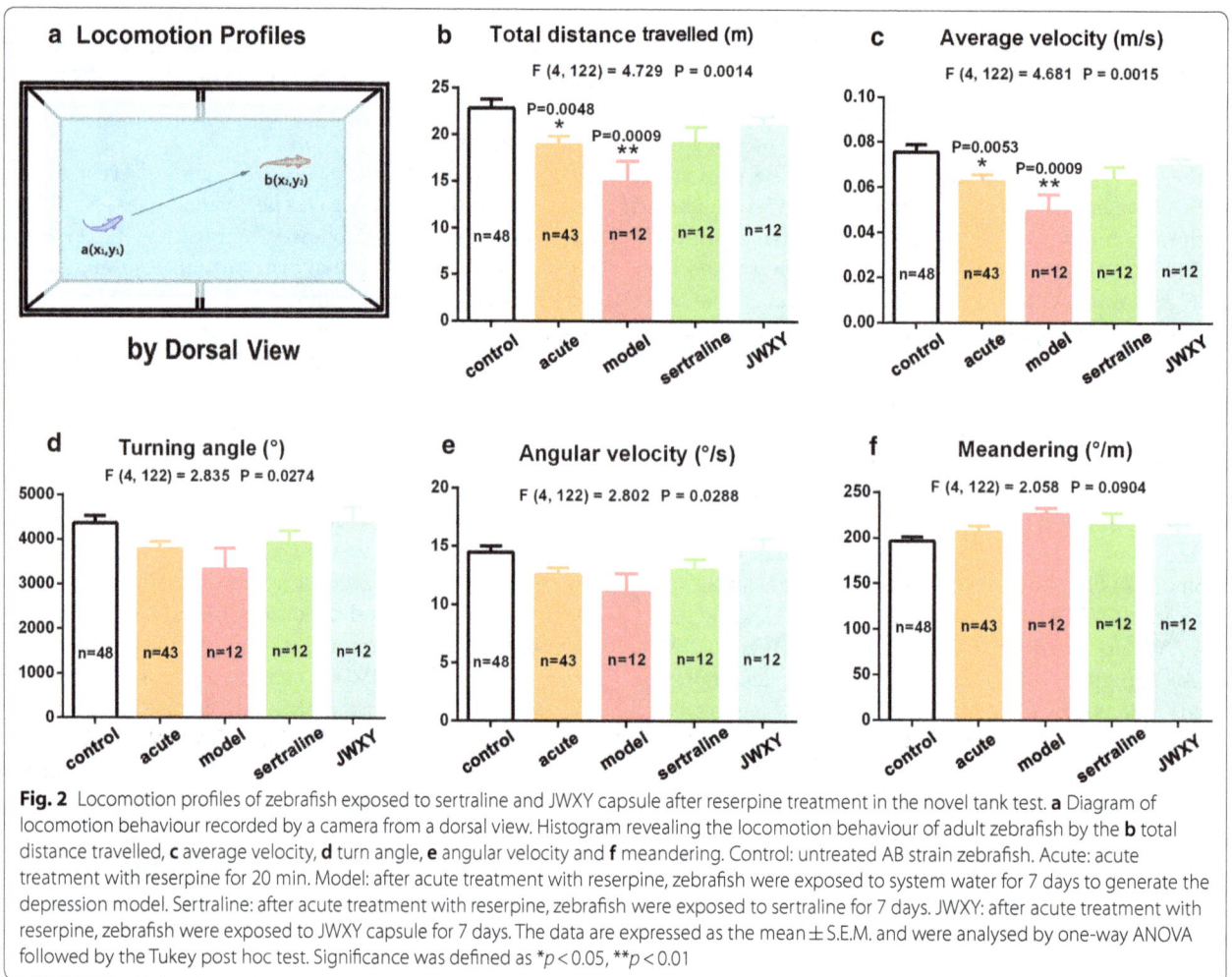

Fig. 2 Locomotion profiles of zebrafish exposed to sertraline and JWXY capsule after reserpine treatment in the novel tank test. **a** Diagram of locomotion behaviour recorded by a camera from a dorsal view. Histogram revealing the locomotion behaviour of adult zebrafish by the **b** total distance travelled, **c** average velocity, **d** turn angle, **e** angular velocity and **f** meandering. Control: untreated AB strain zebrafish. Acute: acute treatment with reserpine for 20 min. Model: after acute treatment with reserpine, zebrafish were exposed to system water for 7 days to generate the depression model. Sertraline: after acute treatment with reserpine, zebrafish were exposed to sertraline for 7 days. JWXY: after acute treatment with reserpine, zebrafish were exposed to JWXY capsule for 7 days. The data are expressed as the mean ± S.E.M. and were analysed by one-way ANOVA followed by the Tukey post hoc test. Significance was defined as *$p < 0.05$, **$p < 0.01$

e). Reserpine slightly increased erratic movements measured by meandering in the novel tank test, and sertraline and JWXY capsule reduced this tendency (Fig. 2f).

JWXY capsule rescued inhibition of exploratory behaviour and reversed the depressive phenotype of zebrafish

Exploratory behaviour, measured by the average entry duration (Fig. 3b), distance travelled in the top (Fig. 3c), time spent in the top (Fig. 3d), time spent ratio of top: bottom (Fig. 3e), distance travelled of top: bottom (Fig. 3f), latency to enter the top (Fig. 3g) and entries ratio of top: bottom (Fig. 3h), was not significantly altered in the treatment groups compared with that in the control group, with the exception of JWXY capsule treatment group. However, exploratory behavioural parameters were decreased in the model group. As shown in Fig. 3, zebrafish treated with JWXY capsule exhibited improvements in exploratory behaviour; the average entry duration, distance travelled in the top, time spent in the top, time spent ratio of top: bottom and distance travelled of

top: bottom were significantly higher in the JWXY capsule group than in the acute group. Reserpine induced an obvious depressive phenotype as shown in Fig. 4. After acute treatment with reserpine, zebrafish did not show changes in their freezing bouts and freezing duration. However, the freezing bouts and freezing duration were enhanced after 7 days. After treatment with of sertraline and JWXY capsule for 7 days, the depressive phenotype was no longer observed. Moreover, the freezing bouts and freezing duration were significantly decreased.

Impact of sertraline and JWXY capsule on the colour preference behaviour of zebrafish after reserpine treatment: JWXY capsule reversed colour preference patterns

Colour preference behaviour was demonstrated by the time spent (Fig. 5) and distance travelled (Additional file 1: Figure S9) in every colour arm using a remoulded offset cross maze (Fig. 5a). The control group (Fig. 5b) spent the most time in the blue area, followed by the

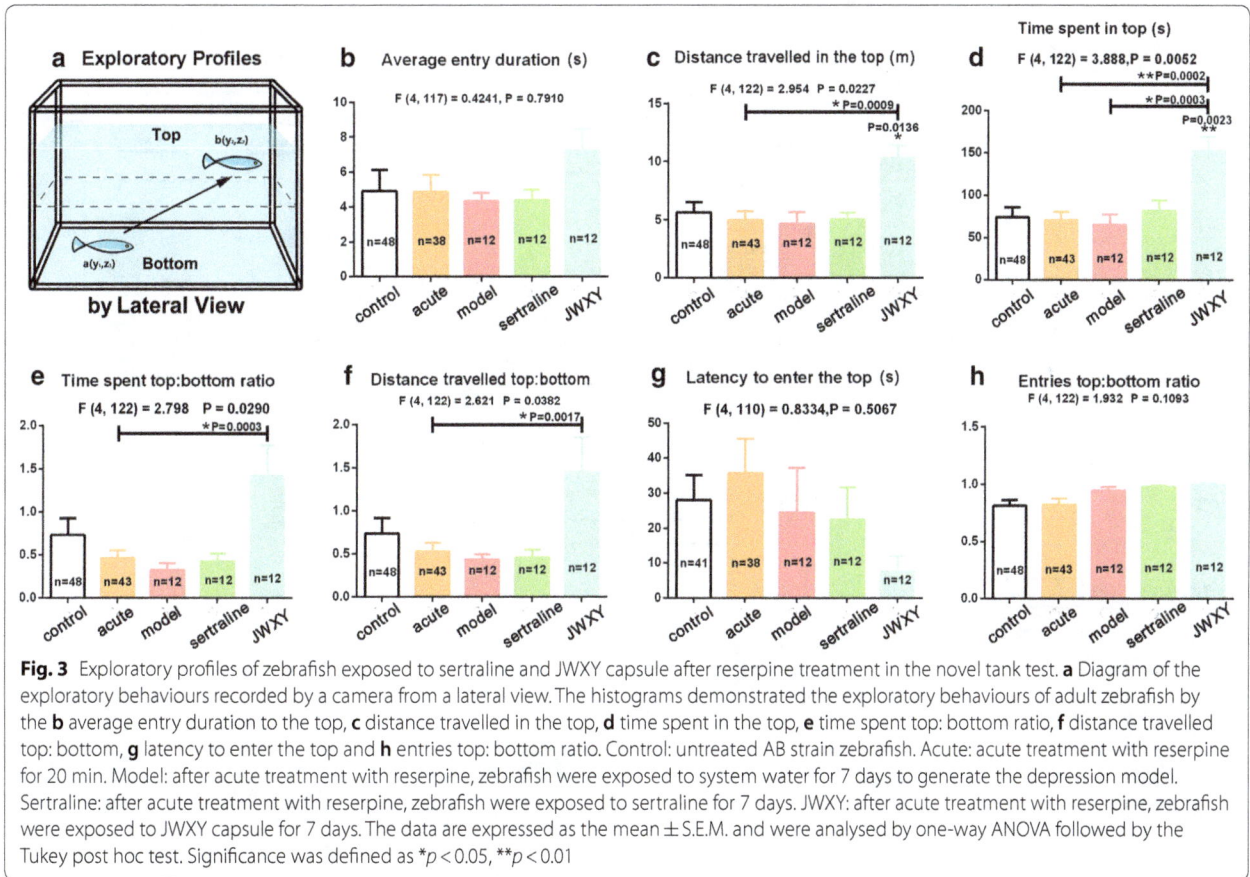

Fig. 3 Exploratory profiles of zebrafish exposed to sertraline and JWXY capsule after reserpine treatment in the novel tank test. **a** Diagram of the exploratory behaviours recorded by a camera from a lateral view. The histograms demonstrated the exploratory behaviours of adult zebrafish by the **b** average entry duration to the top, **c** distance travelled in the top, **d** time spent in the top, **e** time spent top: bottom ratio, **f** distance travelled top: bottom, **g** latency to enter the top and **h** entries top: bottom ratio. Control: untreated AB strain zebrafish. Acute: acute treatment with reserpine for 20 min. Model: after acute treatment with reserpine, zebrafish were exposed to system water for 7 days to generate the depression model. Sertraline: after acute treatment with reserpine, zebrafish were exposed to sertraline for 7 days. JWXY: after acute treatment with reserpine, zebrafish were exposed to JWXY capsule for 7 days. The data are expressed as the mean ± S.E.M. and were analysed by one-way ANOVA followed by the Tukey post hoc test. Significance was defined as *$p < 0.05$, **$p < 0.01$

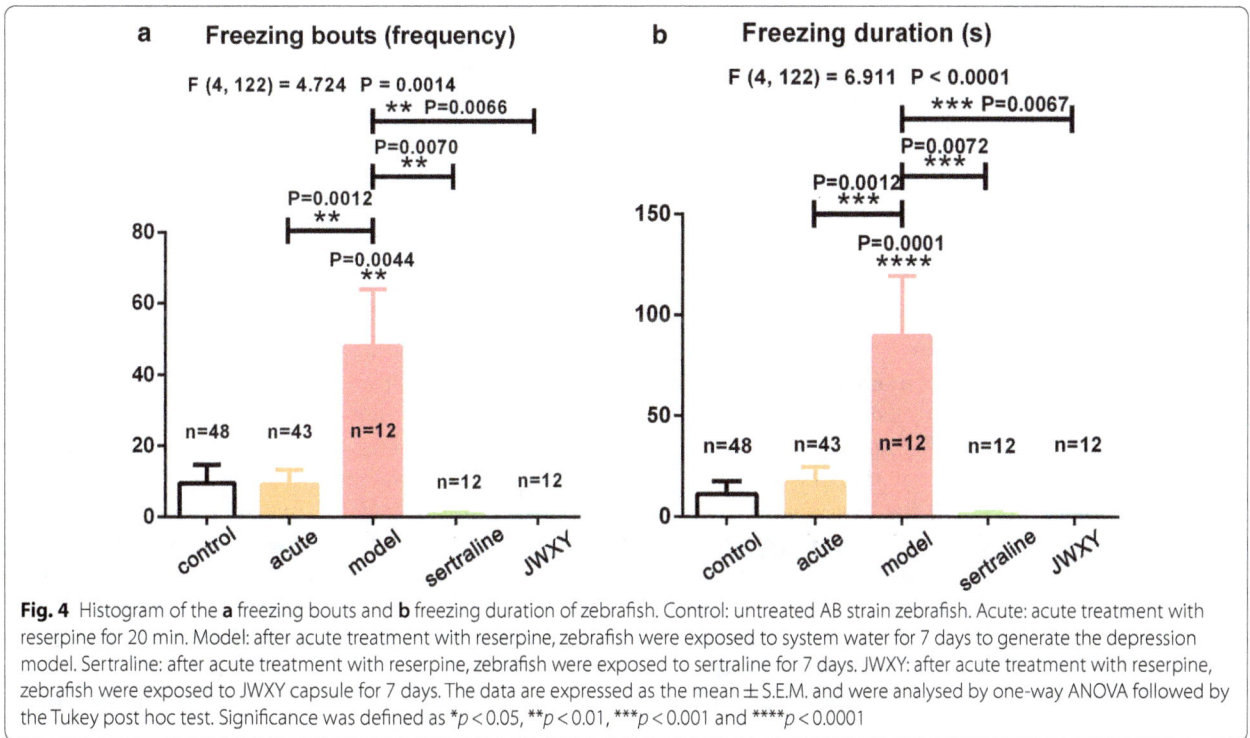

Fig. 4 Histogram of the **a** freezing bouts and **b** freezing duration of zebrafish. Control: untreated AB strain zebrafish. Acute: acute treatment with reserpine for 20 min. Model: after acute treatment with reserpine, zebrafish were exposed to system water for 7 days to generate the depression model. Sertraline: after acute treatment with reserpine, zebrafish were exposed to sertraline for 7 days. JWXY: after acute treatment with reserpine, zebrafish were exposed to JWXY capsule for 7 days. The data are expressed as the mean ± S.E.M. and were analysed by one-way ANOVA followed by the Tukey post hoc test. Significance was defined as *$p < 0.05$, **$p < 0.01$, ***$p < 0.001$ and ****$p < 0.0001$

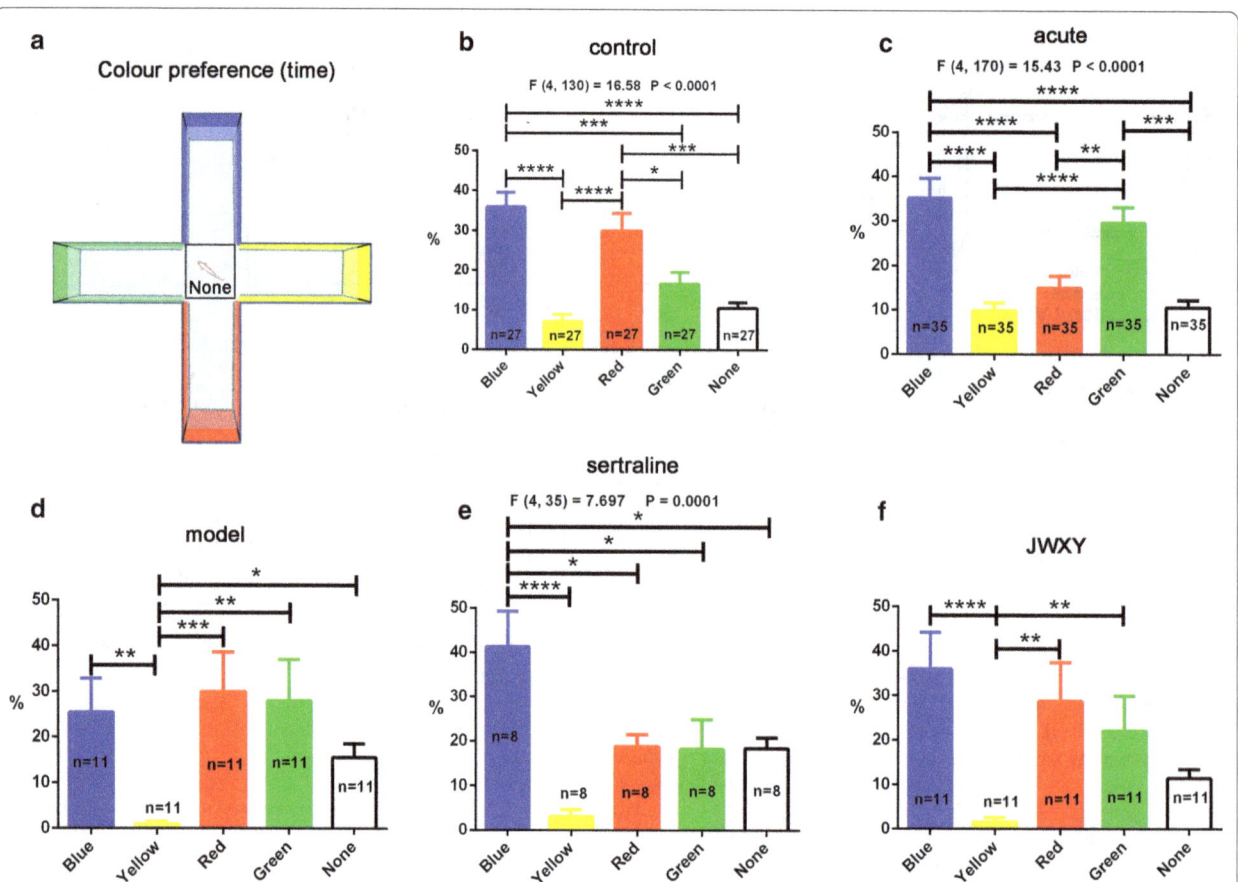

Fig. 5 Colour preference profiles of zebrafish exposed to sertraline and JWXY capsule after reserpine treatment in the remoulded offset cross maze test. **a** Diagram of the remoulded offset cross maze and distribution of colours. The centre of the cross maze was denoted as None, and zebrafish started in that location. **b** The duration (time) of control zebrafish in every colour arm. **c** The duration (time) of zebrafish treated with reserpine for approximately 20 min (acute) in every colour arm. **d** The duration (time) of zebrafish exposed to system water after reserpine treatment (model) in every colour arm. **e** The duration (time) of zebrafish exposed to sertraline after reserpine treatment in every colour arm. **f** The duration (time) of zebrafish exposed to JWXY capsule after reserpine treatment at every colour arm. Control: untreated AB strain zebrafish. Acute: acute treatment with reserpine for 20 min. Model: after acute treatment with reserpine, zebrafish were exposed to system water for 7 days to generate the depression model. Sertraline: after acute treatment with reserpine, zebrafish were exposed to sertraline for 7 days. JWXY: after acute treatment with reserpine, zebrafish were exposed to JWXY capsule for 7 days. The data are expressed as the mean ± S.E.M. One-way ANOVA with post hoc Tukey HSD tests was used to analyse data with a normal distribution, and a nonparametric Kruskal–Wallis test followed by Dunn's multiple comparisons tests was used for data that violated the assumption of normality. Significance was defined as *$p < 0.05$, **$p < 0.01$, ***$p < 0.001$ and ****$p < 0.0001$

red, green, and yellow areas (listed from most to least time spent). The most and least preferred colours were unchanged, but the time spent in green area was higher than that in the red area in the acute group (Fig. 5c). In the model group (Fig. 5d), the amounts of time spent in blue, red and green were not significantly different. Zebrafish continued to spend the least amount of time in the yellow area. After sertraline treatment (Fig. 5e), zebrafish recovered their preference for blue. However, the time spent in the red and green areas was not different. Notably, the JWXY group and control group had the same colour preference (Fig. 5f). The distance (Additional file 1: Figure S9) travelled in every colour arm was the

same over time. Based on the abovementioned results, we concluded that zebrafish preferred blue the most and yellow the least. Following treatment with sertraline and JWXY capsule, the colour preference order was restored, and JWXY capsule was more effective than sertraline in restoring colour preference behaviour.

Based on colour preference behaviour in the remoulded offset cross maze, we chose two colours (blue and yellow) to conduct a concise test using a T-maze. Colour preference behaviour was demonstrated by time (Fig. 6) and distance (Additional file 1: Figure S10) travelled in every colour arm using a T-maze (Fig. 6a). In the control (Fig. 6b) and acute (Fig. 6c) groups, zebrafish spent

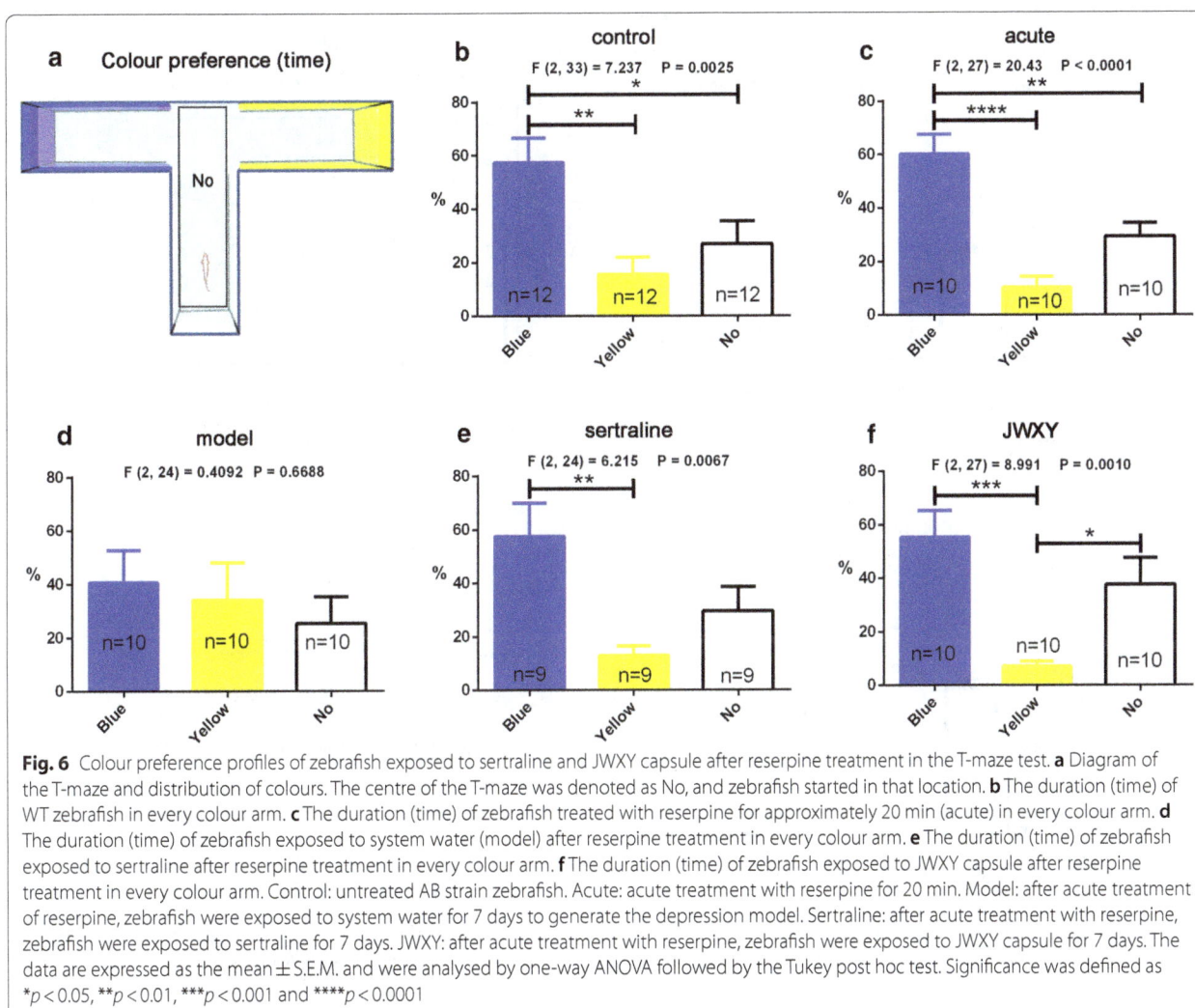

Fig. 6 Colour preference profiles of zebrafish exposed to sertraline and JWXY capsule after reserpine treatment in the T-maze test. **a** Diagram of the T-maze and distribution of colours. The centre of the T-maze was denoted as No, and zebrafish started in that location. **b** The duration (time) of WT zebrafish in every colour arm. **c** The duration (time) of zebrafish treated with reserpine for approximately 20 min (acute) in every colour arm. **d** The duration (time) of zebrafish exposed to system water (model) after reserpine treatment in every colour arm. **f** The duration (time) of zebrafish exposed to JWXY capsule after reserpine treatment in every colour arm. Control: untreated AB strain zebrafish. Acute: acute treatment with reserpine for 20 min. Model: after acute treatment of reserpine, zebrafish were exposed to system water for 7 days to generate the depression model. Sertraline: after acute treatment with reserpine, zebrafish were exposed to sertraline for 7 days. JWXY: after acute treatment with reserpine, zebrafish were exposed to JWXY capsule for 7 days. The data are expressed as the mean $\pm$ S.E.M. and were analysed by one-way ANOVA followed by the Tukey post hoc test. Significance was defined as $*p < 0.05$, $**p < 0.01$, $***p < 0.001$ and $****p < 0.0001$

significantly more time in the blue area than in the yellow area. However, the time zebrafish spent in every colour arm was not different in the model group (Fig. 6d). After sertraline (Fig. 6e) and JWXY capsule (Fig. 6f) treatment, the same colour preference tendency as that of the control was observed. The distance (Additional file 1: Figure S10) travelled in every colour arm was consistent with the time spent.

Cortisol and monoamine levels influenced zebrafish neurobehaviour

Whole-body cortisol, monoamines, including NA, 5-HT, DA, and TH were detected in zebrafish brain tissues after different treatments. The cortisol level in the model group was significantly higher than that in the acute and control groups. After sertraline and JWXY capsule treatments, the cortisol level was markedly decreased, especially in the JWXY group (Fig. 7a). NA in the model group was significantly lower than that in the control and

sertraline group. However, compared with the model and sertraline groups, the JWXY group showed a significant increase in the NA concentration (Fig. 7b). 5-HT was significantly increased in the acute group but increased only slightly in the model group. Sertraline elevated the 5-HT level, but JWXY capsule did not (Fig. 7c). Sertraline decreased TH expression 7 days after acute exposure, and sertraline and JWXY capsule treatments improved TH to a degree (Fig. 7d). However, the DA level did not change after sertraline and JWXY treatments (Additional file 1: Figure S11).

Discussion

JWXY capsule contains nine herbal medicines, and 57 compounds were identified in its extraction by UPLC and Q-TOF-MS. As previously described, TCM posits that depression involves in multiple organs. TCM focuses on the overall effect of medicines contained in a prescription, and it also plays a role in health care and disease

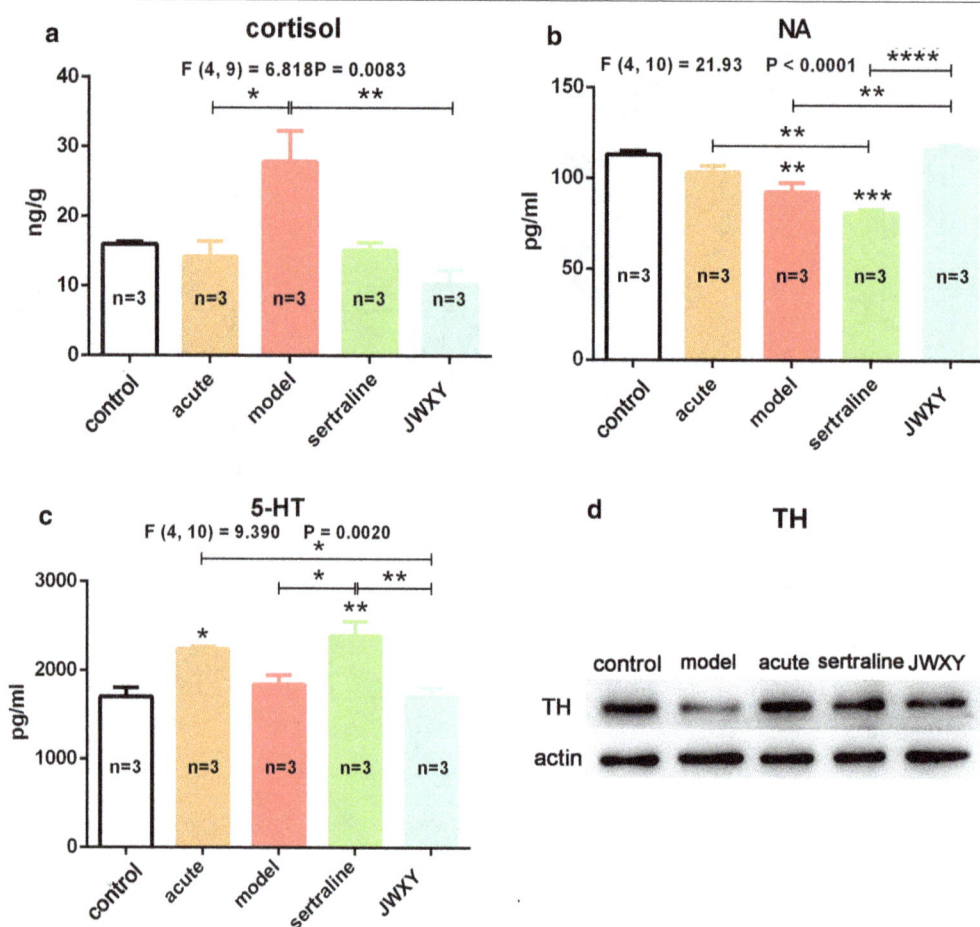

Fig. 7 The effects of sertraline and JWXY capsule treatment on cortisol and monoamines in zebrafish. The levels of cortisol (**a**), noradrenaline (**b**), 5-HT (**c**) and tyrosine hydroxylase (**d**) in zebrafish after different treatments. Control: untreated AB strain zebrafish. Acute: acute treatment with reserpine for 20 min. Model: after acute treatment with reserpine, zebrafish were exposed to system water for 7 days to generate the depression model. Sertraline: after acute treatment with reserpine, zebrafish were exposed to sertraline for 7 days. JWXY: after acute treatment with reserpine, zebrafish were exposed to JWXY capsule for 7 days. The data are expressed as the mean ± S.E.M. and were analysed by one-way ANOVA followed by the Tukey post hoc test. Significance was defined as *$p < 0.05$, **$p < 0.01$, ***$p < 0.001$ and ****$p < 0.0001$

prevention through the treatment of multiple targets. All herbal medicines in the prescription work synergistically and can yield stable and comprehensive curative effects, greatly reducing the side effects of drug treatment. Determining the main components of TCM prescriptions and their mechanisms of action is difficult. However, characterising the multiple constituents, targets and pathways of TCM prescriptions is of greater importance, and requires further research.

We employed a 3D video-tracking system to detect changes in the swimming behaviour of lesioned zebrafish in novel tank. Zebrafish demonstrated long-term depressive symptoms, including elevated baseline whole-body cortisol, social withdrawal and locomotor retardation after reserpine exposure [46]. Reserpine does not induce overt acute behavioural effects but markedly reduces activity after 7 days [5], consistent

with our study. After 20 min of reserpine exposure, zebrafish showed a slight decrease in locomotive activity but did not show obvious changes in exploratory behaviour and freezing behaviour. Zebrafish displayed significantly decreased locomotive activity and a worsened depressive phenotype after 7 days, along with hypoactive exploratory behaviour, which proved that the establishment of zebrafish depression model first introduced by Kyzar et al. was successful in our experiment. However, compared with zebrafish in the model group, zebrafish in the sertraline and JWXY capsule groups treated for 7 days expressed different behaviours. Sertraline treatment increased locomotive activity and rescued the depressive phenotype induced by reserpine. Moreover, JWXY capsule increased locomotive activity, more effectively reversed the depressive phenotype, and improved exploratory behaviour.

The colour preference test could serve as a useful protocol for memory evaluation, cognitive dysfunction, assessment of neurodegenerative disorders, preclinical appraisal of drug efficacy and behavioural evaluation of toxicity [47]. Here, we evaluated cognitive impairment by the colour preference test. Studies have demonstrated the natural colour preference of zebrafish. Zebrafish prefer colours of short wavelengths. Zebrafish exhibit a strong preference for blue relative to all other colours (red, yellow and green), with yellow being less preferred than red and green [26, 48]. In our study, blue was the favourite colour of control zebrafish, and yellow was the least favourite. Control zebrafish exhibited a significantly stronger preference for blue than for red and green. However, compared with control zebrafish, zebrafish exhibiting depressive behaviour lost certain colour preferences. Yellow was the least preferred colour of model zebrafish, but the preference for green and red increased simultaneously and was not significantly different compared with that for blue, indicating that the normal colour preference pattern was disturbed. However, Zebrafish treated by JWXY capsule regained this colour preference pattern. Sertraline also restored the colour preference pattern to a degree, but its efficacy was not as obvious and clear as that of JWXY capsule. To minimize the effects of place preference on the results and further verify this preference in zebrafish, we chose to test blue and yellow in T-maze. All groups except the model group exhibited a preference for blue. However, different from the other groups, the model group also showed an increased preference for yellow and the same preference for all three arms, illustrating the colour preference disorder in depressed zebrafish. In contrast, sertraline and JWXY capsule restored the colour preference pattern. These results showed that the cognitive dysfunction accompanying with depression in zebrafish could be reversed by sertraline and JWXY capsule.

Depression is usually comorbid with anxiety, which leads to behavioural alterations. The effects of chronic depression and anxiety on the hypothalamic–pituitary–interrenal (HPI) axis have been studied previously in zebrafish. Benzodiazepines (anxiolytics) and antidepressants completely prevent increased cortisol levels in zebrafish [49]. The decreases in total distance travelled and velocity in zebrafish are related to the decreased levels of DA and NA [50]. SSRIs were developed and entered clinical trials as a new class of antidepressant in the 1980s. Six SSRIs, including fluoxetine, paroxetine, sertraline, fluvoxamine, citalopram and escitalopram are commonly used for clinical treatment. SSRIs selectively inhibit the reuptake of 5-HT by the presynaptic membrane. SSRIs have little impact on NA and hardly affect the reuptake of DA [51]. In our study, the

reserpine-induced zebrafish model of depression showed increased whole-body cortisol and 5-HT, decreased NA and reduced TH. Compared with the model, sertraline prevented the increase in cortisol and NA and increased 5-HT and TH. However, JWXY capsule prevented the increase in cortisol and 5-HT, consistent with the rescued depressive phenotype. In addition, compared with the model, JWXY capsule improved the levels of NA and TH, consistent with the increased locomotive activity. Interestingly, DA levels in zebrafish brains were unaffected by any treatments. Those changes in monoamine neurotransmitters were related to the colour preference disorder caused by reserpine and were consistent with the restored cognitive ability.

Conclusion

The novel tank test recorded by a 3D method in this experiment revealed the similar anti-depression effects of two treatments for chronic reserpine exposure. This validation was based on the successful establishment of a depressive zebrafish model, which was first introduced by Kyzar et al. The depressive effects of reserpine decrease locomotion, increase erratic movements, reduce exploratory behaviour to the top and enhance depressive phenotype. Furthermore, colour preference testing in a remoulded offset cross maze and T-maze indicated that the natural colour preference pattern (zebrafish prefer blue to red, green and yellow and show a strong aversion to yellow) was disturbed due to depression induced by reserpine. However, sertraline treatment improved depression-like behaviours by increasing locomotion and decreasing erratic movements and the depressive phenotype. Sertraline also restored the colour preference in zebrafish. Notably, JWXY capsule was a more effective treatment than sertraline. JWXY capsule treatment reversed depression-like behaviours by increasing locomotion, decreasing erratic movements, increasing exploratory behaviour to the top and rescued the depressive phenotype. Zebrafish also exhibited their natural colour preference after JWXY capsule treatment.

Depression-like behaviours and cognitive disorder (measured by colour preference) resulted from changes in hormone and monoamine neurotransmitters in the brain. Increased whole-body cortisol and decreased NA and TH were observed in the zebrafish depression model. Sertraline prevented the increase in cortisol, inhibited the reuptake of 5-HT, and improved the expression of TH. Compared with the model, JWXY capsule also prevented the increase in cortisol, recovered NA and improved the expression of TH. Overall, these results show that changes in cortisol and monoamines accounted for the reversal of depressive behaviours and cognitive dysfunction. The high sensitivity of zebrafish to the effects of Western medicine and TCM can help improve our understanding of the psychopharmacological profiles of these drugs and related CNS drugs, as well contribute to further development of TCM as an antidepressant.

Additional file

Additional file 1: Table S1. The composition of JWXY capsule. Figure S1. ESI-MS spectra in the positive and negative ion voltage mode of JWXY capsule (1–30 min). Figure S2. ESI-MS spectra in the positive and negative ion voltage mode of JWXY capsule (15-30min). Table S2. MS data in ($\pm$) ESI modes and the identification results in JWXY capsule. Figures S3–8. The chemical structure of each component identified in JWXY capsule. Figure S9. Colour preference profiles of zebrafish exposed to sertraline and JWXY capsule after reserpine treatment in the remoulded offset cross maze test. Figure S10. Colour preference profiles of zebrafish exposed to sertraline and JWXY capsule after reserpine treatment in the T-maze test. Figure S11. The changes of sertraline and JWXY capsule treatment on dopamine (DA) of zebrafish.

Authors' contributions
XZF, XDL and XL conceived and designed the experiments. XDL, SHZ and XL conducted the zebrafish behavioural assays. SHZ and XDL wrote the manuscript. The video-tracking software was designed by MZS, TL and XZ. XDL and SHZ collected and analysed the behavioural data. QPZ, JX and DYC monitored and evaluated the expression of related hormones and monoamines. All authors discussed the results and implications and reviewed the manuscript at all stages. All authors read and approved the final manuscript.

Acknowledgements
This work was supported by the Special Fund for Basic Research on Scientific Instruments from the Chinese National Natural Science Foundation of China (Grant No: 61327802), the National Basic Research Program of China (2015CB856500) and the Chinese National Natural Science Foundation of China (Grant Nos. 61633012 and U1613220).

Competing interests
The authors declare that they have no competing interests.

References
1. Simon NM. Generalized anxiety disorder and psychiatric comorbidities such as depression, bipolar disorder, and substance abuse. J Clin Psychiatry. 2009;70(suppl 2):10–4.

2. Richelson E. Pharmacology of antidepressants. Mayo Clin Proc. 2001;76(5):511–27.
3. Perrine SA, Ghoddoussi F, Michaels MS, Sheikh IS, Mckelvey G, Galloway MP. Ketamine reverses stress-induced depression-like behaviour and increased GABA levels in the anterior cingulate: an 11.7 T 1H-MRS study in rats. Prog Neuropsychopharmacol Biol Psychiatry. 2014;51(1):9–15.
4. McCarroll MN, Gendelev L, Keiser MJ, Kokel D. Leveraging large-scale behavioural profiling in zebrafish to explore neuroactive polypharmacology. ACS Chem Biol. 2016;11(4):842–9.
5. Kyzar E, Stewart AM, Landsman S, Collins C, Gebhardt M, Robinson K, Kalueff AV. Behavioural effects of bidirectional modulators of brain monoamines reserpine and d-amphetamine in zebrafish. Brain Res. 2013;1527:108–16.
6. Goldstein DS, Eisenhofer G, Mccarty R. Catecholamines: bridging basic science with clinical medicine. Cambridge: Academic Press; 1998.
7. Lillesaar C. The serotonergic system in fish. J Chem Neuroanat. 2011;41(4):294–308.
8. Yamamoto K, Vernier P. The evolution of dopamine systems in chordates. Front Neuroanat. 2011;5(5):1–21.

9. Vignet C, Trenkel VM, Vouillarmet A, Bricca G, Begout ML, Cousin X. Changes in brain monoamines underlie behavioural disruptions after zebrafish diet exposure to polycyclic aromatic hydrocarbons environmental mixtures. Int J Mol Sci. 2017;18(3):560.
10. Levin ED, Kalueff AV, Gerlai RT. Perspectives on zebrafish neurobehavioural pharmacology. Pharmacol Biochem Behav. 2015;139:93.
11. Kalueff AV, Stewart AM, Gerlai R. Zebrafish as an emerging model for studying complex brain disorders. Trends Pharmacol Sci. 2014;35(2):63.
12. Saroya R, Smith R, Seymour C, Mothersill C. Injection of resperine into zebrafish, prevents fish to fish communication of radiation-induced bystander signals: confirmation in vivo of a role for serotonin in the mechanism. Doseresponse Publ Int Hormesis Soc. 2009;8(3):317–30.
13. Fossat P, Bacqué-Cazenave J, De DP, Delbecque JP, Cattaert D. Comparative behaviour. Anxiety-like behaviour in crayfish is controlled by serotonin. Science. 2014;344(6189):1293–7.
14. Maximino C, Puty B, Benzecry R, Araujo J, Lima MG, de Jesus Oliveira Batista E, de Matos Oliveira KR, Crespo-Lopez ME, Herculano AM. Role of serotonin in zebrafish (Danio rerio) anxiety: relationship with serotonin levels and effect of buspirone, WAY 100635, SB 224289, fluoxetine and para-chlorophenylalanine (pCPA) in two behavioural models. Neuropharmacology. 2013;71:83–97.
15. Abril-de-Abreu R, Cruz J, Oliveira RF. Social Eavesdropping in Zebrafish: tuning of Attention to Social Interactions. Scientific Rep. 2015;5:12678.
16. Li X, Liu B, Li XL, Li YX, Sun MZ, Chen DY, Zhao X, Feng XZ. SiO2 nanoparticles change colour preference and cause Parkinson's-like behaviour in zebrafish. Scientific Rep. 2014;4:3810.
17. Khotimah H, Sumitro SB, Widodo MA. Zebrafish Parkinson's model: rotenone decrease motility, dopamine, and increase α-synuclein aggregation and apoptosis of zebrafish brain. Int J Pharmtech Res. 2015;8(4):614–21.
18. Wang YN, Hou YY, Sun MZ, Zhang CY, Bai G, Zhao X, Feng XZ. Behavioural screening of zebrafish using neuroactive traditional Chinese medicine prescriptions and biological targets. Scientific Rep. 2014;4:5311.
19. Anderson HD, Pace WD, Libby AM, West DR, Valuck RJ. Rates of 5 common antidepressant side effects among new adult and adolescent cases of depression: a retrospective US claims study. Clin Ther. 2012;34(1):113.
20. Rascati K, Godley P, Pham H. Evaluation of resources used to treat adverse events of selective serotonin reuptake inhibitor use. J Manag Care Pharm. 2001;7:402–6.
21. Dai Y, Li Z, Xue L, Dou C, Zhou Y, Zhang L, Qin X. Metabolomics study on the anti-depression effect of xiaoyaosan on rat model of chronic unpredictable mild stress. J Ethnopharmacol. 2010;128(2):482–9.
22. Zhou J. Multicenter randomized controlled clinical study of JiaWeiXiaoYao capsule in the treatment of mild to moderate depression with syndrome of qi stagnation transforming into fire. China Academy of Chinese Medical Sciences; 2013.
23. Zhou J, Rui SU, Tao LI, Cao XD, Han ZY, Lin B, Guo RJ, Fan JP. Randomized controlled trial of Jiawei Xiaoyao Capsule in the treatment of mild to moderate depression. China J Trad Chin Med Pharm. 2013;28(9):2804–6.
24. Park JS, Ryu JH, Choi TI, Bae YK, Lee S, Kang HJ, Kim CH. Innate colour preference of zebrafish and its use in behavioural analyses. Mol Cells. 2016;39(10):750–5.
25. Braida D, Ponzoni L, Martucci R, Sparatore F, Gotti C, Sala M. Role of neuronal nicotinic acetylcholine receptors (nAChRs) on learning and memory in zebrafish. Psychopharmacology. 2014;231(9):1975–85.
26. Avdesh A, Martin-Iverson M, Chen M, Groth D, Mondal A, Morgan N, Lardelli M, Martins R, Verdile G. Evaluation of colour preference in zebrafish: a possible potential model for learning and memory disorders. Alzheimers Dementia J Alzheimers Assoc. 2011;7(4):S120–S120.
27. Li X, Li X, Li YX, Zhang Y, Chen D, Sun MZ, Zhao X, Chen DY, Feng XZ. The Difference between Anxiolytic and Anxiogenic Effects Induced by Acute and Chronic Alcohol Exposure and Changes in Associative Learning and Memory Based on Colour Preference and the Cause of Parkinson-Like Behaviours in Zebrafish. PLoS ONE. 2015;10(11):e0141134.
28. Oliveira J, Silveira M, Chacon D, Luchiari A. The zebrafish world of colours and shapes: preference and discrimination. Zebrafish. 2015;12(2):166–73.
29. Robinson J, Schmitt EA, Hárosi FI, Reece RJ, Dowling JE. Zebrafish ultraviolet visual pigment: absorption spectrum, sequence, and localization. Proc Natl Acad Sci USA. 1993;90(13):6009–12.

30. Fadool JM, Dowling JE. Zebrafish: a model system for the study of eye genetics. Prog Retinal Eye Res. 2008;27(1):89–110.

31. Roest CH, Weissenbach J. Fish genomics and biology. Genome Res. 2005;15(12):1675–82.

32. Stewart AM, Ullmann JF, Norton WH, Parker MO, Brennan CH, Gerlai R, Kalueff AV. Molecular psychiatry of zebrafish. Mol Psychiatry. 2015;20(1):2–17.

33. Cheng KC, Xin X, Clark DP, Riviere PL. Whole-animal imaging, gene function, and the Zebrafish Phenome Project. Curr Opin Genet Dev. 2011;21(5):620–9.

34. Rihel J, Prober DA, Arvanites A, Lam K, Zimmerman S, Jang S, Haggarty SJ, Kokel D, Rubin LL, Peterson RT, Schier AF. Zebrafish behavioural profiling links drugs to biological targets and rest/wake regulation. Science. 2010;327(5963):348–51.

35. Bruni G, Rennekamp AJ, Velenich A, McCarroll M, Gendelev L, Fertsch E, Taylor J, Lakhani P, Lensen D, Evron T, Lorello PJ, Huang XP, Kolczewski S, Carey G, Caldarone BJ, Prinssen E, Roth BL, Keiser MJ, Peterson RT, Kokel D. Zebrafish behavioural profiling identifies multitarget antipsychotic-like compounds. Nat Chem Biol. 2016;12(7):559–66.

36. Challal S, Buenafe OEM, Queiroz EF, Maljevic S, Marcourt L, Bock M, Kloeti W, Dayrit FM, Harvey AL, Lerche H, Esguerra CV, de Witte PAM, Wolfender J-L, Crawford AD. Zebrafish bioassay-guided microfractionation identifies anticonvulsant steroid glycosides from the philippine medicinal plantsolanum torvum. ACS Chem Neurosci. 2014;5(10):993–1004.

37. Sourbron J, Smolders I, de Witte P, Lagae L. Pharmacological analysis of the anti-epileptic mechanisms of fenfluramine in scn1a mutant zebrafish. Front Pharmacol. 2017;8:191.

38. Rihel J, Schier AF. Behavioural screening for neuroactive drugs in zebrafish. Dev Neurobiol. 2012;72(3):373–85.

39. Li X, Li X, Chen D, Guo J-L, Feng D-F, Sun M-Z, Lu Y, Chen D-Y, Zhao X, Feng X-Z. Evaluating the biological impact of polyhydroxyalkanoates (PHAs) on developmental and exploratory profile of zebrafish larvae. RSC Adv. 2016;6(43):37018–30.

40. Heilmann S, Ratnakumar K, Langdon EM, Kansler ER, Kim IS, Campbell NR, Perry EB, McMahon AJ, Kaufman CK, van Rooijen E, Lee W, Iacobuzio-Donahue CA, Hynes RO, Zon LI, Xavier JB, White RM. A quantitative system for studying metastasis using transparent zebrafish. Can Res. 2015;75(20):4272–82.

41. Sokolova MV, Fernández-Caballero A, Ros L, Latorre JM, Serrano JP. Evaluation of color preference for emotion regulation. Artificial computation in biology and medicine, vol. 9107. Heidelberg: Springer; 2015. p. 479–87. https://doi.org/10.1007/978-3-319-18914-7_50

42. Pittman JT, Lott CS. Startle response memory and hippocampal changes in adult zebrafish pharmacologically-induced to exhibit anxiety/depression-like behaviours. Physiol Behav. 2014;123:174–9.

43. Macri S, Neri D, Ruberto T, Mwaffo V, Butail S, Porfiri M. Three-dimensional scoring of zebrafish behaviour unveils biological phenomena hidden by two-dimensional analyses. Scientific Rep. 2017;7(1):1962.

44. Kalueff AV, Cachat JM. Zebrafish neurobehavioural protocols. New York: Humana Press; 2011.

45. Li X, Liu X, Li T, Li X, Feng D, Kuang X, Xu J, Zhao X, Sun M, Chen D, Zhang Z, Feng X. SiO2nanoparticles cause depression and anxiety-like behaviour in adult zebrafish. RSC Adv. 2017;7(5):2953–63.

46. Nguyen M, Stewart AM, Kalueff AV. Aquatic blues: modeling depression and antidepressant action in zebrafish. Prog Neuropsychopharmacol Biol Psychiatry. 2014;55:26–39.

47. Jia L, Raghupathy RK, Albalawi A, Zhao Z, Reilly J, Xiao Q, Shu X. A colour preference technique to evaluate acrylamide-induced toxicity in zebrafish. Comp Biochem Physiol C Toxicol Pharmacol. 2017;199:11–9.

48. Bault ZA, Peterson SM, Freeman JL. Directional and colour preference in adult zebrafish: implications in behavioural and learning assays in neurotoxicology studies. J Appl Toxicol JAT. 2015;35(12):1502–10.

49. Marcon M, Herrmann AP, Mocelin R, Rambo CL, Koakoski G, Abreu MS, Conterato GM, Kist LW, Bogo MR, Zanatta L, Barcellos LJ, Piato AL. Prevention of unpredictable chronic stress-related phenomena in zebrafish exposed to bromazepam, fluoxetine and nortriptyline. Psychopharmacology. 2016;233(21–22):3815–24.

50. Anichtchik OV, Kaslin J, Peitsaro N, Scheinin M, Panula P. Neurochemical and behavioural changes in zebrafish Danio rerio after systemic administration of 6-hydroxydopamine and 1-methyl-4-phenyl-1,2,3,6-tetrahydropyridine. J Neurochem. 2004;88(2):443–53.

51. Baldwin D, Buis C, Mayers A. Selective serotonin reuptake inhibitors in the treatment of generalized anxiety disorder. Expert Rev Neurother. 2002;2(5):717–24.

Permissions

The contributors of this book come from diverse backgrounds, making this book a truly international effort. This book will bring forth new frontiers with its revolutionizing research information and detailed analysis of the nascent developments around the world.

We would like to thank all the contributing authors for lending their expertise to make the book truly unique. They have played a crucial role in the development of this book. Without their invaluable contributions this book wouldn't have been possible. They have made vital efforts to compile up to date information on the varied aspects of this subject to make this book a valuable addition to the collection of many professionals and students.

This book was conceptualized with the vision of imparting up-to-date information and advanced data in this field. To ensure the same, a matchless editorial board was set up. Every individual on the board went through rigorous rounds of assessment to prove their worth. After which they invested a large part of their time researching and compiling the most relevant data for our readers.

The editorial board has been involved in producing this book since its inception. They have spent rigorous hours researching and exploring the diverse topics which have resulted in the successful publishing of this book. They have passed on their knowledge of decades through this book. To expedite this challenging task, the publisher supported the team at every step. A small team of assistant editors was also appointed to further simplify the editing procedure and attain best results for the readers.

Apart from the editorial board, the designing team has also invested a significant amount of their time in understanding the subject and creating the most relevant covers. They scrutinized every image to scout for the most suitable representation of the subject and create an appropriate cover for the book.

The publishing team has been an ardent support to the editorial, designing and production team. Their endless efforts to recruit the best for this project, has resulted in the accomplishment of this book. They are a veteran in the field of academics and their pool of knowledge is as vast as their experience in printing. Their expertise and guidance has proved useful at every step. Their uncompromising quality standards have made this book an exceptional effort. Their encouragement from time to time has been an inspiration for everyone.

The publisher and the editorial board hope that this book will prove to be a valuable piece of knowledge for researchers, students, practitioners and scholars across the globe.

List of Contributors

Jenni Puurunen, Sini Sulkama, Katriina Tiira, Cesar Araujo and Hannes Lohi
Department of Veterinary Biosciences and Research Programs Unit, Molecular Neurology, University of Helsinki and Folkhälsan Research Center, Biomedicum Helsinki, 00014 Helsinki, Finland
The Folkhälsan Research Center, Helsinki, Finland

Marko Lehtonen
School of Pharmacy, University of Eastern Finland, Kuopio, Finland

Kati Hanhineva
Institute of Public Health and Clinical Nutrition, University of Eastern Finland, Kuopio, Finland.
LC–MS Metabolomics Center, Biocenter Kuopio, Kuopio, Finland

Espen A. Sjoberg
Department of Behavioral Sciences, Oslo and Akershus University College of Applied Sciences, St. Olavs Plass, 0130 Oslo, Norway

Kevin Lloyd and Peter Dayan
Gatsby Computational Neuroscience Unit, 25 Howland Street, London, UK

Shinya Kinoshita, Tetsufumi Kanazawa and Hiroshi Yoneda
Department of Neuropsychiatry, Osaka Medical College, 2-7, Daigaku-Cho, Takatsuk, Osaka 569-8686, Japan

Hiroki Kikuyama
Department of Neuropsychiatry, Osaka Medical College, 2-7, Daigaku-Cho, Takatsuk, Osaka 569-8686, Japan
Department of Psychiatry, Shin-Abuyama Hospital, Osaka Institute of Clinical Psychiatry, Osaka, Japan

Thelma Beatriz González-Castro and Yazmín Hernández-Díaz
División Académica Multidisciplinaria de Jalpa de Méndez, Universidad Juárez Autónoma de Tabasco, Jalpa de Méndez, Tabasco, Mexico

Isela Esther Juárez-Rojop and Mariela Alpuin-Reyes
División Académica de Ciencias de la Salud, Universidad Juárez Autónoma de Tabasco, Villahermosa, Tabasco, Mexico

María Lilia López-Narváez
Secretaría de Salud, Hospital General de Yajalón, Yajalón, Chiapas, Mexico

Carlos Alfonso Tovilla-Zárate
División Académica Multidisciplinaria de Comalcalco, Universidad Juárez Autónoma de Tabasco, Ranchería Sur, Cuarta Sección, C. P. 86650 Comalcalco, Tabasco, Mexico

Alma Genis-Mendoza
Secretaría de Salud, Instituto Nacional de Medicina Genómica (INMEGEN), Servicios de Atención Psiquiátrica (SAP), Ciudad de México, Mexico

Jenni Puurunen
Institute of Public Health and Clinical Nutrition, University of Eastern Finland, Kuopio, Finland

Kati Hanhineva
Institute of Public Health and Clinical Nutrition, University of Eastern Finland, Kuopio, Finland
LC–MS Metabolomics Center, Biocenter Kuopio, Kuopio, Finland

Marko Lehtonen
LC–MS Metabolomics Center, Biocenter Kuopio, Kuopio, Finland

Aquiles Luna-Rodriguez and Thomas Jacobsen
Experimental Psychology Unit, Helmut-Schmidt-University/University of the Federal Armed Forces Hamburg, Holstenhofweg 85, 22043 Hamburg, Germany

Mike Wendt
Faculty of Human Sciences, Medical School Hamburg, Hamburg, Germany

Nan Wu, Feng Wang, Zhen Zhang, Lian-Kun Wang, Chun Zhang and Tao Sun
Ningxia Key Laboratory of Cerebrocranial Disease, Incubation Base of National Key Laboratory, Ningxia Medical University, Yinchuan, Ningxia, China.
Department of Neurosurgery, General Hospital of Ningxia Medical
University, Yinchuan, Ningxia, China

Zhe Jin
Department of Neuroscience, Uppsala University, Uppsala, Sweden

En-Zhao Cong, Gai-Ling Xu, Ting-Ting Lv, Ying-Li Zhang, Qiu-Fen Ning and Ji-Kang Wang
Department of Psychiatry, The Second Affiliated Hospital of Xinxiang Medical University (Psychiatric hospital of Henan province, China), Xinxiang 453002, Henan, China

Chang-Hong Wang and Cong Liu
Department of Psychiatry, The Second Affiliated Hospital of Xinxiang Medical University (Psychiatric hospital of Henan province, China), Xinxiang 453002, Henan, China

Hui-Yao Nie
Department of Psychiatry, The Second Affiliated Hospital of Xinxiang Medical University (Psychiatric hospital of Henan province, China), Xinxiang 453002, Henan, China

Yan Li
Department of Child and Adolescent, Public Health College, Zhengzhou University, 100 Kexue Road, Zhengzhou 450001, Henan, China

Jianqin Cao, Yang Li and Jun Yang
Department of Nursing, Harbin Medical University, Daqing, Heilongjiang Province, China

Quanying Liu
Laboratory of Movement Control and Neuroplasticity, KU Leuven, 3001 Louvain, Belgium. Neural Control of Movement Laboratory, ETH Zurich, 8057 Zurich, Switzerland

Ruolei Gu, Jin Liang, Yanyan Qi, Haiyan Wu and Xun Liu
CAS Key Laboratory of Behavioral Science, Institute of Psychology, Chinese Academy of Sciences, 16 Lincui Road, Chaoyang District, Beijing 100101, China
Department of Psychology, University of Chinese Academy of Sciences, Beijing 100101, China

Matthew T. Sutherland and Jessica S. Flannery
Department of Psychology, Florida International University, AHC-4, RM 312, 11200 S.W. 8th St, Miami, FL 33199, USA

Michael C. Riedel
Department of Psychology, Florida International University, AHC-4, RM 312, 11200 S.W. 8th St, Miami, FL 33199, USA
Department of Physics, Florida International University, Miami, FL, USA

Angela R. Laird
Department of Physics, Florida International University, Miami, FL, USA

Julio A. Yanes
Department of Psychology, Auburn University, Auburn, AL, USA

Peter T. Fox
Research Imaging Institute, University of Texas Health Science Center, San Antonio, TX, USA.
South Texas Veterans Health Care System, San Antonio, TX, USA.
State Key Laboratory for Brain and Cognitive Sciences, University of Hong Kong, Hong Kong, China

Elliot A. Stein
Neuroimaging Research Branch, National Institute on Drug Abuse, Intramural Research Program, NIH/DHHS, Baltimore, MD, USA

Saleh N. Maodaa, Jamaan Ajarem, Mostafa A. Abdel-Maksoud and Gadah I. Al-Basher
Department of Zoology, College of Science, King Saud University, Riyadh 11451, Saudi Arabia

Ahmed A. Allam
Department of Zoology, Faculty of Science, Beni-Suef University, Beni-Suef, Egypt

Zun Yao Wang
State Key Laboratory of Pollution Control and Resources Reuse, School of the Environment, Nanjing University, Nanjing 210023, Jiangsu, People's Republic of China

Noémi Ágnes Varga, Klára Pentelényi, Péter Balicza, Viktória Reményi, Vivien Hársfalvi, Renáta Bencsik, Anett Illés and Mária Judit Molnár
Institute of Genomic Medicine and Rare Disorders, Semmelweis University, Tömő Str. 25-29, Budapest 1083, Hungary

András Gézsi
Institute of Genomic Medicine and Rare Disorders, Semmelweis University, Tömő Str. 25-29, Budapest 1083, Hungary
Department of Genetics, Celland Immunobiology, Semmelweis University, Nagyvárad tér 4, Budapest 1089, Hungary

Csilla Prekop
Vadaskert Foundation for Children's Mental Health, Lipótmezei Str. 1-5, Budapest 1021, Hungary

Jacqueline S. Womersley, Bafokeng Mpeta, Jacqueline J. Dimatelis, Lauriston A. Kellaway and Vivienne A. Russell
Department of Human Biology, Faculty of Health Sciences, University of Cape Town, Anzio Road, Observatory, Cape Town 7925, South Africa

Dan J. Stein
Department of Psychiatry and Mental Health, Faculty of Health Sciences, University of Cape Town, Groote Schuur Hospital, Observatory, Cape Town 7925, South Africa

Simon Baijot
Center for Research in Cognition and Neurosciences (CRCN), Université Libre de Bruxelles (ULB), Campus du Solbosch CP 191, Avenue F.D. Roosevelt 50, CP 151, 1050 Brussels, Belgium
Research Unit in Cognitive Neurosciences (UNESCOG), Université Libre de Bruxelles (ULB), 1050 Brussels, Belgium
Department of Neurology, Queen Fabiola Children's University Hospital (HUDERF), Université Libre de Bruxelles (ULB), Avenue Jean-Joseph Crocq, 15, 1020 Brussels, Belgium

Cécile Colin
Center for Research in Cognition and Neurosciences (CRCN), Université Libre de Bruxelles (ULB), Campus du Solbosch CP 191, Avenue F.D. Roosevelt 50, CP 151, 1050 Brussels, Belgium
Research Unit in Cognitive Neurosciences (UNESCOG), Université Libre de Bruxelles (ULB), 1050 Brussels, Belgium
Laboratory of Cognitive and Sensory Neurophysiology, CHU Brugmann, Université Libre de Bruxelles (ULB), Place Van Gehuchten, 4, 1020 Brussels, Belgium

Hichem Slama
Center for Research in Cognition and Neurosciences (CRCN), Université Libre de Bruxelles (ULB), Campus du Solbosch CP 191, Avenue F.D. Roosevelt 50, CP 151, 1050 Brussels, Belgium
Research Unit in Cognitive Neurosciences (UNESCOG), Université Libre de Bruxelles (ULB), 1050 Brussels, Belgium
Neuropsychology and Functional Neuroimaging Research Group (UR2NF), Université Libre de Bruxelles (ULB), 1050 Brussels, Belgium
Department of Clinical and Cognitive Neuropsychology, Erasme Hospital, Université Libre de Bruxelles (ULB), Route de Lennik, 808, 1070 Brussels, Belgium

Nicolas Deconinck
Department of Neurology, Queen Fabiola Children's University Hospital (HUDERF), Université Libre de Bruxelles (ULB), Avenue Jean-Joseph Crocq, 15, 1020 Brussels, Belgium

Bernard Dan
Department of Neurology, Queen Fabiola Children's University Hospital (HUDERF), Université Libre de Bruxelles (ULB), Avenue Jean-Joseph Crocq, 15, 1020 Brussels, Belgium
Inkendaal Rehabilitation Hospital, Vlezenbeek, Belgium

Paul Deltenre
Laboratory of Cognitive and Sensory Neurophysiology, CHU Brugmann, Université Libre de Bruxelles (ULB), Place Van Gehuchten, 4, 1020 Brussels, Belgium

Göran Söderlund
Faculty of Teacher Education and Sports, Sogn og Fjordane, University College, Sogndal, Norway

Hina Abid
Quaid-e-Azam University, Islamabad, Pakistan

Fayyaz Ahmad and Iftikhar Ahmad
University of Gujrat, Gujrat, Pakistan

Soo Y. Lee, Hyun W. Park and Dongmi Im
Korea Advanced Institute of Science and Technology, Daejeon, South Korea

Safee U. Chaudhary
Lahore University of Managment Sciences, Lahore, Pakistan

Jamaan Ajarem and Naif G. Altoom
Department of Zoology, College of Science, King Saud University, Riyadh 11451, Saudi Arabia

Ahmed A. Allam
Department of Zoology, College of Science, King Saud University, Riyadh 11451, Saudi Arabia
Department of Zoology, Faculty of Science, Beni-suef University, Beni-Suef, Egypt

Billy KC. Chow
School of Biological Sciences, University of Hong Kong, Hong Kong, China

Christina Artemenko
LEAD Graduate School and Research Network, University of Tuebingen, Tuebingen, Germany
Department of Psychology, University of Tuebingen, Tuebingen, Germany

Ann-Christine Ehlis and Thomas Dresler
LEAD Graduate School and Research Network, University of Tuebingen, Tuebingen, Germany
Department of Psychiatry and Psychotherapy, University of Tuebingen, Tuebingen, Germany

Hans-Christoph Nuerk
LEAD Graduate School and Research Network, University of Tuebingen, Tuebingen, Germany
Department of Psychology, University of Tuebingen, Tuebingen, Germany
Leibniz-Institut für Wissensmedien, Tuebingen, Germany

Mojtaba Soltanlou
Department of Psychology, University of Tuebingen, Tuebingen, Germany

Graduate Training Centre of Neuroscience/IMPRS for Cognitive and Systems Neuroscience, Tuebingen, Germany
Leibniz-Institut für Wissensmedien, Tuebingen, Germany

Julia Kerner auch Koerner
Educational Psychology, Helmut-Schmidt-University/University of the Federal Armed Forces Hamburg, Hamburg, Germany
Center for Individual Development and Adaptive Education of Children at Risk (IDeA), Frankfurt, Germany

Caterina Gawrilow
School Psychology, Eberhard Karls Universität Tübingen, Tübingen, Germany
Center for Individual Development and Adaptive Education of Children at Risk (IDeA), Frankfurt, Germany

Yi-Tzu Chang
Department of Educational Psychology and Counseling, National Taiwan Normal University, Taipei, Taiwan
Department of Occupational Therapy and Graduate Institute of Behavioral Science, Chang Gung University, Taoyuan, Taiwan

Ching-I Wang
Department of Occupational Therapy and Graduate Institute of Behavioral Science, Chang Gung University, Taoyuan, Taiwan

Hsiang-Yu Chen
Department of Occupational Therapy and Graduate Institute of Behavioral Science, Chang Gung University, Taoyuan, Taiwan
Faculty of Psychology, Technische Universität Dresden, Dresden, Germany

Ling-Fu Meng
Department of Occupational Therapy and Graduate Institute of Behavioral Science, Chang Gung University, Taoyuan, Taiwan
Division of Occupational Therapy, Department of Rehabilitation, Chiayi Chang Gung Memorial Hospital, Chiayi, Taiwan

Yuan-Chieh Huang
Department of Clinical Psychology, Fu Jen Catholic University, New Taipei, Taiwan

Wan-Yu Shih
Institute of Neuroscience, National Yang-Ming University, Taipei, Taiwan

Hsiao-Lung Chan
Department of Electrical Engineering, Chang Gung University, Taoyuan, Taiwan

Ping-Yi Wu
Division of Occupational Therapy, Department of Physical Medicine and Rehabilitation, Center for Neural Regeneration, Taipei Veterans General Hospital, Taipei, Taiwan

Chen-Chi Chen
Health Center, Taipei Fuhsing Private School, Taipei, Taiwan

Julia Mock, Stefan Huber, Julia F. Dietrich and Elise Klein
Leibniz-Institut für Wissensmedien, Schleichstraße 6, 72076 Tuebingen, Germany

Johannes Bloechle and Johannes Rennig
Leibniz-Institut für Wissensmedien, Schleichstraße 6, 72076 Tuebingen, Germany
Division of Neuropsychology, Hertie-Institute for Clinical Brain Research, Otfried-Müller-Straße 27, 72076 Tuebingen, Germany

Julia Bahnmueller and Korbinian Moeller
Leibniz-Institut für Wissensmedien, Schleichstraße 6, 72076 Tuebingen, Germany
Eberhardt-Karls University Tuebingen, 72074 Tuebingen, Germany

Shuhui Zhang, Xiaodong Liu, Xiang Li and Xizeng Feng
State Key Laboratory of Medicinal Chemical Biology, The Key Laboratory of Bioactive Materials, Ministry of Education, College of Life Science, Nankai University, Tianjin 300071, China

Qiuping Zhang, Jia Xu and Dongyan Chen
Tianjin Key Laboratory of Tumor Microenvironment and Neurovascular Regulation, Department of Histology and Embryology, School of Medicine, Nankai University, Tianjin 300071, China

Mingzhu Sun, Teng Li and Xin Zhao
The Institute of Robotics and Automatic Information Systems, Nankai University, Tianjin 300071, China

Index

www.ingramcontent.com/pod-product-compliance
Lightning Source LLC
Chambersburg PA
CBHW061314190326
41458CB00011B/3805